Toba Schwaber Kerson
and Associates

Social Work
in Health Settings
Practice in Context
Second Edition

Pre-publication
REVIEWS,
COMMENTARIES,
EVALUATIONS . . .

"**S**ocial work departments in hospitals and medical centers are under attack and in some cases are being dismantled. Toba Kerson has put together a volume that should be read by every hospital administrator, every director of a managed care organization, and every legislator who has any concern for what happens to sick people. This book tells in graphic detail what social workers do every day in thirty-odd health care settings from burn to renal dialysis clinics, from emergency rooms to oncology departments, from hospice care to well-baby clinics. Every social worker, student, faculty member, line worker, or administrator will feel proud of his or her profession after reading this volume."

Harold Weissman
Executive Officer,
DSW Program,
Hunter College School
of Social Work

"**S**ocial Work in Health Settings provides practitioners with a remarkably diverse and rich collection of state-of-the-art essays. A particularly appealing feature is the use of a common outline and framework for the analysis of social work with various populations in acute care, long-term care, rehabilitation, community-based, and mental health settings. The book's generalist approach and simultaneous focus on relevant clinical, policy, organizational, and technological features of social work practice enhance its instructional value. The authors' detailed descriptions of professional life in specific health settings make relevant practice theories and concepts come alive."

Frederic G. Reamer, PhD
Professor, School of Social Work,
Rhode Island College

"**A**uthors in mature and developing professions typically struggle with the emphasis one should place on practice ('the real world') and theory. Even authors who recognize the artificiality of splitting these [concepts] are often short of the skills and the knowledge required to keep practice and theory integrated and thereby serve the needs of both.

This second edition of the Kerson book displays the enormous scope of health social work, as well as the skills and scholarship of its major author and many other distinguished people who contribute to the work. Despite the fact that chapters are contributed by 49 authors in addition to Kerson, the material flows smoothly—a tribute to the controlled and consistent use of the conceptual framework that forms the theoretical basis for the book. Noteworthy, too, is its potential for the practice of beginners and advanced clinicians, as well as the possibilities it offers for doctoral students taking work in theory building.

Social Work in Health Settings: Practice in Context, Second Edition is a first-class document, worthy of perusing quickly, and of detailed, thorough study. It will be found among the steadier and lasting documents in the social work aspects of American health care."

Hans S. Falck, PhD
Professor Emeritus,
Former Chair,
Health Specialization
in Social Work,
Virginia Commonwealth University

"**S**ocial Work in Health Settings: Practice in Context, Second Edition, is the most creative and inclusive text of it's kind on the market today. Rather than attempting an overview, skim-the-surface approach, each chapter presents social work practice in a focused manner, usually through an in-depth description of a specific program. This is an excellent way to stimulate discussion by graduate social work students and provides an opportunity to move them from the specific to more generally applicable principles through the careful selection of additional readings. While Kerson suggests the text may be used as a casebook, as a professor, I would recommend its use as the primary text given the breadth and depth of the book."

Dianne Garner, DSW, ACSW
Professor and Chair,
Department of Social Work,
Washburn University,
Topeka, KS

The Haworth Press, Inc.

Social Work in Health Settings
Practice in Context

Second Edition

HAWORTH Social Work Practice
Carlton E. Munson, DSW, Senior Editor

New, Recent, and Forthcoming Titles:

Gerontological Social Work Supervision by Ann Burack-Weiss and Frances Coyle Brennan

Group Work: Skills and Strategies for Effective Interventions by Sondra Brandler and Camille P. Roman

If a Partner Has AIDS: Guide to Clinical Intervention for Relationships in Crisis by R. Dennis Shelby

Social Work Practice: A Systems Approach by Benyamin Chetkow-Yanoov

Elements of the Helping Process: A Guide for Clinicians by Raymond Fox

Clinical Social Work Supervision, Second Edition by Carlton E. Munson

Intervention Research: Design and Development for the Human Services edited by Jack Rothman and Edwin J. Thomas

Forensic Social Work: Legal Aspects of Professional Practice by Robert L. Barker and Douglas M. Branson

Now Dare Everything: Tales of HIV-Related Psychotherapy by Steven F. Dansky

The Black Elderly: Satisfaction and Quality of Later Life by Marguerite M. Coke and James A. Twaite

Building on Women's Strengths: A Social Work Agenda for the Twenty-First Century by Liane V. Davis

Family Beyond Family: The Surrogate Parent in Schools and Other Community Agencies by Sanford Weinstein

The Cross-Cultural Practice of Clinical Case Management in Mental Health edited by Peter Manoleas

Environmental Practice in the Human Services: Integration of Micro and Macro Roles, Skills, and Contexts by Bernard Neugeboren

Basic Social Policy and Planning: Strategies and Practice Methods by Hobart A. Burch

Fundamentals of Cognitive-Behavior Therapy: From Both Sides of the Desk by Bill Borcherdt

Social Work Intervention in an Economic Crisis: The River Communities Project by Martha Baum and Pamela Twiss

The Relational Systems Model for Family Therapy: Living in the Four Realities by Donald R. Bardill

Feminist Theories and Social Work: Approaches and Applications by Christine Flynn Saulnier

Social Work Approaches to Conflict Resolution: Making Fighting Obsolete by Benyamin Chetkow-Yanoov

Principles of Social Work Practice: A Generic Practice Approach by Molly R. Hancock

Nobody's Children: Orphans of the HIV Epidemic by Steven F. Dansky

Social Work in Health Settings: Practice in Context, Second Edition by Toba Schwaber Kerson and Associates

Social Work in Health Settings
Practice in Context
Second Edition

Toba Schwaber Kerson
and Associates

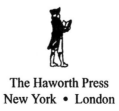

The Haworth Press
New York • London

The Haworth Press, Inc., 10 Alice Street, Binghamton, NY 13904-1580

Cover design by Marylouise E. Doyle.

Library of Congress Cataloging-in-Publication Data

Kerson, Toba Schwaber.
 Social work in health settings : practice in context / Toba Schwaber Kerson and associates.–2nd ed.
   p. cm.
 Includes bibliographical references and index.
 ISBN 0-7890-6019-1 (alk. paper).
 1. Medical social work–United States. 2. Public health–United States. I. Title.
HV687.5.U5K48 1997
362.1′0425–dc21

                                                                          96-51915
                                                                             CIP

CONTENTS

ABOUT THE EDITOR

Toba Schwaber Kerson, DSW, PhD, is Professor in the Graduate School of Social Work and Social Research at Bryn Mawr College in Pennsylvania. She is the author of the books *Medical Social Work: The Pre-Professional Paradox* and *Understanding Chronic Illness: The Medical and Psychosocial Dimensions of Nine Diseases* and the editor of *Field Instruction in Social Work Settings.* She serves on the editorial boards of *Women & Aging* and *Arete* and is the Book Review Editor of *Social Work in Health Care.* She received her master's degree from the Columbia University School of Social Work and her DSW and PhD in sociology from the University of Pennsylvania.

Contributors

Sherri Alper, MSS, is associated with The Spicer Group of Otter Creek in Manchester, Vermont.

Margo Regan Bare, MSW, LSW, is an Assistant Professor at Cabrini College, Radnor, Pennsylvania.

Betsy C. Blades, MSW, LCSW, is a Social Worker at Bon Secours Hospital in Baltimore, Maryland.

Edward Blanchard, MSW, LCSW, is a Social Worker for the Shalom House, Inc., in Portland, Maine.

Bonnie Carolan-McNulty, RN, MSN, CHRN, is Hospice Client Service Manager at Community Health Affiliates in Ardmore, Pennsylvania.

Perry H. Charley is Director of the Navajo Abandoned Mine Land Reclamation Program, Shiprock Field Office, Shiprock, New Mexico.

Maria DeOca Corwin, PhD, is an Assistant Professor in the Graduate School of Social Work and Social Research at Bryn Mawr College, Bryn Mawr, Pennsylvania.

Genevieve S. Coyle, MSW, is a Family Therapist at the New England Rehabilitation Hospital in Woburn, Massachusetts.

Susan E. Dawson, PhD, is Associate Professor of Social Work in the Department of Sociology, Social Work, and Anthropology, at Utah State University, Logan, Utah.

Carey Donovan, MSS, is the Guidance Counselor at the Mount Desert Elementary School in Northeast Harbor, Maine.

Elisabeth Doolan, MSS, is in private practice in Philadelphia, Pennsylvania.

Carol Appolone Ford, ACSW, is a Pediatric Neurology Social Worker in the Comprehensive Epilepsy Program, Bowman Grey School of Medicine, Winston-Salem, North Carolina.

Zelda Foster, MS, LCSW, is Chief of the Social Work Service for the Veterans Administration Medical Center in Brooklyn, New York.

Diane Frankel, MSS, LSW, BCD, is in private practice in Chestnut Hill, Pennsylvania.

Susan B. Freeman, MS, LCSW, is a Social Worker for the Home, Health, and Counseling Agency in the East Bay Area, Contra Costa County, California.

Randee Morose Gallo, MSS, is a Program Director for Resources for Human Development in Philadelphia, Pennsylvania.

George S. Getzel, DSW, is a Professor in the Hunter College School of Social Work, New York, New York.

Tina Powell Green, MSW, is Social Worker II, Child Service Coordinator at the Franklin County Health Department in Lewisburg, North Carolina.

Danielle L. Hammer, MSW, LSW, ACSW, is Director of Case Management for Montgomery Hospital in Norristown, Pennsylvania.

Lyne Iris Harmon, MSW, PsyD, is a psychologist for the Northwest Corporation, Philadelphia, Pennsylvania.

Phyllis Braudy Harris, PhD, ACSW, is Associate Professor of Sociology and Director of the Gerontology Program at John Carroll University, in Cleveland, Ohio.

Phillip Harrison Jr. is an advocate and owner of a construction firm on the Navajo Nation.

Mary Ellen Hass, MSW, LCSW, is Executive Director of Student Health Services of Stamford, CT, Inc., Stamford, Connecticut.

Lesley Sharp Haushalter, MSS, LSW, is a Social Worker in the Delaware Hospice, Wilmington, Delaware.

Judith F. Hirschwald, MSW, LSW, is Director of Social Services at Magee Memorial Rehabilitation Center, Philadelphia, Pennsylvania.

Debra Katz, MSW, LCSW, is a School-Based Health Center Consultant, Student Health Services of Stamford, CT, Inc., and AIDS Program Coordinator, City of Stamford, Stamford, Connecticut.

Robin S. Johnson, DSW, is a partner in The Constantine Group, a health options management company in Columbus, Ohio.

Nancy V. Lotz, MSS, is a Medical Social Worker at Community Home Health Services, Philadelphia, Pennsylvania.

James A. Martin, PhD, is an Associate Professor in the Graduate School of Social Work and Social Research at Bryn Mawr College, Bryn Mawr, Pennsylvania.

Judy Mason, MSW, is a Preceptor in Social Work at the Mt. Sinai Medical Center, New York, New York.

Susan O. Mercer, DSW, is a Professor in the Graduate School of Social Work at the University of Arkansas, Little Rock, Arkansas.

Renee Weisman Michelsen, MSS, is Director of Senior Services for the Center for Geriatric Care, at Morristown Memorial Hospital, Morristown, New Jersey.

Martin B. Millison, DSW, is a Professor in the School of Social Administration at Temple University, Philadelphia, Pennsylvania.

Nancy Nelson, MSW, is a Program Supervisor at the Ohio Youth Advocate Program, Columbus, Ohio.

Mary O'Neill, MSS, is Director of Social Services at St. Edmond's Home, Rosemont, Pennsylvania.

Joyce Preisinger, MSW, is a Clinical Social Worker in Obstetrics and Gynecology at the Mt. Sinai Medical Center, New York, New York.

Elizabeth Read, ACSW, LCSW, is a Program Supervisor at Catholic Charities, Trenton, New Jersey.

Betsy Robinson, MSW, is a Geriatric Clinical Social Worker at Riley's Oakhill Manor South in Little Rock, Arkansas.

Kathleen Rounds, PhD, is an Associate Professor in the School of Social Work at the University of North Carolina, Chapel Hill, North Carolina.

Wendy Schmid, MSW, LSW, is Coordinator of Outpatient Social Work Services, Children's Hospital of Philadelphia, Philadelphia, Pennsylvania.

Mary Ann Shanahan, MA, MSW, LCSW, is Director of Public Health Education for the City of Stamford, Stamford, Connecticut.

Carol Silbergeld, LCSW, BCD, is in private practice in Santa Monica, California.

Janet L. Taksa, MSW, LSW, is a Social Work Supervisor at Thomas Jefferson Hospital, Philadelphia, Pennsylvania.

Virginia Walther, MSW, is Senior Assistant Director of Social Work at the Mt. Sinai Medical Center, New York, New York.

Mona Wasow, MSW, is a Clinical Professor in the School of Social Work, University of Wisconsin, Madison, Wisconsin.

Carolyn S. Weiss, MSS, is Executive Director of the Planned Lifetime Assistance Network of Pennsylvania, Wayne, Pennsylvania.

Beth Wrightson, MSW, is a Social Worker at the Regional Center of the East Bay, Oakland, California.

Irene Nathan Zipper, MSW, is a Clinical Instructor in the School of Social Work, University of North Carolina, Chapel Hill, North Carolina.

Sylvia Ziserman, MSS, BCD, is a Social Worker for the Palliative Care Service/Hospice at the Fox Chase Cancer Center in Philadelphia, Pennsylvania.

Acknowledgments

I would like to thank all of the superb practitioners, educators, and researchers who contributed to this volume. Several of the authors have been involved with this enterprise since 1979 when the first edition was conceived. Now, with the second edition, written 17 years later, we can see the evolving chapters as individual practice examples of the maturation of social work in health care. Lorraine-Orlady-Wright remains the best editor I know, and Peg McConnell is unsurpassed as a computer consultant and General Trouble-shooter. Special thanks to Helen Rehr and Hans Falck for their vision of my career. Eventually, I hope to match their expectations of my capabilities. Most of all, I thank Larry Kerson and Jennie Kerson for their devotion to me and respect for my work.

Introduction

The Framework

Social Work in Health Settings: Practice in Context uses a decision-making model to explore a wide range of social work services in health care settings. Although the cases and settings in this book are all health related, the framework is generic and, therefore, suitable for teaching direct practice in any setting. The framework proposes, first, that social workers understand the context in which their work with clients occurs in order to be able to interpret and influence important dimensions of context. Second, the framework encourages social workers to understand the decisions that structure the helping relationship so that they can evaluate and, when necessary, alter the decisions to meet the needs of each client.

Context is a set of circumstances or facts that surround and constrain a particular event or situation. Three elements of context that influence and often limit the nature and conditions of the helping relationship are policy, technology, and organization. Policy refers particularly to laws; technology, to means for diagnosis, treatment, and monitoring; and organization, to systems involved in the delivery of health services. Within context, the practice decisions that structure the helping relationship are (1) the definition of the client; (2) goals; (3) contract; (4) meeting place; (5) use of time; (6) interventions and strategies; (7) stance of the social worker; (8) use of resources outside of the social worker/client relationship; (9) reassessment; and (10) transfer or termination. After the termination of each client case, the social worker conducts a differential discussion reviewing and evaluating each practice decision in order to decide whether to follow the structure for the next similar client or to alter some elements in order to further the work. The differential discussion can be a kind of mental review similar to one an athlete carries out after a particular play or game, or a chef thinks about as he or she develops a new recipe, or it can be made a regular part of the supervisory process in which the social work student or supervisee uses a printed grid to review each practice decision and make notes for the next similar case.

The Casebook

The framework will be applied to 32 settings drawn from (1) services to children and/or families; (2) acute and high-technology care; (3) rehabilitation; (4) long-term intervention and advocacy; (5) mental health; and (6) care for the frail elderly and hospice care. In each chapter, the practitioner has chosen a particular case to demonstrate the framework's utility. Thus, *Social Work in Health Settings* can be used as a casebook for understanding particular techniques and interventions; a means of introducing students to a range of clients; an overview of many social work settings and services in the health arena; and, perhaps most important, a way to help students to consider practice and policy issues and interventions as a whole. In this framework, as in reality, practice and policy are inextricably intertwined.

CONTEXT

Policy

Unlike many other countries, the United States has no clearly demarcated and defined health policy. Primarily, health care is considered the responsibility of individual states. Specific federal health policies are directed toward particular populations for which the U.S. government has decided it must assume some responsibility, such as present and past members of the armed services and the elderly. Examples among the "Practice in Context" chapters are those dealing with emphysema patients in a Veterans Administration Medical Center, the chapters related to renal dialysis, and the chapter that has as its focus interventions in a combat environment. Chapters related to early interventions for children at risk for delay and case management services for the frail elderly reflect more recent federal policy concerns.

Health policy relates also to shifts in the value orientation in the history of the United States. Between 1935 and 1944, when the United States was recovering from the Great Depression and participating in World War II, many categorical programs such as Maternal and Child Health were developed through the Social Security Act of 1935. The years from 1945 to 1960 saw an investment in and expansion of health resources, facilities, manpower, and research, with many hospitals being built or expanded and large numbers of social workers, physicians, nurses, and a range of therapists being trained through the auspices of the federal government. The technological possibilities of diagnosis and treatment were embraced and supported as never before. The years from 1960 to 1970 focused on equity of access, in part through the passage of Medicare, Medicaid, and Community Mental Health Center legislation. The 1970s saw the concern with the national allocation of resources, the concomitant building of an infrastructure for planning and regulation, and the concern for cost containment. Deinstitutionalization was highly valued.

Competition and regulation were the themes of the 1980s, with the federal government regulating costs on the one hand and enhancing free-market competition on the other hand. Deinstitutionalization continued with an increased number of services having cost containment as a prime objective. Hospice, home care, and home services for the frail elderly are meant to cost less than their institutional alternatives. Cheaper cost will probably ensure the future of such services. The 1990s have raised the stakes for cost containment and have seen the ascendancy of managed care in many guises. Through managed care, federal and state governments are shifting a great deal of financial risk to companies who promise that they can deliver high-quality health care for predetermined amounts of money. In turn, those companies are shifting much of the financial risk to institutional and professional providers. Some highlights of the redefinition that the system is experiencing are the following: (1) completely moving as many services as possible out of institutions, (2) delivering health care through an elaborate continuum of services and organizations linked in many different ways; and (3) redefining the nature and extent of mental health care. Notions of inpatient and outpatient are no longer ways to codify health care systems. Anyone who can possibly be helped in the community is being treated outside the walls of costly institutions, and institutional and agency relationships seem to be shifting daily. For social workers, the very tight restrictions imposed by managed care companies on psychotherapy are being felt deeply, but the increased use of clinical or advanced case managers to work with the severely mentally ill and other groups is presenting new opportunities.

Often, policies determine restraints or entitlements. For example, specific pieces of legislation entitle those with developmental disabilities to many educational and training programs (See the chapters titled "Family-Centered Care: Life Span Issues in a Spina Bifida Specialty Care Program" and "Residential Care Facility: Treatment of a Child with Severe Disabilities"), while other pieces of legislation restrict driving for those with uncontrolled epilepsy or dementia. Policies regarding specific issues evolve over time, reflecting the values of a particular period of a society. At present, for example, fines and restrictions have become heavier for those arrested for driving under the influence of alcohol. Policies related to family planning seem to remain in flux. For example, the use of abortion remains prominent and controversial in the political arena.

Finally, the policy often determines which professionals will be part of a specific service. The inclusion or exclusion of social work in areas such as renal dialysis, hospice, home care, community mental health, and health maintenance organizations is critical for the future of the profession. To be excluded removes social work from policy-making as well as from service delivery; neither the profession nor its clientele can afford exclusion.

Technology

Technology is the sum of the ways in which social groups provide themselves with the material objects of their civilization. It is the branch of knowledge that deals with applied science. Examples of technology include life support systems, diagnostic machinery, and computer systems for monitoring foster children or the chronically mentally ill. Technology seems most applicable to health settings, though it is important in all social service delivery. Chapters that focus on high-technology combinations of machinery and medication are the following: "Psychological Recovery from Burn Injury: Regional Burn Center," "Beyond Survival by Machine: Reflections of a Spouse," "Confronting a Life-Threatening Disease: Renal Dialysis and Transplant Program," "Rehabilitation of a Quadriplegic Adolescent: Regional Spinal Cord Injury Center," "Intensive Case Management for People with Serious and Persistent Mental Illness," and "Premature Babies in the Intensive Care Nursery." Medication is also a critical element in chapters such as "Epilepsy in Childhood: Pediatric Neurology Clinic" and "Adult Oncology: Helping a Terminally Ill Woman to Plan and Cope."

The chapter "He's Schizophrenic and the System Is Not Helping: Reflections of a Troubled Parent and Professional" allows one to examine a situation in which political and technological solutions conflict. A young man who is very ill cannot be hospitalized or medicated without his consent. To do so inhibits his freedom, and the state protects this freedom. Without medication, the young man cannot manage the activities of daily living, so his life is wretched, primitive, and painful but free.

Technological solutions are not only valued but expected in the United States. Thus, while spending for public health and nutrition programs has decreased, spending for "high-tech" medicine such as organ transplantation and diagnostic imaging has increased. Also, as a society, we are loath to deny or end treatment; that is to say that someone's life quality is so poor, he or she should be allowed to die. The absence of a technological solution is also important for social work because our services are often valued more in those situations where there is no effective medical treatment (See the chapters titled "A Community-Based Response to the HIV/AIDS Pandemic," "Alzheimer's Disease: Intervention in a Nursing Home Environment," and "Advocacy and Social Action Among Navajo Uranium Miners and Their Families").

The meaning of technological intervention varies according to the individual. This is evident in the example of the young man with schizophrenia who would not allow medication. At times, in renal dialysis, patients and family members name their machine, thus anthropomorphizing it. Sometimes patients refuse to return to facilities because the apparatus reminds them of their pain or vulnerability. Often, people are concerned that they will be kept alive beyond the time when they can control their futures. Thus, technology presents increased opportunities and dilemmas.

Organization

An organization can be defined as a body of persons brought together to accomplish some end or work, or the personnel or apparatus of an agency, business, or institution. Size, hierarchy or its lack, rules and expectations regarding behavior of workers and clients or customers, and ethos and values shape the entity and create parameters for work. Contrasting a very large organization with a very small one helps one understand the importance of the size of the organization. The Veterans Administration, for example, sets very different work parameters from Shalom House, the transitional residence for the mentally ill. In the former, an elaborate and rigid hierarchy is probably necessary for managing a huge, complex, multifacted program. In the latter, small size and a simpler program allow professionals flexibility. Creative and excellent practice is obviously possible in both organizations, but size and complexity set different parameters. Of all of the organizational arrangements described, one which presents the practitioner with the greatest freedom is private practice because the organization and the relationship between social worker and client are the same. The rules for the individual relationship are the rules of organization.

Ethos, the underlying character or spirit of an organization, is also important. This sustaining sentiment carries the assumptions and informs the beliefs, customs, and practices of a group. To be unaware of ethos is like swimming against the tide: One may be using the proper techniques, but using too much energy and getting nowhere. One wonders what will happen in a situation where the ethos of the service delivery agency and social worker differ from that of the funding agency. For example, if funding agencies for in-home services assume a certain low level of cost, and in-home service agencies assume that clients should be kept out of institutions at all costs, even if those costs exceed allocation, will service cease?

The strong mission of organizations such as the Gay Men's Health Crisis and Navajo Abandoned Mine Reclamation Program sets certain expectations for work. More than in other kinds of organizations, the agency, social workers, and clients share purpose. In organizations such as acute care hospitals, while everyone might agree that the ultimate purpose is health, work objectives may vary and even be conflicting for different constituencies.

DECISIONS ABOUT PRACTICE

Within the constraints of context, the social worker and client make decisions that structure their relationship. Practice decisions include the definition of the client, goals, contract, meeting place, use of time, treatment modality, stance of the social worker, use of outside resources, reassessment, and transfer or termination. At times, some of these decisions are determined through policy or organization. For example, the number of days for which a person can be hospitalized is determined by insurance coverage. To a great extent, the number of days for which an elderly person can be hospitalized for an acute condition is set through Medicare's System of Diagnosis-Related Groups. The Gay Men's Health Crisis has the policy of helping clients for the rest of their lives. Generally, however, practice decisions are left to the social worker and client.

Definition of the Client

One first step in practice is to determine who the client will be. Sometimes, as in the chapter "Would You Abandon Your Child?", that decision is immediately clear. The person in pain who comes for the service remains the client. In "Psychological Recovery from Burn Injury," since the patient is at first too ill for social work intervention and his wife needs help, the wife is the client. As the patient recovers physically, his need for social work intervention becomes greater, and he becomes the primary client. In the chapter "Epilepsy in Childhood," the patient is the child, but the primary client is his mother. She must understand her noncompliance with the medical regimen and address her own problems before her son's illness can be controlled. The child is also the client because he, too, must learn to understand his illness. In "Would You Abandon Your Child" and "Placement of a Developmentally Disabled Man," the patient and her mother are both clients. In some cases, such as those described in "Social Work in a Parental AIDS Program," and "Discharge Planning in a Community Hospital," the patient is not available for direct work. Instead, relatives become the focus of intervention. At other times, the patient is too ill and the social worker must reevaluate the person's capacity to relate as he or she recovers.

Goals

Generally, goals are related to the health or mental health problems for which the patient sought treatment. Maintaining independence, avoiding social isolation, and continuing to carry one's responsibilities are general goals towards which much work is directed. In the "Epilepsy in Childhood" case, the goal can be helping the family adhere to the medical regimen. In cases such as those described in "Rehabilitation of a Quadriplegic Adolescent," the "Family Centered Care," "Family House/Womanspace," "Social Work in a Perinatal AIDS Program," or "Placement of a Developmentally Disabled Man," people learn to manage profound disabilities that can affect every part of their lives. The general goal for "A Support Group in a Home for the Elderly" was to understand and accept the aging process. In the chapters "Hospital-Based Case Management for the Frail Elderly," and "Home Care," a goal was to maintain clients in their homes. For the school-based program, a goal was to have the young woman be able to learn in the school environment and live positively in her home. In the case of "Mental Health Care in a Combat Unit," the goal was for the men to continue to soldier.

Goals can also be highly specific, as in brief treatment, or general, as in the private practice chapter, "A Woman Addresses Her Recurrent Depression in Psychotherapy." They can be about life's beginnings as in the chapters on "Premature Babies in the Intensive Care Nursery" and "Social Work Interventions on Behalf of a Burned Child," or about life's endings as in the chapters on "Hospice Care for a Widowed Mother of Six Children" and "Adult Oncology: Helping a Terminally Ill Woman to Plan and Cope." When there are as many goals as there are in the chapter on the residential program for mothers and their children, and the spina bifida clinic, the social worker helps the clients to determine priorities and to pace the work to avoid overwhelming the clients and making the work more difficult. Primarily, goals are about the shared definition of a problem, shared expectations regarding the resolution of problems, and the means for reaching resolution. Thus, goals relate directly to contract, the next decision area, which explicates expectations.

Use of Contract

A contract is an agreement between two or more parties for the doing or not doing of something specified. A contract can be an agreement between parties such as social worker and client, client and agency, social worker and agency, agency and mandating body, or agency and funding source. To some extent, all work with clients involves many contracts on various levels of relationship including clients, relatives, social workers, agencies, larger funding and oversight bodies, and law-making entities. An explicit contract lessens the risk of misunderstanding. Clients and social workers each often wish that the other would be or do something different or more. Contract avoids the disappointment and retreat that can result from failed but unspoken expectations. When used well, contract is flexible and changing. It should enhance rather than confine the work.

In the psychiatric halfway house chapter ("A Transitional Residence for the Mentally Ill"), the client who enters Shalom House also enters into an elaborate set of agreements involving many aspects of behavior. In the private practice chapter ("A Woman Addresses Her Recurrent Depression"), the client contracts only to attend the session and to pay for the service. In the chapter on the "Mutual Help Group for Emphysema Patients," the contract is to help each other to manage their illness. Thus, contract depends on the broad purpose of the service. The degree to which it is explicated seems to depend on the social worker and the agency's expectations of the clients. Contract is the linchpin of this framework. If it is well-drawn, it will specify goals, definition of the client, modality, use of time, meeting place, use of outside resources, and perhaps even the conditions of termination. Therefore, all parties can refer to it to reassess their work.

Meeting Place

Meeting place refers to the physical space in which the relationship occurs. The most obvious distinction is between the institution and the client's home. Issues regarding privacy, space, turf, control, and comfort are important here. In institutional work, the conditions of a private conversation between social worker and client must often be created in the most public of spaces. In the emergency room, or in intensive care, for example, often the patient begins to think that even his or her body is public property. Often, as in an institution, the social worker's office is too far from the patient's bedroom to make office interviews possible. If other personnel undervalue the special quality of the social work relationship, what space the social worker can construct may be fraught with interruption. Although social workers soon learn to take the problems of space and privacy for granted, the creative and innovative social worker produces a feeling of intimacy and importance for the client, whatever the physical circumstances.

The issue of control is especially powerful in the description of the spinal-cord-injured young man who has so little control over his body ("Rehabilitation of a Quadriplegic Adolescent"). The social worker decided that they should meet on the client's turf in the institution as much as was possible. In another interesting solution to meeting place, the being-old group ("A Support Group for the Elderly") met in the board room of the home–a place denoting high status, with a conference table and chairs in which serious business takes place. Some excellent relationship work in the chapter titled "Family House/Woman Space" occurred on the telephone. In another view of place, the "School-Based Health Care Centers" encouraged the students to drop in and to see the space as a refuge from much else in their lives.

Use of Time

To a certain extent, the structuring of time–that is, the spacing and duration of meetings and the length of the relationship–determines the nature of the work. The consultative function described in the chapter concerning the emergency room ("Social Work Interventions on Behalf of a Burned Child") demonstrates that important work may be accomplished with brief interaction. The work described in the "Brief Treatment" and "Rehabilitation with a Chronic Pain Patient" chapters was also brief and powerful. However, the depth of relationship achieved in the spina bifida clinic ("Family Centered Care"), intensive case management ("Intensive Case Management for People with Serious and Persistent Mental Illness," and "Children's Intensive Case Management in an Urban Community Mental Health Center"), residential care facilities, private practice, and renal dialysis ("Confronting a Life-Threatening Disease") chapters was due, in part, to a relationship of longer duration. Little has been written in social work about the length of an individual interaction. Certainly, any experienced clinician can point to a time when he or she helped someone in 15 minutes and another time when he or she and the client spun their wheels for an hour and 15 minutes. There must be meaning for relationship in the concepts of too much or too little time. This is an area for further investigation.

Strategies and Interventions

The selection of particular methods of help involves choices regarding orientation, modality, intervention, and technique. When questioned, social workers in health care generally describe themselves as eclectic and practical. They say their methods are determined by the needs of the clients. Interventions and strategies are also sometimes determined by the agency or funding source. For example, in the chapter describing the developmental disabilities center ("Placement of a Developmentally Disabled Man"), the state designed, instituted, mandated, and monitored the case management system. In the psychiatric halfway house ("A Transitional Residence for the Mentally Ill"), all methods of intervention were clearly presented to social worker and client as one aspect of the contract. Again, the most effective choices depend on fine interpretation of the demands of context, the needs of the client, and the continued flexibility of the social worker. Interventions are adapted to the needs of the client. Thus, the emphysema patients in the Veterans Hospital ("Mutual Help Group for Emphysema Patients") needed peer support, so the social worker instituted a mutual support group. The nursing home resident with Alzheimer's Disease required redefined involvement from her relatives, therefore the social worker educated and supported the relatives in order to enable them to help the patient.

Stance of the Social Worker

The stance of the social worker implies that the social worker has sufficient awareness and discipline about his or her use of the self to choose how to relate and behave in any particular client situation. Of course, this is not always the case even with highly experienced, well-trained, and self-aware clinicians. Increasingly in social work in health care, stance has to do with the social worker as advocate. In the discharge planning chapter ("Discharge Planning in a Community Hospital"), the social worker and the client's mother became the client's chief advocate with almost all of the organizations they looked to for help. The chapters concerning the Navajo uranium miners ("Advocacy and Social Action Among Navajo Uranium Workers and Their Families") and the Gay Men's Health Crisis ("A Community-Based Response to the HIV/AIDS Pandemic") have advocacy as perhaps their primary stance. However, advocacy plays a part in almost every "Practice in Context" chapter in the book.

Outside Resources

Outside resources are services located outside of the relationship and often outside of the agency, which further the work of the relationship. The use of outside resources is perhaps most clear in situations involving case management such as wraparound services, intensive case management, developmental disability, and geriatric outreach. One also sees the importance of these kinds of services in the chapters on the spinal cord injury center ("Rehabilitation of a Quadriplegic Adolescent") and the Gay Men's Health Crisis ("A Community-Based Response to the HIV/AIDS Pandemic"). As will be explained in the richer discussion of the framework, making use of an ecomap is most helpful in thinking about outside resources.

Reassessment

Reassessment allows participants to judge their work before it has concluded. This is particularly important in the case-management situations in the book, which can continue for a long time. Also, certainly, the work with the young man with spina bifida and his family was reassessed many times in the years in which he was part of the clinic. The social worker in the chapter on patients with emphysema describes reassessment as the beginning of the termination process. Reassessment is a time to decide what is working, to alter direction if necessary, and to let a client know that he or she is doing good work.

Transfer and Termination

Case transfer and termination mark an end of the social worker and client's access to each other. If they work together again, the difference in time and perhaps circumstances will change the nature of the relationship. In settings such as renal dialysis and hospice, only death means termination. In other situations, as in the chapters on discharge planning, community mental health, and the being-old group, termination occurs when the goals of the relationship have been reached.

Case Conclusion

Case conclusion refers to the outcome of the work and the current functioning of the client. Reading case conclusions first is a slightly different way of conducting the discussion of a case. First being informed of a client's current functioning and then learning about the work involved in helping the client to reach that level of functioning exposes one to a larger understanding of the work of referring agencies.

Differential Discussion

Differential discussion helps the social worker to evaluate the work with the present client and to generalize to a category of similar clients. One may use a chart such as the one included in this introduction.

In the differential discussion of the being-old group, the social worker decided that the next time she led such a group, she would change the meeting time and reach out more to clients who had dropped out, but would otherwise follow the same structure. The social worker who wrote about epilepsy in childhood noted she would have defined the client differently by involving the father as well as the mother and child, and she may have been more confrontational with the mother. Often, the differential discussions suggest that more family members should have been involved earlier for optimal results. The utility of this exercise increases with experience.

Differential Discussion Form

Client_____Similar Client Group_____

	Retain	Alter	Specific Alterations
Context			
Policies			
Technology			
Organization			
Practice Decisions			
Definition			
Goals			
Contract			
Meeting Place			
Use of Time			
Treatment Modality			
Stance			
Outside Resources			
Reassessment			
Termination			

THEMES EMERGING FROM THE FRAMEWORK

Use of this framework raises many additional themes. For example, in terms of context, mission-oriented agencies such as Family House/Womanspace and the geriatric outreach services help social workers to feel part of the purpose. Other organizations that have mixed purposes find the social worker sometimes siding with the client or protecting the client from the rest of the staff. Also, the many technological innovations that allow clients to live longer but that do not necessarily guarantee fine life quality raise many ethical and moral dilemmas for social workers. Perhaps, because social workers are concerned with the social roles of patients and clients after discharge, they are more caught in these dilemmas than are other professionals. Another theme related to technology is how little medical or psychiatric diagnosis informs social work practice. It is much more helpful for social workers to understand a client's functional ability and the course of his or her disease or disability than it is to be able to name it. Another theme related more to practice decisions is how difficult it is to acknowledge and write about failure. The old adage, "We learn from our mistakes," somehow does not find its way into scholarly meetings and publications. Finally, the power of the payer is a theme throughout the book. Today, social workers in health care are dealing with this predominantly from managed care companies, but it is always a part of the work. Over the years, some payers have allowed the professional more latitude and autonomy in setting the conditions of work. The current environment requires more savvy and more creativity on the part of the social work practitioner than ever. Finally, a critical theme that emerges is the power of relationship to support, to expand options, and to make a difference in the life of the client. In many of the situations described, the social work relationship sustained the clients in the most trying and difficult circumstances.

In retrospect, each chapter reaffirms the utility of the framework. The context of social work in health care has three primary dimensions: policy, technology, and organization. Together, these elements provide parameters for the practice decisions that social workers and clients make to determine the structure of their work together. In sum, a large measure of the art of social work is the ability to structure the relationship between social worker and client in ways that maximally support the work. To do this, the social worker must be able to understand, influence, and alter many dimensions of practice in context.

Practice in Context: The Framework

Toba Schwaber Kerson

Social Work in Health Settings presents a framework called "practice in context," which has been developed and used by the author for the past 20 years as a tool for teaching and evaluation. This approach is called a framework as opposed to a model or paradigm because it is composed of elements the author has framed together for their utility in learning and progressing in the rich and expansive art of social work practice. The primary subject of the framework is the relationship between social worker and client (Allphin, 1982). As a concept, relationship bears considerable, intense, and diverse meaning. It is an association or involvement, a connection by blood or marriage, or an emotional or other connection between people. Synonyms for relationship are connection, association, dependence, alliance, kinship, affinity, or consanguinity; yet, each of these words suggests a different meaning based on a different bond and duration. People can be related who have never met and never will; for example, people who have a common membership in a religious or fellowship group or a common profession may feel or act more "related" than first cousins.

The concept of relationship has many dimensions. Borrowing from and building with the dimensions described by several theorists will lead us to the definition of the social worker/client relationship used for this framework. The sociologist, Erving Goffman, and the anthropologist, Gregory Bateson, have theorized about some of the structural dimensions of relationship such as the interactional focus, the connection of a relationship to its milieu, and the rules that inform or govern a relationship. Bateson uses the word "interaction" and Goffman, the word "encounter" to be as precise as possible about their subjects. For this framework, "interaction" and "encounter" are seen as aspects of the broader concept of "relationship."

Goffman suggests that when studying interaction, the proper focus is not on the individual and his or her psychology, but rather the syntactical relations among the acts of different persons mutually present to one another (Goffman, 1981, p. 2). To understand interaction, one must understand not the separate individuals but what occurs between them. Goffman further alludes to the special mutuality of immediate interaction:

"When two persons are together, at least some of their world will be made up out of the fact (and consideration for the fact) that an adaptive line of action must always be pursued in this intelligently helpful or hindering world. Individuals sympathetically take the attitude of others present, regardless of the end to which they put the information thus acquired." (Goffman, 1966, p. 16)

Thus, in interaction, there is always a shared sense of situation and of an ability to, in some way, be in the other individual's place, no matter what each participant's purpose in the interaction.

Goffman places relationship in context when he develops the notion of a "membrane" that "wraps" the interaction and, to some extent, separates it from its surroundings. "Any social encounter," he writes, "any focused gathering is to be understood, in the first instance, in terms of the functioning of the 'membrane' that encloses it cutting it off from a field of properties that could be given weight" (Goffman, 1961b, p. 79). Still, while the relationship can be viewed and defined in its own right, it remains intimately related to the world outside of it. Thus, Goffman says, "An encounter provides a world for its participants, but the character and stability of the world is intimately related to its selective relationship to the wider one" (Goffman, 1961b, p. 80).

The rules that inform a relationship and the uses the participants make of those rules are also part of Goffman and Bateson's analyses of relationship. According to Bateson, interaction is the "process whereby people establish common rules for the creation and understanding of messages" (Bateson, n.d., p. 3). Goffman adds to this definition by noting that in encounters, rules are considered and managed rather than necessarily followed: Rules may shape interaction, but they also may be influenced by the participants. He writes, "Since the domain of situational proprieties is wholly made up of what individuals can experience of each other while mutually present, and since channels of experience can be interfered with in so many ways, we deal not so much with a network of rules that must be followed as with rules that must be taken into consideration, whether as something to follow or carefully to circumvent" (Goffman, 1966, p. 42).

Helen Harris Perlman adds a psychological dimension to the more structural views of relationship posed by Goffman and Bateson. She defines relationship as "a person's feeling or emotional bonding with another" (Perlman, 1979, p. 23). Elaborating on the psychological dimension, Perlman says the relationship between social worker and client is "a catalyst, an enabling dynamism in the support, nurture, and freeing of people's energies and motivations toward problem solving and the use of help" (Perlman, 1979, p. 2). The relationship affirms and motivates the client (Perlman, 1982). To these dimensions, Carol Meyer adds *purpose*. The social worker/client relationship, she says, is not an end in itself but a tool for moving the problem situation forward (Meyer, 1976). It is formed for the purpose of meeting goals.

Thus, for this framework, the relationship between social worker and client is defined with the help of both sociological and psychological ideas. The sociological contributions have to do with structure; the focus is on interaction rather than on individual participants, on the use of rules, on the relationship's connection to (or separation from) its surroundings, or context. The psychological contributions are the purposive, feeling, catalytic, and enabling dimensions. Here, the relationship of social worker and client means one or more purposive encounters intended to be catalytic and enabling. It also means that its structure and the rules for interaction are set by dimensions of context as well as by decisions made by the participants (Kerson, 1978).

PRACTICE-IN-CONTEXT FRAMEWORK

According to this framework, then, the two basic elements that structure the relationship between social worker and client are (1) the "context" in which the relationship occurs, and (2) the "practice decisions," which social worker and client make about the nature and form of the relationship. Context and practice decisions act as a matrix for the relationship. By determining many of the rules by which the work of social worker and client proceed, context and practice decisions define the possibilities for relationship. Although elements such as personality, nature and degree of illness, psychosocial assessment, and cultural background contribute to the social worker/client relationship, they are characteristics of the individuals involved and not the interaction.

This approach or framework is not a generic practice theory because it is not a system of ideas meant to explain certain phenomena or relations. Nor is it a model, because it does not show proportions or arrangements of all of its component parts. Here are described elements of context and practice, which structure the relationship between social worker and client. The framework has three overarching purposes: (1) to help the social worker to clarify the work, (2) to understand alterable and unalterable dimensions of practice and context, and (3) to be able to evaluate work in light of these dimensions. An artist decides which medium is most suitable for a subject. In the same way, with client participation, the social worker understands and tries to influence context and constructs the relationship in ways that will help meet client goals. Thus, *Social Work in Health Settings* is about the craft of social work, that is, the skill with which the social worker manages dimensions of practice.

CONTEXT

To a great extent, dimensions of context determine many of the rules for the helping relationship (Germain, 1981). To assume that possibilities are completely determined within the relationship is unrealistic, and may contribute to disappointment and a sense of failure on the part of the participants, evaluators of service, and funding sources. Context means the set of circumstances or facts that surround a particular event or situation. Gregory Bateson defines context as a "collective term for all those events which tell the organism among what set of alternatives he must make his next choice" (Bateson, 1975, p. 289). He adds, ". . . however widely *context* be defined, there may always be wider contexts a knowledge of which would reverse or modify our understanding of particular items" (Bateson, n.d., p. 16). Therefore, context is a limitless concept, and focusing on certain dimensions means ignoring others. To some extent, social scientists and social workers disagree about the most salient elements for the context of health care. For example, Strauss and his colleagues describe four features in the larger context of where work takes place: contemporary prevalence of chronic illness, images of acute care, medical technology and its impact on hospitals, and the hospital as a set of work sites (Strauss, Shizuko, Sagerhaugh, Suczek, and Weiner, 1985). In her discussion of the context of social work practice in health care, Germain includes the health care system, the health care organization, illness and the sick role, and the professional frame of reference (Germain, 1984). The present framework addresses three dimensions of context that are thought to have the most direct and describable consequences for the relationship between social worker and client: policy, technology, and organization. These three elements are considered most important because of the ways in which each contributes to the structure of the social worker/client relationship. Policies increasingly provide rules specifying the services clients may receive, and under what conditions. Organizations are also rule makers, defining the nature of service often at the behest of policymakers. Finally, in the cases of many illnesses and traumatic situations, dependence on technological intervention has contributed to the conditions of relationship. Such interventions contribute to the content of the relationship and also often constrain it. The salience of each dimension and the ways in which dimensions are related depend on the particular setting. In effect, these contextual factors contribute to the rules of the game, and as they change, the constraints and possibilities for action are altered as well.

Policy

A policy is a definite course of action that a government, an organization, or a group has decided to take in order to function in a certain situation. Charles Schottland defines social policy as "a statement or social goal or strategy, or a settled course of action dealing with the relations of people with each other, the mutual relations of people with their government, the relations of governments with each other, including legal enactments, judicial decisions, administrative decisions, and mores" (Gil, 1982, p. 6). Kahn says that policy "is the implicit or explicit core of principles that underlies specific programs, legislation, priorities" (Kahn, 1979, p. 67). Richan adds that policy "is more than a single program. It is the set of principles guiding a range of actions in a particular sphere" (Richan, 1988, p. xi). As Moroney argues, social policy is tightly linked to and often determined by the political economy (Moroney, 1991). The place of the populations with which social work is most concerned and the place of the social profession itself is to a great extent reflected in the social policies of any particular period in U.S. history. Peter Drucker notes that "within a few short decades, society rearranges itself–its world view; its basic values; its social and political structure; its arts; its key institutions" (Drucker, 1993). Thus, social policy is dynamic, fluid, and responsive to many powerful forces within and outside of a particular community or society.

The base for policy is law; and law, in the form of legislation, administrative regulations, and/or court decisions, affects every dimension and nuance of social work practice in any health setting (Dickson, 1995; Dobelstein, 1990; Wing, 1985). Dickson identifies the following aspects of the health and human services to be permeated by the law:

1. The entrance into and exit from health and human services delivery systems
2. The criteria used to determine eligibility for treatment, benefits, or services
3. The rights to which patients and clients are entitled
4. The rights to which professionals and staff are entitled
5. The way in which health and human services programs are administered and regulated

6. The relationship between the professional and the patient or client
7. The practice of the health and human services professional (p. 3)

Therefore, in order to understand the policies that shape their practice, social workers must be able to understand the laws that affect the policies. There is no way to ensure that clients receive all services and protections to which they are entitled without understanding the law.

No matter whether they work on the individual, group, community, or policy level, social workers must be able to contribute to, interpret, and influence policy in order to advocate for their clients and the profession ("Commission," 1986; Dear and Patti, 1981). Decisions regarding which populations to serve, allocation of resources, planning, and programming are too often made before social work practitioners become involved, and it is far easier to affect the structure of a program before it is instituted rather than after. These activities are also most beneficial to clients when clients and social workers advocate together. In addition, involvement in policy formulation helps the social work profession to broaden and strengthen its influence (Cayner, 1996b; "Social Work," 1985). When policy has a negative effect on clients or the profession, a united and concerted lobbying effort can stem the tide (Cayner, 1996a; Cohen, 1996; "Rebuff Urged," 1996; "Therapy Parity," 1996; Carlton, 1985).

Historically, the presence of social work has been strongest in areas such as maternal and child health, as well as services to veterans, where social workers have been involved in developing policy on national, state, and local levels (Smith, 1996; Skocpol, 1992; Trattner, 1989; Kerson, 1985a; Kerson, 1980). With regards to two contemporary examples, the Mental Health Project at the School of Social Welfare, State University of New York at Stony Brook, and the Sayville Community Support System Program, professionals said, "Our challenge is to invite people to join us in their own struggle, a task that requires us to understand the stakes/benefits/costs involved for the person acting out mental patienthood as a survival, as a way of life" (Rose and Block, 1985). Thus, patients are empowered through advocacy. In another example, the Tennessee Conference on Social Welfare describes the strategies and actions it used to obtain governmental approval for increases in the Aid to Families with Dependent Children standard of need and level of payment (Granger and Moynihan, 1987).

Diagnosis-Related Groups

One example of a policy that has directly affected the relationship of social worker and client is the federal creation of the Diagnosis-Related Group or DRG (for a discussion of DRGs, see Hammer and Kerson's chapter titled "Discharge Planning in a Community Hospital"), in which Medicare and participating insurers pay hospitals according to case diagnosis rather than cost (Fein, 1986). Formerly, the hospital charged the insurer what it had cost the hospital to care for the patient. Now, the insurer pays the hospital based on the patient's diagnosis. According to the DRG classification, if the diagnosis indicates four days of hospitalization, the hospital will be paid for four days of hospitalization only, even if the patient stays in the hospital longer. When the patient is hospitalized beyond the number of days indicated in the schema, the hospital must absorb the extra cost. Consequently, there is great pressure on the hospital to discharge the patient and great pressure on the social worker to make prompt and appropriate arrangements for the patient to return to the community. Thus, a social worker who previously may have had weeks to develop a relationship with and an adequate discharge plan for a patient, now may have a matter of days to accomplish the same task.

Managed Care

For the late 1990s, a focal point for influencing policy formulation and advocating for clients and the profession is managed care and especially managed behavioral health care (Iglehart, 1996; Shore and Beigel, 1996; Goldman and Mukherjee, 1995; Minkoff, 1994). It is critical that social workers in health care see this current panacea-like solution as a series of complex strategies viewed by important and powerful interest groups as ways to control the costs of health care (Jackson, 1996; Jackson, 1995; Kissick, 1994; Cornelius, 1994; Mizrahi, 1993; Newhouse, 1993; Stoline and Weiner, 1993). Managed care is not the enemy of social work, nor is it a simple way to solve deep, complicated problems; in fact, it is not even an *it*. At this point, the term managed care is used for almost any strategy or structure put forth to manage the quality or cost of health care (Freeborn and Pope, 1994).

> Broadly defined, (managed care) encompasses any measure that, from the perspective of the purchaser of health care, favorably affects the price of services, the site where the services are received, or their utilization. As such, it represents a continuum–from plans that, for example, do no more than require prior authorization of inpatient stays, to the staff model HMO that employs its doctors and assumes risk for delivering a comprehensive benefit package. Ideally managed care should not simply seek to reduce costs; rather it should strive to maximize value, which includes a concern with quality and access. (Fox, 1990, p. 1)

Iglehart includes the following characteristics of most managed care approaches: (1) contracts with providers who supply a comprehensive set of health services to enrolled members, generally for a predetermined monthly premium; (2) patient financial incentives to use providers who have contracted with the plan; (3) quality and utilization controls, which contracting providers have accepted; and (4) the assumption of a varying degree of financial risk by the providers (Iglehart, 1992, p. 742).

In many settings, managed care is altering roles and tasks for social workers (Kadushin and Kulys, 1995). In one example of advocating for its clients and the profession, the Connecticut chapter of the National Association of Social Workers (NASW) is pressing for the enactment of a law that will regulate the ways in which managed care companies can conduct business in the state. A letter written by the executive director of the state chapter to one insurance company raised concerns regarding patient confidentiality and also about the amount and length of mental health sessions allowed ("Managed Care Eyed," 1995; "Managed Care Sparks," 1996). Also, among others, social workers in Louisiana, Oklahoma, New York, Rhode Island, and Massachusetts have been active in shaping their states' Medicaid managed care plans to advocate for care recipients (Landers, 1995). "Practice and politics mix," as Bailis said, ". . . solid health policy makes for strong social work practice in health care and those . . . concerned with practice issues must focus on the objective of improving policy. Politics is the vehicle for getting there" ("Health Experts," 1984). Thus, interpreting and advocating are prime social work tasks. Policy is a key element in the context of social work in health care.

Technology

Technology is applied science—the ways in which a social group satisfies its material needs. In the broadest sense, technology means the concrete, practical solutions people invent or discover. In the present framework, technology primarily refers to medical/scientific inventions that are used for diagnosis or treatment: medication, surgical techniques, life-sustaining machinery, or ways of viewing or measuring bodily functions (Abramson and Black, 1985). In addition, technology increasingly means information management, the rise of electronic recordkeeping, and the computerization of all imaginable kinds of data (Parks, 1996; Drucker, 1993). Current concerns about confidentiality stem from these technological developments. Determining who has the right to access to information—the individual or group paying for the care, the individual receiving the care, the individual with access to the computer system, etc.—has yet to be resolved satisfactorily. These same tools also allow for new learning techniques such as interactive video, video conferencing, and social work rooms on the World Wide Web (Landers, 1996; Resnick, 1995).

For contemporary health care, the development and cost of technology relate directly to policy formulation. Technology and the organizations that house and/or distribute it account for a good deal of the astronomical costs of medical care today (Lee and Estes, 1994; Fox, 1993; Rutten and Bonsel, 1992; Aaron, 1996; Aaron and Schwartz, 1984; Reiser and Anbar, 1984). The United States' passion for, rapid acceptance of, and diffusion of "high-tech" solutions means that hospitals, health professionals, patients, and families want the best available to them no matter what the cost (Russell, 1979). From the end of World War II until very recently, the federal government spent massive sums of money to develop medical technology, train health professionals, and build facilities. From the 1960s until the mid-1970s, the purpose of much federal health policy such as Medicare, Medicaid, and the Community Mental Health Centers Act was to ensure access to health care and expensive technology. Since the beginning of the 1980s, most federal health policies have been generally directed toward controlling health care costs with specific attention to expensive technological interventions.

For social workers, sometimes the very lack of medical means to intervene in an illness creates opportunities for psychosocial intervention. Historically, social workers had important roles in the care of people with venereal diseases and tuberculosis, in part because medical interventions were inadequate to treat the illnesses. Before the discovery of penicillin permitted treatment of syphilis at an early stage with a single injection, treatment required many outpatient visits over a period of eighteen months. The social worker's role was to ensure that patients returned for prolonged outpatient treatment and to educate patients and others in their social circles who might have been infected. Now, the task might be purely epidemiological or educational (Kerson, 1980). Contemporary situations provide similar opportunities. With diseases such as AIDS and Alzheimer's, for which there are not yet adequate medical treatments, social workers help garner the social support needed to live with the illness. With other conditions, such as end-stage renal disease and severe burns, technology provides life support, and the social worker helps the patient and family to live with both the illness and the technology.

The development of life-sustaining technology has also raised perplexing ethical and legal problems in health care (Reamer, 1995; Reamer, 1994; Callahan, 1986; Reamer, 1985; Elliott, 1984; President's Commission, 1983). Sometimes, the extension of life can mean greatly diminished life quality. In other situations, medical solutions may be dehumanizing and/or produce negative side effects. Each of these circumstances provides opportunities for social work intervention. Thus, the presence or absence of technological solutions shapes the parameters of the relationship between social worker and client.

Organization

An organization is defined here as a body of people structured for some end or work, and the administrative personnel or apparatus of an agency, business, or institution (French, Bell, and Zawacki, 1989). Increasingly, to understand organizational context means to be knowledgable about multiple, complex systems involving varied funding streams, auspices, professional and nonprofessional providers, and public, not-for-profit, and for-profit agencies with varied degrees of authority (Gitterman and Miller, 1989; Maynard-Moody and McClintock, 1987; Gortner, Mahler, and Nicholson, 1987). Even the simplest organization, in the grand scheme of the delivery of health care, must be closely related to very large and complex networks of service. To compete in today's health care arena, most health care organizations are in the midst of transforming themselves in order to become more efficient (Kotter, 1995; Duncan, Ginter, and Kreidel, 1994; Minkoff, 1994; Gustafson and Allen, 1994; Cooper and Williams, 1994; Mintzberg, 1981). For professional social workers, there can be no more hiding out in an office, seeing individual clients, and acting as if there is no world encroaching from outside. Organization also structures practice (Patti, 1985). The role of a social worker in a prison for the criminally insane is necessarily different than it is in a community mental health center. Prison walls, guards, and garb must affect the relationship with the client. Even in a prison, the social worker is likely to be working for a behavioral health company that has contracted with the state-owned prison to provide treatment for drug and alcohol abuse. In the community mental health center, the social worker may be working with clients whose care is paid for by a range of managed care alternatives, each of which has different rules about who is entitled to service and the conditions of the service itself.

Formal dimensions of organization are size, division of labor, degree of bureaucratization, degree of centralization of control, and role structure (Flynn, 1992; Hasenfeld, 1992; Drucker, 1990). Changes in structure and design carried out in the name of efficiency and cost-effectiveness can restrict services and creativity (Gortner, Mahler and Nicholson, 1987; Lynn, 1980). For example, when told to spend less money, one county agency fired all of its first-line supervisors, saying their tasks could be carried out by two or three administrators. The following year, problems with staff morale and poor, undirected practice caused almost a 100 percent turnover in line staff.

Informal dimensions include mores, the unwritten rules about behavior, which people know implicitly but rarely discuss, such as ways in which to relate to members of other professions or whether it is acceptable to have a meal at a client's home (Farmer, 1996; Cooper and Williams, 1994). Also important are the networks that people develop outside the formal organizational structure in order to accomplish tasks. Often, the establishment of such a network means being able to enlist those with expertise or power regarding matters that are critical to clients (Levinson, 1992; Tichy and Charan, 1992; Shapiro, 1992; Rogers and Roethilsberger, 1991; Havassy, 1990). Such power does not necessarily reside with high office. Sometimes it can be held by a chief of service, other times by a clerk. Although it is generally easier to make exceptions or bend the rules in a smaller organization, those who work for large, highly bureaucratized organizations also learn to develop informal networks. Intimate knowledge of an organization increases the possibility of making it more responsive to clients' needs (Germain and Gitterman, 1996; Gortner, Mahler, and Nicholson, 1987).

DECISIONS ABOUT PRACTICE

Within the constraints of context is located the relationship between social worker and client. The framework maintains that specific elements in the context (policy, technology, and organization) structure the relationship between social worker and client. Similarly, the framework suggests that specific elements within the relationship, which are to a degree determined by the participants in that relationship, provide structure and regulate interaction (Goffman, 1981). In the framework, the elements are called practice decisions because they are often determined by decisions made by social worker and client, which set the pattern for their relationship. Practice decisions means that the participants themselves have the power to create the vehicle that will enable them to accomplish their goals. The term stresses the dimensions of activity, judgment, and responsibility implicit in such choices.

In some situations, practice decisions may be constrained by elements of context. For example, in order to receive funding, an organization may have to adhere to policies set by a funding source regarding use of time or even goals. The organization would therefore constrain its social workers in those ways. Also, practice decisions are not always discrete and can recur as the relationship evolves. Alterable, they act as a flexible structure that can guide the relationship and help the participants to judge the quality of their work. The ten practice decisions in this framework are (1) definition of the client; (2) goals, objectives, and outcome measures; (3) use of contract; (4) meeting place; (5) use of time; (6) strategies and interventions; (7) stance of the social worker; (8) use of outside resources; (9) reassessment; and (10) transfer or termination.

Definition of the Client

Defining the client involves the choice of a client unit; that is, deciding with whom one works in a situation. The client can be any unit, such as an individual, family, couple, parent and child, group, committee, housing project, or clinic. While a case is open, the definition of the client can change as needs change. Sometimes, one may intervene with the most troubled people in the situation, and in other instances, the social worker may work on the client's behalf because that person is not available for work (Chetnik, 1980). For example, the person who is most dependent or most troubled may be too young, demented, or ill to be directly involved. At times, broadening the definition of the client from an individual to a larger unit enhances the social support of the ill person and strengthens the whole (Pilisuk and Parks, 1986).

Goals, Objectives, and/or Outcome Measures

Goals refer to solutions that the social worker and client work to attain. In the literature, these points of attainment are referred to by various terms such as treatment objectives or outcomes (Woods and Hollis, 1990; Hepworth and Larsen, 1986; Germain, 1984; Carlton, 1984b). Primarily, goals reflect the needs and desires of the client (Goldstein, 1983; Leader, 1981). Of all of the practice decisions, goals are owned primarily by the client, with whom the social worker collaborates to help to articulate those goals. With the client's help, the social worker uses the rest of the practice decisions to structure the relationship in ways that will support the work. If the goals have been formulated by the social worker, family members, or other staff, and not by the client, they are less likely to be attained.

The relationship between social work goals and diagnosis is important in that diagnosis is often made by another profession, usually medicine, with which social work collaborates. In some ways, when a diagnosis is imposed, it becomes part of context, an organizational issue that informs social work practice. Often, a diagnostic term such as schizophrenia, arthritis, or epilepsy is a label that provides very little information about functional capacity. If the social worker employs this kind of information to limit the use that he or she thinks a client can make of the relationship or even to discard certain clients into a category that receives no service, he or she is allowing diagnosis to restrict his or her work.

Goals may be as concrete as obtaining an apartment or a prosthesis, or as intangible as feeling better about oneself or feeling happier. If some of the goals in each client situation are concrete, then they are measurable, and the social worker and client are provided with a means of assessing progress. To be measurable, they must be objectifiable; that is, they must be able to be described in concrete terms. Being able to call attention to some success such as "arriving at work on time nearly every day" or "screaming at the children less than five times a week" is helpful in encouraging a client to continue to work in the relationship. Increasingly, funding sources are asking social workers and other helping professionals for outcome measures, which are the concrete means they will use to evaluate their work and the work of the clients. Through outcome measures, social workers will be able to prove their results and their economic value to the organization and the funding sources.

Additionally, goals should be separated from wishes or dreams of client and social worker. Goals are realistic and attainable aims rather than fantasies one would hope for in the best of all possible worlds. However, while setting realistic expectations for work, the social worker must also "lend a vision," that is, help the client to envision a more satisfying life (Gitterman and Shulman, 1994; Schwartz and Zalba, 1971).

Use of Contract

Contract means agreement between social worker and client about the means used to obtain goals, as well as the description of the goals themselves (Neugeboren, 1995; Rothary, 1980; Seabury, 1976; Mallucio and Marlow, 1974). It is the keystone, cynosure, and linchpin of the social worker/client relationship and of this framework. Comprised of mutually agreed-upon obligations and expectations, a contract is a way of establishing norms for the relationship (Goffman, 1972). Norms also exist for the relationship between client and agency (Stewart, 1984; Weissman, Epstein, and Savage, 1983). Increasingly, there are contracts between funding source, agency, and client. For example, many drug-abuse treatment centers require that clients sign agency-formulated contracts stipulating the conditions of treatment.

Whether verbal or written contracts are more effective remains a matter for debate and most probably depends on the nature of the agency, work, and clients (Klier, Fein, and Genero, 1984). Certainly, written form clarifies the agreement, and having all participants sign adds formality and perhaps importance to the matters at hand. Some would argue that this very formality stultifies the interaction, interfering with creativity, transference, or other aspects of the relationship. Because contract requires that each party articulate goals and norms, it includes each of the elements of relationship structure. Participants in a helping relationship always have some expectations of each other. Use of the dimensions of contract allows the expectations of all parties to be made explicit and helps prevent misunderstanding.

Meeting Place

Meeting place refers to the physical space in which the relationship happens. Most work occurs in the institution/agency or in the client's home. Increasingly, meeting place is determined by the organization rather than by the needs of the clients. The major portion of some services such as home care, foster care, and hospice is dispensed in the home, while other services such as dialysis, discharge planning, and community mental health are most often offered within the institution. There is a renewed trend to place social work services back in the community with the increase in a range of case managment and intensive case management services occurring wherever the client is (Simmons, 1994; Raiff, 1993; Vourlekis and Greene, 1992).

Meeting place can influence assessment by limiting or increasing the amount of information made available about the client. One's social scene provides some information about his or her identity (Goffman, 1972). When meetings take place outside of the client's habitat, the social worker relies on the person's appearance and the details he or she provides about his or her life. The sight of an institutionally gowned person lying in bed in a hospital room provides no clues to individual identity. Personality, memories, experiences, and style are all obscured. Often in such situations, the social worker assumes information which he or she does not have.

When the client is seen at home, the social worker learns something about the client's means, organizational abilities, values, neighborhood, and, perhaps, his or her relationships with family members and neighbors (Hodges and Blythe, 1992; Markowitz, 1992; Bloom, 1983; Cohen and Egen, 1981). No other means compare to home visits for assessing the life of a client or, sometimes, for empowering him or her (Whittington, 1985; Bregman, 1980; Moynihan, 1974). One sees the impact of problems, illnesses, and disabilities on daily living. Through home visits, social workers can help collaborating professionals and aides to understand a client's life and problems. Many organizations think that home visits are too expensive and as a result do not allow them; however, denying social workers the opportunity to see their clients in their home environments, if the clients are willing, limits the ability of the social workers to assess client capacities and resources.

Two important aspects of meeting place are space and privacy, which in many institutional or agency settings are at a premium. Where none exists, social workers can create private space for themselves and their clients by using undivided attention, eye contact, voice quality, and body language. When other professionals ignore the need for privacy, social workers have to educate them in order to protect their clients and foster the work.

The telephone is another "place" in which to help people who cannot come to the organization and whom the social worker cannot visit. It has proven effective as a means of support and treatment for isolated clients (Shepard, 1987; Stein and Lambert, 1986; Ranan and Blodgett, 1983). Again, decisions about meeting place are determined to a degree by the rules of the setting and the needs of the clients.

Use of Time

Decisions about time relate to the duration of the relationship and the duration and spacing of each meeting. Since use of time is a means of structuring the relationship, sharing this information with clients empowers them (Lemon and Goldstein, 1978). In the broadest sense, orientation in time and space "is felt as a protection rather than a straitjacket, and its loss can provoke extreme anxiety" (Mead and Bateson, 1942). The importance of time is no less diminished in single-encounter work in a hospital emergency room than it is in group work or long-term psychotherapy (Budman and Gurman, 1988; Alissi and Casper, 1985). In many instances, the use of time is determined by the organization or funding source. For example, policy may determine the duration of a session, how many sessions a client may be seen, or the number of days for which a patient is hospitalized. Time is also an important dimension of contract. No matter who determines duration, using time to structure the relationship and having the client participate in the structure aids the work (Perlman, 1979; Smalley and Bloom, 1977).

Strategies and Interventions

Strategies and interventions refers to the selection of particular methods of care that are most appropriate for specific clients in particular situations (Germain and Gitterman, 1996; Hanrahan and Reid, 1984; Carlton, 1984b; Rushton and Davies, 1984; Hartman, 1983; Lemon, 1983; Meyer, 1983). In every situation, the social worker makes decisions about the ways in which the client can best be helped. These decisions involve choices about orientation, modality, technique, and intervention.

To some degree, choice of strategies and interventions relates to definition of client and client unit. Thus, designating an individual as the client might indicate that one would do individual work, while designating the family as the client would indicate family work. However, the more general decision to work with a certain client unit opens the possibility for a plethora of decisions regarding particular theoretical orientations such as a psychodynamic, cognitive, or behavioral approach (Woods and Hollis, 1990; de Shazer, Berg, and Lipchik, 1986; Hepworth and Larsen, 1986; Turner, 1986; Carlton, 1984a; Germain, 1984; Rosenblatt and Waldfogel, 1983; Birdman, 1981). Such orientations often reflect beliefs and world views of the social worker, which may relate little to particular client problems (Germain and Gitterman, 1996). For example, because it is common in our society to believe that elderly people are not amenable to psychodynamic work, these approaches are unusual in work with the elderly; yet, programs for the elderly report excellent psychodynamic work (Lewis, 1987; Milinsky, 1987; Kaminsky, 1985). This practice decision cautions social workers to choose treatment modalities that reflect needs and goals of clients rather than their own worldviews or beliefs.

In turn, choice of a particular theoretical orientation and treatment modality brings one to decisions regarding specific techniques or interventions, such as the use of ritual, life story, or sculpting (Laird, 1984; Fox, 1983; Jefferson, 1978). Techniques such as these are tools to bring a theoretical model into action. Monitoring their use offers the social worker another way to assess ongoing work because strategies such as these tend to have specified outcomes (Hanraham and Reid, 1984; Russell et al., 1984). At times, interventions that are used are different from ones that had been anticipated, because a client's needs may be redefined as the work progresses (Rosen and Mutschler, 1982). Articulating practice interventions enhances the social worker's control of his or her medium. Treatment method is also sometimes determined by dimensions of context such as organization or funding policy. For example, one facility may extol a particular form of family therapy to treat an illness such as bulimia and another may use a specific form of individual therapy to treat the same illness. These choices seem to arise from differing beliefs about etiology and/or cure.

At times, the nature of the illness or disability affects the choice of modality (Mailick, 1979). For example, an illness or disability that leaves an individual physically dependent, such as advanced rheumatoid arthritis or emphysema, may require that the social worker work with family members as well as the ill person. In the case of advanced Alzheimer's disease or with a seriously ill infant, the social worker may work only with family members. Use of time, another practice decision, sometimes may be a dimension of treatment modality. Since the 1960s, short-term, brief, and crisis-oriented work have been conventional, but within each of these orientations there are a myriad of practice decisions regarding modality and specific technique (Reid, 1992; Turner, 1986; Carlton, 1984b; Rosenblatt and Waldfogel, 1983; Kanter, 1983; de Shazer, Berg, and Lipchik, 1982).

Case Management

One modality that has resumed its important place in social work practice is case management, which is sometimes referred to as advanced or intensive case managment (Hagen, 1994; Wolk, Sullivan, and Hartmann, 1994; Raiff, 1993; Harris and Bachrach, 1993; Dinerman, 1992; Vourlikis and Greene, 1992: Weil, Karls, and Associates, 1985; Rubin, 1983). Developed for client groups such as the frail elderly, chronically mentally ill, the developmentally disabled, and foster children, this modality is one response to the complexity of service delivery systems (Johnson and Rubin, 1983; Weissman, Epstein, and Savage, 1983; Lamb, 1980). Bachrach says case management rests on the notions of comprehensiveness, that is, a full array of services; on longitudinality, that is, service over a relatively long period of time; and on a special, dependable, therapeutic relationship with another individual (Bachrach, 1992). It can be used to organize the services of an entire agency, a national program of immense proportions, or a single caseload; but, properly defined, case management should never exclude clinical work. In fact,

> case management is both a concept and a process. As a concept, it is a system of relationships between direct service providers, agency administrators, and clients. As a process, case management is an orderly, planned provision of services intended to facilitate a client's functioning at as normal a level as possible and as economically as possible. (Weil, Karls, and Associates, 1985)

There are many approaches to case management as a strategy or intervention for the social work practitioner. These approaches vary in terms of the direct involvement of the social worker. They range from a broker-ing role, in which the social worker links clients to services, advocates for clients, and moniters client activities, to clinical or advanced case man-agement, in which the managers act as primary therapists as well as monitors, advocates, and brokers (Harris and Bachrach, 1993). In these latter positions, the social workers carry a great deal of authority in the system of services that the client requires. Especially with those with serious and persistent chronic mental illness, such clinical case managers work in teams, although the special one-to-one relationship of clinical case manager and patient continues to be paramount. Case management has a special appeal to managed care approaches because such services are generally community-based rather than being based in institutions, and they can serve a utilization review function if given the authority to authorize or deny services to prevent their unreasonable or unnecessary use (Wolk, Sullivan, and Hartmann, 1994; Brennan and Kaplan, 1993).

Pragmatic and Eclectic Approaches

Practitioners generally suggest that their approach is both pragmatic and eclectic; that is, they do what they must depending on the circum-stances, needs, and capabilities of their clients, and they tend to draw from many modalities and techniques. Sometimes, it is difficult to distin-guish between the style of the social worker and the choice of treatment modality. Social workers who are more comfortable in a listening and supporting mode may report their orientation as Rogerian or psychoana-lytic. Those who are highly structured and/or directive may say they use crisis intervention or a task-oriented approach. In some ways, this is like self-typecasting. One plays the ingenue or bad guy because it is comfort-able. Again, the allusion to an art form is meant to underscore the notion that conscious decisions about modality are more likely based on the client need than in the style of the social worker.

Stance of the Social Worker

Stance of the social worker is closest to the old-fashioned term "con-scious use of self," which is an understanding of one's self, motivations, and place in and impact on relationships (Baldwin and Satir, 1987; Lam-mert, 1986; Robinson, 1978). It implies that the social worker has suffi-cient self-awareness, experience, and discipline to be able to choose how to behave in a particular client situation. Unlike some other practice decisions shared with the client, the social worker is totally responsible for this choice. Experience and self-awareness provide the social worker greater mastery of stance so that, within realistic limits, the social worker can be what the client and situation need him or her to be. Just as an actor learns to assume a role, the social worker adapts and refines his or her stance according to the needs of the client situation.

Some elements of stance are the worker's degree of activity or passivity, amount of advice-giving, use of authority, self-disclosure, and touch (Philip, 1993; Palombo, 1987; Borenzweig, 1983; Lackie, 1983; Reynolds and Fischer, 1983; Leader, 1983; Gourse and Cheschier, 1981; Ewalt and Katz, 1976; Goffman, 1961). Other elements such as transference and counter-transference, prejudices, and false assumptions, which may support action that is different from the needs of the client situation, are part of the stance of the social worker as well (Saari, 1986; Biggs, 1979; Brown, 1984; Carlton, 1984a; Googins, 1984; Atwood, 1982; Hardman, 1975).

Use of Outside Resources

Outside resources are the services used by client and social worker, which are outside of the relationship, often external to the agency, and which further the work of the relationship (Woods and Hollis, 1990; Germain, 1983). These services can range from the protective work of a state or county child welfare agency to assistance with obtaining an apartment, walker, or prosthesis. Determination of the client's ability to broker his or her own services is an issue in the use of outside resources. Sometimes, the client and/or family can grow stronger by managing outside resources themselves; in some instances, the social worker can enhance the relationship by arranging services; and at other times, the social worker must procure outside resources because the client/family is unable to manage (Bates, 1983).

Ecomap

Many of the chapters in this book include an ecomap that illuminates the interactions of clients with some individuals, institutions, and agencies in their lives (Compton and Galaway, 1994; Hartman and Laird, 1983). This graphic representation is useful for assessment, evaluation, and helping clients to set priorities and make decisions about altering relationships with individuals and organizations. Because it allows one to lay out very complicated relationships on a single page, it gives client and social worker a greater feeling of control of a situation. In the ecomap, a large center circle is generally comprised of the client's nuclear family, with circles surrounding that one which represents people and organizations with whom the client interacts. In this book, a strong relationship is drawn as an unbroken line. The flow of energy is either depicted as going back and forth between both parties, with an arrow at either end, or as going from only one to the other, with an arrow pointing at the party who is receiving the energy. A tenuous relationship is depicted as a light, broken line, while a stressful relationship is drawn as a heavy, broken line. A circle with a name in it and no line drawn to it means that there is no relationship between the client and the person or agency named in the circle. For example, in the sample ecomap that was borrowed from the chapter "Children's Intensive Case Management in an Urban Community Mental Health Center," there are stressful relationships between the client and his sister, the foster mother and the foster care agency, and between the foster father and his work situation, while the foster mother is shown as having an energizing relationship with her work, and the whole family relates positively to church. Like a snapshot, an ecomap captures a one-time period in the life of the client. Updated regularly, the ecomap shows the client and social worker where they might make changes, can demonstrate progress, and can be used for evaluation.

Reassessment

Reassessment presents an opportunity for social worker and client to evaluate their work during the course of the relationship. Like artists, they are asked to step back from their work and examine it. Reassessment is the process of reexamining the dimensions of the framework as well as other issues that participants have deemed important. It can be made part of the pattern of each meeting or set aside to be brought into the work at certain intervals. The technique can be as simple as discussing how the work is going or as sophisticated as using standardized measures of success (Corcoran, 1987; Ivanoff, Blythe, and Briar, 1987; Thomlinson, 1984; Reid and Hanrahan, 1982; Bloom and Fischer, 1982; Levitt and Reid, 1981). Also, reassessment can be a way to reactivate a stalled relationship or to slow one that seems to be speeding along almost out of control. Schwartz's questions, "Are we working?" and "What are we working on?" are helpful here (Schwartz and Zalba, 1971). Finally, reassessment provides the social worker an opportunity to assess and obtain feedback about his or her performance (Gummer, 1984).

Transfer or Termination

Transfer and termination mark the end of the relationship between client and social worker, that is, the fact that they will not be meeting in

FIGURE 1.1. Ecomap for Charles Williams

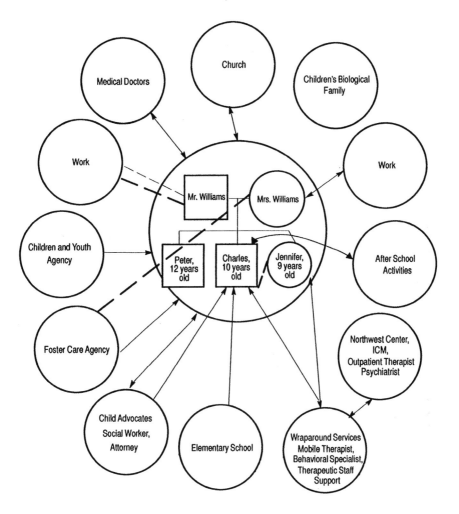

this way any longer (Woods and Hollis, 1990; Hepworth and Larsen, 1986; Sanville, 1982; Hollis and Woods, 1981; Levinson, 1977). Goffman noted that greetings and farewells are ritual displays that mark a change in degree of access (Goffman, 1972). Here, social worker and client will not have the same kind of access to each other as they would have had if the work continued. Ideally, termination is a decision that social worker and client have made together because goals have been accomplished and their work is finished. Often, when clients terminate before the social worker is ready, it is because the client has perceived work more positively than the social worker (Toseland, 1987). Even when the client wants to terminate before the social worker thinks work is finished, it is important to end the relationship positively so that the client may return to the agency (or to another one) if he or she needs further help. Sometimes, termination signals the end of the relationship between client and agency. At other times, the social worker is leaving the organization, and the client will continue with another social worker (Super, 1982). Vacations also evoke issues about termination (Webb, 1983). Often a difficult period, termination has great potential for growth through the use of the relationship (Fortune, Pearlingi, and Rochelle, 1992, 1991; Fortune, 1987; Fortune, 1985).

Case Conclusion

Conclusion refers primarily to outcome and current functioning of the client. Client and social worker summarize their work together so that each can leave the relationship with knowledge of accomplishments. In addition, they finish in a positive manner that will allow the client to seek help again, if necessary.

Differential Discussion

In a differential discussion, all of the previous framework decisions are reviewed in order for the social worker to analyze his or her work. Differential discussion allows the social worker to be a "Monday night quarterback," that is, to look back on the case to decide which elements would remain the same the next time he or she worked with a client with similar capacity, personality, and problems. Differential discussion encourages the social worker to generalize from a specific client to a category of like cases with which he or she can use similar structure and techniques. For example, in retrospect, the social worker may decide he or she was too confrontational with a client, the coldness of the meeting place might have been a detriment, or the client may have been asked to coordinate more resources than he or she was able to manage. Emphasis on the social worker's ability to (1) generalize from a particular case and (2) alter elements in the relationship between social worker and client makes differential discussion the most useful dimension of the framework. This step moves the social worker out of the present relationship and on to the next.

PRACTICE IN CONTEXT

A review of the overarching conception of practice in context brings the framework full circle. The first chapter is a summary that reviews the framework and provides examples from the setting chapters. Here, themes drawn from setting articles are developed for a broad discussion of social work in health settings. Constraints on the setting, the influence that these constraints have had on the relationship, and the series of decisions that determine the structure of the relationship enable social workers to map their work and, as a result, enhance action. This review also helps to identify areas of advocacy and social action for the social worker (Ashord, Macht, and Mylym, 1987; Haynes and Mickelson, 1986; Sosin and Caulum, 1983; Sosin, 1979).

Using the framework described above, *Social Work in Health Settings* acts as a casebook, a collection of real cases in settings described by and reflecting the style of each experienced social work practitioner. Altogether, 33 health and mental health settings demonstrate "the cadence and pattern" of social work in health (Mead, 1973). Each setting article follows the practice-in-context framework as its outline.

The settings are presented in five broad-based sections based on related settings:

1. Services to children and/or families,
2. Acute and high-technology care,
3. Rehabilitation, long-term intervention, and advocacy,
4. Mental health care, and
5. Care for the frail elderly and hospice care.

These sections are not discrete. As a matter of fact, many of the settings overlap into two or more sections. For example, renal dialysis is a treatment for end-stage renal disease, which has acute episodes but requires long-term care. The chapter titled "Premature Babies in the Intensive Care Nursery" describes a service to children and families, but it is also an example of acute and high-technology care. Similarly, the spina bifida program could be part of services to children and families, acute and high-technology care, and rehabilitation. Other settings include

1. a premature nursery,
2. a perinatal AIDS program,

3. an emergency room,
4. a rural health department,
5. a school-based health center,
6. a pediatric neurology clinic,
7. a spina-bifida program,
8. a residential program for women and their children,
9. a residential care facility for treatment of children with severe disabilities,
10. discharge planning in a community hospital,
11. a regional burn center,
12. a renal dialysis and transplant program,
13. adult oncology,
14. treatment of chronic pain in a rehabilitation hospital,
15. a regional spinal cord injury center,
16. a mutual help group for emphysema patients in a veterans administration medical center,
17. an advocacy program for uranium miners and their families,
18. a self-help program for persons with AIDS,
19. brief treatment in a community mental health center,
20. an inpatient psychiatric unit,
21. a center for developmental disability,
22. a transitional residence for the mentally ill,
23. case management for the seriously and persistently mentally ill,
24. wraparound services for a mentally ill child,
25. mental health care in a combat zone,
26. treatment of recurrent depression in private practice,
27. hospital-based case management for the frail elderly,
28. home care,
29. a support group in a home for the elderly,
30. Alzheimer's disease intervention in a nursing home, and
31. hospice care.

As well, there are two special chapters providing an insider's view of social work in health settings. These chapters, "He's Schizophrenic and the System Is Not Helping: Reflections of a Troubled Parent and Professional," and "Beyond Survival by Machine: Reflections of a Spouse," are written by social workers who have personal and professional interests in a particular setting. The first is written by a social worker with many years of experience as a practitioner, educator, and advocate for the chronically mentally ill and whose son has chronic schizophrenia. The author of the second is a social worker whose husband was maintained on renal dialysis for almost 20 years, has been the social worker in a dialysis unit, and is a consultant to several organizations having to do with renal disease.

Ideally, the format for this book would be a three-ringed notebook in which case/setting articles and dimensions of context and practice could be arranged and rearranged for teaching purposes. One could then use these case/settings to discuss issues around settings and populations, such as short-term and long-term care; institutional and home care; physical and mental health; services for children, adults, and the elderly; or trauma and disease. In addition, one can examine a particular practice decision, such as use of contract or stance of the social worker, across 33 practice settings. Overall, *Social Work in Health Settings* has one primary purpose: to help the social worker to clarify and explicate practice in context in order to best ply his or her craft.

The chapters that follow are generally written in the first person, although some chapters have multiple authors. This format was used to enhance the notion that the practitioner is speaking about his or her work. The names of all clients have been changed in order to preserve confidentiality.

REFERENCES

Aaron, H. J. (1991). *Serious and unstable condition: Financing America's health care.* Washington, DC: The Brookings Institution.

Aaron, H. J. (1996). *The problem that won't go away: Reforming U.S. health care financing.* Washington, DC: The Brookings Institution.

Aaron, H. J. and Schwartz, W. V. (1984). *The painful prescription: Rationing health care.* Washington, DC: The Brookings Institution.

Abramson, M. and Black, R. B. (1985). Extending the boundaries of life: Implications for practice. *Health and Social Work, 10*(3), 165-173.

Alissi, A. S. and Caspar, M. (1985). Time as a factor in group work. *Social Work in Groups, 8*(2), 3-16.

Allphin, C. (1982). Envy in the transference and countertransference. *Clinical Social Work Journal, 10*(3), 151-164.

Ashford, J., Macht, M. W., and Mylym, M. (1987). Advocacy by social workers in the Public Defender's office. *Social Work, 32*(3), 199-203.

Bachrach, L. L. (1992). Case management revisited. *Hospital and Community Psychiatry, 43*(3), 209-210.

Baldwin, M. and Satir, V. (Eds.). (1987). *The use of self in therapy.* Binghamton, NY: The Haworth Press.

Bates, M. (1983). Using the environment to help the male skid row alcoholic. *Social Casework, 64,* 276-282.

Bateson, G. *The natural history of an interview.* Unpublished manuscript.

Bateson, G. (1975). *Steps to an ecology of mind.* New York: Ballantine.

Birdman, S. (Ed.). (1981). *Forms of brief therapy.* New York: Guilford Press.

Birdwhistell, R. L. (1970). *Kinesics and context: Essays on body motion communication.* Philadelphia, PA: University of Pennsylvania Press.

Bloom, M. (1983). Usefulness of the home visit for diagnosis and treatment. *Social Casework, 54*, 67-75.

Bloom, M. and Fischer, J. (1982). *Evaluating practice: Guidelines for the accountable professional.* Englewood Cliffs, NJ: Prentice-Hall.

Borenzweig, H. (1983). Touching in clinical social work. *Social Casework, 64*, 238-242.

Bregman, A. (1980). Living with progressive childhood illness: Parental management of neuromuscular disease. *Social Work in Health Care, 5*(4), 387-407.

Brennan, J. P. and Kaplan, C. (1993). Setting new standards for social work case management. *Hospital and Community Psychiatry, 44*(3), 219-222.

Briggs, D. (1979). The trainee and the borderline client: Countertransference pitfalls. *Clinical Social Work Journal, 7*, 1-20.

Brown, F. (1984). Erotic and pseudoerotic elements in the treatment of male patients by female therapists. *Clinical Social Work Journal, 12*(3), 244-257.

Budman, S. H. and Gurman, A. S. (1988). *Theory and practice of brief therapy.* New York: Guilford Press.

Callahan, D. (1986). How technology is reframing the abortion debate. *Hastings Center Report, 16*(1), 33-42.

Carlton, T. O. (1984a). *Clinical social work in health settings.* New York: Springer.

Carlton, T. O. (1984b). Understanding and choice of treatment procedures. In *Clinical social work in health settings.* New York: Springer, pp. 422-445.

Carlton, T. O. (1985). Highlights of a decade. *Health and Social Work, 10*(4), 308-312.

Cayner, J. J. (1996a, February). Reclaiming the high ground in policy. *NASW News, 41*(2), 2.

Cayner, J. J. (1996b, June). Health reform back on front burner. *NASW News, 41*(6), 2.

Chetnik, M. (1980). The treatment of a preschooler via the mother. In J. Mishne (Ed.), *Psychotherapy and training in clinical social work.* New York: Gardner Press, pp. 135-149.

Cohen, R. (1996, May). Owning up to tomorrow's promise. *NASW News, 41*(5), 2.

Cohen, S. and Egen, B. (1981). The social work home visit in a health care setting. *Social Work in Health Care, 6*(4), 55-67.

Commission allies with lobby seeking healthy budget policy. (April 1986). *NASW News*, p. 6.

Compton, B. R. and Galaway, B. (1994). *Social work processes.* Pacific Grove, CA: Brooks/Cole.

Cooper, C. L. and Williams, S. (1994). *Creating healthy work organizations.* New York: John Wiley & Sons.

Corcoran, K. (1987). *Measures for clinical practice: A sourcebook.* New York: The Free Press.

Cornelius, D. S. (1994). Managed care and social work: Constructing a context and a response. *Social Work in Health Care, 20*(1), 47-63.

Dear, R. B. and Patti, R. I. (1981). Legislative advocacy: Seven effective tactics. *Social Work, 26,* 289-296.

de Shazer, D., Berg, I. K., and Lipchik, E. (1986). Brief therapy: Focused solution development. *Family Process, 20*(3), 281-289.

Dickson, D. T. (1995). *Law in the health and human services: A guide for social workers, psychologists, psychiatrists and related professionals.* New York: The Free Press.

Dinerman, M. (1992). Managing the maze: Case management and service delivery, *Administration in Social Work, 16*(1), 1-9.

Dobelstein, A. (1990). *Social welfare policy and analysis.* Chicago: Nelson-Hall.

Drucker, P. (1990). *Managing the nonprofit organization.* New York: HarperCollins.

Drucker, P. (1993). *Post-capitalist society.* New York: Harper Business.

Duncan, W. J., Ginter, P. M., and Kreidel, W. K. (1994). A sense of direction in public organizations: An analysis of mission statements in state health departments. *Administration & Society, 26*(1), 11-27.

Ehrenreich, J. (1985). *The altruistic imagination: A history of social work and social policy in the United States.* New York: Cornell University Press.

Elliot, M. W. (1984). *Ethical issues in social work: An annotated bibliography.* New York: Council on Social Work Education.

Ewalt, P. and Katz, J. (1976). An examination of advice-giving as a therapeutic intervention. *Smith College Studies in Social Work, 47,* 3-19.

Farmer, B. C. (1996). *A nursing home and its organizational climate: An ethnography.* Westport, CN: Auburn House.

Fein, R. (1986). *Medical care: Medical costs.* Cambridge, MA: Harvard University Press.

Flynn, J. (1992). *Social agency policy: Analysis and presentation for community practice.* Chicago: Nelson-Hall.

Fortune, A. E. (1985). Planning, duration, and termination of treatment. *Social Service Review, 59,* 647-661.

Fortune, A. E. (1987). Grief only? Client and social worker reactions to termination. *Clinical Social Work Journal, 15*(2), 159-171.

Fortune, A .E., Pearlingi, H., and Rochelle, C. (1991). Criteria for terminating treatment. *Families in Society, 22,* 366-370.

Fortune, A. E., Pearlingi, H., and Rochelle, C. (1992). Reactions to termination of individual treatment. *Social Work, 37,* 171-178.

Fox, D. M. (1993). *Power and illness.* Berkeley, CA: University of California Press.

Fox, P. D. (1990). Forward: Overview of managed care trends. In National Health Lawyers Association, *The Insider's Guide to Managed Care.* Washington, DC: National Health Lawyers Association.

Fox, R. (1983). The past is always present: Creative methods for capturing the life story. *Clinical Social Work Journal, 11,* 368-378.

Freeborn, D. K. and Pope, C. R. (1994). Promise and performance in managed care: The prepaid group practice model. Baltimore, MD: The Johns Hopkins University Press.

French, W. H., Bell, C. H., and Zawacki, R. A. (1989). *Organization development: Theory, practice and research* (Third Edition). Plano, Texas: BPI/Irwin.

Germain, C. (1981). The ecological approach to people-environment transactions. *Social Casework, 62*(1), 67-76.

Germain, C. (1984). *Social work in health care*. New York: Free Press.

Germain, C. (1983). Using social and physical environments. In A. Rosenblatt and D. Waldfogel (Eds.), *Handbook of clinical social work*. San Francisco: CA: Jossey-Bass, pp. 26-57.

Germain, C. and Gitterman, A. (1996). The life model of social work practice (Second Edition). New York: Columbia University Press.

Gil, D. (1982). *Unravelling social policy: Theory, analysis and political action towards social equality* (Second Edition). Cambridge, MA: Schenkman.

Gitterman, A. and Miller, I. (1989). The influence of the organization on clinical practice. *Clinical Social Work Journal, 17*(2), 151-164.

Gitterman, A. and Shulman, L. (Eds.). (1994). *Mutual aid groups: Vulnerable populations and the life cycle*. New York: Columbia University Press.

Goffman, E. (1959). *Presentation of self in everyday life*. New York: Doubleday.

Goffman, E. (1961a). *Asylums: Essays on the social situation of mental patients and other inmates*. New York: Doubleday & Co.

Goffman, E. (1961b). *Encounters: Two studies in the sociology of interaction*. New York: Macmillan.

Goffman, E. (1966). *Behavior in public places*. New York: The Free Press.

Goffman, E. (1972). *Relations in public*. New York: Harper and Row.

Goffman, E. (1981). *Interaction ritual: Essays in face to face behavior*. New York: Pantheon.

Goldman, R. L. and Mukherjee, S. K. (1995). *Managed service restructuring in health care: A strategic approach in a competitive environment*. Binghamton, NY: The Haworth Press.

Goldstein, H. (1983). Starting where the client is. *Social Casework, 64*, 267-275.

Googins, B. (1984). Avoidance of the alcoholic client. *Social Work, 29*(2), 161-166.

Gortner, H. F., Mahler, J., and Nicholson, J. B. (1987). *Organization theory: A public perspective*. Chicago, IL: The Dorsey Press.

Gourse, J. E. and Cheschier, M. W. (1981). Authority issues in treating resistant families. *Social Casework, 62*(2), 60-68.

Granger, B. P. and Moynihan, L. (1987). Successful engagement in social legislation. *Administration in Social Work, 11*(1), 37-45.

Gummer, B. (1984). How'm I doing?: Current perspectives on performance appraisals and the evaluation of work. *Administration in Social Work, 8*(2), 91-101.

Gustafson, L. and Allen, D. (1994). A new management model for child welfare. *Public Welfare, 52*(1), 31-40.

Hagen, J. L. (1994). JOBS and case management: Developments in 10 states. *Social Work, 39*(2), 197-205.

Hanrahan, P. and Reid, W. (1984). Choosing effective treatment interventions. *Social Service Review, 58*, 244-258.

Hardman, D. S. (1975). Not with my daughter you don't. *Social Work, 20*(4), 278-285.

Harris, M. and Bachrach, L. L. (Eds.). (1993). *Clinical case management: New directions for mental health services.* San Francisco, CA: Jossey-Bass.

Hartman, A. (1983). Theories for producing change. In A. Rosenblatt and D. Waldfogel (Eds.), *Handbook of clinical social work.* San Francisco, CA: Jossey-Bass, pp. 97-279.

Hartman, A. and Laird, J. (1983). *Family-centered-social work practice.* New York: The Free Press.

Hasenfeld, Y. (Ed.). (1992). *Human services as complex organizations.* Newbury Park, CA: Sage.

Havassy, H. M. (1990). Effective second-story bureaucrats: Mastering the paradox of diversity. *Social Work, 35*(1), 103-109.

Haynes, K. S. and Mickelson, J. S. (1986). *Affecting change: Social workers in the political arena.* New York: Longman.

Health experts take policy to task. (1984, July). *NASW News, 1*(10), 3.

Hepworth, D. H. (1986). Negotiating goals and formulating a contract. In *Direct social work practice: Theories and skills.* Chicago, IL: Dorsey Press, pp. 300-335.

Hepworth, D. H. and Larsen, J. A. (1986). The final phase: Termination and evaluation. In *Direct social work practice: Theory and skills.* Homewood, IL: Dorsey Press, pp. 319-342.

Hodges, V. S. and Blythe, B. J. (1992). Improving service delivery to high-risk families: Home-based practice. *Families in Society, 73*(5), 259-265.

Hollis, F. and Woods, K. M. (1981). *Casework: A psychosocial therapy.* New York: Random House.

Iglehart, J. K. (1992). The American health care system: Managed care. *New England Journal of Medicine, 327*, 742-747.

Iglehart, J. K. (1996). Managed care and mental health. *The New England Journal of Medicine, 334*(2), 131-135.

Ivanoff, A., Blythe, B., and Briar, S. (1987). The empirical clinical practice debate. *Social Casework, 68*(5), 290-298.

Jackson, V. H. (Ed.). (1995). *Managed care resource guide for social workers in agency settings.* Washington, DC: NASW Press.

Jackson, V. H. (Ed.). (1996). *Managed care resources guide for social workers in private practice.* Washington, DC: NASW Press.

Jansson, B. and Simmons, J. (1986). The survival of social work units in host organizations. *Social Work, 31*, 339-343.

Jeffersen, C. (1978). Some notes on the use of family sculpture in therapy. *Family Process, 17*, 69-75.

Johnson, P. and Rubin, A. (1983). Case management in mental health: A social work domain. *Social Work, 28,* 49-55.

Kaminsky, M. (1985). The arts and social work: Writing and reminiscing in old age. In R. Dobrof (Ed.), *Gerontological Social Work in the Community.* Binghamton, NY: The Haworth Press, pp. 225-246.

Kadushin, G. and Kulys, R. (1995). Job satisfaction among social work discharge planners, *Health and Social Work, 20*(3), 174-186

Kahn, A. (1979). *Social policy and social services* (Second Edition). New York: Random House.

Kanter, J. S. (1983). Reevaluations of task-centered social work practice. *Clinical Social Work Journal, 11*(3), 228-244.

Kerson, T. S. (1978). The social work relationship: A form of gift exchange. *Social Work, 23,* 326-327.

Kerson, T. S. (1980). *Medical social work: The pre-professional paradox.* New York: Irvington.

Kerson, T. S. (1985a). Responsiveness to need: Social work's impact on health care. *Health and Social Work, 10*(4), 300-307.

Kerson, T. S. (1985b). *Understanding chronic illness: The medical and psychosocial dimensions of nine diseases.* New York: The Free Press.

Kissick, W. L. (1994). *Medicine's dilemmas: Infinite needs versus finite resources.* New Haven, CN: Yale University Press.

Klier, J., Fein, E., and Genero, C. (1984). Are written or verbal contracts more effective in family therapy? *Social Work, 29,* 298-299.

Kotter, J. P. (1995). Leading change: Why transformation efforts fail. *Harvard Business Review,* (March/April), 59-67.

Kadushin, G. and Kulys, R. (1995). Job satisfaction among social work discharge planners, *Health and Social Work, 20*(3), 174-186.

Lackie, B. (1983). The families of origin of social workers. *Clinical Social Work Journal, 11,* 309-322.

Laird, J. (1984). Sorcerers, shamans and social workers: The use of ritual in social work practice. *Social Work, 29*(2), 123-129.

Lamb, H. (1980). Therapist-case managers: More than brokers of services. *Hospital and Community Psychiatry, 31,* 762-764.

Lammert, M. (1986). Experience as knowing: Utilizing therapist self–awareness. *Social Casework, 67,* 369-76.

Landers, S. (1995). Managed Medicaid: Care in the balance. *NASW News, 40*(4), 3.

Landers, S. (1996). High-tech brings rapid, radical change. *NASW News, 41*(4), 3.

Leader, A. (1981). The relationship of presenting problems to family conflict. *Social Casework, 62*(8), 451-457.

Leader, A. (1983). Therapeutic control in family therapy. *Clinical Social Work Journal, 11*(4), 351-361.

Lee, P. R. and Estes, C. L. (1994). *The nation's health.* Boston, MA: Jones and Bartlett.

Lemon, E. C. (1983). Education and methods for clinical practice. In A. Rosenblatt and D. Waldfogel (Eds.), *Handbook of clinical social work.* San Francisco, CA: Jossey-Bass, pp. 281-548.

Lemon, E. and Goldstein, S. (1978). Use of time limits in planned brief treatment. *Social Casework, 59*(19), 588-596.

Levinson, H. (1977). Termination of psychotherapy: Some salient issues. *Social Casework, 58*(10), 480-489.

Levinson, H. (1992). Fads, fantasies and psychological management. *Psychology Journal,* (Winter), 1-12.

Levitt, J. L. and Reid, W. (1981). Rapid-assessment instruments for practice. *Social Work Research and Abstracts, 17*(1), 13-19.

Lewis, M. (1987). Is sex bias dangerous to women's mental health? *Perspectives on Aging, 16*(2), 9-11.

Lynn, L. (1980). *The state and human services: Organizational change in a political context.* Cambridge, MA: MIT Press.

Mailick, M. (1979). The impact of severe illness on the individual and family: An overview. *Social Work in Health Care, 5*(2), 117-128.

Mallucio, A. and Marlow, W. (1974). The case for contract. *Social Work, 19*(1), 28-35.

Managed Care Eyed in Report on Insurer Pay. (October 1995). *NASW News, 40*(9), 7.

Managed Care Sparks Action by 2 Chapters, (May 1996). *NASW News, 41*(5), 7.

Markowitz, L. M. (1992). Making house calls. *Family Therapy Networker,* (July/August), 26-27.

Maynard-Moody, S. and McClintock, C. (1987). Weeding an old garden: Toward a new understanding of organizational goals. *Administration and Society, 19*(1), 125-142.

Mead, M. (1973). *An anthropologist at work.* New York: Equinox Books.

Mead, M. and Bateson, G. (1942). *Balinese character.* New York: Academy of Sciences.

Meyer, C. (1976). *Social work practice.* New York: The Free Press.

Meyer, C. (1983). Selecting important practice methods. In A. Rosenblatt and D. Waldfogel (Eds.), *Handbook of clinical social work.* San Francisco, CA: Jossey-Bass, pp. 731-749.

Milinsky, T .S. (1987). Stagnation and depression in the elderly group client. *Social Casework, 68,* 173-179.

Minkoff, K. (1994). Community mental health in the nineties: Public sector managed care. *Community Mental Health Journal, 30*(4), 317-321.

Mintzberg, H. (1981). Organizational design: Fashion or fit. *Harvard Business Review,* (January/February), 103-116.

Mizrahi, T. (1993). Managed care and managed competition: A primer for social work. *Health and Social Work, 18*(2), 86-91.

Moroney, R. M. (1991). *Social policy and social work: Critical essays on the welfare state.* New York: Aldine deGruyter.

Moynihan, S. K. (1974). Home visits for family treatment. *Social Casework,* *55*(12), 612-617.

Neugeboren, G. (1995). Organizational influences on management information systems in the human services. *Computers in the Human Services 12*(3-4), 295-310.

Newhouse, J. P. (1993). *Free for all? Lessons from the RAND health insurance experiment.* Cambridge, MA: Harvard University Press.

Palombo, J. (1987). Spontaneous self-disclosures in psychotherapy. *Clinical Social Work Journal, 15*(2), 107-120.

Parks, B. (1996). Under review: Billing, management software. *NASW News, 41*(6), 5.

Patti, R. (1985). In search of purpose for social welfare administration. *Administration in Social Work, 9*(3), 1-15.

Perlman, H. H. (1979). *Relationship: The heart of helping people.* Chicago, IL: University of Chicago Press.

Perlman, H. H. (1982). The helping relationship: Its purpose and nature. In H. Rubenstein and M. Bloch (Eds.), *Things that matter.* New York: Macmillan, pp. 7-27.

Philip, C. (1993). Dilemmas of disclosure to patients and colleagues when a therapist faces life-threatening illness. *Health and Social Work, 18*(1), 13-19.

Pilisuk, M. and Parks, S. H. (1986). *The healing web.* Hanover, NH: University Press of New England.

President's Commission. (1983). *Summing up: Final Report on studies of the ethical and legal problems in medicine and biomedical and behavioral research.* Washington, DC: U.S. Government Printing Office.

Raiff, N. R. (1993). *Advanced case management: New strategies for the nineties.* Newbury Park, CA: Sage.

Ranan, W. and Blodgett, A. (1983). Using telephone therapy for unreachable clients. *Social Casework, 64*(1), 39-44.

Reamer, F. G. (1985). The emergence of bioethics in social work. *Health and Social Work, 10*(4), 271-281.

Reamer, F. G. (1994). *Social work practice and liability: Strategies for prevention.* New York: Columbia University Press.

Reamer, F. G. (1995). *Social work values and ethics.* New York: Columbia University Press.

Rebuff Urged for Governors' Reform Plans. (1996, April). *NASW News, 41*(4), 1,10.

Reid, W. (1992). *Task strategies: An empirical approach to clinical social work.* New York: Columbia University Press.

Reid, W. and Hanrahan, P. (1982). Recent evaluation of social work: Grounds for optimism. *Social Work, 27,* 328-340.

Reiser, S. and Anbar, M. (Eds.). (1984). T*he machine at the bedside: Strategies for using technology in patient care.* New York: Cambridge University Press.

Resnick, H. (Ed.). (1995). *Electronic tools for social work practice and education.* Binghamton, NY: The Haworth Press.

Reynolds, C. and Fischer, C. (1983). Personal versus professional evaluations of self-disclosing and self-involving counselors. *Journal of Counseling Psychology, 30,* 451-454.

Richan, W. C. (1988). *Beyond altruism: Social policy in American society.* Binghamton, NY: The Haworth Press.

Robinson, V. P. (1978). *The development of a professional self-teaching and learning in professional helping processes.* New York: AMS Press.

Rogers, C. R. and Roethilsberger, F. J. (1992). Barriers and gateways to communication. In Gabarro, J. (Ed.), *Managing people and organizations.* Boston, MA: HBS Publications, pp. 105-111.

Rose, S. and Block, B. L. (1985). *Advocacy and empowerment.* Boston: Routledge and Kegan Paul.

Rosen, A. and Mutschler, E. (1982). Correspondence between the planned and subsequent use of interventions in treatment. *Social Work Research and Abstracts, 18,* 28-34.

Rosenblatt, A. and Waldfogel, D. (1983). *Handbook of clinical social work.* San Francisco: Jossey-Bass.

Rothary, M. A. (1980). Contracts and contracting. *Clinical Social Work Journal, 8,* 179-186.

Rubin, A. (1983). Case management in mental health: A social work domain? *Social Work, 28*(1), 49-56.

Rushton, A. and Davies, P. (1984). Social work methods in health settings. In *Social Work and Health Care.* London: Heineman Educational Books, pp. 48-63.

Russell, L. B. (1979). *Technology in hospitals: Medical advances and their diffusion.* Washington, DC: The Brookings Institution.

Rutten, F. F. H. and Bonsel, G. J. (1992). High cost technology in health care: A benefit or a burden? *Social Science and Medicine, 35*(4), 567-577.

Saari, C. (1986). The created relationship: Transference, countertransference and the therapeutic culture. *Clinical Social Work Journal, 14*(1), 39-51.

Sanville, J. (1982). Partings and impartings: Towards a non-medical approach to interruptions and terminations. *Clinical Social Work Journal, 10*(2), 123-130.

Schwartz, W. (1971). On the use of groups in social work practice. In Schwartz, W. and Zalba, S. *The practice of group work.* New York: Columbia University Press.

Seabury, B. (1976). The contract: Uses, abuses and limitations. *Social Work, 21,* 16-21.

Shapiro, B. S. (1992). Functional integration: Getting all the troops to work together. In Gabarro, J. (Ed.), *Managing people and organizations.* Boston, MA: HBS Publications, pp. 353-369.

Shepard, P. (1987). Telephone therapy: An alternative to isolation. *Clinical Social Work Journal, 15*(1), 56-65.

Shore, M. F., and Beigel, A. (1996). The challenges posed by managed behavioral health care. *The New England Journal of Medicine, 334*(2), 116-118.

Simmons, J. (1994). Community based care: The new health social work paradigm. *Social Work in Health Care, 20*(1), 35-46.

Simos, B. (1979). *A time to grieve.* New York: Family Service America.

Skocpol, T. (1992). *Protecting soldiers and mothers: The origins of social policy in the United States.* Cambridge, MA: Harvard University Press.

Smalley, R. and Bloom, T. (1977). Social casework: The functional approach. In J. Turner (Ed.), *Encyclopedia of social work.* New York: National Association of Social Workers, pp. 1280-1290.

Smith, R. (1996, January). VA hospital shake-up signals a role shift. *NASW News, 41*(1), 3.

Social services in the year 2000. (1985). Washington, DC: U. S. G. P. O.

Social work in hospitals expanding. (1985). *NASW News* (October), 14.

Sosin, M. (1979). Social work advocacy and the implementation of legal mandates. *Social Casework, 60*(3), 265-273.

Sosin, M. and Caulum, S. (1983). Advocacy: A conceptualization for social work practice. *Social Work, 28*(1), 12-17.

Steidl, J. (1977). What's a clinician to do with so many approaches to family therapy? *The Family, 4*(2), 60-65.

Stein, P. M. and Lambert, M. J. (1986). Telephone counseling and crisis intervention: A review. *American Journal of Community Psychology, 12*(1), 101-126.

Stewart, R. (1984). Building an alliance between the family and the institution. *Social Work, 29,* 386-390.

Stoline, A. M. and Weiner, J. P. (1993). *The new medical marketplace: A physician's guide to the health care system in the 1990's.* Baltimore, MD: Johns Hopkins University Press.

Strauss, A., Shizuko, S., Sagerhaugh, F., Suczek, B., and Weiner, C. L. (1985). *Social organization of medical work.* Chicago, IL: University of Chicago Press.

Super, S. (1982). Successful transition: Therapeutic interventions with the transferred client. *Clinical Social Work Journal, 10*(2), 113-121.

Therapy parity in senate bill wins backing. (June 1996). *NASW News, 41*(6), pp. 1, 10.

Thomlinson, R. (1984). Something works: Evidence from practice effectiveness studies. *Social Work, 29,* 51-56.

Tichy, N. and Charan, R. (1992). Speed, simplicity, self-confidence: An interview with Jack Welch. In Gabarro, J. (Ed.), *Managing people and organizations.* Boston, MA: HBS Publications, pp. 432-446.

Toseland, R. (1987). Treatment discontinuance: Grounds for optimism. *Social Casework, 68*(4), 195-204

Trattner, W. (1989). *From poor law to welfare state: A history of social welfare in America* (Second Edition), New York: The Free Press.

Turner, F. (Ed.). (1986). *Social work treatment: Interlocking theoretical approaches.* New York: The Free Press.

Vourlekis, B. S. and Green, R. R. (Eds.). (1992). *Social work case management.* Hawthorne, New York: Aldine de Gruyter.

Webb, N. (1983). Vacation separations: Therapeutic implications and clinical management. *Clinical Social Work Journal, 11*(2), 126-138.

Weil, M., Karls, J. M., and Associates. (1985). *Case management in human service practice*. San Francisco, CA: Jossey-Bass.

Weissman, H., Epstein, I., and Savage, A. (1983). *Agency-based social work: Neglected aspects of clinical practice*. Philadelphia: Temple University Press.

Whittington, R. (1985). House calls in private practice. *Social Work, 30*(3), 261-264.

Wing, K. E. (1985). *The law and the public's health*. Ann Arbor, MI: Health Administration Press.

Wolk, J. L., Sullivan, W. P., and Hartmann, D. J. (1994). The managerial nature of case management. *Social Work, 39*(2), 152-159.

Woods, M. and Hollis, F. (1990). *Casework: A psychosocial therapy*. New York: McGraw-Hill.

PART I:
SERVICES FOR CHILDREN
AND/OR FAMILIES

Chapter 1

Premature Babies
in the Intensive Care Nursery

Janet L. Taksa

CONTEXT

Description of the Setting

The Intensive Care Nursery (ICN) of Thomas Jefferson University Hospital is a 24-bed facility in a general teaching hospital in the heart of Philadelphia. The hospital itself has a capacity of 610 beds, including an 18-bed unit called the Transitional Care Nursery, which serves as a step-down unit for the ICN, as well as a unit where less seriously ill babies are admitted. The ICN is a level-III nursery, which means it can offer treatment for the most seriously ill newborn infants (Manginello and DiGeronimo, 1991). Newborn babies who need advanced technology and the services of physicians who specialize in neonatology are admitted here from the hospital's delivery room, or are transferred from other hospitals in a wide geographical area. During the past academic year, 684 babies were admitted to the ICN. All socioeconomic groups were represented. Over 50 percent of the babies were covered by managed care insurance, either commercial or Medical Assistance. An additional 24 percent were covered by non-managed-care Medical Assistance.

The ICN is composed of seven large rooms that form a rectangle around two nursing desks. One room is divided into five smaller units for patients requiring isolation. Another, known as the Special Care Unit, is geared to providing a quieter, slower-paced environment for chronically ill babies who have been in the ICN for at least one month. Directly outside the ICN is a lounge designated for parents of the ICN babies. It contains a comfortable couch and chairs, TV, phone, and toys for patients' siblings. There is also a small room on the unit with two electric breast pumps, where mothers of the ICN babies can pump their breasts. There is no designated space for parents to stay overnight, but campus housing can be arranged in a former student dormitory across the street from the hospital.

In addition to the expenses of the hospitalization itself, parents often incur many associated expenses: transportation to and from the ICN, meals, phone bills, housing for those who live far away. Reduced meal tickets for the hospital's cafeteria and reduced parking vouchers are provided, and there is limited financial assistance for campus housing available through a special memorial fund designated by the hospital for this purpose. A baby may stay in the ICN for several weeks, or for many months, depending on his or her condition and progress. For premature babies, the discharge date is estimated to be around the original due date. However, this date is only a general guideline and is not accurate in many cases.

Policy

Many of the policies affecting patients in the ICN and their families are financial ones. A baby with a birthweight under 1200 grams (two pounds and eight ounces) is automatically eligible for Supplementary Security Income (SSI), a program under the social security administration that provides financial assistance and a Medical Assistance card. Babies with higher birthweights may still be eligible if their conditions meet the medical eligibility requirements, as determined by the Social Security Administration. While the baby is in the hospital, all parents meet the financial criteria for SSI, as only the baby's "income" is considered. A baby whose hospitalization is being paid by public assistance is eligible for $30 a month while in the hospital and $490 after discharge. A baby covered by commercial insurance receives $490 a month while in the hospital. However, after discharge, the parents' income is considered, and most parents who work become ineligible for SSI.

There have been several problems concerning SSI for newborn infants. First of all, benefits are retroactive only to the date of the initial application, which can be filed by phone (an 800 number is provided) or in person at the parents' local social security office. If the social worker delays in telling the parents about this program, the parents can lose benefits. On the other hand, it is not an optimal time to discuss this program with parents who have suddenly been confronted with the overwhelming situation of having a very sick infant. Usually, depending upon the baby's progress and the needs of the parents, the social worker tells the parents about SSI within the first two weeks of the baby's hospitalization.

Another problem has been that this program is significantly different from other SSI programs for older children or adults; and the difference is not always known to the Social Security intake workers, particularly those who answer the toll-free customer service line. Often, parents are erroneously told that they are not eligible to apply for SSI because they make too much money, the baby has no social security number, etc. Occasionally, even when the application is taken, the intake information is not transferred to the local social security office. Parents are told when they call later that there is no record of their application, and, therefore, benefits cannot be retroactive to that date. The social worker tries to prevent these situations by providing accurate information to parents, and by encouraging them to apply in person, when possible, as fewer problems occur. The social worker's attempts to intervene directly with social security staff when a mistake has been made have not proved effective.

Parents who receive Public Assistance are eligible for reimbursement for transportation to visit their babies. Parents who do not receive Public Assistance are not eligible for this program. As already noted, parents who do not receive Public Assistance usually do not qualify for SSI when the baby is discharged. However, in Pennsylvania, due to a little-known loophole identified by the Pennsylvania Development Law Project, parents with a "disabled child" may be able to receive Medical Assistance regardless of their income. New Jersey also has a financial aid program called the "Catastrophic Fund," which can provide financial assistance for medical bills if the medical expenses exceed a certain percentage of the family's income (currently, 15 percent, plus 20 percent of any income over $100,000).

The increased appearance of managed care insurances, which usually contain the requirements of preapproval for hospitals and services, and are contracted with specific hospitals and agencies, has had a major effect on the ICN as it has in all areas of health care. For example, a baby may be transferred after birth from a hospital approved by the family's managed care insurance to Thomas Jefferson as an emergency admission for treatment not provided by the original hospital. As soon as that emergency treatment is over, however, there is pressure from the insurance company to transfer the baby back to the contracted hospital. This can be very difficult for parents who have formed trusting relationships with the staff and gained familiarity with the hospital. Discharge planning for premature babies has also been completely changed by the advent of managed care, and the case manager of the insurance company has become a powerful, if unseen, member of the discharge planning team. In the past, premature babies were usually considered ready for discharge when they weighed about four and one-half pounds and could take all feedings by mouth. However, with the advent of managed care, an increasing number of babies are being discharged much earlier, often with various home nursing services in place. Some parents have expressed anxiety about being responsible for medical procedures such as nonoral feedings and failing to do them properly, even when they are assured that home nurses will visit to assist them. Others have expressed feelings of disappointment and anger that they will be functioning as part-time nurses instead of full-time mothers. The effects of earlier discharges on the premature infants themselves are not accurately known. Jefferson's ICN staff are currently participating with a neonatal/pediatric home health agency in a research project whose stated goal is to decrease the length of hospital stays for premature infants by discharging them at significantly lower weights with in-home skilled nursing care, and physician supervision.

One particular discharge plan, which used to be almost automatic–that is, the transfer of the premature baby to a rehabilitation center for intensive services prior to going home–is now rarely an option. Most insurance companies are refusing to pay for this type of care, which they believe can be done at home. Many other recommendations from hospital physicians are also being challenged, and often denied, by managed care staff.

Technology

Each year, approximately 4,000,000 infants are born in the United States. Over 7 percent of these newborns are premature. A baby is usually considered to be a mature or "term" infant within the range of 37 to 42 weeks gestation (Ensher and Clark, 1994). Over the past twenty years, advances in medical science and technology have resulted in increasing survival of even extremely premature babies. Treatment for babies with birthweights as low as 500 grams (one pound, two ounces) and/or those born as early as 24 weeks gestation, is now accepted practice (Gottwald and Thurman, 1995; Hack et al., 1994). The development of artificial surfactant, which helps keep babies' lungs from collapsing; improvements in respirators; and the development of laser surgery, which helps to prevent detached retinae, and therefore blindness, are among the most important contributions to both survival and quality of life for premature babies (Krollman et al., 1994). For a complete overview of the medical course and complications of prematurity, see *Your Premature Baby* (Manginello and DiGeronimo, 1991).

When a baby is born prematurely, his or her development in utero is suddenly stopped. The basic task of the neonatologist and other intensive-care nursery staff is to help the baby survive and grow with as few complications as possible in what is essentially a hostile environment, until she or he can live in the normal world outside the nursery. In order to grow in this environment, the baby needs to breathe, in spite of small, stiff lungs; stay warm without having the ability to regulate body temperature; and receive nourishment, in spite of an immature digestive tract that isn't ready to accept food.

Immediately following the birth of a premature baby, the medical team begins a series of procedures designed to help the baby survive. The baby is first placed on a warming bed (a small, open bed with a heat source overhead); connected to a ventilator, if necessary; and transported to the intensive care nursery in an incubator, which is temperature-controlled. In the nursery, the baby is again placed on a warming bed. A full physical examination is completed; weight, length, and head circumference are measured and blood samples are drawn. To allow for the monitoring of necessary functions, at least five wires that are connected to read-out monitors through small electrodes (sensors) are secured to the baby's skin, to provide instant information about body temperature, oxygen level, and heart and breathing rates. These are the numbers that so often become the object of the parents' focus.

Most premature babies who require admission to an intensive care nursery have breathing problems at birth. If these respiratory problems are mild, an oxygen hood may be placed over the baby's head. The hood is a plastic box that allows oxygen to be administered to the baby through a tube. Babies with more severe breathing problems may require another method of receiving oxygen, which is called continuous positive airway pressure (CPAP) and which consists of a tube providing a constant flow of air by forcing air into the lungs through the baby's nostrils. Babies with the most severe breathing problems require placement on a respirator, which is a machine that supplies a flow of air, oxygen, and air pressure through a tube in the baby's nose or mouth into the trachea. These are the primary methods of respiratory management used during the baby's progress toward the goal of breathing without assistance.

Many premature babies do not have enough body fat or energy reserves at birth to maintain a stable body temperature. As noted, they are first placed in warming units. As soon as they are more stable, they can be transferred to incubators, which are enclosed, clear boxes that are temperature-controlled. Eventually, when the baby grows enough to be able to sustain a normal body temperature without assistance, he or she is transferred to a crib. Nutrition is a major focus in the ICN. Most premature babies, born with immature digestive tracts, cannot tolerate oral feedings. Young preemies cannot coordinate sucking, swallowing, and breathing. In these cases, nourishment is provided through intravenous lines. Oral feedings are slowly introduced, usually at first through a tube threaded through the nose (nasogastric or NG feeding) or through the mouth (orogastric or gavage feeding.) Gradually, the baby is helped to take feedings from bottle and/or breast.

All along this progression toward growth and stability, the baby faces complications that can result in severe, often life-threatening problems. These include bronchopulmonary dysplasia, a scarring of the lungs caused, in part, by long periods of mechanical ventilation; infections, which can overwhelm the baby's immature immune system; intraventricular hemorrhages, or bleeding from veins in and around the brain, which can cause brain damage; and retinopathy of prematurity, or scarring from bleeding into the eye, which can result in severe vision problems including blindness. Even when babies do well, progress is rarely consistent (Cusson and Lee, 1994).

Organization

The Department of Pediatrics is part of a large, general teaching hospital, with a staff of 44 physicians, including both general pediatricians and pediatric subspecialists. The intensive care nursery is staffed by 11 neonatologists, 9 neonatogy fellows, 7 neonatal nurse practitioners, and 65 nurses. Respiratory therapists, radiology technologists, and other specially trained health care professionals are assigned to the ICN. Since Thomas Jefferson is a teaching hospital, pediatric residents and students in the allied health sciences rotate through the ICN as part of their training. The physicians also staff intensive care nurseries in other hospitals affiliated with Thomas Jefferson and participate in research.

The Department of Social Work has a staff of 40 Master's-prepared social workers, 3 social work technicians, and 3 clerical workers. Social workers are assigned to specific clinical services. Three social workers have responsibility for social work services to the pediatric clinical area, which includes the 18-bed pediatric unit, 5-bed pediatric intensive care unit, 6-bed adolescent inpatient unit, the outpatient pediatric clinic, and the outpatient pediatric sexual abuse project, as well as the 40-bed transitional and intensive care nurseries. All ICN patients are considered to be of high acuity since they are in an intensive care setting. All patients are assessed by a social worker, and the progress of most is followed. The pediatric social workers are assigned patients according to a daily schedule: each worker has an "assignment day," in which he or she follows all patients admitted to any of the pediatric units on that day. If a baby is admitted to another unit following discharge from the ICN, the same social worker will be assigned.

Until recently, the hospital was governed by a vice president for health services, who reported to the president of the university and an appointed board of trustees. In response to the major changes taking place in health care, the hospital and the Main Line Health System signed agreements that officially established a new corporate entity known as the Jefferson Health System, which includes several community hospitals, a rehabilitation center, and an agency that provides home care and hospice. The president of Thomas Jefferson University was named the chairman of the board of the Jefferson Health System, and the president of the Main Line Health System was named the new organization's president and chief executive officer. The administration also hired a consulting firm to "help identify areas where [the organization] could reduce costs" (Jefferson Hospital, 1995). The effects these changes will have on both the pediatric and the social work departments are not yet known.

Although Jefferson's ICN, like any other level-III nursery, may appear highly technical to parents (Thurman and Korteland, 1989), the staff is committed to family-centered care (Plaas, 1994). Visiting times, and rules in general, are flexible to allow families to spend as much time with their infants as possible. Siblings are allowed and even encouraged to visit. The ICN nurses support the system of primary nursing, which is a team approach designed to promote the assignment of the same nurses to individual babies. The nurses' attitude is clearly that the babies belong to the parents, and they actively encourage parents to participate in care.

Even with family-centered care, however, many parents feel overwhelmed by the number of people involved with their baby. Parents often seek information from a variety of staff members, and become frustrated and at times angry when the replies are inconsistent. The change of attending neonatologists covering the ICN, which occurs every three weeks, can also be very frustrating for parents. Parents sometimes complain that the physicians leave the unit just when they get to know their baby. Explanations that the neonatologists are partners and that each is very familiar with every baby are not always effective. However, the knowledge that the large number of neonatologists guarantees that one is on site 24 hours a day is very reassuring to parents.

DECISIONS ABOUT PRACTICE

Client Description

Lori Anne Reynolds was born at Jefferson Hospital on March 3, 1994. Her mother had gone into premature labor during her twenty-fourth week of pregnancy, and had been transferred from her community hospital to Jefferson's antenatal unit two days prior to delivery. Efforts to stop premature labor were unsuccessful, and when the fetal monitor indicated problems, an immediate caesarian section was performed. Lori Anne, weighing 690 grams (one pound, eight ounces), was immediately connected to a respirator and admitted to the ICN. She was placed in a warming bed, and the necessary sensors and tubes were attached.

Lori Anne is the younger of two children. Her brother Daniel was three years old at the time of her birth. Mr. and Mrs. Reynolds, ages 30 and 28 respectively, are college graduates. Mr. Reynolds is an accountant, employed by the same firm for six years. Mrs. Reynolds, a former grade school teacher, had elected to become a full-time homemaker and mother following Daniel's birth. The family lives in a four-bedroom house in a Philadelphia suburb approximately 30 miles from the hospital.

Definition of the Client

In concrete terms, of course, the client is the premature baby, as all efforts are geared toward his or her welfare. However, the birth of a premature baby is a devastating experience for the entire family (Siefert et al., 1983). The parents are overwhelmed by their emotions and by the tasks confronting them. They feel isolated from their usual supports, as relatives and friends often either avoid them or overwhelm them with advice. Mothers and fathers cope differently (Hughes, et al., 1994; Thurman and Korteland, 1989), and parents often feel isolated from each other. Siblings experience feelings of guilt, anger, and jealousy, as well as feelings of abandonment (Oehler and Vileisis, 1990). Thus, the parents and siblings of the premature baby are also seen as primary clients. In the Reynolds' case, both parents were seen for support and help in discharge planning. Daniel was also encouraged to visit, and interviews were at times centered on him. (Daniel was seen twice on an individual basis.)

Goals, Objectives, and/or Outcome Measures

The social worker's ultimate goal is to help the family provide the best possible environment, both emotional and physical, for the baby at the time of discharge. This goal requires helping the family complete a lengthy and difficult adjustment process. The initial step in this process is for the parents to attach to the baby, by visiting and spending as much time with him or her as possible. To help accomplish this, the social worker tries to remove barriers, both concrete and emotional, that may prevent parents from visiting. On the practical side, the social worker may help provide campus housing, transportation reimbursement, reduced meal and parking vouchers, babysitting for siblings, letters to employers validating the need for parents to be with the baby, and other concrete services, depending on individual needs. In my experience, emotional factors are more likely to limit parental visitation than practical ones, even though parents may focus on concrete difficulties. Parents are often overwhelmed by feelings of fear, guilt, anxiety, anger, and helplessness (Bernbaum and Hoffman-Williamson, 1991; Cobiella, Mabe, and Forehand, 1990). By helping them to express and cope with these feelings, the social worker helps the parents become more comfortable in being with their baby.

The initial emotional adjustment of parents of a baby in an intensive care nursery has been likened to the grieving process: parents mourn the loss of the ideal baby they anticipated in much the same way as parents mourn the actual death of their newborn (Minde et al., 1978; Benfield, Lieb, and Reuter, 1976). Many expectant parents begin the attachment process at the time the pregnancy is confirmed. Indeed, in these days of high technology, the first picture in the baby album may well be a prenatal ultrasound. The birth of a premature baby means that parents do not experience the last part of that preliminary process. They miss part or all of the last trimester–a time noted for an increasing emotional attachment to the baby, as well as for preparation for the birth and the reality of parenthood (Bernbaum and Hoffman-Williamson, 1991; Davis, Richards, and Robertson, 1983). Parents need encouragement to express their feelings of anger and disappointment, which may be associated with having been "cheated" out of these experiences. Mrs. Reynolds spoke of feeling overwhelming anger and envy every time she saw a woman who was obviously in the last trimester of pregnancy.

Feelings of guilt, particularly those experienced by mothers, are common, and may interfere with the attachment process. In many cases, physicians are unable to identify the exact cause of a premature delivery. Parents, in trying to find causes, construct their own theories, which often result in self-blame (Affleck, Tennen, and Rowe, 1991). When a cause cannot be found, this kind of guilt may actually be beneficial, as an *identified* cause may give parents a sense of control. Often, however, this guilt is destructive and should be diminished as much as possible. Mrs. Reynolds initially expressed guilt feelings because she had gone to an aerobics class several weeks before Lori Anne was born. She also felt very guilty that she didn't love her baby "the way mothers should" and the way she had loved her first child. She found it difficult to even look at her baby, who like other neonates of the same gestation, looked more like a fetus than the beautiful baby she had expected (Manginello and DiGeronimo, 1991). She was relieved to learn that attachment to an infant who could not give clear behavioral emotional signals was known to be very difficult (Seligman, 1995), and she could not expect herself to feel the same way as she had with her full-term son.

Parents' feelings of helplessness are increased by the initial reality of having a baby they cannot hold, fondle, or, if their baby is on a respirator, even hear cry. Often, this is their first experience of feeling so completely without control. Mr. and Mrs. Reynolds, like many others of their generation, had been able to plan the most important parts of their lives: they had chosen their colleges, careers, marital partners, and even the time to have children. With Lori Anne's premature birth, all sense of control vanished.

Parents are also helped to recognize that they have a major role in their baby's care. Studies have shown that parents' interaction with their babies has a positive impact on the baby's progress (Zeskind and Iacino, 1984; Minde et al., 1983, 1978). This kind of information often helps the parents to feel less helpless. Mrs. Reynolds had expressed concern that her baby would "bond with the nurse," and she was relieved to learn that she was unique to her newborn baby: the only source of familiarity to her (Manginello and DiGeronimo, 1991).

As the baby's hospitalization continues, parents begin to lose some of their fears that the baby will not survive, and begin to realize they are confronting a chronic situation. The social worker's goal is now to help parents participate in their baby's care as much as possible (Shellabarger and Thompson, 1993), and become more involved in the preparations for taking their baby home. It is often at this time that parents' anxieties about what their baby will be like begin to emerge. Also, when the threat of the baby's survival is much less, family problems that have been dormant may begin to surface. The social worker helps the parents to cope with these feelings and problems, and may refer them for outside counseling, if appropriate.

Use of Contract

Parents are not given a choice about seeing a social worker, and sometimes feel that there must be something especially wrong with their baby or with themselves to require social services. Usually, once the social worker explains that all parents of babies in the ICN are seen by a social worker, they are receptive. Providing the parents with concrete services like reduced cafeteria and parking vouchers or campus housing, often helps to establish the relationship (Guillemin and Holmstrom, 1986).

In the beginning of the relationship between parents and social worker, the social worker is often seen as connected to the physicians and nurses and thus as a possible source of information about the baby's medical course (Able-Boone, Dokecki, and Smith, 1989). Parents are terrified that their baby will die and often seek concrete and specific information about the management of the baby (Perlman et al., 1991). Mr. Reynolds and, to a lesser extent, Mrs. Reynolds, focused on numbers; they carefully watched the monitors and repeatedly asked questions about ventilator settings, oxygen percentages, and heart rates. They often asked me if I had heard the latest statistics and watched me carefully (as they did all staff) to see my reaction. As the baby improves, and the parents realize the baby will survive, the relationship changes. At this point, the social worker is seen more as a counselor, as well as the resource for referrals to community agencies and concrete services.

Meeting Place

Finding an appropriate place in the ICN for the social worker and the family to talk is always a problem. Space is limited and, therefore, so is privacy. The social worker's office is in another building across the street from the ICN, and parents are usually reluctant to go that far away from the baby. Sometimes, meetings can take place in the parents' lounge, but the lounge is often occupied by other parents, and therefore not appropriate. The same problem applies to meetings in the breast-feeding room. Crises can occur at any time and precipitate a need for immediate discussion. At such times, any available space may be utilized. Many spontaneous interviews with the Reynolds' took place in the hallway by the elevators or in the ICN, with all its distractions.

Use of Time

Because an individual premature baby's progress cannot be accurately predicted, there is no way to know what the length of the relationship between the parents and the social worker will be. In the beginning of the baby's hospitalization, the family is usually seen every day. The length of interviews varies with the needs of the family, and, increasingly in the world of phone and form-intensive managed care, with the time available by the social worker. Length and number of interviews tend to be reduced as the baby progresses; but may go up again if the baby's condition deteriorates. Interviews usually also increase in length and frequency as the baby's discharge date approaches. Near discharge time, the parents' anxiety often increases, and plans for post-discharge services must be finalized.

Interventions

During the first part of the baby's hospitalization, when the parents are struggling with the overwhelming situation of having a premature baby, the social worker's most effective treatment technique is crisis intervention. As the baby's condition improves, the social worker functions more as a case manager, arranging necessary services and acting as a coordinator in helping parents prepare both emotionally and practically for the baby's discharge. Case management is an optimal treatment technique in this area, as the parents of premature babies are usually competent, and will able to be, eventually, independent (Hepworth and Larson, 1993).

Stance of the Social Worker

In the beginning of the hospitalization, when parents feel helpless and are often convinced that their baby will die, the social worker is very supportive. Parents are encouraged to express feelings and concerns, and are often more comfortable in revealing what they feel to the social worker, who is not directly responsible for their baby's medical care. As the baby progresses, the social worker continues to be supportive, but becomes more direct in encouraging parents to become more independent as they prepare for the eventual discharge of their baby. Although the social worker is still active in discharge planning, it is now appropriate for the parents to make some of the phone calls or investigate resources involved in specific plans. This direct encouragement toward independence may raise the parents' anxiety level, but it is necessary to help them gain confidence in themselves as primary caretakers of their baby.

Use of Outside Resources

The establishment of agencies to help families of premature babies has not kept up with the technology that is allowing so many more of these infants. Most of the outside resources used at the present time involve early intervention services. Even babies who do well have had to complete a long, hazardous stay in a difficult environment. Their development is rarely equal to that of a term baby at the same gestational age (Gottwald and Thurman, 1995). Most premature babies are referred for early intervention services that usually consist of physical therapy and speech therapy. Most of these services are provided on an outpatient basis, since intensive, inpatient services are rarely approved by insurance companies. Often, services can take place in the baby's home. There are now agencies that can act as clearing houses for helping parents locate and access early intervention services. Still, there are often waiting lists for these services, and it may take weeks or months until an early intervention program can be implemented. The Reynolds' insurance approved three home visits from a physical therapist between Lori Anne's discharge from the hospital and her acceptance to an early intervention program three months later. Many other insurance companies may not have approved these visits.

Some premature babies will have residual problems and will require a great many services after discharge (Hack et al., 1994). If the baby has a recognized condition such as cerebral palsy or blindness, referrals can be made to the agencies specifically designated for these conditions. However, for the babies with feeding problems or other common problems associated with prematurity, and even in babies with ultimately good prognoses, resources are limited. (Allen, 1993). At times, even when an appropriate agency is identified, the family's insurance company will not approve the referral because the insurance company is contracted with another, sometimes less appropriate, agency.

Reassessment

Because the course of a premature baby is unpredictable, reassessment of the relationship between the family and the social worker is frequently necessary and is often related to the physicians' medical reassessment of the baby. When the baby is doing well, the social worker and the family tend to have a more relaxed, friendly relationship. If the child's condition deteriorates, it may become necessary to reactivate the relationship to a more directly therapeutic one.

Transfer or Termination

Ideally, termination of the relationship between the social worker and the family would be determined through an assessment of the individual situation. Realistically, however, in most cases, the relationship ends artificially with the baby's discharge from the hospital or shortly thereafter. Time and staffing limitations, including the increasingly time-consuming demands of insurance companies, make longer-term follow-up impossible. As parents often continue to have anxieties when the baby goes home, and as continued implementation of even the best-planned services may become problematic, it is unfortunate that the relationship cannot be extended. In many cases, referrals to community agencies are made. However, as noted previously, many more resources to help families are needed *after* the baby is discharged from the hospital.

Case Conclusion

Lori Anne Reynolds was in the ICN for almost four months. She has been fortunate. At 18 months, she has almost caught up to her chronological peers in motor and speech development, and her prognosis appears excellent. Mr. and Mrs. Reynolds are very grateful for the medical knowledge and technology that made her recovery possible, and are happily planning to show her off at Jefferson's biannual ICN reunion. The cost of this technology, however, is high in both human and economic terms. Annually, the estimated cost of neonatal intensive care in the United States is approximately $4 billion (Ensher and Clark, 1994). The development of artificial surfactant alone, which dramatically increases the survival rate of babies with low birth weights, raised the mean cost of care $100,000 for each "extra" survivor (Eidelman, 1993). Statistics about the outcomes of premature infants vary, but it is generally acknowledged that many babies with birth weights as low as Lori Anne's may well have ongoing motor and/or neurological problems ranging from mild to very severe (Gottwald and Thurman, 1995; Hack et al., 1994; Jakobi, Weissman, and Paldi, 1993). In addition to the enormous emotional consequences for these children and their families, the expenses for continuing medical care will be high (Eidelman, 1993). Unfortunately, at the time of delivery, it is not possible to predict accurately which babies will do well. In this era of cost-effective health care, and with the possibility of rationing medical care in the future, it may well be economic factors as well as medical and ethical ones, which decide the fates of the lowest birth weight babies like Lori Anne.

REFERENCES

Able-Boone, H. D., Dokecki, P. R., and Smith, M. S. (1989). Parent and health care provider communication and decision making in the intensive care nursery. *Children's Health Care, 18*, 133-141.

Affleck, G., Tennen, H., and Rowe, J. (1991). *Infants in crisis: How parents cope with newborn intensive care and its aftermath.* New York, NY: Springer-Verlag.

Allen, M. C. (1993). An overview of long-term outcome. In F. R. Witter and L. Cheat (Eds.), *Textbook of Prematurity: Antecedents, treatment, and outcome.* Boston, MA: Brown and Company, pp. 371-383.

Benfield, D. G., Leib, S., and Reuter, J. (1976). Grief response of parents after referral of the critically ill newborn to a regional center. *The New England Journal of Medicine, 294*, 975-978.

Bernbaum, J. C. and Hoffman-Williamson, M. (1991). *Primary care of the preterm infant.* St. Louis, MO: Mosby-Year Book.

Cobiella, C. W., Mabe, P. A., and Forehand, R. L. (1990). A comparison of two stress-reduction treatments for mothers of neonates hospitalized in a neonatal intensive care unit. *Children's Health Care, 19*, 93-100.

Cusson, R. M. and Lee, A. L. (1994). Parental interventions and the development of the preterm infant. *Journal of Obstetrics, Gynecologic and Neonatal Nursing, 23*, 60-68.

Davis, Richards, R. and Robertson, S. (Eds.). (1983). *Parent-baby attachment in premature infants.* New York, NY: St. Martin's Press

Eidelman, A. I. (1993). Economic consequences of surfactant therapy. *Journal of Perinatology, 13*, 137-139.

Ensher, G. L. and Clark, D. A. (1994). *Newborns at risk: Medical care and psychoeducational intervention.* Gaithersburg, MD: Aspen Publishers, Inc.

Gottwald, S. R. and Thurman, K. (1995). Parent-infant interaction in neonatal intensive care units: Implications for research and service delivery. In Blackman, J. A. (Ed.), *Infant development and mental health in early intervention.* Gaithersburg, MD: Aspen, pp. 26-37.

Guillemin, J. H. and Holmstrom, L. L. (1986). *Mixed blessings: Intensive care for newborns.* New York: Oxford University Press.

Hack, M., Taylor, H. G., Klein, N., Eiben, R., Schatschneider, C., and Mercuri-Minich, N. (1994). School-age outcomes in children with birth weights under 750g. *The New England Journal of Medicine, 331*, 753-759.

Hepworth, D. H. and Larsen, J. (1993). *Direct social work practice: Theory and skills.* Pacific Grove, CA: Brooks/Cole.

Hughes, M., McCollum, J., Sheftel, D., and Sanchez, G. (1994). How parents cope with the experience of neonatal intensive care. *Children's Health Care, 23*, 1-14.

Jakobi, P., Weissman, A. and Paldi, E. (1993). The extremely low birth weight infant: The twenty-first century dilemma. *American Journal of Perinatology, 10*, 155-159.

Jefferson Hospital. (1995). On the horizon, author.

Krollmann, B., Brock, D. A., Nader, P. M., Neiheisel, P. W., and Wissmann, C. S. (1994). Neonatal transformation: Thirty years. *Neonatal Network, 13*, 17-20.

Manginello, F. P. and DiGeronimo, T. F. (1991). *Your premature baby.* New York, NY: John Wiley & Sons.

Minde, K., Trehub, S., Corter, C., Boukydis, C., Celhoffer, L., and Marton, P. (1978). Mother-child relationships in the premature nursery: An observational study. *Pediatrics, 61*, 373-379.

Minde, K., Whitelaw, A., Brown, J., and Fitzhardinge, P. (1983). Effect of neonatal complications in premature infants on early parent-infant interactions. *Developmental Medicine and Child Neurology, 25*, 763-777.

Oehler, J. M. and Vileisis, R. A. (1990). Effect of early sibling visitation in an intensive care nursery. *Developmental and Behavioral Pediatrics, 11*, 7-12.

Perlman, N. B., Freedman, J. L., Abromovitch, R., Whyte, H., Kirpalani, H., and Perlman, M. (1991). Informational needs of parents of sick neonates. *Pediatrics, 88*, 512-518.

Plaas, K. M. (1994). The evolution of parental roles in the NICU. *Neonatal Network, 13*, 31-33.

Seligman, S. (1995). Concepts in infant mental health: Implications for work with developmentally disabled infants. In Blackman, J. A. (Ed.) *Infant development and mental health in early intervention.* Gaithersburg, MD: Aspen, Inc., pp. 1-13.

Shellabarger, S. G. and Thompson, T. L. (1993). The critical times: Communication needs throughout the NICU experience. *Neonatal Network, 12,* 39-44.

Siefert, K., Thompson, T., Bensel, R. W. T., and Hunt, C. (1983). Perinatal stress: A study of factors linked to the risk of parenting problems. *Health and Social Work,* 107-121.

Thurman, S. K. and Korteland, C. (1989). The behavior of mothers and fathers toward their infants during neonatal intensive care visits. *Children's Health Care, 18,* 247-251.

Zeskind, P. S. and Iacino, R. (1984). Effects of maternal visitation to preterm infants in the neonatal intensive care unit. *Child Development, 55,* 1887-1893.

Chapter 2

Social Work in a Perinatal AIDS Program

Virginia Walther
Judy Mason
Joyce Preisinger

CONTEXT

Description of the Setting

The Maternal-Child Health AIDS Prevention and Treatment Program at The Medical Center was initiated in 1986 in recognition of the rising number of HIV-infected women and their perinatally infected newborns (Stuntzner-Gibson, 1991). The state in which the program is located has an HIV seroprevalence rate among childbearing women of .67–the highest in the United States (Novick et al., 1989). AIDS is the leading killer of women ages 25 to 34 years. Sixty percent of the female cases with AIDS are attributable to intravenous drug use and an additional 30 percent to sexual contact with an infected man. In women under the age of 25, however, the predominant mode of transmission is heterosexual contact. Black and Hispanic women make up 83 percent of all AIDS cases in women, a distribution that has remained constant since 1989. Minority women in the state have rates of infection 13 to 17 times greater than white women, although the annual rate of infection among females has been increasing for all racial groups. Women in this city account for almost one-third of the Centers for Disease Control's reported AIDS cases for ages 13 to 24. Data from the ongoing State Department of Health's anonymous newborn survey revealed that 1.23 percent of childbearing women in the city are HIV infected (Novick et al., 1989). In 1987, an anonymous seroprevalence survey using cord blood samples from newborns revealed a 2.7 percent HIV antibody positivity rate among women receiving care in the hospital's prenatal program (Sperling et al., 1989).

Composed of a school of medicine and a 1,100-bed tertiary care hospital, the Medical Center is fully accredited by the Joint Commission on the Accreditation of Hospitals, and is approved for internship and residency training by the Council on Medical Education and Hospitals of the American Medical Association and 20 medical specialty boards. A full range of inpatient services is offered including medicine, surgery, pediatrics, psychiatry, obstetrics-gynecology, and rehabilitation. As well, there is an ambulatory care department that consists of over 150 specialty clinics; a primary care unit; a large narcotics rehabilitation center that enrolls over 600 people annually; a hemophilia center caring for over 400 patients with congenital clotting disorders; an adolescent health care center; an emergency medicine department with over 40,000 patient visits per year; and an AIDS treatment center. Treatment at the hospital is provided by full-time attending physicians, voluntary physicians, interns and residents, and fellows, as well as by professionals in social work, nursing, nutrition, child life, genetics, and human resources. Outreach to the surrounding community–a very low income, multicultural area with many socioeconomic and medical problems–is facilitated by a large, active community medicine department.

Approximately 5,200 births occur here each year; 1,750 of these occur to women who receive care in the institution's prenatal clinic, which provides continuity care to predominantly poor, minority women, of whom 36 percent are African American and 55 percent are Latina. The population is drawn from communities collectively identified as an AIDS epicenter, which, although comprising approximately 1.4 percent of the city's population, accounts for 13.5 percent of its adult cases of HIV infection. As noted, although 60 percent of the city's female AIDS cases are intravenous drug users, the proportion of women infected through heterosexual contact has increased over time. Accompanying this trend is the accelerated rate of HIV infections in newborns. As a result, social workers provide HIV preventive programs for all pregnant women registering for prenatal services, regardless of individual risk behaviors. Voluntary HIV testing is also offered within the clinic, and pregnant women who are identified as HIV positive and who elect to continue their pregnancies are followed by the Department of Obstetrics and Gynecology's Perinatal Infectious Disease Team, which comprises team physicians, nurses, and social workers. Following delivery, the mother's primary care is provided by the AIDS Treatment Center, while the newborn is referred immediately to the center's Pediatric AIDS Team. Women delivering at the hospital who have received minimal or no prenatal care also receive HIV counseling and testing, if requested. An intensive community follow-up effort that includes home visits helps those who choose to be tested for HIV to receive post-test counseling and medical services following discharge.

Policy

As the AIDS epidemic enters its third decade, conflicts between public health priorities and individual civil liberties have continued to have profound implications for women of childbearing ages. The greatest dilemmas that challenge the infected perinatal patient, her potential children, and those who deliver health and social services are confidentiality versus disclosure; voluntary versus mandatory testing; and capitation of services under managed care versus free, unrestricted access to routine, urgent, and emergent multidisciplinary care. In view of the stigmatization associated with an AIDS diagnosis, federal, state, and local governments have policies to protect patients' privacy. On the federal level, the Centers for Disease Control (CDC), which recommend guidelines for treatment to state and local departments of health, mandate that all states report collected, coded AIDS information to them. This gathered, anonymous information assists states in their understanding of the pathogenesis and epidemiology of the disease. In spite of regulatory efforts to protect confidentiality, however, cases of discrimination against HIV-infected persons and loss of confidentiality have been widely documented (New York City Commission on Human Rights: The AIDS Discrimination Division, 1987), and social workers find themselves daily advocating for patients who experience loss of confidentiality with resulting loss of jobs and housing, restriction of interpersonal activities, and discrimination in accessing health-related services. To avoid the persistent dangers of stigmatization, many states have passed laws specifically protecting patients' privacy. Public Health Law provides civil penalties for disclosing unauthorized information that identifies an individual's serostatus in this state. Additional laws prohibit all health and social service providers from refusing to serve or discriminate in the provision of service to people who have or are perceived to have any HIV-related condition. These laws include the City Human Rights laws, the 1990 Federal Americans with Disability Act, and the Federal Fair Housing Amendment Act of 1988.

By 1995, the CDC had received reports of over 58,000 AIDS cases among adult and adolescent women and over 5,500 cases among children who acquired HIV perinatally (Centers for Disease Control, 1995). With an ever-increasing incidence of perinatal transmissions, the CDC, the American College of Obstetricians and Gynecologists, and the Pediatric AIDS Foundation recommended that all women, especially those who are pregnant, be given the opportunity to learn of their HIV-infection status through voluntary HIV testing and counseling (Kurth, 1995). In this state, all newborns are tested for the prevalence of HIV antibodies. The seroprevalence results, which are blinded (not linked with an individual identity), are sent to the CDC for the purpose of measuring the incidence of HIV infection in women who have given birth. Thus, pregnant women are tested for HIV by proxy through their newborns, yet these results are not made known to women unless specifically requested. In 1993, a bill (A6747) that sought to reveal the identities of participants in the state's anonymous newborn seroprevalence study and their HIV test results was introduced in the state legislature (Cooper and Powerly, 1995). The bill was eventually tabled. A similar bill was introduced in the House of Representatives by Bill Ackerman (Ackerman, Bill, H.R. 4507, 103D Congress, 2D Session). Unblinding the study is tantamount to mandatory testing, which raises ethical and legal issues about identifying the serostatus of mothers. Many social workers, among others, have argued that mandatory testing would discourage pregnant women from seeking prenatal care rather than face the perceived discriminatory or real consequences of HIV testing.

The fact that AIDS is sexually transmitted has also shaped these conflicts. Private acts carrying public consequences or conflicts between individual rights and social imperatives have come to the forefront as public health authorities strive to develop methods of epidemic control. These ethical problems that we face are not problems of success but are more problems of failures–failure to prevent and failure to cure. Public safety versus individual rights to privacy, treatment, and nontreatment of HIV youngsters; entry of women and children into clinical trials; and maternal-child screening programs have all provoked ethical debate and thought among those in the medical community, in government and, indeed, in society at large. While public measures were never intended to be in conflict with individual civil liberties, they have in fact been accompanied by ethical concerns for privacy, autonomy, and justice. Of special concern to social work practice, mandatory testing could transform a joyous event into a traumatic one. In its worst form, this traumatizing event could possibly create domestic violence if the status is disclosed to a partner. In addition, mandatory testing programs of pregnant or parturient women, or of their newborns, will rightly be viewed as selective and repressive by women and will therefore be counterproductive to the goal of increasing the use of health care services for women and their children (Cooper and Powderly, 1995).

In these changing times of health care, where Medicaid Managed Care will regulate the practice of all providers, carved-out services may be in contrast to the complex and comprehensive biopsychosocial treatment needs of HIV-infected individuals. In 1991, the state passed the Statewide Managed Care Act, under which the city is required to enroll 50 percent of its Medicaid recipients in managed care plans by 1998. This policy decision was designed to cut costs and provide preventive health care. In 1990, Medicaid was estimated to cover approximately 25 percent of the total national cost of AIDS-related health services (Scitovsky, 1990). While many infected women and children are dependent on Medicaid payments for a gamut of services, and more importantly because their survival time is continuing to rise, the cost of direct and indirect services will rise (Merzel, 1992). Thus, the implications for the delivery of medical and psychosocial care are multiple. Studies have indicated that many women are diagnosed late in the course of HIV illness. Therefore, the need for access to "sickness" care rather than preventive care will not be uncommon (Centers for Disease Control, 1995). From a psychosocial perspective, perinatal transmission in high prevalent areas is compounded by existing problems of poverty, homelessness, and substance abuse, which will require additional and intensive service for women and children. The continuum of counseling needs and services related to mental health, entitlements, affordable housing, and treatment for drug dependence may not be reimbursable or cost-effective for institutions who receive a fixed monthly fee per person.

Funding in this clinical program has made it both possible and imperative that all women entering prenatal care are offered pretest counseling and education as a condition of care and hospital cost reimbursement. Patients who opt for HIV testing and HIV-related services must sign very specifically regulated informed consents (in essence, legal contracts) and they must be offered an array of mandatory services and protections. The intent of most of the legal and regulatory contracts in perinatal HIV/AIDS programs is to guide the behavior of the health care institution and its employees who provide care rather than to regulate the behavior of the consumer.

In summary, many of the social debates and recent policy changes related to the HIV-infected mother and child may be well-intended regulatory efforts. However, it is equally important for policy-makers to address and enhance the delivery of coordinated services with the biopsychosocial model of care. These measures will be at the core of improving prevention and better care of the infected mother and child.

Technology

The extent to which technological solutions are available to counteract disease processes impacts the relational dimensions that are formed between social worker and client. The boom in high-tech medical therapies over the past several decades has driven specialization in fields of social work practice in health care settings, especially in perinatology. In this area, past problems encountered by women in reproductive health settings have been largely combatted by biomedical advances in technology. Assisted reproductive technologies to combat infertility, intrauterine surgery, and the human genome project offered promise to countless women of reproductive age. As the weight of intervention has been increasingly directed toward the biological component of our biopsychosocial framework of practice, social workers have correspondingly developed high levels of specialized skills and knowledge to enable women to cope with the impacts of these developments. In the midst of this technological explosion, AIDS appeared–a disease for which there exists no cure and only limited medical treatment options. This epidemic has sent social workers back to their historic roots in public health practice with a focus on education and prevention directed toward broad-based populations. Prevention and education, rather than biotechnical intervention directed at the individual, have become the key strategies in curbing the spread of this disease; and, providing and brokering supportive services is a central component in working with individuals and their families who are learning to live with the impact of having been infected with HIV. A parallel development in social work practice–case management–reflects the needs to manage complex resources and services to serve those confronted with a modern epidemic.

AIDS is also the first epidemic to emerge in the era of the computer, with its unprecedented information explosion linking social workers across the country working in similar practice areas and enabling them to tap into each others' expertise and knowledge. In fact, the technologies most often utilized to assist those with HIV infection as well as their providers have been related to computers and information exchange rather than the traditional biomedical technologies. Expanded databases, e-mail, teleconferences, and the information highway have enhanced the rapid transmission and accessibility of scientific and practice information in the field of HIV/AIDS. Computer technology has enhanced our ability to track patients and their course of illness, to provide continuity of care, as well as to educate and empower broad populations. This has been of central importance, given the horizontal and vertical transmission of HIV.

Such technological advances have also demanded that social workers develop computer literacy and skill in order to expand their knowledge base and to best serve their clients. Direct consumer access to on-line information has also served to empower a population that is at constant risk of disenfranchisement and has enabled the consumer to enter a partnership of advocacy for the needs of this special population. While social workers and advocacy groups alike must be vigilant against the potential abuses of computer technologies, the gains they have produced are remarkable.

Organization

Clinical practice in perinatal AIDS demands a biopsychosocial treatment approach and knowledge about legal and regulatory issues, viral transmission, pathogenesis, testing, treatment options, and prevention. Social workers must also develop a repertoire of collaborative and brokerage skills and a fine-tuned understanding of resources and their management. Many clients who learn they are infected with HIV are already dealing with a multitude of environmental and sociological stressors such as homelessness, substance use, limited financial resources, child care demands, and family violence. In these situations, during the initial prenatal visit, social work involvement targets early identification of stressors. In view of the multigenerational nature of HIV infection and the overwhelming impact this disease has on the family unit, it is clear that maintaining a family-centered approach to the delivery of health care services is crucial. Family-centered clinical case management consists of rapid assessment, crisis and short-term treatment, psychiatric consultation, resource management, and outreach services to all family members, with a flexible definition of family provided by the consumer. Family-centered case approaches place the social worker in the role of case manager on an interdisciplinary team and protect integrated, continuous care.

Consideration of racial, cultural, ethnic, and socioeconomic diversity is essential in planning and implementing programs (Mitchell, 1988). Bilingual educational materials, social workers, and other staff members are essential, given the demographic makeup of the clinic population. Because diversity among staff and clients influences service utilization, staff has been hired who represent the diverse populations served in the program. For example, many community resident clinic staffs bring local concerns to clinic care. In addition, Latino social workers help minimize language barriers and provide culturally attuned continuing education for social workers and staff (Walther, 1994). Program communication is maintained through a biweekly, multidisciplinary staff meeting led by the medical director. Content includes scientific updates and staff education, and planning and discussion of patient care (Mason et al., 1991).

This model supports cooperation in planning, patient care, and administration. In order to ensure optimal continuity of care for mothers and newborns, a coordinated, cross-specialty approach is utilized to form linkages needed in the delivery of quality services. A pediatric nurse

specialist is on site in the Obstetrics Infectious Disease Clinic to familiarize patients with the various pediatric services and treatment options and
to provide education about the care of newborns as it relates to HIV.
Patients are visited by a pediatric infectious-disease social worker postpartum, and during that time they are also seen by a member of the Adult
Infectious Disease Medical Care Team. These contacts help to ease the
transition from pregnancy-focused care to appropriate after-care services.

DECISIONS ABOUT PRACTICE

Description of the Client

Ana Sanchez is a 31-year-old woman of Puerto Rican descent. She was
born in New York City and raised by her parents in a stable family as the
oldest of four girls. In addition, there are some half-siblings from her
father's earlier marriage with whom the patient has had little contact. The
patient described close relationships with both parents, particularly her
father who died when Ms. Sanchez was 25 years old. Her mother, a
trained nurse, relocated to Puerto Rico where she now cares for her sick
father. Ms. Sanchez dropped out of high school in the tenth grade, later
earning her GED and completing a year of college.

Ms. Sanchez tested HIV seropositive in 1985. She was prompted to
take the test when the sister of her college boyfriend informed Ms. Sanchez that she knew the boyfriend to have a history of some high-risk
behaviors, including criminal activity, which resulted in a prison term,
and some homosexual relationships. The patient reacted to her HIV-sero-
positive status with anger, despair, hopelessness, and thoughts of hurting
herself. Ms. Sanchez reported that she nearly ran herself off the road
while driving her car. She suddenly slammed on the breaks after seeing a
vision of her young son, then a year old, living without a mother, and she
realized that she could not do this to him. The patient denied having any
thoughts of suicide since that time. According to Ms. Sanchez, she
refused to deal with her HIV-positive status for a long time, and it was not
until 1990 that she began to accept her situation and deal with health-
related matters in a more direct manner.

This patient had a second child in 1992, who was found to be virus-
free. Ms. Sanchez was referred to the Prenatal Infectious Disease Clinic
from the AIDS Center when she was six weeks pregnant with her third
child. At the time of referral, her son was 16 years old, and the younger
child, a daughter, was 4 years old. Ms. Sanchez has been in a relationship

with her 42-year-old common-law husband for one and one-half years. He earns his living as the owner and operator of a small candy store. Ms. Sanchez has been employed as a driver for a package courier company for the past seven years. The father of the baby has known of Ms. Sanchez's HIV status from the onset on their relationship. They are both members of the Santeria religion in which he was a priest. Ms. Sanchez has stated that she and her husband believe that one day she will be free from the virus and that the husband will be protected from exposure to the virus. This belief has prevented the husband from utilizing safe-sex measures and has resulted in his refusal to test for the HIV antibody. Despite ongoing efforts to involve the husband in counseling and testing services offered in the perinatal program, he has never accompanied Ms. Sanchez to her many medical appointments and he has remained at a distance.

General Client Definition

In the perinatal AIDS program, with its emphasis on education and screening as well as treatment, the client unit is largely defined as the pregnant woman, her partner, and her unborn child. This client unit may change if and as the patient identifies certain risk behaviors that may enlarge that network of at-risk individuals. Clearly in the area of perinatal HIV and AIDS, the mother's HIV status is inextricably linked to that of her fetus. This fact drives much client behavior in the perinatal practice arena from the decision for HIV testing, to decisions about pregnancy continuation and family planning, to medical treatments, especially those available through clinical trials. For the social worker in the Perinatal AIDS Program, the need to merge the priorities of both mother and unborn child is paramount.

At the point of entry, the HIV Perinatal Program client is generally a woman of reproductive age who has recently registered in the Prenatal clinic or has not registered in a clinic but has delivered her baby in this hospital. She is usually married or in a stable relationship, of minority status, from East Harlem or the South Bronx, and is the mother of other children. This prototypical woman tends to be unemployed and to have a limited educational background. During an initial social work evaluation, 50 percent of this population presents with major psychosocial stressors. This client is usually in her second trimester of pregnancy at the time of her clinic enrollment and does not identify herself as having HIV-related high-risk behaviors. Some clients are more chronically dysfunctional–homeless, drug users, involved with child welfare authorities, seeking late or no prenatal care–and discover that they are HIV positive. Other clients come to prenatal care already knowing that they are HIV infected.

The definition of client broadens at the time of HIV-antibody pretest counseling when testing is also made available to sexual partners. The scope of client definition expands further when a pregnant woman is identified as HIV-infected. Involving this client's larger network of social supports is an important aspect of the early diagnosis phase of HIV illness, as well as later through the adjustment stages of disease progression. The verticle and horizontal nature of HIV transmission makes it imperative to further expand the definition of client to include past and present partners, and children who may be in need of counseling, testing, and HIV-related services. Implicit in this work is the recognition of the implications of HIV on the unborn fetus.

Goals, Objectives, and Outcome Measures

In the perinatal setting, the social worker's goals with the client must also be congruent with those of the perinatal medical program. While the individual needs and wishes of the pregnant woman are of paramount importance to any comprehensive treatment plan, social work goals are also lodged in population-based program mandates to provide primary and secondary HIV education and prevention service to all pregnant women. This context drives the provision of HIV pretest counseling and individual risk assessments provided by social workers to all women as they begin their care in a prenatal program. Following this broad-based intervention, the individual woman will, with the assistance of the social worker, articulate goals for her continued medical and social interventions in the arena of perinatal AIDS, such as choices for testing, further counseling, and case management. In the case of pregnancy, a diagnosis of HIV or AIDS forms a powerful context under which the patient's goals for herself and her unborn child are developed. These may be as focused as making decisions as to whether or not to be tested and as broad-based as coming to emotional and pragmatic terms with a life-threatening diagnosis, with its potentially dire consequences for the future of the unborn child. It is particularly important, given the uncertainties of the course of HIV progression for both mother and baby, that the social worker set treatment goals based on the client's ability to tolerate the realities and multiple implications of the diagnosis within her own social context and in keeping with her capacities to use a variety and wide range of available services, which may change over the course of pregnancy. It must also be always considered that the majority of perinatal patients have come to our attention not originally for services related to HIV/AIDS but rather for pregnancy care. Thus, their responses to diagnosis are categorically different from a client who initiates HIV care based on a specific set of HIV concerns, and our goals will be shaped by this contextual issue. The pregnancy itself demands a family focus to all goal setting as even the definition of client is shifted from the individual woman to the maternal child dyad. The effectiveness of social work service delivery is measured by an increase in knowledge of HIV issues geared to maternal transmission on the part of an entire population of pregnant women; the ability to engage patients and families in an individually focused counseling process; and the coordination of specialized medical and case management services opted for by patients, based on their goals.

Use of Contract

Within the perinatal HIV/AIDS program, the contract is defined by traditional parameters of agreement between client and social worker, which guide their relationship and which determine the objectives that they will identify to meet mutually agreed upon goals. The contract in this field of practice is also determined by written, legal contracts between a variety of regulatory agencies and funding sources and the hospital, which seek to protect the consumer and to influence the conditions of her treatment. For social work practitioners, formal written, as well as verbal, contracts with women are driven by the ethics of the social work profession.

At the time of her first prenatal appointment, Ms. Sanchez went through the same triage evaluation process provided to all clinic patients. Building upon the information provided by referring colleagues, a more in-depth assessment was completed. The patient revealed that this was a planned pregnancy, and she went on to say that she and her partner also want to have a second child together sometime in the future. Ms. Sanchez had used holistic treatment measures and was very resistant to the use of conventional medication in her treatment regimen. Despite this strong antimedicine bias, she did agree to AZT therapy for herself and baby in the face of compelling scientific evidence that rates of maternal-child transmission could be significantly reduced. At the time of referral, the patient's CD4 count was 90. Tests repeatedly showed her to have a very high level of viral burden throughout the pregnancy.

Besides the husband, the only other person aware of Ms. Sanchez's HIV status was her mother, with whom she maintained a close and supportive long-distance relationship. The patient had shared her HIV situation years before with one other person, a half-sister who had such a difficult time dealing with this information that she severed all contact with Ms. Sanchez. The patient spoke of having strained relationships with other family members, and she has been adamant about not disclosing to them any information regarding her HIV status.

Meeting Place

The meeting place in which social work with pregnant women takes place is generally within the confines of the medical center's prenatal clinic setting. The clinic has a special infectious disease program incorporating HIV/AIDS so that all care of the HIV-infected pregnant woman is centered in this continuity clinic. The social worker has a private office, which provides a further assurance that transactions will be confidential and private. Home visits are provided by community liaison workers who work closely with and are supervised by the social worker on the service. The social worker may at times also visit the client in her own environment. Much telephone counseling is a part of this program, given the multiple family obligations, social service, and health care demands experienced by these women. Because all pregnant women are triaged by a social worker and are provided HIV counseling at program entry, the meeting place does not become stigmatized as a woman obtains additional HIV-related services from the social worker.

Ms. Sanchez worked into her twelfth week of pregnancy. Due to the discomfort associated with pregnancy and heavy lifting required on her job, the patient applied for and was granted a disability leave. She was somewhat erratic with regard to keeping scheduled medical appointments but was generally conscientious about maintaining telephone contact when she did not show up in person.

This patient had medical insurance in connection with her job, but was reluctant to use it, fearing discrimination or dismissal if her HIV status were discovered by her employer. The patient also received medical coverage through the New York State HIV Universal Care Programs (ADAP Plus). Ms. Sanchez's intention was to return to work after the birth of her baby. A contract for work was established during the initial contact and revised later, as changing circumstances indicated. It was agreed that Ms. Sanchez's confidentiality would be maintained and protected, that she would refrain from using her private insurance, and that the social worker and she would meet on a regular basis for supportive counseling sessions. As the patient began keeping her clinic appointments more sporadically, the agreement was necessarily revised to include regular telephone contacts between clinic visits, which was more tolerable to this patient from both an emotional need to maintain some distance from her HIV concerns as well as a pragmatic and logistical stance given her other life responsibilities.

Use of Time

The clinical manifestations and emotional and social needs engendered by perinatal AIDS heightens the use of time in the patient and social work relationship. Perinatal social work by its very nature is chronologically limited by the gestation of pregnancy and its immediate postpartum period. The use of time may either be constricted or structured. This depends on the gestational stage of the patient as she enters care, regulatory and insurance requirements, and individual medical and social needs corresponding to the stage of HIV/AIDS disease progression. If the patient begins obstetric care late in the pregnancy, the engagement process and social work interventions are compromised and constricted by time factors inherent in late initiation of prenatal care. Furthermore, the majority of AIDS programs are supported by federal, state, and foundation funding. Each funding source is chronologically finite, with various mandates and time lines for accomplishment of program goals, including those with individual patients. Therefore, regulatory issues have in many ways structured the continuum of care in a perinatal AIDS program. At their best, they have enhanced the focus and timeliness of interventions in relation to counseling, testing, and case management services. At worst, they make it difficult for successful programs to continue beyond the provision of "soft" monies. Finally, each stage of the infection has its own set of psychosocial stressors, and the social work services offered will be in response to the severity of medical and psychosocial needs, which will advance with time and disease progression.

The ambulatory care portion of the work with Ms. Sanchez was restricted by the duration of her gestational period, which was 37 weeks. We worked with this patient from her sixth week of pregnancy, for a total of 31 weeks. In addition, the obstetrics care team typically remains involved for a minimum of six weeks postpartum.

Interventions

In considering the most appropriate method of care for clients dealing with HIV infection and related illness, it is important to keep in mind the nature of HIV transmission, the manner of HIV disease progression, and the psychosocial characteristics of the client population. Those women hardest hit by this epidemic are poor, urban women of color whose lives may already be compromised by violence, social isolation, and chemical dependency. The actual or potential transmission of HIV to sex partners and children make a family-centered approach to care an imperative. The myriad social and psychological stressors confronting these families, as well as the chronic and progressive nature of HIV illness, make case management the modality of choice. This is a useful means by which to organize needed services for family members infected, as well as affected, since the multiple needs of each individual interfaces with what is often a complex service delivery system. Case management can provide a framework by which to coordinate and sustain interconnecting relationships between clients, direct service professionals, and ancillary service providers.

Given the unpredictable nature of HIV disease, there is no one prescribed model of treatment for persons infected with HIV. Effective modalities can run the gamut from individual, couples, and family counseling, to psychoeducational and psychodynamic treatment groups. Special issue-focused counseling programs related to topics such as bereavement and drug abuse are available to clients and their support systems. The social worker is called upon to empower clients, enhance coping skills, provide medical psychosocial education, advocate, coordinate medical services, and identify social service needs. In addition, the social work case manager is essential in the establishment and maintenance of linkages between family members and other involved providers within and outside the medical center setting. (See Figure 2.1.) The time-limited nature of an obstetric service is conducive to short-term focused treatment models. Depending on the stage of illness and the needs of individual clients, social work involvement may be either intensive and continuous or crisis-focused and episodic.

Stance of the Social Worker

Deliberation about value and ethical dilemmas is inherent in social work practice in a perinatal AIDS program setting. A social worker's conscious or unconscious behavioral, cognitive, or emotional responses to the circumstances, emotions, or behaviors presented by clients can cause blurring of ethical and professional boundaries. Social workers are required to manage complex, ambiguous questions and must be aware of their own and others' biases. For example, they must contend with health providers' overt or subtle opinions about infected women's continuation or termination of pregnancy. Providers may promote the use of sterilization to guard against future pregnancies without regard to values important to the client in her own context. Since providers have variable understanding of infected women's pregnancy-related decisions, social workers must be comfortable in exploring issues, options, and resources to support the client's decisions. HIV infection linked to maternal substance abuse raises complex legal and ethical questions for the professional, especially as related to issues of child welfare

FIGURE 2.1. Case Management Linkage and Referral System

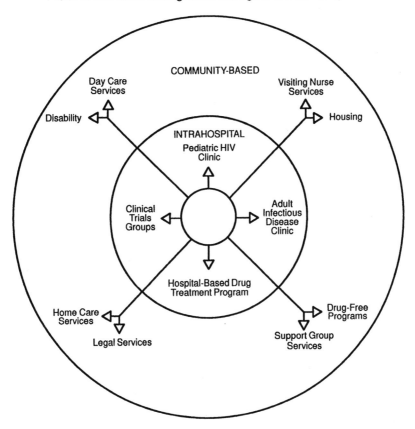

and protection. While working with HIV-infected mothers and children can evoke anxiety, touch deep feelings, and challenge deeply rooted attitudes and professional beliefs, the social worker is challenged to intervene in a positive, creative, and nonjudgmental manner.

Reassessment

HIV is a continually changing and evolving medical illness that necessitates ongoing assessment of the social and emotional needs of those persons whose lives it touches. During every clinical encounter, the levels of physical, social, and emotional functioning of the client need to be assessed, as well as the existing environment stressors and familial supports. As the case is reevaluated, new contracts should be established accordingly.

Transfer and Use of Outside Resources

Pregnancy and the progressive nature of the infection require the social worker and the patient to establish from the onset the need for further coordinated medical and social service care postdelivery. The medication regimens, eligibility for entitlements, and counseling needs must be met on a continual basis. As the woman approaches her expected date of delivery, a review of counseling focuses on affective responses, strengths, progress, and reactions to rearing a child who potentially is infected with the HIV virus. At the time of delivery, the infected mother is introduced to the pediatric and adult infectious disease medical and social work providers. To maximize utilization of services for mother and baby, appointments are consolidated on the same day. Over the next several weeks, the perinatal social worker maintains contact with the patient until appropriate linkages and transitions of care are made and solidified.

Due to various medical concerns, Ms. Sanchez was induced at 37 weeks gestation. Postdelivery, the patient continued to express significant discomfort in her lower back and abdomen, and further testing revealed a large growth on her liver. This required that Ms. Sanchez be transferred to a medical/surgical service and that her primary medical care and case management be shifted to the Adult Infectious Disease Team. The obstetrical social worker remained involved to help ensure a smooth transition and to coordinate the discharge planning needs of the infant. After enduring serious discomforts of a high-risk pregnancy and childbirth, the patient then had to deal with the news that her illness was rapidly progressing, and the increasing realization that her medical prognosis was poor. Ms. Sanchez's immediate response to these unfolding developments was that she would be feeling fine and that she and new baby would be returning home soon. As this dream and denial began to break down, the patient continued her attempts to hold onto the idea that she and her baby would go home together. Initially, she would change the subject whenever the future plans for the baby were raised, as if protecting herself from more disappointment and loss. Ms. Sanchez continued to be firm in her decision not to disclose her condition to family members who lived in the area, and she also insisted that her husband had his hands full taking care of his business and other family demands, including supervising the care of the four-year-old child. As Ms. Sanchez gradually began to accept her changing medical condition and the implications in terms of her health, her family situation, and child care planning needs, she began to use counseling to address these issues. Ms. Sanchez spoke with her mother in Puerto Rico, and arrangements were made for her to come to New York to take care of the two youngest children. Once this was arranged, the patient expressed great relief. She then raised the subject of a health care proxy and permanency planning for the children. Along with a team of volunteer attorneys, the processes were begun. Ms. Sanchez was also able to accept the fact that she would not be returning to work and agreed to assistance to explore eligibility with regard to entitlements. This would make it possible for future home health needs to be met.

Throughout the postpartum period, the transition of Ms. Sanchez's care to the Adult Medicine AIDS Designated Center and its multidisciplinary team was facilitated by the perinatal social worker who took great care to assure that the transition would not be abrupt nor perceived as an abandonment of her or her family. Continuity of care remained the focus of work as did family-centered care. At this time, Ms. Sanchez is treated in the AIDS Designated Center as is her child. She is working well with that team, yet still maintains informal, cordial relations with her perinatal providers. Figure 2.2 is an ecomap for Ana Sanchez.

Case Conclusion and Differential Discussion

Ms. Sanchez is an intelligent and strong-willed woman who is highly knowledgeable about her medical condition. She was quite assertive in the articulation of how she wanted to utilize both medical and social work services. Reflecting upon the work done with Ms. Sanchez perinatally, and with the benefit of hindsight, a number of questions present themselves for review. Should the case manager have been more aggressive in working to reach consensus on a mutually agreed upon treatment plan? Would it have been more beneficial to the patient if greater effort had been made to break through her denial with regard to the progression of her illness? Or was it the very firmly held defensive structure that enabled her to take control of her personal destiny? After all, since her infection was diagnosed in 1980, Ms. Sanchez had married, given birth to two additional children, and worked as a full-time parcel delivery person for seven years. Should this patient have been helped to better anticipate her emotional reaction and behavioral response when her physical condition began to deteriorate? Had this been done, would the patient have been able to more realistically consider the feasibility of employment, insurance, entitlements, and other needed services?

FIGURE 2.2. Ecomap for Ana Sanchez

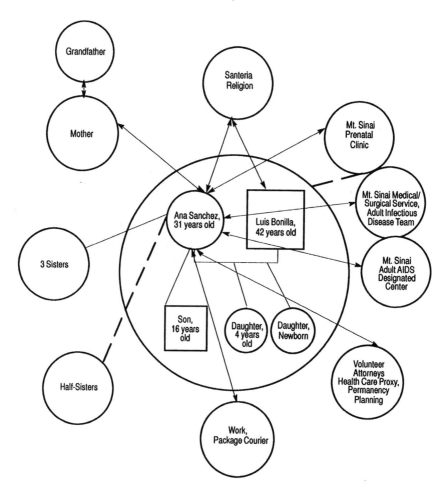

REFERENCES

Centers for Disease Control. (July 1995). Recommendation for human immunodeficiency virus counseling and voluntary testing for pregnant women. *Morbidity and Mortality Weekly Report, 44,* no. RR-7.

Cooper, E. and Powerly, K. (1995). Ethical, legal, and policy considerations. In P. Kelly (Ed.), *Primary Care of Women and Children with HIV Infection.* Boston: Jones & Bartlett Publishers, pp. 245-257.

Kurth, A. (1995). HIV disease and reproductive counseling. *Focus: A Guide to AIDS Research and Counseling, 10*(7), 14.

Mason, J., Preisinger, J., Sperling, R., Walther, V., Berrier, J., and Evans, V. (1991). Incorporating HIV education and counseling into routine prenatal care: A model program. *AIDS Education and Prevention, 3,* 118-123.

Merzel, C. (1992). New Jersey's Medicaid waiver for acquired immunodeficiency syndrome. *Health Care Financing Review, 13,* 27-44.

Mitchell, J. L. (1988). Women, AIDS, and public policy. *AIDS and Public Policy Journal, 3,* 50-52.

New York City Commission on Human Rights: The AIDS Discrimination Division. Report on discrimination against people with AIDS and people perceived who have AIDS. January 1986-June 1987.

Novick, L., Berns, D., Stricof, R., Stevens, R., Pass, K., and Wethers, J. (1989). HIV seroprevalence in newborns in New York State. *Journal of the American Medical Association, 261,* 1745-1750.

Scitovsky, A. (1990). Studying the cost of HIV related illness: Reflections on the moving target. *Milbank Quarterly, 67,* 318-344.

Sperling, R., Sacks, H., Mayer, L., Joyner, M., and Berkowitz, R. (1989). Umbilical cord blood seroprevalence for human immunodeficiency virus in parturient women in a voluntary hospital in New York City. *Obstetrics and Gynecology, 73,* 179-181.

Stuntzner-Gibson, D. (1991). Women and HIV disease: An emerging social crisis. *Social Work, 36,* 22-28.

Walther, V. and Mason, J. (1994). Social work field instruction in a perinatal AIDS setting. *The Clinical Supervisor, 12*(1), 33-52.

Chapter 3

Social Work Interventions on Behalf of a Burned Child: Children's Hospital Emergency Room

Robin S. Johnson
Nancy Nelson
Toba Schwaber Kerson

CONTEXT

Description of the Setting

Children's Hospital is a pediatric, regional, tertiary-care hospital and level-I trauma center. A major teaching institution, it houses the department of pediatrics of a large land-grant public university. This not-for-profit hospital is one of five divisions of an umbrella corporation that includes a fund-development corporation for all charitable contributions, pediatric community-based mental health centers, a research foundation that conducts clinical research in diseases of childhood, and a home care and hospice division. Rapid development of a new ambulatory services division, which unites outpatient care with community medical clinics, is underway. A strong continuum of care is essential to weather stiff competition for pediatric patients as managed care grows steadily in this conservative midwestern market.

The Children's Hospital system describes itself as a strong alliance of expert personnel, facilities, and other specialty resources dedicated to the care of children, which is directed by community leaders and supported by volunteer auxiliary organizations and individuals. Its mission is to provide children and their families with the highest levels of quality care, advocate for children's health, and conduct research and education. Promoting and enhancing a health care delivery system dedicated to the ideals of availability, accessibility, quality, continuity, and efficiency has been the historic goal of the hospital. This is proving to be an increasing challenge as competition for managed care contracts and pressure from adult care systems and payer panels shakes this hospital's autonomy.

The hospital serves patients and families from its surrounding neighborhoods, as well as patients throughout the county in which it is situated. A large number of patients present from primarily rural outlying counties, as well as adjoining states. Little more than one-half of all inpatient admissions are male, and four-fifths are Caucasian, with the remainder predominantly African American. Half of all patients are under four years old, over a quarter are between four and ten years old, and the remainder are 11 years old and older.

Primary, secondary, and tertiary care are provided for acute and chronic diseases and conditions. This hospital is one of the largest pediatric hospitals in the country, with 15,400 inpatient admissions in 1994. It currently has 313 beds and is authorized for an additional 26. Trends toward increased outpatient care, driven by aggressive insurer utilization management, have driven down the length of stay. This, in turn, has led to decreased average daily census and bed utilization. A large ambulatory program of 200,000 outpatient visits in 1994 included 6,000 outpatient surgery admissions, 54,000 outpatient diagnostic visits, and 102,000 specialty clinic visits. An additional 38,000 visits were made to the five community-based primary care clinics. The hospital's Emergency Department, which houses a level-I trauma center, saw nearly 80,000 patients in 1994 and was the busiest emergency department in the county, fourth in the state, and second nationally in pediatric emergency room visits.

Policy

This hospital is a not-for-profit organization under the federal Internal Revenue Service Code. It is licensed to provide health care services and is subject to government regulation including Medicaid and Medicare (Wilson and Neuhauser, 1985). Laws that significantly affect social work practice are documented in the hospital policy manual and are reviewed during orientation. Of particular interest is the State Revised Code, which mandates all health care professionals to report suspicions of child abuse or neglect to the appropriate county protective service agency. Children's Hospital treats and often admits an unfortunate array of abuse and neglect cases, and social workers are frequently confronted with cases that require close understanding of related laws, hospital policy, and protocols. These demand strong ethical, clinical, and organizational judgment to balance the sometimes conflicting rights of children, parents, professionals, and payers. Social workers also have to be familiar with a variety of other relevant laws, including those mandating early intervention programs for children with developmental disabilities (Bishop, Rounds, and Weil, 1993).

Clinical social work in Ohio is regulated by the State Counselor and Social Worker Board. In 1984, the Counselor and Social Worker Law was enacted by the General Assembly of the State of Ohio. This bill provided for the licensing or registration of counselors and social workers, and created a Board to develop, monitor, and regulate professional standards. Licensure is established for two levels of social work practice. The Licensed Social Worker must possess a degree in a program closely related to social work, and must show evidence of coursework in three core social work areas. The Licensed Independent Social Worker must possess a master's or doctoral degree in Social Work from an institution accredited by the Council on Social Work Education, and have two years of paid, supervised employment in social work after completion of the MSW degree. Social work clinicians at Children's Hospital are Licensed Independent Social Workers whose scope of practice in the provision of brief social psychotherapy without supervision ensures a level of clinical excellence necessary to effectively manage complex medical cases.

In the 100 years since its foundation, Children's Hospital has consistently served children and families regardless of their ability to pay and has annually underwritten significant amounts of uncompensated care (Rosenbaum, 1992; Rosenbaum and Johnson, 1986; National Center for Children in Poverty, 1990). It is significant that the hospital receives over half of its revenues from Medicaid. Reimbursement cuts for outpatient services have continued steadily since 1988, and further reimbursement reduction seems inevitable in the near future. Following national trends, this state has applied for a federal waiver that would permit enrollment of all Medicaid patients into managed care programs. The effect of this proposal for a capitated system is expected to be a further significant drop in reimbursement to Children's Hospital from the public sector.

The private sector presents a similar challenge. As in the adult markets, insurance coverage by Blue Cross/Blue Shield and traditional group policies declined considerably nationwide after 1965. Health maintenance organizations (HMOs), preferred provider organizations (PPOs), and a host of self-insured and prepaid managed care plans rose to fill the gap, in some cases even purchasing the individual not-for-profit Blue Cross/Blue Shield agencies. This market change and its rapid pace have demanded comparable changes in price structure and service delivery systems to remain competitive. Children's Hospital has taken a proactive stance toward contracting with HMOs, though simply at the level of discounted fees for service. The impending shift toward a fully capitated market, aggressive competition from local adult and regional pediatric providers, and networked systems of organized provider/payer relationships may leave Children's Hospital at a disadvantage. It does not presently enjoy affiliation with other systems, believing that a go-it-alone stance is appropriate to the only dedicated pediatric provider in this part of the state.

Recognizing the extent to which reimbursement trends demand draconian cost curtailment measures, several far-reaching measures have been taken. The Physician Hospital Organization has been developed, tightening the relationship between medical staff and hospital administration, and laying the groundwork for dramatic shifts in medical practice at both the clinical and teaching levels. Increased incentives for community pediatricians to join the Physician Hospital Organization is an integral part of this plan. Significant reorganization of clinical services has occurred to reduce costs by reducing clinical staff, including nursing and allied health professions. In this process the Department of Social Work has been eliminated, and social work clinicians absorbed with clinical nurse specialists and continuity of care personnel to form the Department of Case Management. The wisdom of this choice may take some time to become apparent.

While now organized to provide continuity within a managed care continuum, social workers are also eligible for reimbursement from third-party payers including Medicare and Medicaid. Within the hospital, social workers practice in a variety of reimbursed settings. Of significance to its Emergency Department is the Family Development Program, which provides a range of medical and psychosocial support services to victims of child abuse and receives partial reimbursement from the county Child Protective Service agency. LISW licensure permits Medicaid reimbursement. Social work clinicians in the Emergency Department may also bill for counseling services, although revenues generated accrue to that department. Hospital administration has historically resisted establishing a dedicated social work cost center.

Technology

Children's Hospital is a level-I pediatric regional trauma center. The state within which it is located divides emergency medical services (EMS) districts along county lines, and the service area of this setting includes both urban and rural populations. This catchment area includes the central and southeastern part of the state and adjoining states also. As may be expected, state-of-the-art medical technology is available to meet the wide range of problems presenting, which range from trauma, including physical and sexual abuse, to primary care for the indigent populations that live adjacent to the hospital. The Emergency Department is a newly constructed area of the hospital and includes an EMS squad room. Located within the department is an emergency communications center, which is the communications link with the outside for all incoming calls linking EMS personnel, referring physicians, and referring hospitals. In 1994, there were 8,800 communications through this center.

The Emergency Department has ten full-time pediatric emergency medicine physicians. Pediatric anesthesia, neurosurgery, radiology, and pediatric rehabilitation are integral parts of the trauma team, as are laboratory technicians, and blood bank and radiology technicians. There is intensive nursing coverage. Clinical social work has members on the trauma team, some of whom are also members of the hospital abuse team. Social work is well-positioned to manage both critical care and abuse and neglect issues, as well as to provide early intervention with patients and families managing chronic conditions such as cancers, cystic fibrosis, or end-stage renal disease, who may present in crisis to the emergency department.

Incoming trauma patients are categorized primarily according to physiologic data and to a lesser extent by mechanism of injury information. The two categories of trauma alerts are level I (highest) and level II. Once the patient is categorized, the trauma team is notified and is expected to present to the Emergency Department within five minutes. This occurs virtually 100 percent of the time. Members of the team carry two-way radios with which to communicate with the emergency communications center as well as incoming helicopters and pre-hospital ground transport vehicles. Patients are met by the team, including social workers, immediately as they arrive at the emergency room.

Two large rooms are dedicated for trauma resuscitations in the Emergency Department. These can easily handle three simultaneous trauma patients, and can be expanded to six patients if necessary. Each room has dedicated equipment, including end-tidal CO_2 monitors and oxygen saturation monitors. The remainder of the equipment, including a level-I fluid warmer, is also state-of-the-art. The contiguous operating room is adequately staffed seven days a week, 24 hours a day, and has a suite always kept available for trauma patients. Two Pediatric Intensive Care Units with 16 and 11 beds respectively are the primary recovery rooms. A blood bank and clinical laboratory are close, as is a dedicated burn unit. Spinal cord injuries are managed by neurosurgery and orthopedic surgery.

The hospital maintains a vigorous continuous quality improvement process with pre-hospital personnel and actively tracks its populations using a variety of research and clinical evaluation tools. It is an active participant in the maintenance and design of the statewide pre-hospital program. All data are entered into the Trauma Base Registry. This is a sophisticated database that allows not only basic data monitoring, but provides a platform for clinical research and for regular mortality and morbidity review (American College of Surgeons, 1995).

Prior to elimination, the Department of Clinical Social Work maintained the Clinical Social Work Information System, a relational database linking clinicians practice records with all hospital databases, including lab, pharmacy, patient records, and human resources. This database similarly allowed basic practice monitoring and provided a research platform. As with all social work staff, emergency room clinicians recorded practice on this system and used it to access data on presenting patients where necessary.

Organization

Children's Hospital is responsible to a board of trustees that is comprised of leading business and community figures in the city and county where the hospital is located. Board membership ostensibly reflects community commitment to the health and well-being of children. Increasingly, hospital administration has struggled with the reorganization and clinical prioritization necessary to survive in the present local market, and has been fortunate to convince the board of trustees of the wisdom of its unaffiliated stance at a time when adult hospitals are merging to ensure their stability. An additional threat is mounting from for-profit surgery centers and aggressive acquisition of local hospitals by out-of-state for-profit chains. At this point, the board of trustees continues to endorse the leadership of its long-standing hospital executive group.

Nested within the Children's Hospital campus, and some miles from the university itself, is the School of Medicine's Department of Pediatrics of the major land-grant public university located in this city. The chair of the Department of Pediatrics is the medical director of Children's Hospital, and is half of a unique dual reporting arrangement at this hospital, in which the chief executive officer and the medical director both report directly to the Board of Trustees. This relationship is intended to ensure an appropriate balance between clinical excellence and fiscal responsibility, and to encourage participatory management. While laudable in its intended goal, this arrangement has left academic physicians vulnerable to the reverberations of politics within the School of Medicine on the distant campus, while contributing to a perception that a clinically unsophisticated administration dictates clinical practice to a demoralized medical staff. Whether or not this is true, this leadership arrangement works well in communicating fiscal conservatism to the Board of Trustees and to the community, a city dominated by insurance interests. It has, however, been argued that fiscal conservatism for its own sake has resulted in diminished attention to clinical practice, and that this has contributed to a decline in the competitive edge of the hospital in the regional pediatric market. Lacking the economies of scale that affiliation and membership in a larger system can provide, the hospital is having difficulty dropping costs to the level required for healthy managed care contracts. This challenge is common to the hospital industry, especially academic medical centers throughout the nation at this point in time.

Children's Hospital is large by pediatric standards, with nearly 3,000 employees, including more than 500 physicians on the medical staff. Administrative concern for the well-being of patients and families, without regard to ability to pay, and commitment to employee satisfaction are cornerstone values at Children's, and together combine to project a competent caring organization. These sentiments are routinely articulated through in-house publications, marketing materials, in management meetings, employee forums, and other institutional meetings including board meetings, and are more formally coded in the hospital values statement. The hospital values statement is prominently posted around the institution, including the Emergency Department, and describes five core values: quality, teamwork, compassion, innovation, and leadership. These are framed to focus service provision and organization for hospital and staff, and were developed after a hospital-wide process. They combine knowledge, skill, ethical standards, and service with effective responsible use of all resources.

Ironically, it is the weight of commitment within the values statement that is a source of skeptical comment on the part of some hospital employees. Reorganization and aggressive restructuring have led to considerable attrition of the workforce, including termination of employment due to position redefinition. The redefinition of job descriptions has, in many cases, the effect of deprofessionalizing care as multipurpose staff are developed. This trend toward deprofessionalization as a means of permanently reducing cost is particularly difficult for employees to manage. Where high-quality clinical service has historically been synonymous with highly trained and credentialed professionals, the present trend is perceived by many staff as sacrificing quality for short-term institutional financial benefit. There is widespread belief that the present-day changes in health care are in fact no more than the swing of a pendulum in a particular direction, reflecting a self-serving trend on the part of hospital administration to sweeten the bottom line at the expense of quality patient care through elimination of clinical staff. Whether this belief is true or not, hostility toward hospital administration is reflected in a decrease in the tendency to "go the extra mile," which formerly typified the value set of those who work in medical centers of last resort. This, in turn, further conflicts with the values systems of those staff who remain. Accustomed to providing often heroic support to children and families, personnel often find themselves spread thinly on the inpatient units and staffed at levels that do not permit anything beyond essential medical care. Education, counseling, grief work, and family support are often unavailable or presumed to be available in other agencies beyond the hospital. In fact, community support resources beyond the hospital are already strained, and furthermore are not reimbursed for on-the-spot educational and psychosocial support that is clinically indicated and most economically provided in-house. Patients who are members of minority groups are often the first to suffer as a result of this lack of resources.

Discharge planning and medical care conferences are similarly reduced. As they struggle with their interpretations of what is and is not available to patients under their insurance policies, clinicians also struggle with the notion that their practice is dictated by the terms of the patient's medical coverage under an insurance plan, rather than by what is clinically indicated. Especially in a teaching hospital, medical staff are keenly exercised around what are reasonable definitions of appropriate medical care. Where medical outcome measurement has enjoyed so little common agreement, it is understandable that a financial model of clinical management would come to provide an acceptable substitute.

With a clear universal commitment to excellence in providing care to children, the common theme–open communication–is encouraged at every organizational level at Children's Hospital and is articulated as a common value. Unfortunately, despite commitment to this value, job insecurity and shifts in professional roles and functions have considerably eroded relations between medical staff, administration, clinical staff, and support staff, and this is reflected in a high degree of suspicion and fear at different levels of the organization. Increasingly, staff are unwilling to speak their minds openly on clinical and organizational issues. Often erroneously, staff assume that clinical decision-making is driven by external case managers employed by the insurance companies. Organizational decision-making is believed to be similarly externally driven such that clinical care and staffing for it are no longer related to clinical need but are driven solely by the need to reduce costs. This phenomenon adds additional strain to already stressed professionals. Particular stress is placed on nursing and social work personnel who have been used to working in close harmony. Nurses, perceiving themselves understaffed and compromised by increased numbers of temporary agency nurses in their midst, ask more support from social workers. Social workers, with increased spans of responsibility, have found it harder to provide consistent levels of support as caseloads have risen and numbers of clinicians dropped.

Three self-directed work teams are organized by practice areas: crisis and critical care, medical, and ambulatory. Social workers form subteams within these areas to support specialty and unit-based services, and are assigned to provide crisis intervention and support to patients and families with acute, life-threatening conditions. The Crisis and Critical Care Team is primarily responsible for assessment, crisis intervention, treatment, and referral for the Emergency Department, and child abuse, failure-to-thrive, and trauma services, and has additional responsibility for all intensive care units and cardiology, neurology, and neurosurgery. Referrals are generated through active case finding, screening, rounds, from nursing and medical staff, and, as in the case of Shakeela (the client discussed later in the chapter) from membership on the Trauma Team. External child abuse referrals largely originate from child protection agencies requesting medical and psychosocial evaluations.

The values of the Department of Clinical Social Work were historically congruent with those of Children's Hospital in the provision of excellence in clinical practice, teaching, and research, and have been substantively maintained despite the change from a centralized department to a decentralized entity where social workers functioned in self-directed work teams as members of a case management division (Plavnick, 1995). A combination of social workers with master's degrees from accredited graduate schools across the United States, who are state licensed and funded through managed care programs, as well as direct patient revenues, State and Federal grants, and fee-for-service programs have been able to maintain the participative, open-practice style favored by previous departmental leadership. Strong interdisciplinary relations with administration, nursing, and medicine continue to be maintained while fostering collegial decision-making between staff and others, despite the limitations above. Social work clinicians have taken leadership roles in specialty areas and interdisciplinary teams within the hospital which requires specialized service-specific clinical training in addition to generic social work knowledge and skills, and these persist despite organizational change. This is not to deny, however, the additional stress placed on clinicians in managing the high anxiety of colleagues as well as their complex caseloads. Their own mixed feelings about changes in health care, which may make their own future uncertain, are an additional stressor.

As noted above, Children's Hospital is a corporation in the multicorporate entity know as Children's Hospital Incorporated. A home care division is part of this corporate structure. This is both a benefit and a challenge to families, because care at Children's Hospital does not automatically determine that children can use Children's home care services. While this would seem illogical, regulation demands strict enforcement of consumer choice. Making the right choice can be a test of the relationship between hospital staff and the social worker, as well as the family when home care is required.

Children's Hospital is a freestanding corporate body. Social work connection with other agencies is, however, routine, with particular connection to Child Protective Services; home care; home health equipment and durable goods companies; visiting and public health nurses; police forces; disease-specific agencies related to conditions such as epilepsy, end-stage renal disease, or cystic fibrosis; county welfare, housing, and assistance agencies; schools; mental health, mental retardation, and drug and alcohol programs. Children's Physician Hospital Organization has contractual agreements with some community pediatric providers and maintains strong links with both private for-profit and state-supported insurers. Any agency that has children as a constituent may be included by a social worker in a patient treatment plan. Additionally, as the child's parents and often grandparents are centrally involved in care, the domains of interagency involvement may be considerably larger.

PRACTICE DECISIONS

Description of the Client

Shakeela is a three-year-old African-American female child brought into the Emergency Department with second- and third-degree burns to her face, head, torso, and hands, received from a house fire. A level-I trauma alert was called as Shakeela was transported by emergency medical technicians of the city fire department to the hospital, with an estimated arrival time of three minutes. Social work was alerted for family support and crisis intervention, and met the patient on arrival.

Family and extended family members arrived at the Emergency Department 15 minutes after Shakeela, in an appropriate state of crisis. These included her 23-year-old aunt, who claimed to be the legal guardian of the child, and the patient's 19-year-old mother, who appeared with alcohol on her breath and was somewhat unsteady in her gait and demeanor. She also claimed to have legal custody of the patient. Additional family members present were the patient's six-year-old brother, Otha, and the mother's brother, who claimed to be physically disabled as result of an injury sustained in the construction industry. The initial history presented on arrival to the social worker in the Emergency Department waiting area by the mother was that Shakeela's brother was playing with matches, and that this led to her catching on fire. The patient's aunt reported that the children live with her, as their mother is addicted to crack cocaine.

As noted above, Children's has an exceptionally busy Emergency Department. After taking the initial history and further assessing the emotional status of all parties, the social worker was obliged to assess a second, unrelated trauma that arrived soon after. It is commonplace for social work clinicians to manage several of these cases concomitantly, and to take an initial triage history prior to returning for detailed assessment and intervention.

While working on the second case–a near drowning of a 16-year-old Caucasian male–the social worker was informed by staff that Otha had been overheard in the waiting room "bragging" to his aunt and other family members who had subsequently arrived, that he had "set Shakeela on fire." When this occurred, the aunt had become physically aggressive toward the boy. Physical restraint was required by Emergency Department staff, as well as the intervention of hospital security before she regained her composure. Significantly, off-duty city police officers are employed as security officers in the Emergency Department. This is a reflection of the number of cases presenting that have violent components to them. As noted above, Children's is located in a socially disadvantaged area of the city, and has increasingly become the admission site for pediatric gunshot wounds and other trauma stemming from the vagaries of drug-related violence. The hospital and neighborhood lie adjacent to the intersection of north-south and east-west major freeways, and the combination of poverty and accessibility to key transportation routes has led to a significant increase in drug trading and violence in the last three years.

While the aunt was loudly expostulating that she would not take Otha home with her ever again because he is "sick and crazy," Shakeela was admitted from the Emergency Department to the Pediatric Intensive Care Unit in critical condition (Dungan et al., 1995; Weinberg and Miller, 1983).

Definition of the Client

From a medical, critical care standpoint, the client was necessarily Shakeela herself. She was "the patient" admitted to the hospital by the Emergency Department attending physician and was transferred to the care of the intensivists in the Pediatric Intensive Care Unit. She required comprehensive medical care and a range of supportive therapies, including social work, before she was discharged, and thereby generated a wide range of charges for the hospital. The social work component of her bill was paid from charges bundled together under the daily bed rate.

From a social work perspective however, each of the family members present benefited from intervention individually and as a group. This occurred at different times over the course of Shakeela's hospitalization and her post-hospital course to ensure maximization of her medical care and full adjustment to the trauma and its sequelae. It is of note, however, that no reimbursement was provided for this work on the family system, and that psychosocial support of the burned child only persisted during the course of her inpatient hospitalization. No social work support is funded by Children's Hospital in the outpatient clinics to which the child returned for follow-up after discharge from the hospital, nor did her insurance coverage provide for such services.

Goals and Expectations

The initial goal was to immediately ensure the protection and safety of Otha from his aunt's harm in the waiting room during the crisis of his sister's stabilization in the Emergency Department. Second, the family system was quickly assessed to clarify the legal relationships between all parties. An emergent reason for this was the need for appropriate documentation of consents for procedures and for insurance reimbursement for Shakeela's care. A further goal was an immediate referral to Child Protective Services and to the city police, as the sibling was assessed as being at risk of harm while in the hospital and after the family returned home. Child Protective Services planned to release the sibling to the custody of the mother and began court action to get an emergency court order transferring custody from the aunt back to the mother, reversing the legal arrangement the agency had originally initiated some time prior to this event. While provision of crisis intervention and anticipatory grief work toward the possibility that Shakeela would die in the Emergency Department or during the Pediatric Intensive Care Unit transfer was indicated, the chaos of the situation, which was exacerbated by the impaired judgment of the aunt and mother, made this an impossibility.

Fortunately, despite her considerable injuries, Shakeela responded favorably to treatment. As soon as this became apparent, further social work goals were developed. The family support system was assessed, as well as all additional resources for discharge planning. This included family member's ability to learn and provide burn care. A further goal was to initiate and develop collaboration between the interdisciplinary team and the third-party payer, which in this case was the Medicaid health maintenance organization. Improving communication between the health maintenance organization's nurse case manager and the team was facilitated by the social worker to ensure timely authorization of indicated services. Further streamlining the match between payer and indicated clinical services was ensured by the consistent inclusion of the Child Protective Services caseworker in the medical management as it unfolded. In this way, the ongoing protection and safety of both children in a somewhat problematic social situation was secured, with an additional benefit to the third-party payer. This was the shift of costs from the payer to the Child Protective Service agency, which through its legal custody of, by this point, both children, became liable for a significant contribution to Shakeela's medical expenses. This, in turn, became an inducement to the original payer to be lenient in authorizing additional days of care thought necessary by the medical team. The implications of this cost shift from the original for-profit payer to the county tax payers who underwrite the Child Protective Service agency is beyond the scope of discussion in this chapter. In summary, all of the above goals reflect a coordinated discharge planning strategy of a kind typical in ensuring optimal outcomes for complex medical and psychosocial cases such as this.

Use of Contract

In the heat of events and the forceful intervention of hospital security at admission, no immediate contract was deemed advisable. As the subsequent three-month hospitalization of Shakeela progressed, and especially when she was transferred from the Pediatric Intensive Care Unit to the calm and order of the Rehabilitation Unit, family rhythms resumed a more measured beat. It then became possible to initiate a contract with the aunt to visit her niece as often as she was able, and to agree to support her sister by learning Shakeela's burn care. Multiple care conferences and synchronized interprofessional and interagency communication initiated and facilitated by the social worker led to a further series of contracts, namely the agreements to proceed with strategies for discharge planning by coordinating principals from the hospital's interdisciplinary treatment teams, the patient's health maintenance organization, the hospital's home-care services, and the family and the Child Protective Service agency.

More specific illustration of the above activity will further reveal some dimensions of the successful social work case management activity that ensued. While hospital staff, primarily nursing, began to teach burn care to both mother and aunt, the social worker facilitated the teaching schedule with family members, and provided supportive counseling while so doing. She assessed the capacity of the family to provide care, and empowered members to become supportive of each other in the service of Shakeela's health and well-being. Post-discharge, the social worker negotiated with Child Protection Services to provide transportation for Shakeela to daily physical therapy and medical appointments at the hospital outpatient clinics, and obtained in-home aid for additional assistance to the family in the home. Negotiation with the health maintenance organization resulted in twice-daily skilled-nursing visits to Shakeela's home to assist the family with bathing and painful dressing changes. Referrals were then made for assessment for counseling and psychotherapy for Shakeela and for her younger brother, who was also enrolled in the Juvenile Firestarters program. Shakeela's mother was offered support to enter a program for her addiction but refused, saying she needed to be available to help care for her daughter. While some might question this response, it is of note that this mother was not observed by staff either in the hospital or in the home as evidencing frank signs of her addiction after the initial presentation to the Emergency Department of her daughter.

Meeting Place

Predictably, the initial meeting place for this case was the Emergency Department. Remarkable for its total focused attention to saving life using the most sophisticated medical technology, and typically managing a number of high-risk cases simultaneously, this environment lends itself simply to elicitation of information and interaction essential to save life. The atmosphere is often tense and fearful. It is in the emergency rooms of the United States that the awful contrast between the unpredictability of life and the medical means to fix it is most clearly on display. Basic issues of information, safety, protection, and crisis intervention were first managed here by the social worker.

The family became a little less tense when Shakeela was admitted to the Pediatric Intensive Care Unit, knowing she would recover from her injuries if all went well. But the unit shares some of the technology of the Emergency Department, and matters here are exacerbated by the large number of critically ill children being managed on the unit. Here, too there is tension and an uneasy sense of unpredictability, despite the calm professionalism of the unit staff. While the waiting areas of the Emergency Department are bustling and sometimes violent, the waiting rooms for this unit are more controlled in their activity. The family had weathered the first wave of shock and disbelief with its concomitant emotional lability, and was now hunkered down to hope for the best outcome that medicine could offer while witnessing around them the sad results when things have not worked out. They saw other families rehearsing the same scenarios they were themselves experiencing, and also those they hoped they never would. Against this background, where communication is driven by the hour-by-hour status of critically ill children, the social work clinician dealt with the family regarding medical information and its interpretation;

management of the effects of that information; and fortunately in the case of Shakeela, where things were improving, planning was begun for the long inpatient stay and the hoped-for discharge. Here, the groundwork was laid for post-discharge care: assessing and reinforcing family capacity to perform home care and to manage the long period of adjustment to perhaps diminished function against the certain knowledge that once a traumatic event has occurred in a family, its world view is irretrievably changed (Bowlby, 1961). A full family conference took place against this background, with medicine, nursing, social work, and the family represented, but this meeting was professionally controlled: the family learned its options and received information that confirmed a major change had taken place. As in the Emergency Department, the identities of family and of staff were diminished by the technology and the architecture that contained it.

Step-down to the Rehabilitation Unit provided a sometimes unexpected contrast to the above. In the Rehabilitation Unit, there is a large team of a variety of disciplines with the time and resources to capitalize on the work already performed on the child. Visiting hours are uncontrolled, individual care plans include the family, and relationships have room to flourish (Goffman, 1972). Here the emotional reaction to what had taken place became more fully integrated, and the social worker facilitated that process with longer meetings in which education took place around the normal reactions of normal people to abnormal events (Mitchell and Bray, 1989), as well as to prepare the family to assist in Shakeela's care in the home.

After the child was discharged from the hospital, the Home Care Team became involved, and case management responsibility was transferred. The social worker followed up with the family to support as required. A medical setback at home often triggers recollection of the inpatient course and its precipitants in unexpected and dramatic ways. Telephone contact with the social worker who walked through the hospitalization with the family was particularly helpful at that time (Shepard, 1987).

Use of Time

Decisions about time are driven almost exclusively by the shape of the medical course of the patient and the availability of the treatment teams for interaction with the family, irrespective of their locations. This phenomenon in concert with the facts of the trauma, may be a major contributor to the disorientation experienced by families in such circumstances. Deprived of regular habits of control over time, they experience an increase in anxiety (Mead and Bateson, 1942) even above what the medical facts of their situation might evoke.

Recognizing the importance of time, both in the adjustment process of patient and family and in the particular number of days authorized for treatment by the payer, is an essential aspect of working in the emergency room and with patients who transfer from it. Reconciling these two sometimes conflicting elements to the extent possible requires a high degree of clinical skill. The reimbursed time frame of the hospital course with the medical events that punctuate it may not coincide with the time frames necessary for family members to adjust to them. The social worker was sensitive to this mismatch and used education and crisis intervention techniques to manage family affect and assist coping and adaptation over time. Appreciation of these dynamics and of the degree of change that even a single intervention can accomplish went far to ensure a reasonable outcome (Alissi and Caspar, 1985). In cases such as this, the skillful clinician must pace his or her interventions with child and family accordingly. While the hospital setting invites careful therapeutic intervention, management of dramatic medical events must be the primary consideration (Horn, Feldman, and Ploof, 1995). It is after discharge, when the safety of the hospital is relinquished, that referral for counseling may be most effective. Review of the goals set for working with Shakeela above, and of the interventions outlined below will reveal the systematic sensitivity of the clinician to the restraints and opportunities of time in the medical setting.

Interventions

Crisis Intervention

Management of the initial crisis of trauma required judicious crisis intervention when Shakeela presented to the Emergency Department. Elicitation of basic information to clarify the custodial parent required an empathetic but clear and focused approach to join with the family in their shock, and to maintain control of the situation, establishing the boundaries of expression of affect. When the altercation between Shakeela's brother and aunt took place, it required the intervention of security to establish control, and the social worker had no difficulty in following on from security. Again, calm and nonconfrontational direct communication was required, with acknowledgment of the medical facts and the capacity to witness and be present at the family's response to them.

Child Protective Services

Engaging child protective services to ensure the safety of Shakeela's brother was in fact an act of advocacy for the 6-year-old boy. Remaining connected to the perpetrating adults at such a time requires professional restraint and a clear sense of clinical priority (Moncher, 1995). It does not require disengaging from the adults, and it is surprising how clinician's mixed feelings about calling Child Protective Services can rob them of a better understanding of the extent to which it is very possible to advocate for a child while continuing to build a useful relationship with the parents.

Case Management and Education

Case management began with the activity on behalf of the interdisciplinary team to ensure legal guardianship for consent purposes and to confirm insurance coverage. Continued liaison with the Medicaid insurer and with Child Protective Services by the interdisciplinary care team on the Rehabilitation Unit was a further dimension of the complex management of this case. Subsequent dimensions of case management included early inclusion of the home care social worker to facilitate a smooth transition and maintain a social work role after discharge; liaison with all agencies to ensure that commitments for care and treatment are honored; and coordination of communication with outpatient medical providers, surgeons, and occupational and physical therapies to ensure continuity of care. Education about phases of medical care, statement of expectations of the interdisciplinary team and the medical course, available community resources, and the psychosocial effects of trauma were significant intervention techniques that normalized the shifting context of care for the family to the extent possible.

Advocacy

Shakeela and her family required continued advocacy on the part of the social worker. First, the social worker advocated for the family with the interdisciplinary team, especially during early phases of care, where the altercation in the Emergency Department, the suspicion of alcohol dependency, and apparent lack of supervision of the children conspired to lower the sympathies of the team toward the family (Mitchell and Bray, 1990). Second, she advocated for multiple support resources so that the patient's family could be provided with intensive home medical burn care. This involved facilitating the interaction of family, care team, the insurer's nurse case manager, Child Protective Services, medical unit personnel, the hospital's billing office, and home care personnel. It also meant that the social worker had to treat Shakeela's as a special case, rather than one in a busy caseload from which she might at any time be distracted by another trauma alert. Thus, the choices of clinical modality, in this case, were driven by the hospital context, the role of the social worker within that context, and the medical needs of the child. While the social worker was able to make subtle choices within the interventions as to time, place, and principals, either physically present or on conference telephone calls, predictably the practice was driven primarily by the clinician's function within the agency (Smalley and Bloom, 1977).

Stance of the Social Worker

Managing trauma and possible abuse and/or neglect in a busy emergency room demands considerable discipline, calm, and confidence in professional authority, as well as the knowledge and skill requisite to intervene appropriately and strategically. Prior identification of the clinician's own feelings about sudden traumatic events and their sequelae is essential to professional practice, especially when there are similarities between the case and the events in the clinician's personal experience. Common issues for which to be alert are the identifications caused when a presenting patient is the same age or gender as children of the worker, when the parent or family is "familiar" to the clinician for reasons such as class or geographical location, or when transference and countertransference issues are unexpectedly present. Another risk is when the event occurs on the anniversary either of a significant event in the life of the professional or another family member. In this case, the social work clinician had children of approximately the same age as those in this case, and additionally was managing the catastrophic illness of another family member. Forthright identification of these issues and discussion with colleagues went far to regaining the perspective necessary for optimal work on this difficult case.

Professional attitudes toward violence and abuse demand training and experience to work to the best advantage of child, family, and professional. To experience the full gamut of emotions, including extreme anger, violence, and abuse, maintaining a calm, nonthreatening, professional demeanor is essential (Foster, 1995). Management of drug and alcohol issues in the family also can challenge staff in the emergency room. Training is the best solution; this clinician had no difficulty in matter-of-factly interviewing the crack-addicted mother or managing the family after security was called. Long experience of managing families while bringing in Child Protective Services was helpful also in taking steps necessary to protect the brother and establish legal custodial responsibility.

Use of Outside Resources

This case illustrates clearly the extent to which medical management of the medically and psychosocially complex child demands collaboration with outside agencies. Systematic interaction with Child Protective Services, homecare, home aid, and the nurse case manager at the primary insurer was a primary function of the social work clinician. In the early stages of Shakeela's course, the social worker dealt directly with principal agencies, but informed the family every step of the way. As Shakeela stabilized and the family regained its composure and increasingly invested in the details of her care, the worker increasingly shifted from direct contact with the agencies to supporting the mother and aunt in accessing needed services, and following through with ongoing communication with the agencies. Teaching the family to establish relationships with contact people in the agencies was an accomplishment that signaled the readiness of the family to take full responsibility for Shakeela on discharge. Figure 3.1 illustrates Shakeela's ecomap and the relationships already existing, as well as those formed because of the trauma.

Reassessment

Each shift and change in the medical course of the child entry to the Emergency Department, transfer to the Pediatric Intensive Care Unit, transfer to the Rehabilitation Unit, discharge and transfer to homecare, visits to the outpatient clinics, and ultimate discharge from the system itself, all provided ongoing opportunity for reassessment. This was especially true at each transition point where change in location demanded relinquishing some relationships and building new ones. Each discharge to the next level of care raised questions. Was Shakeela receiving care as directed by the attending physician? Were medical and occupational therapy appointments being kept? Was the family meeting the needs of the child and her brother? Were all necessary supports in place?

Several points are of interest in this regard. More help was required from Child Protective Services for provision and payment of transportation to and from the clinics after discharge. Less home nursing care was required than estimated, and the insurer began to withdraw home nursing supports, and finally refused to pay. Assessment of the family's ability to provide adequate care with less nursing support required further communication with Child Protective Services on the one hand and attending physicians on the other. As crisis intervention theory would indicate (Aguilera and Messick, 1974), the relationship of the social work clinician with all members of the family except Shakeela was well set from the initial interaction. This social worker presented a calm, consistent, informed, and informing professional presence, tempered with empathy and compassion, yet firm enough to mobilize services within the hospital and community. Unafraid to honestly manage hard facts, and with a sense of humor through which to filter some of the bureaucratic details of care, such as treatment authorization issues with the payer,

FIGURE 3.1. Ecomap for Shakeela

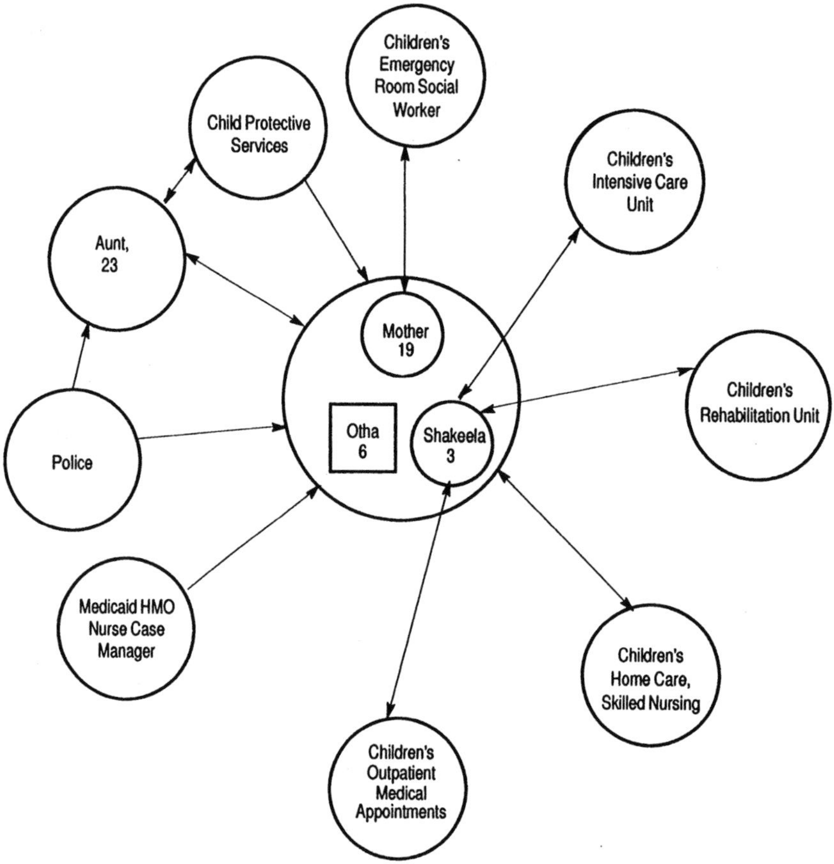

the worker was equally unafraid to confront the family with its options and to advocate on its behalf to ensure it received the best care assistance.

Transfer or Termination

Consistent with the plans above, the social worker terminated all but telephone contact with the family when Shakeela was discharged from the hospital. At that point, social work management of Shakeela was transferred to the Child Protective Service agency. As no social work is provided in the

Plastic Surgery Clinic, involvement would have been expected to end unless Shakeela was again admitted to the hospital; however, confident of the relationship with the worker, and grateful for the excellent care Shakeela had received, the family requested ongoing telephone contact after discharge. The clinician promised to call on Shakeela's birthday, and did so. She received news of the patient from a receptionist in the office of Shakeela's plastic surgeon and from informal contacts with colleagues in the Child Protective Service agency.

Case Conclusion

Shakeela has limited range of motion in her left arm and facial disfigurement that is expected to respond to plastic surgery. She will have the first of the reconstructive procedures in spring of the year following the event. Her outcome and current functioning are well within normal limits. Her legal custody and that of her brother is with her mother, who has attended a drug rehabilitation program. Her mother says it took Shakeela's accident for her to "go straight." Shakeela's brother has shown no further documented inclination to play with fire.

Differential Discussion

Review of this case revealed little the clinician could control that she wished had been done otherwise. Clearly, the necessity of physically leaving this family soon after initial contact to deal with another trauma was problematic; ironically, the unfolding of matters in the waiting room precipitated a sequence of events that brought structure to the family early in Shakeela's medical course. Early mobilization of support agencies ensured early stabilization of the family system just as the three-year-old's medical course was stabilizing. She was thus empowered to enjoy a more trouble-free environment on discharge than she had experienced prior to her trauma.

This case illustrates the power of early intervention in trauma and critical care where psychosocial complexity is also present. Psychosocially challenged families may sometimes experience the horror of trauma in addition to their other misfortunes. Ready and available professional social work services are an essential support to family, child, and hospital staff at such unhappy times.

REFERENCES

Aguilera, D. C. and Messick, J. M. (1974). *Crisis intervention*. St. Louis, MO: C. V. Mosby.

Alissi, A. S. and Caspar, M. (1985). Time as a factor in group work. *Social Work in Groups, 8(2)*, 3-16.

American College of Surgeons Committee on Trauma Verification. (1995). Consultation Programs for Hospitals. *Reverification regional pediatric trauma center (level I)*, 2-10.

Bishop, K. K., Rounds, K., and Weil, M. (1993). P. L. 99-457: Preparation for social work practice with infants and toddlers with disabilities and their families. *Journal of Social Work Education, 29*, 36-45.

Bowlby, J. (1961). The process of mourning. *International Journal of Psychoanalysis, 4*(37).

Dungan, S. S., Jaguay, T. R., Reznik, K. A., and Sards, E. A. (1995). Pediatric Critical Care Social Work: Clinical Practice with Parents of Critically Ill Children. *Social Work in Health Care, 21*(1), 69-80.

Foster, J. (1995). Child Abuse. In A. M. Dietrich and S. Shaner (Eds.), *Basic trauma life support international,* 104-107.

Goffman, E. (1972). *Relations in public.* New York: Harper & Row.

Horn, J. D., Feldman, H. M., and Ploof, D. L. (1995). Parent and Professional Perceptions about Stress and Coping Strategies During a Child's Lengthy Hospitalization. *Social Work in Health Care, 21*(1), 107-127.

Mancher, F. J. (1995). Social Isolation and Child Abuse Risk. Families-in-Society, 76(7), 421-433.

Mead, M. and Bateson, G. (1942). *Balinese character.* New York: New York Academy of Sciences.

Mitchell, J. T. and Bray, G. P. (1989). *Emergency service stress: Guidelines for preserving the health and careers of emergency services personnel.* Englewood Cliffs, NJ: Brady Publishing.

National Center for Children in Poverty. (1990). *Five million children: A statistical profile of our poorest young children.* New York: Author.

Plavnick, C. (1995). Centralized vs decentralized: Rationale for a blended model. *Social Work Administration, 21*(4), 1-4.

Rosenbaum, S. (1992). Child health and poor children. *American Behavioral Scientist, 35,* 275-289.

Rosenbaum, S. and Johnson, K. (1986). Providing health care for low income children: Reconciling child health goals with child health financing realities. *Milbank Quarterly, 64,* 442-478.

Shephard, P. (1987). Telephone therapy: An alternative to isolation. *Clinical Social Work Journal, 15*(1), 56-65.

Smalley, R. and Bloom, T. (1977) Social casework: The functional approach. In J. B. Turner (Ed.), *Encyclopedia of Social Work.* New York: National Association of Social Workers, pp. 1280-1290.

Weinberg, N. and Miller, N. J. (1983). Burn Care: A Social Work Perspective. *Health and Social Work, 8*(2), 97-105.

Wilson, F. and Neuhauser, D. (1985). *Health sciences in the United States.* New York: Ballinger.

Chapter 4

Social Work Practice in Early Intervention: Child Service Coordination in a Rural Health Department

Kathleen Rounds
Irene Nathan Zipper
Tina Powell Green

CONTEXT

Description of the Setting

Rural County, North Carolina is a large agricultural county with a population of approximately 37,000, and is located within a one-hour drive of a metropolitan area. More than 40 percent of the employed adults work outside the county; many commute to the nearest metropolitan area for work. The median household income in 1989 was $25,049 (U.S. Bureau of the Census, 1990). There is no public transportation in the county; however, a van service is available to transport Medicaid-eligible residents to medical appointments if it is arranged several weeks in advance.

The Rural County Health Department is the only provider of obstetric and pediatric care in the county. It is located in a complex that houses the county's Department of Social Services and the local mental health center. This physical arrangement promotes client access to a range of services and fosters interagency collaboration. Residents with private insurance usually seek obstetrical and pediatric care out of county, whereas individuals who have no medical insurance and those who have Medicaid coverage use the County Health Department. Resident doctors from a large university medical center (hereafter referred to as "UMC") that is located within sixty miles provide obstetric and pediatric medical services at the County Health Department, and a pediatrician who recently completed her residency at UMC is in clinic three days a week. The collaborative agreement between the County Health Department and UMC also permits women who receive prenatal care at the health department to deliver at the UMC. Pediatric patients with problems that cannot be handled at the health department are referred and/or transported to the UMC.

Policy

In 1986, Congress passed Public Law (P.L.) 99-457, amending the Education of the Handicapped Act (EHA), which was passed in 1970 (now referred to as P. L. 102-119, Individuals with Disabilities Education Act or IDEA). The amendment created, among other things, Part H, the Handicapped Infants and Toddlers section, which authorizes the federal government to provide financial assistance to states to establish a "statewide, comprehensive, coordinated, multidisciplinary, interagency program of early intervention services for handicapped infants and toddlers and their families" (IDEA Amendments of 1986, sec. 671b[1]). The passage of the amendment was the result of approximately 25 years of activity at the federal level in early childhood special education (Hebbeler, Smith, and Black, 1991) and reflected growing empirical evidence that early intervention is effective in improving child development and minimizing the effects of disabilities (Silverstein, 1989; Shonkoff and Hauser-Cram, 1987).

The underlying intent of the legislation emphasized the belief that (1) families play a central role in the development of young children and therefore services should be designed and delivered in a family-centered way that stresses family/professional collaboration (Shelton and Stepanek, 1994; Bishop, Woll, and Arango, 1993); and (2) the existing service system needs to promote interagency collaboration and interdisciplinary collaboration to reduce fragmentation in order to effectively meet the needs of young children with developmental disabilities and their families (McNulty, 1989).

The concepts of family-centered care and family/professional collaboration were operationalized by requiring that all eligible children and their families be assigned a service coordinator and that services be provided in accordance with an Individualized Family Service Plan (IFSP). The plan outlines the family's goals, concerns, resources, and priorities; activities to meet these goals; and specific responsibilities of the various service providers and of family members. The IFSP should be developed by a multidisciplinary team in which a family member plays a key role (McGonigel, Kaufmann, and Johnson, 1991). To deal with the issues of service-delivery fragmentation, P. L. 99-457 required that states designate a lead agency and state-level interagency coordinating council (ICC). The role of the state ICC initially included advising and working with the lead agency to develop a state system of interagency programs and to promote interagency agreements (McNulty, 1989). In many states, local ICCs or consortiums were established to address local service-delivery problems and gaps to develop mechanisms for interagency collaboration.

Families are eligible for services under Part H if they have a child below the age of three who has a developmental delay or is diagnosed with a physical or mental condition that will result in developmental delay or disability. A number of states have also included infants and toddlers who are "at risk for delay" in their eligibility criteria. The definition of "at risk" varies from state to state (Silverstein, 1989).

P. L. 99-457 delineated which services can be provided under Part H and to whom. Services listed include many that social workers might typically provide when working with a family; for example, family counseling and training, early identification, screening and assessment, home visits, and case management, which is now referred to as "service coordination" (Bishop, Rounds, and Weil, 1993). In many early intervention systems, social workers function in the role of service coordinator and are responsible for facilitating the development of the IFSP and for coordinating services (Zipper, Weil, and Rounds, 1993).

The financing of medical care and early intervention services for infants and toddlers with special needs is of ongoing concern, given proposed changes in health care financing, the rapid growth of managed care, and the shift in financial responsibility from the federal government to state and local governments. The authors of Part H wrote the legislation to make the federal government the payer of last resort for early intervention services, thus encouraging states to optimize alternative funding sources, both public and private. Medicaid, through the Early and Periodic Screening, Diagnosis, and Treatment Program (EPSDT) may be the most important funding stream for services for Part H-eligible infants and toddlers (Perkins and Zinn, 1995; Fox, Freedman, and Klepper, 1989). Of the infants and toddlers receiving Part H services, it is estimated that from 30 percent to 60 percent are also eligible for Medicaid (Shanahan and Cunningham, 1993).

Other legislation has been passed that supports the implementation of Part H. For example, P. L. 99-272, the Consolidated Omnibus Budget Reconciliation Act (COBRA), allows states to include "targeted case management" as a Medicaid-reimbursable service. The Child Care and Development Block Grant legislation requires coordination among agencies, and names children with special needs as one of two target populations for services. Amendments to Title V, the Maternal and Child Health Block Grant Program regulations encourage states to develop coordinated systems of care and mandate case management for children with special health care needs (Fox, Freedman, and Klepper, 1989).

In North Carolina, state legislation was passed that identified the Division of Mental Health, Developmental Disabilities, and Substance Abuse Services in the Department of Human Resources as the lead agency for Part H. Other state agencies included in the Part H system in North Carolina are: Maternal and Child Health, Services for the Blind, and Services for the Deaf and Hard of Hearing. The Division of Maternal and Child Health was designated as the coordinative agency for the Child Service Coordination Program (CSCP). The division contracted with local county health departments to implement the program and established an interagency data collection and reporting system to monitor program implementation. Each county health department maintains a Child Service Coordination Log, listing all children enrolled in the program. In North Carolina, the CSCP is available to families with children under the age of three who have a developmental delay, are at risk for delay, or demonstrate atypical (emotional or behavioral) development. Families of children with a diagnosed developmental disability may receive child service coordination services up until the age of five, at which time they are referred to the public school system for services.

Technology

Many families receiving early intervention services may deal with various forms of technology. For families with a history of genetic or chromosome disorders, the initial experience with technology may be with prenatal screening (ultrasonography) and prenatal diagnosis, for example, amniocentesis and chorionic villi sampling (CVS) during pregnancy (Black, 1992; Adler, Keyes, and Robertson, 1991). Amniocentesis is a method of prenatal testing that is usually conducted between 13 and 16 weeks of pregnancy. Using a needle and syringe, the physician does a transdominal puncture of the amniotic sac and removes amniotic fluid, which is then examined to detect genetic and biochemical disorders. CVS is a newer method of prenatal diagnosis conducted between the ninth and eleventh week of pregnancy. A plastic catheter is inserted transcervically or a needle is inserted transabdominally under real-time ultrasound guidance to aspirate 10 to 20 mg of corionic villi. Many of the infants who are referred for early intervention services are born at low birth weight, with medical complications, and/or have been exposed to drugs or alcohol in utero. Thus, these infants and their families have experienced the multiple technological interventions that are present in a neonatal intensive care unit (Affleck, Tennen, and Rowe, 1991). In addition, depending upon the cause of the infant's/toddler's disability, some families will have to learn how to use complicated technology in the home, such as a ventilator, apnea monitor, or tracheostomy or gastrostomy tube. Some young children with multiple disabilities or communication disorders benefit from the use of assistive technology.

Many young children who are receiving early intervention services have survived as the result of highly sophisticated technology that in itself may raise a number of difficult and complex ethical and psychosocial issues for individual families. Social workers, along with other health care providers, play an important role in explaining the reasons for and uses of technology to families. This requires an ability to translate complex technical information into understandable and usable language for families, as well as the skill to help families begin to make sense of the ethical and psychosocial issues with which they are coping. Social workers also need to understand how the family's cultural values and beliefs influence their perception of and experience with medical interventions that use complex technology (Rounds, Weil, and Bishop, 1994).

Most states have developed a data-management system for tracking service delivery to families receiving services under Part H. Social workers in early intervention programs, such as child service coordination, must understand and be skilled at using the computer technology and the database systems for tracking and monitoring service delivery. Social workers can use these systems to track service delivery for individual clients and as a "tickler" system to remind them of contacts and reassessments with families. Data from these information management systems can also provide important information to social workers for evaluating programs and advocating for policy and program change at the state and local level (Farel, Fraser, and Kegg, 1995).

Organization

The Rural County Health Department provides obstetric, gynecologic, family planning, and pediatric services. Providers from within the health department, other community agencies, and hospitals refer infants and toddlers to the Child Service Coordination Program (CSCP), which is staffed by social workers (referred to as child service coordinators or CSCs). The CSC is a member of a multidisciplinary team at the health department and a member of the county's Interagency Consortium. The CSC's active involvement on the consortium and his or her skill at collaborating with providers in other agencies, enables him or her to tap into a range of resources for clients.

Like other health departments throughout North Carolina, pregnant and postpartum women are followed by a maternity care coordinator (MCC) as part of the Baby Love Program, a state-wide program to prevent infant mortality and promote healthy birth outcomes. MCCs are likely sources of referrals because they provide case management and counseling to pregnant women and postpartum follow-up, and are therefore likely to be aware of situations in which an infant is born with a known developmental disability or is at risk for developmental delay.

When the CSC receives a referral, he or she typically follows up with the infant's or toddler's mother or primary caregiver to conduct an initial psychosocial assessment. The CSC's primary responsibilities include ensuring that developmental assessments and evaluations to determine the child's eligibility for services are conducted in a timely and family-centered way; participating in and arranging for child developmental assessments and evaluations; facilitating the IFSP process; coordinating and monitoring service provision; providing counseling; preparing periodic status reports on each enrolled child; and facilitating the transition to a different service system when the child reaches three or five years of age, whichever is appropriate.

DECISIONS ABOUT PRACTICE

Client Description

Lakia is an 18-month-old African-American female who was referred to the CSCP at the Rural County Health Department by a child health nurse, when she was ten weeks old. The nurse had observed that her 16-year-old mother, Sandra, frequently brought Lakia to the health department with a variety of problems and "didn't seem to have a clue as to how to care for her." The child health nurse noted the mother's quiet, withdrawn behavior and flat affect, and was concerned that Lakia might be at risk for developmental delay.

Sandra's pregnancy was uncomplicated; she started prenatal care at the County Health Department in her twenty-fifth week of pregnancy. As a client of the Baby Love Program, she was followed by a Maternity Care Coordinator, who provided case management services during her pregnancy. Lakia was born prematurely at 34 weeks with a birth weight that placed her in the twenty-fifth percentile for weight. Lakia had one-minute and five-minute APGAR scores of 9. The APGAR (American Pediatric

Growth Assessment Record) score tests a newborn's general status at one and five minutes after delivery. The score is based on a nurse's or physician's assessment of the newborn's color, heart rate, respiratory effort, muscle tone, and reflex irritability. The highest APGAR score that a newborn can receive is a 10; a very low score suggests that the newborn must be closely observed. Lakia's head circumference was disproportionately large (in the seventy-fifth percentile) relative to her height and weight. Head circumference in relationship to weight and length is one indicator used in assessing infant development. If the head circumference is unusually small or large there may be reason for concern. At this checkup, Lakia's head circumference was disproportionately larger relative to her height and weight than it was at birth. She did not seem to have any medical difficulties and was discharged home with her mother within 24 hours of being born.

At ten weeks, Sandra brought Lakia to the Health Department because Lakia had diarrhea, was not eating, and had a low-grade fever. She was transferred to University Medical Center (UMC) by ambulance, and after a week of evaluation was diagnosed with metabolic renal acidosis, tachypnea (excessively rapid breathing), and hematuria (blood in the urine), in addition to viral respiratory illness. She was also referred to the CSCP. The Rural County Consortium conducted an initial assessment to determine if Lakia met the criteria for the CSCP, and found that Lakia had developmental lags and that her medical problems placed her at high risk for further developmental delays. She was referred for a complete multidisciplinary evaluation by the regional Developmental Evaluation Center (DEC).

Following her discharge from UMC, Lakia was seen for monthly follow-up visits at the Health Department, and her condition seemed to improve. At her four-month checkup, Lakia was found to be in the ninety-fifth percentile for head circumference, and she was immediately referred back to UMC for a CAT scan to rule out hydrocephaly, a condition commonly known as "water on the brain," which refers to the increased accumulation of cerebrospinal fluid within the ventricles of the brain. Results of the scan indicated the presence of bilateral subdural hematomas, which the physicians felt could have been caused by trauma resulting from severe shaking, or Shaken Baby Syndrome, a condition which results from violent, whiplash-type shaking of an infant. This syndrome can include serious bleeding in the brain, hemorrhages, and in some cases, skull fractures that cause motor and mental impairments and sometimes death. A social worker from the Child Protection Team at UMC immediately reported suspected child abuse to Child Protective Services at the Rural County Department of Social Services.

Lakia stayed at UMC for three weeks while her condition was further assessed. Multiple pediatric specialists evaluated Lakia, including an endo-crinologist, neurosurgeon, ophthalmologist, nephrologist, and geneticist. Finally, Lakia was diagnosed as having rickets, probably caused by a cal-cium deficiency, and metabolic renal acidosis. Rickets is a childhood defi-ciency condition that leads to inadequate deposition of lime salts in develop-ing cartilage and newly formed bone, causing abnormalities in the structure and shape of bones. It was determined that her macrocephaly (unusally large head size) and bilateral subdural hematomas were secondary to rickets; she had not been severely shaken as earlier suspected. Lakia was discharged home to her mother on several medications and with a plan for follow-up visits with UMC and the Rural County Health Department for close monitoring. At one year of age, Lakia was diagnosed with reactive airway disease (asthma) and was started on medication and nebulizer treatments three times per day. A nebulizer is an apparatus that produces a mist or fine spray and is used in the treatment of ashtma.

Sandra and Lakia live with Sandra's 35-year-old mother, who is pregnant, and her grandparents, who are in poor health. Her father died when she was very young. Sandra's 21-year-old brother lives in an apartment nearby, but has limited contact with the family, although he and Sandra maintain a positive relationship. The family is supported by Social Security Survivor Benefits and by the mother's income, although she works sporadically. They currently live in a trailer park, which is known as a transient community where drugs are used and sold. Service providers do not generally go to the trailer park unescorted, and certain times are particularly dangerous because of drug-dealing activity. Sandra's relationship with her mother is very strained due, in part, to her mother's alcohol abuse and her inconsistent parenting and support. The household is frequently without electricity and heat due to the mother's failure to pay the bills. The family has no telephone and no dependable means of transportation. All of the adults in the house-hold smoke, which concerns Sandra because of Lakia's continuing problems with reactive airway disease. She has had several severe asthma or reactive airway disease attacks.

Sandra was always an excellent student and was placed in classes for academically gifted children until her junior year, when Lakia was born. She tried to return to school, but found that she couldn't keep up with her schoolwork while taking care of Lakia. Sandra was ambivalent about placing Lakia in day care because she was afraid that her medical and developmen-tal needs would not be adequately met. Although her mother offered to care for Lakia, Sandra did not feel comfortable with this arrangement because of her mother's drinking habits. Lakia's 17-year-old father is unemployed.

Sandra is adamant about wanting him to remain involved with Lakia and would prefer that he take care of Lakia when she needs child care. However, they have difficulty arranging for transportation and she cannot always take Lakia to her father. The lack of access to affordable and dependable child care has contributed to Sandra's decision not to return to school and has made it difficult for her to maintain employment.

Definition of the Client

Early intervention policy recognizes the family as the central and most consistent influence in a child's life; therefore, the focus of decision-making and service delivery is on the family, not the child. The client system in this case includes Lakia and her mother Sandra. Because of conflicts within the family and Sandra's desire for independence, Sandra has decided not to include other family members in making decisions about Lakia.

Goals

Sandra's goals center primarily on her desire to be independent of her own mother, and to be a "good mother to Lakia." She wants to do whatever is necessary to ensure Lakia's good health and optimal development. In order for Sandra to become independent at the age of 16, she needs to be declared an "emancipated minor." In order to do so, she will need to retain a lawyer to petition the court. The district court judge could declare her an "emancipated minor" based on evidence that Sandra is able to support herself and has a place to live. Then she will be able to receive direct financial assistance for herself and Supplemental Security Income (SSI) for Lakia. This financial support will enable her to obtain affordable and safe housing and a reliable means of transportation. With an adequate income and dependable transportation, her options for securing safe and developmentally appropriate child care are greatly expanded, although the lack of child care in the county means that Lakia will be placed on a waiting list. With child care, Sandra can continue her education, thus increasing the likelihood of her obtaining satisfactory employment. One of Sandra's long-range goals is to get a job that pays enough so she can support herself and Lakia.

Because of risk factors related to her prematurity, her medical history, and her social situation, Lakia was evaluated by a multidisciplinary team from the DEC at the Health Department. It was determined that Lakia's psychosocial development was age-appropriate, but she evidenced moderate delays in receptive language and fine motor skills. There was also some concern about her gross motor skills, as it was felt that she had increased muscle tone in her lower extremities. It was recommended that she receive physical therapy, occupational therapy, and developmental stimulation through the Parent and Child Training (PACT) Program from the local mental health center. Because the PACT Program does not meet the federal guidelines for home-bound services financed through Medicaid, Lakia was not able to receive the physical and occupational therapy that were recommended by the DEC. She was, however, able to receive developmental stimulation from a PACT team member.

The CSC worked closely with Sandra to help her articulate her goals. In addition, various service providers including the infant/toddler specialist from the DEC worked with Sandra and the CSC to develop an Individualized Family Service Plan (IFSP) so that services could be provided based on their evaluation of Lakia's developmental needs and Sandra's concerns, resources, and priorities.

In preparation for the IFSP meeting, the CSC met with Sandra to explain the process, to inform her of her rights, and to discuss her options for involvement in the process. The IFSP meeting was facilitated by the CSC and held at Sandra's mother's trailer. It included Sandra, her mother, the PACT worker from the area mental health program, and the infant/toddler specialist from the DEC. Based on Sandra's goals, the IFSP called for a variety of services for both Lakia and Sandra. Transportation assistance would be provided so that Lakia's medical condition could be monitored by the Rural County Health Department in collaboration with the pediatric specialists at UMC. It was agreed that the PACT worker would work with Lakia on learning to stand and walk, and with Sandra on activities to stimulate her cognitive development. When Sandra returns to school or begins to work on her GED, she will be eligible to participate in the Adolescent Pregnancy Prevention Program, which will involve her in monthly support group meetings and other services. Sandra decided to retain the social worker from the Health Department as her CSC even though the PACT worker could have taken on this role.

Contract

The IFSP serves as the contract between Sandra and Lakia and the CSC and other community service providers. The plan includes information on Lakia's development, strengths, and needs; Sandra's concerns, priorities, and resources; expected outcomes; strategies and activities to accomplish these outcomes; and timelines and criteria for evaluating outcomes. The IFSP is reviewed every three months or as needed, based on changes in Sandra's or Lakia's situation; a meeting is held annually to evaluate and rewrite the IFSP plan.

Meeting Place

Whenever Sandra comes to the Health Department for appointments, the CSC tries to meet with her, even if only briefly. When possible, the CSC contacts clients by telephone on a regular basis, but is unable to do this with Sandra because she does not have a telephone. She prefers to meet with clients in their own environments, so she makes home visits when possible. On several occasions, she has met with Sandra at her mother's trailer, but these visits have to be carefully scheduled due to safety concerns in the trailer park.

Use of Time

The duration of involvement is defined by Sandra's continued desire for services, as well as by state guidelines for eligibility for early intervention services. The frequency of involvement varies, depending on Sandra's concerns and Lakia's needs. Because of the rural nature of the county and the difficulty in arranging for transportation, it is important that service providers be flexible in scheduling appointments. Sandra's CSC tries to meet with Sandra whenever she has appointments at the Health Department or the Department of Social Services, located in the same complex. The length of these meetings varies, depending on Sandra's and Lakia's situation at that time. Contacts range from brief "check-ins" to more lengthy planning sessions.

Treatment Modality

The CSC engages in case management that is focused on helping Sandra define her goals, develop a plan of action to reach those goals, and negotiate the service system. The CSC utilizes a problem-solving approach and crisis intervention techniques in her work. The PACT team provides physical therapy, occupational therapy, and developmental stimulation for Lakia, as well as parent education for Sandra. The CSC also advocates with the service system to ensure that appropriate services are available and accessible, and that they are provided as mandated in the IFSP. The CSC facilitates the IFSP meetings and sees that services are coordinated. In addition, she participates in the local Interagency Consortium, made up of families with eligible young children and representatives of local agencies providing early intervention services. The Interagency Consortium responds to the needs and concerns of families who have young children who are at risk for or have established developmental delays or disabilities, and addresses identified service gaps.

Stance of the Social Worker

The CSC works from a family centered and empowerment perspective to build on family strengths (Dunst, Trivette, and Deal, 1988). Before the initial IFSP meeting, the CSC told Sandra that she "was the ball club owner: she owned the ball park, the ball, and the ball players." Therefore, decisions regarding services for Lakia were Sandra's decisions. Working from an empowerment approach, the CSC also teaches Sandra how to assert herself with medical care professionals and how to negotiate the local service system.

Outside Resources

Despite the paucity of resources in Rural County, the level of collaboration among agencies within the county and with agencies in adjoining counties assures the availability of a much broader array of services than could be provided locally in most rural communities. Because of these strong formal and informal connections, services have been provided, for the most part, in a coordinated and collaborative manner. The Health Department has collaborative agreements with the closest tertiary care center, UMC, to provide specialty pediatric care and hospitalization. The multidisciplinary team from the regional Developmental Evaluation Center (DEC), located in a neighboring county, schedules evaluations at the Health Department, making these much more accessible to local families. The team from the DEC works closely with the CSC, and the PACT Program from the local mental health center. Through the local mental health center's PACT Program, a practitioner trained in infant and toddler development comes to the home weekly to provide information and assistance with addressing Lakia's developmental needs. The PACT team will continue working with Lakia and her mother until she is three years old.

The Department of Social Services Adolescent Pregnancy Prevention Program provides services to pregnant and parenting adolescents to help them remain in school. A social worker from this program was working with Sandra during her pregnancy but is currently no longer providing services. The program will be available once Sandra is ready to return to school or complete a GED.

Because this is a rural community, many of the service providers in various agencies have strong informal working relationships. The relationships among staff at the mental health, social services, and public health agencies are further enhanced because they are all located in the same complex, making it easier to have frequent face-to-face contact. The fact that this county is relatively rural shapes the relationships between service providers and clients. Services are provided in a personal manner and service providers know Lakia, Sandra, and other family members. Figure 4.1 is an ecomap of Sandra's immediate support structure.

Reassessment

The IFSP is formally reviewed and updated every three months to reflect the family's concerns, resources, and priorities, and Lakia's developmental needs. At least every six months, the PACT Team assesses Lakia's developmental progress, and the CSC together with Sandra assess the family's resources and service needs. If at any time Sandra decides to discontinue her involvement with the CSCP or change service coordinators, she has this option.

Transfer or Termination

Because eligibility criteria for Child Service Coordination change at age three, Lakia will undergo a comprehensive multidisciplinary evaluation at thirty months of age by the team from the DEC. If there is documented evidence of developmental delay, she will be eligible for Preschool Handicapped Services, including Child Service Coordination, until she is five years old. At that time, the CSC will refer Lakia to the local mental health program, where she will be assigned a case manager who works with individuals with developmental disabilities.

It is likely that because of Lakia's complex medical condition and related developmental needs, she and Sandra will continue working with the CSC until she reaches age five. At that point, the focus of intervention and service provision will narrow from the family to the child, and only Lakia's needs will be addressed through the Individualized Education Program (IEP), which will be developed by the school system with input from Lakia's mother. Because the Health Department is the only provider of pediatric medical care in this community, Lakia will continue to be followed by staff at the Health Department and specialists at UMC until she reaches adulthood, allowing for continuity of care in dealing with her chronic medical condition.

FIGURE 4.1. Ecomap for Lakia

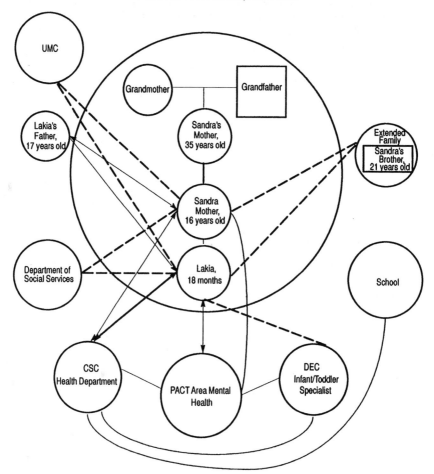

Case Conclusion

Sandra has not been able to rely on consistent family support in meeting Lakia's medical and developmental needs or her own needs. Nonetheless, Sandra is firmly committed to Lakia's well-being and to managing her care. Sandra prides herself in taking good care of Lakia. For example, when she brings Lakia to the health department, she brings toys and things for her to do, as well as diapers, formula, and snacks, knowing that a visit to the clinic can involve a long day. Through her determination to ensure that Lakia's needs are met and with the support of the CSC and numerous other service providers, Sandra has developed a sense of efficacy remarkable in a person of her age. She has become assertive about defining goals for herself and Lakia, and about enlisting agencies and service providers to support her in meeting her goals.

Sandra has matured remarkably since Lakia's birth; she has fairly realistic and well-articulated goals for herself and for her daughter. She is determined to finish high school or complete the requirements for a GED, although she does not yet know when this will be possible. Sandra firmly believes that Lakia's father must remain involved in her life, and has taken actions to ensure that he will continue to see and spend time with Lakia. Sandra has not been able to realize her goal to live independently from her mother as she had hoped. Her attempts to be declared an "emancipated minor" have not been successful in part due to her inability to stabilize her situation, making it extremely difficult for her to establish her own place of residence. However, she has arranged to be the payee of Lakia's SSI checks, rather than her mother, which affords her some degree of financial independence.

Staff at the Health Department describe Lakia as a particularly engaging child. She laughs responsively, likes to play with adults, and is calm and easygoing. They have come to know her well and look forward to seeing her. Although Lakia looks like a typical, active, healthy toddler now, her chronic medical problems will gradually lead to noticeably short stature, fragile bones, and failure to thrive. She may eventually develop renal failure. Her chronic medical situation will continue to put her at risk for developmental delay. Lakia will need ongoing access to specialty medical care and developmental services. Sandra will need the support of professionals who can help her understand and cope with her daughter's medical condition and developmental needs and assist her in negotiating complex service systems. Sandra's determination and a well-integrated service system combine synergistically to increase the likelihood that Lakia will reach her full potential despite her chronic medical condition and physical and developmental delays.

Differential Discussion

In reviewing her work with Sandra , the CSC noted that she wished she had become involved with Sandra and Lakia earlier in the process. The MCC did not refer Lakia and Sandra to the CSCP at the time of Lakia's birth because she did not have any medical problems, and Sandra's social situation had improved and seemed to be stable. The first time that the

CSC met with Sandra was during a crisis, when Lakia was referred to the emergency room at UMC. At that time Sandra was overwhelmed and lacked confidence in her ability to parent Lakia and negotiate a complex medical system. Had she had a CSC prior to her initial medical crisis, Sandra would have been able to turn to someone with whom she had established a relationship and might have felt more confident in her ability to deal with the situation. Also, the CSC's initial impression of Sandra might have been different if she had first seen her in other circumstances.

The school system did not offer Sandra the homebound services that might have enabled her to complete her junior year. Perhaps, if the CSC had involved the school system early on and advocated for homebound services, they might have been made available to Sandra. It is not unusual for school systems to be "left out of the loop" when services are planned and implemented; this situation underscores the critical need for including the schools in collaborative interagency efforts.

PRACTICE IN CONTEXT

Families with young children who are at risk for or have a developmental delay or disability require additional support and resources from their community in order to ensure their child's optimal development. Research demonstrates that when support and resources are provided early in the child's life in a comprehensive, coordinated, and consistent manner, they have a positive impact on child health and development (Ramey and Ramey, 1992; Shonkoff and Hauser-Cram, 1987). The case presented in this chapter illustrates how federal and state (North Carolina) early intervention policies and service systems guide the social work practice of a child service coordinator. The CSC uses his or her social work practice skills to assess and evaluate child and family needs and strengths, help families identify their priorities and goals, ensure that families have access to services, monitor service delivery, and advocate with and for families. The CSC also participates in a locally organized consortium to improve collaboration and coordination among agencies and service providers, and to respond to gaps in the service system. The efforts of this consortium clearly make a difference in the CSC's ability to work effectively with and for families.

Federal early intervention policy is based on the belief that families are central to their young child's development and that they should play a critical role in decision-making, service planning, and implementation. This belief, which is consistent with social work values, guides family centered models of service coordination in early intervention. The family's needs, concerns, and priorities must be taken into account to ensure an environment that promotes child health and development. When working with young, low income, single mothers such as Sandra, the CSC needs to support the mother's efforts at coping with and managing the problems that she faces in her everyday life in order to promote the development of her young child. These problems may include conflicts with her own mother or other family members, concerns about finances and her educational and vocational future, fears about personal safety, and problems with her relationship with the father of their baby (Bry, 1987). As illustrated by the case presented in this chapter, the CSC focused on helping Sandra identify her own goals and meet her own needs in order to ensure that she develop the capacity to meet her daughter's health and developmental needs.

Part H of the Individuals with Disabilities Education Act Amendments of 1986 has made a difference in ensuring that infants and toddlers and their families receive needed early intervention services. The future institutionalization and effectiveness of early intervention services will depend upon a number of factors. Part H will come up for Congressional reauthorization in the near future; the outcome of this reauthorization is difficult to predict given the current political climate. In addition, the provision of many Part H services relies heavily on other financing mechanisms, some of which (for example, Medicaid) are experiencing major structural changes and funding cutbacks. It is also important to note that early intervention services are provided in the context of larger health and human service systems, and the effectiveness of early intervention is greatly determined on how well the larger system is functioning. For example, in the case presented here, Sandra's ability to return to school and eventually be self-supporting and live independently of her family is highly dependent upon her receiving subsidized housing, child care, and higher education or advanced vocational training. The existence of and funding for these larger health and human service systems, which provide a safety net to many families like Sandra's, are currently being challenged by Congress. While Sandra is highly motivated to accomplish her goals to be independent and self-supporting and to ensure that her daughter receive needed medical care and early intervention services, her ability to do so will largely be determined by the existence of a well-coordinated early intervention service system and a health and social welfare system that supports her move toward independence.

REFERENCES

Adler, N. E., Keyes, S., and Robertson, P. (1991). Psychological issues in new reproductive technologies: Pregnancy-inducing technology and diagnostic screening. In J. Rodin and A. Collins (Eds.), *Women and new reproductive technologies: Medical, psychosocial, legal, and ethical dilemmas.* Hillsdale, NJ: Lawrence Erlbaum, pp. 111-133.

Affleck, G., Tennen, H., and Rowe, J. (1991). *Infants in crisis: How parents cope with newborn intensive care and its aftermath.* New York: Springer-Verlag.

Bishop, K. K., Rounds, K., and Weil, M. (1993). P. L. 99-457: Preparation for social work practice with infants and toddlers with disabilities and their families. *Journal of Social Work Education, 29*(1), 36-45.

Bishop, K. K., Woll, J., and Arango, P. (1993). *Family/professional collaboration for children with special health needs and their families.* Burlington, VT: Family/Professional Collaboration Project.

Black, R. B. (1992). Seeing the baby: The impact of ultrasound technology. *Journal of Genetic Counseling, 1,* 45-54.

Bry, T. (1987). The importance of cooperation among child health professionals and agencies in an inner city infant mental health service. *Infant Mental Health Journal, 8*(2), 166-180.

Dunst, C. J., Trivette, C. M., and Deal, A. (1988). *Enabling and empowering families: Principles and guidelines for practice.* Cambridge, MA: Brookline Books.

Farel, A. M., Fraser, J. G., and Kegg, C. L. (1995). *North Carolina child service coordination program* (Report for Contract No. E5086). Raleigh, NC: North Carolina Department of Environment, Health and Natural Resources, Division of Maternal and Child Health.

Fox, H. B., Freedman, S. A., and Klepper, B. R. (1989). Financing programs for young children with handicaps. In J. J. Gallagher, P. L. Trohanis, and R. M. Clifford (Eds.), *Policy implementation and PL 99-457: Planning for young children with special needs.* Baltimore, MD: Paul H. Brookes, pp. 169-182.

Hebbeler, K. M., Smith, B. J., and Black, T. L. (1991). Federal early childhood special education policy: A model for the improvement of services for children with disabilities. *Exceptional Children, 58*(2), 104-112.

McGonigel, M. J., Kaufmann, R. K., and Johnson, B. H. (Eds.) (1991). *Guidelines and recommended practices for the individualized family service plan* (Second Edition). Bethesda, MD: Association for the Care of Children's Health.

McNulty, B. (1989). Leadership and policy strategies for interagency planning. In J. J. Gallagher, P. L. Trohanis, and R. M. Clifford (Eds.), *Policy implementation and PL 99-457: Planning for young children with special needs.* Baltimore, MD: Paul H. Brookes, pp. 147-167.

Perkins, J. and Zinn, S. (1995). *Toward a healthy future: Early periodic, screening, detection, and treatment for poor children.* Washington, DC: National Health Law Program.

Ramey, S. L. and Ramey, C. T. (1992). Early educational intervention with disadvantaged children: To what effect? *Applied and Preventive Psychology, 1*, 131-140.

Rounds, K. A., Weil, M., and Bishop, K. K. (1994). Practice with culturally diverse families of young children with disabilities. *Families in Society, 75*(1), 3-15.

Shanahan, T. E. and Cunningham, L. E. (1993). Part H and EPSDT: Helping at-risk infants and toddlers. *Clearinghouse Review, 27*(1), 2-10.

Shelton, T. L. and Stephanek, J. S. (1994). *Family-centered care for children needing specialized health and developmental services.* Bethesda, MD: Association for the Care of Children's Health.

Shonkoff, J. P. and Hauser-Cram, P. (1987). Early intervention for disabled infants and their families: A quantitative analysis. *Pediatrics, 80*(5), 650-658.

Silverstein, R. (1989). A window of opportunity: P. L. 99-457. In *The intent and spirit of P. L. 99-457.* Washington, DC: National Center for Clinical Infant Programs, pp. A1-A7.

U.S. Bureau of the Census. (1990). Census of population and housing summary. Washington, DC: U.S. Government Printing Office.

U.S. Congress. (1986). *Public Law 99-457, Individuals with Disabilities Education Act Amendments of 1986.*

U.S. Congress. (1991). *Public Law 102-119, Individuals with Disabilities Education Act Amendments of 1991.*

Zipper, I. N., Weil, M., and Rounds, K. (1993). *Service coordination for early intervention: Parents and professionals.* Cambridge, MA: Brookline Books.

Chapter 5

School-Based Health Centers: A Multisystem Approach to the Delivery of Primary Health Care

Mary Ellen Hass
Debra Katz
Mary Ann Shanahan

CONTEXT

Description of the Setting

School-Based Health Centers (SBHCs) deliver comprehensive primary health care to students. Staffed by multidisciplinary teams and located on site, in schools, these health centers provide a broad array of medical and psychological services (Newton-Logsdon and Armstrong, 1993; Irigon et al., 1981). The first comprehensive SBHCs were established in the early 1970s in Dallas, Texas and St. Paul, Minnesota. During the ten-year period of 1985 to 1994, SBHCs have grown from 40 to well over 600 nationwide (Schlitt et al., 1994).

Over the past 30 years, adolescents have been the only age group in the country whose health status has not improved. Adolescents are surrounded by a host of health threats, including poverty, sexually transmitted diseases, and violence. More than one in four adolescents live in poverty or near poverty. Fifty-four percent of high school students have engaged in sexual intercourse. Each year, 3 million teens are infected with a sexually transmitted disease (STD) and more than 1,100,000 become pregnant. Today, injury and violence account for three out of four adolescent deaths (Robert Wood Johnson Report, 1993). These statistics do not even begin to touch upon the issues of substance use, depression and suicide, lack of primary medical care, physical and sexual abuse, and other community problems that impact on the lives of youth.

In response to these health problems and risks, SBHCs have become a successful model of care, addressing many of the serious physical and emotional health problems facing young people today (Weist et al., 1995). Services provided in SBHCs include treatment of acute illnesses and injuries, management of chronic health problems, physical examinations, nutritional counseling, dental care, reproductive health care, pregnancy testing, HIV testing, STD treatment, mental health counseling, support groups, substance abuse assessments, health education, and other crisis intervention services. The goals of the centers include coordinating and delivering accessible primary health care, improving the health of today's youth, and enabling students to learn to make good decisions about their own health. SBHCs, originally located in high schools, have been expanded to include middle or junior high schools and elementary schools. These centers are located in over forty states across the nation.

SBHCs were piloted in Connecticut in 1986. Over time, Connecticut has become one of the most successful states in the nation in building a statewide system designed to increase access to care for school-aged youth. Over 40 such centers now exist in the state, with the city of Stamford having three. Two are located in the public high schools, and the third, which is in a middle school, also serves the connecting elementary school. Stamford's first SBHC opened in 1989 and the most recent one in 1995. Also in 1995, a full-service dental clinic, available to all youth attending Stamford's public schools, opened as a component of one of the centers. Stamford's centers presently have 3,200 students registered, who make over 4,200 visits to the centers each year.

In Stamford, all SBHCs are located within school buildings, and space is leased at no cost to the managing agency, Student Health Services of Stamford, Inc., which is a not-for-profit community organization. Neither owned nor operated by the school system, each center is distinct in ambience, yet has much in common with the others. Every facility includes a waiting room, two medical examination rooms, a counseling room, a bathroom, and a group/meeting room. The health centers are warm and inviting to the students, convey a feeling of respect and caring, and are easily accessible, well-integrated, and linked with other support services in the school. In one center, students' artwork is displayed prominently to further reinforce the idea that the health center belongs to students.

Staffing of each health center includes a nurse practitioner, social worker, receptionist, and consulting physician. Many middle and elementary school health centers also have an outreach worker who actively encourages the involvement of families (Pacheco et al., 1991). Managed by coordinators who report to community advisory boards, the SBHCs receive the majority of funding from the State of Connecticut with additional funds coming from foundations, corporations, and the United Way. SBHCs will be sustained and grow only if public/private partnerships and third-party reimbursements are maintained and fostered.

Policy

SBHCs provide a holistic approach to wellness and treat both medical and mental health problems of adolescents and youth through a team approach. The complex policy issues related to the treatment of minors in SBHCs have emerged from many distinct and sometimes conflicting arenas. They include legal statutes; federal, state and local mandates; medical protocols; professional ethics; and the emerging world of managed health care (National Association of Social Workers, 1990; Reamer, 1988).

State Statutes

Each state has explicit statutes that define treatment of minors with and without parental consent. Most students who use these health centers are under the age of 18 and considered minors in the eyes of the law. Although the law generally requires parental consent when health care is provided to minor children, there are many exceptions to this requirement, which are based on either the minor's status or the specific services sought. Every state has a law that enables minors to consent to diagnosis and treatment of sexually transmitted diseases. At least 13 states have statutes that specifically allow minors to consent to HIV testing without parental consent. Laws in most states enable minors to consent to treatment for other conditions including mental health problems, drug or alcohol problems, rape or sexual assault, and pregnancy. In particular, minors' independent access to family planning services is protected by the constitutional right of privacy. Minors have a right to obtain family planning services without parental consent in federally funded Title X programs in a majority of the states in this country (English, 1995). Most SBHCs have tried to avoid potential conflicts by having a consent form signed by a parent or guardian before access to the health center is available to a student.

State Grant Initiatives

Policy development in SBHCs was initially the domain of the health centers' advisory committees. As states' financial involvement has grown, their attention to policy and program issues has increased. Now, most states have used grant initiatives as opportunities to establish program goals, define service and staffing standards, and outline prototypes for replication. The common denominator across most state guidelines is the desire to strike a careful balance between ensuring a standard of care and allowing for community flexibility in program development. Required components most often include mandatory parental consent and broad-based community input into planning and operations (Schlitt et al., 1994).

Managed Care

The managed care revolution that is sweeping across this country will ultimately affect SBHCs. Policy planning initiatives and strategies must be in place to meet, accept, and integrate this new challenge. SBHCs are in the early stages of negotiating a relationship with managed care providers. While this relationship is yet to be determined, clearly SBHCs will seek out participation with Medicaid as well as with other managed care initiatives as a part of a long-term viable financial strategy. Additionally, they will secure a clear role within this managed care if they are to receive reimbursement for their services.

Forty-two states have opted for managed care plans to implement their Medicaid programs. If the estimated savings to these states of 5 to 15 percent is accurate, it is feasible to predict that most, if not all, states will adopt mandatory Medicaid managed care plans in the near future (Department of Children and Families Hartford, 1995). At the same time, Medicaid support for health centers has been limited. In 1991, Medicaid provided only two percent of the operating costs of SBHCs. A survey of these health centers, conducted from 1992 to 1993 by the Robert Wood Johnson Foundation, reported that 13 percent of their operating budgets were supported by patient care revenue, primarily Medicaid (Schlitt et al., 1994).

The State of Connecticut is in the unique position of developing a Medicaid managed care program in the presence of an already established statewide network of SBHCs. This new program will require that the managed care providers contract directly with the health centers in their service catchment areas (Schlitt et al., 1994). The viability of School-Based Health Centers will depend on the outcome of efforts to design a long term funding strategy in the midst of significant changes affecting both the public and private health care systems (Polster, Dryfoos, and Lear, 1995; Rienzo and Button, 1993).

Technology

Immediate Test Results

The presenting complaint for many students entering the health center is medical. The advanced technology of primary health care enables the nurse practitioner of an SBHC to assess a number of medical concerns immediately without having to wait for test results from outside laboratories. At the SBHC, the results of the following are immediately available: pregnancy, strep, mono-spot and hemoglobin tests, and routine urinalysis. The ability to perform these laboratory tests in the health center enables the nurse practitioner or physician to immediately involve the social worker when the results of a student's laboratory tests present emotional consequences. Negative test results might indicate psychosomatic complaints resulting from underlying mental health concerns. A positive pregnancy test presents many counseling needs, while a negative pregnancy test indicates sexual activity and brings up the need for counseling on issues of HIV, birth control, and relationships. Technology has enabled SBHCs to deliver primary health care efficiently and to optimize the collaboration of the multidisciplinary team and the vital role of mental health services.

Data Collection

Data collection through the use of computers has significantly increased the capacity of SBHCs to track the care and need of students. Citywide tracking of conditions such as tuberculosis has enabled the local health department to contact an SBHC if a student in that school is not following up with his or her treatment regimen. SBHC staff can then call the student from class and work with him or her by providing the medication on site. This type of tracking of communicable diseases helps the health centers play a vital role in enhancing students' compliance with treatment protocols.

Data are entered at SBHC into each student's record. They note the date of and reasons for the visit, procedures used, and the staff. This database directly enhances the delivery of care. If the social worker in the health center wants to run a support group on a specific issue, he or she can get a computerized list of all students who have presented with that concern. The social worker on the team can also access a student's record and review his or her presenting complaints. The pattern of these visits might indicate an underlying mental health issue that goes beyond the presenting medical problem. Data collection has direct implications for both service and funding. The ability to track the number and demographics of students using the health centers, the reasons for visits, and treatments provided has enabled SBHCs to prove to funders that these programs fill a vital need in the community.

Organization

Teamwork

SBHCs epitomize the concepts of collaboration and teamwork. This organizational framework is evident within the health center and as it extends into the school and community. One of the exciting aspects of working in an SBHC is being part of a multidisciplinary team. The team approach allows staff to maximize the skills of the individual providers and gives access to a broader range of services. Collaboration works best when providers feel confident about their own professional roles and are willing to draw on the expertise of others on the team. Multidisciplinary staff take the time to understand each other's language and get past the turf issues within the school. Everyone has a chance to be heard and to focus on the common purpose, that is, the needs of the student (Robert Wood Johnson Foundation, 1993). The team shares a genuine appreciation for children and adolescents and advocates for their needs, which often extend far beyond the scope of health care. Routine staff meetings are crucial to foster true collaboration.

The social worker is a critical member of the multidisciplinary team, since in contrast to the infectious diseases of childhood, many problems of youth are behaviorally related (Balassone, Bell, and Peterfreund, 1991). Thus, the program provides not only traditional medical care but also mental health services that address behaviors and the underlying emotions that drive them (Harold and Harold, 1993; Harold and Harold, 1991).

Guests in a School Setting

SBHCs are often considered guests in a school setting because they are in the school by invitation, not by mandate. SBHCs become part of a setting with a host of players, and instant harmony is not easily achieved. Tension can occur as a result of space issues as well as professional competition (Robert Wood Johnson Foundation, 1995). Special attention is given to working out role clarity between school nurses and the health center's nurse practitioner as well as the school social worker and the health center's social worker. School-Based Health Centers do not lead to unnecessary duplication and confrontation, but rather to the enhancement of support services for students. SBHC staff also foster relationships with school administrators and teachers, since most student referrals to the health center come from school staff. Health centers are active participants in the school, holding open houses, teaching health education in the classroom, attending faculty meetings, and helping out in the cafeteria. In a collaborative spirit, nurse practitioners consult with faculty on their health concerns and health center social workers serve on school crisis teams.

Vital team members in SBHCs are both the students and their families. Students actively participate in decisions made regarding their own health and become the most vocal advocates for SBHCs, referring friends and seeking out care as the need arises. Written parental consent is required before students can use the services of the health center. Families choose to allow their child to use a convenient and competent source of health care, yet need to feel confident that the health center will not interfere in their relationships and decisions regarding their child. Staff is trusted by students to protect their confidentiality while strongly encouraging family communication. SBHC staff members take great pride in helping students share even the most private problems with their families. The goal is to achieve open communication in families. Family members are often invited into the health center to attend counseling sessions with the social worker and their child. Home visits are offered whenever a situation warrants such an intervention. SBHCs are designed to make things easier for a family by collectively and collaboratively keeping students physically and emotionally healthy.

Community Support

Community support is the underlying foundation for SBHCs. Advisory groups and the board of directors provide the network of strength behind the program. Community agencies provide the link for successful referrals. Advisory boards made up of vital community members serve as the backbone of these health centers. They are the connection between the health center and the community, providing positive public relations efforts, strategic planning, strengthening alliances, securing funds, and developing policies (Robert Wood Johnson Report, 1993). SBHCs depend on the network of agencies that provide services on and off site to the students of the health center. The health center social worker might have a provider from a community agency come to the center to meet with the student to help with the referral process. This often occurs in situations of rape and substance abuse. In other situations, the health center social worker might bring the student to a community agency to be evaluated when there is a concern regarding a student's mental status or suicidal ideation. Some other community services that are involved with SBHCs and that receive referrals are child protective services, local mental health agencies, medical specialty services, youth shelters, and local hospitals.

Without the collaboration of local medical and social service agencies, the SBHC staff would be unable to meet the needs of many of the students. The health centers do not work in a vacuum but are parts of an intricate and complicated web of services. School-Based Health Centers hold the unique responsibility of being the spoke of the wheel, responsible for making the referral and providing the follow-up for the student. Without collaboration, the wheel would not turn.

Decisions about Practice

Case Description

Ella Bogarden is a 15-year-old female who came with her father and siblings to the United States three years ago from the West Indies (Brice, 1982). Ella is the second youngest of seven children. Since Ella's mother remained in the West Indies, the two oldest children, aged 23 and 21, functioned as surrogate parents for the younger siblings. With the promise of employment, Ella's father and the children moved to Connecticut. During a routine school physical examination at the SBHC, Ella tested positive for tuberculosis. Although she did not actively have the disease, her tuberculosis exposure required treatment. Ella was referred to the health center nurse and was placed on a six-month course of prophylactic medication. When Ella did not return to the health center for her one-month follow-up appointment, the nurse practitioner located her in school and found that she was not taking the medication. Ella appeared depressed, made no eye contact, and exhibited poor hygiene. The nurse practitioner resumed her tuberculosis medication and referred Ella to the health center social worker.

An assessment by the social worker revealed that Ella felt hopeless, displayed flat affect, and was moderately depressed with suicidal ideation. She reported feeling very isolated and having few friends. While she had no specific plan, Ella reported feeling no desire to live. A psychiatric consultation at the Teen Crisis Center was arranged immediately and Ella's family was notified. Her family was unresponsive and refused to accompany her to the evaluation. The psychiatric evaluation confirmed Ella's depression and recommended outpatient counseling for her and her family at the Teen Crisis Center (Adelman and Taylor, 1993; Barker and Adelman, 1994; Levy and Land, 1994). The SBHC social worker continued to provide support to Ella in school, and the nurse practitioner provided the necessary medical intervention.

Definition of the Client

The task of separation is crucial to the development of the adolescent. School-Based Health Centers provide adolescents with the opportunity to learn to access services that are important to their well-being. Equally important is a relationship between adolescent and family that supports this development and encourages social and emotional maturation (Zastrow and Kirst-Ashman, 1987). Ella struggled with the developmental issues of adolescence. As a member of the SBHC, Ella was viewed as the client. When it became clear that her family had great difficulty in relating to her and understanding her emotional reactions to life, the family was also viewed as clients.

Goals and Contracts

Social workers are continually faced with the challenge of providing an accurate assessment of the client and, in concert with the family, mutually develop a treatment plan. In implementing the assessment, it is crucial to the success of the treatment plan that the family be understood within the context of its environment (Holman, 1988). During the assessment phase, the social worker identifies the systems with which the family interacts and then determines their relevance to the identified client. An ecological perspective serves as a cornerstone for the social worker and a framework through which the assessment will be evaluated.

Using this theory, goals are continually redefined based on the progress made by the client within each system. SBHCs provide the social worker with the unique opportunity to interact with the client on a daily or weekly basis. In assessing Ella's needs, the first goal for the social worker was to gather information regarding her functioning in school. While she seemed to be having no difficulty with her academic performance, it became clear that Ella had few friends and was not well-known by her teachers. Described as quiet and isolated, Ella had occasionally shared some of her feelings of isolation and sadness with a few school personnel. Her poor hygiene had also been noticed by several teachers, but they reported being uncertain of how to approach her with these observations. Designing a team approach to working with Ella in school became one of the first goals in helping her.

In using an ecological framework, goals are defined concurrently. Engaging a client in a relationship that results in the accomplishment of these identified goals is referred to as the working alliance (Goldstein, 1984). As the task of gathering information about school functioning continued, the social worker began to engage Ella in coming to the SBHC. It was important to allow Ella to set the pace for this alliance, supporting the gradual exploration of her feelings. Ella's father and older siblings were angry with her for seeking help at school and discussing "family business." They refused involvement with the center, the school, and the Teen Crisis Center. Over time, Ella became increasingly wary of her contact with professionals in the school and withdrew from the health center social worker. She also began to exhibit multiple somatic complaints such as headaches, stomachaches, and leg cramps, and sought relief from these symptoms from the nurse practitioner at the health center. The nurse practitioner gently urged her to resume her relationship with the social worker.

Another goal was to help Ella's family understand her feelings and her need for help outside of the family. Ella's older sister was also a member of the health center and confirmed that Ella's mother was planning a visit to the United States at the end of the school year. It was agreed, with Ella's consent, that the social worker and the nurse practitioner would make a home visit to the family following her mother's arrival. The goals for the visit were to introduce themselves, discuss Ella's need for outpatient counseling, and define strategies for successful medication compliance to prevent tuberculosis. Ella and her sister were pleased with this idea and were anxious for the health center staff to meet their mother.

Cultural issues emerged quickly during the home visit. While all the children spoke English fluently, Ella's parents did not. This resulted in the older siblings, acting as translators. Ella's father was not present during the visit because he was at work. Her mother and older siblings did not respond when told of Ella's emotional difficulties and her inability to function without feeling depressed. They were aware of the recommendation for counseling at the Teen Crisis Center but were uncomfortable with the notion that others would be involved intimately with their family.

Following the home visit, Ella came to school having been severely beaten by her older brother. Her family was furious with her for talking to the health center staff. This crisis necessitated an immediate referral to Child Protective Services and emergency medical treatment at the local hospital. The extent of Ella's injuries and her reluctance to return home resulted in her placement in a youth shelter until a full assessment could be made. After several days, the youth shelter staff became concerned about Ella's emotional state and recommended that she receive a full psychiatric evaluation in an inpatient setting. She was admitted to the hospital and placed in the psychiatric unit.

This development caused two major changes in the work with the family. The first was the entrance of two new systems, the hospital and the protective services agency. The second was the reaction of the family to further intrusion into their lives. It was at this point that all the systems involved with the family had to mobilize. Cultural issues played a major role in understanding the family's reactions to Ella, which resulted in the use of physical punishment for disclosing family information. The hospital arranged for weekly case conferences with a representative from each agency, Ella, and her family. Interpreters provided clarity and support to the family at these meetings. Slowly, it became apparent that this family had little understanding of Ella's psychological needs and were quite frightened by the intrusion of several professionals in their lives. Ella was placed on Prozac for depression and received daily individual and group therapy sessions within the hospital. In this therapeutic milieu, her symptoms diminished rapidly and she emerged as an advocate for herself, able to clearly express her thoughts and needs to the hospital staff. The SBHC social worker visited Ella regularly. Ella's family gradually accepted her difficulties and agreed to support her need for outpatient counseling following her discharge from the hospital. The Bogarten family was referred to the Intensive Family Preservation Program for outreach services. Workers from all these programs were invited to the hospital team meeting. The team identified the role each agency would have in Ella's treatment following her discharge. The SBHC social worker would act as a daily support to Ella at school and would monitor her progress.

Ella returned to school following a four-week hospitalization and seemed to function well for several weeks. The health center staff then noticed that her somatic complaints gradually returned. The social worker was also concerned about the deterioration in Ella's appearance. Further exploration revealed that Ella's Prozac prescription had not been filled since her discharge from the hospital and that she had failed to attend any of the outpatient counseling appointments scheduled at the Teen Crisis Center. The plan that was developed before Ella's discharge had slowly unraveled. The health center social worker reconvened the team and the roles of each member were clarified with the health center social worker as the case coordinator. Working in close contact with Child Protective Services and Intensive Family Preservation Program, the health center social worker helped Ella get back on track by making certain she and her family stayed connected to each of the agencies. To facilitate the transition to the Teen Crisis Center, the health center social worker accompanied Ella to several appointments. These sustained interventions from multiple systems provided necessary solutions.

This case is an example of what can occur when families are dependent on multiple systems and communication is not consistent (Shulman, 1979). Systemic failure can result in clients being stereotyped as "resistant" and providers becoming frustrated over who is primarily responsible for the client. As a result, more time and energy must be devoted to increasing the communication between the systems. If the agencies involved cannot communicate effectively with each other, the client will not be able to benefit from the treatment plan.

Meeting Place

Accessibility and confidentiality are two major issues that are important to adolescents when seeking help for a problem. They need to trust the adult from whom they are seeking help before they will reveal their concerns. The School-Based Health Center provides the adolescent with a safe, comfortable, accessible environment. Because the center is located within the school, students can drop in, meet the staff, and become comfortable before seeking help. In fact, many students accompany a friend to the health center before seeking services for themselves. Students are invited to give feedback to the staff on how to be most helpful. During a student's initial visit, the social worker explains the center's confidentiality policy. This helps students understand how confidential information will be handled and under what emergency circumstances information must be shared. For Ella, the center's familiar, comfortable setting allowed her to use its services. Since she was having difficulty in expressing her feelings of sadness and depression, it was easier for her to be seen initially for physical complaints. It became the task of the social worker to engage her in such a way that she would feel comfortable in talking about her feelings as well.

Use of Time

Adolescents enrolled in an SBHC are able to use the services for as long as they attend the school. For example, in a high school health center, an adolescent can enroll while in ninth grade and use services any time until graduation. Typically, an adolescent will come to the health center with a particular issue or crisis. Following the resolution of the identified issue, the visits to the center will stop until another precipitating event brings him or her back to the health center. In addition to counseling, the health center social worker also interacts with the students in a less formal way through classroom presentations or during chance meetings in the hallway. Informal contacts can be very important in the development of the relationship with the social worker and help to build a comfort level that enables the student to ask for assistance. Ella used these contacts to build her trust in the staff at the health center to a level that allowed her to seek help.

Treatment Modality

A variety of treatment modalities are available at the SBHCs. The most common of these, crisis intervention, requires the mobilization of school, family, and community supports to alleviate the symptoms of the adolescent and to find a solution to the problem. Usually, treatment is short-term in nature. If long-term treatment is indicated, the student is referred for services to an appropriate community agency. Transition can be difficult for students who already feel comfortable with the School-Based Health Centers. Seeking help from a community agency can be both intimidating and stigmatizing. Helping students make the transition becomes an important part of the clinical work of the health center social worker. This is demonstrated by the work involved in helping Ella become connected to the Teen Crisis Center. Once a relationship had developed between Ella and the SBHC social worker, she had difficulty making the transition to the Teen Crisis Center social worker. Transitional visits with Ella and both workers helped her to feel more comfortable.

An understanding of the development of the adolescent reveals the importance of the peer group and the need for acceptance and approval. The social worker offers a variety of groups in which students' needs can be met. Within the structure of each group, a range of techniques such as role play are used to allow for the expression of feelings, to encourage coping skills, and to work toward a solution to the problem. When needed, the nurse practitioner will join the group to provide health information on issues relating to the focus of the particular group. Outside agencies with expertise in specific areas are also asked to share information on a specific issue and to introduce the adolescents to community resources.

Stance of the Social Worker

Working with adolescents in a school setting requires the social worker to be available, flexible, and supportive. Staff members have to balance their time between scheduled appointments and attending to students in crisis. Team work is essential in this setting for a variety of reasons. Working as a team within the health center provides the students with a valuable didactic approach to their development as young adults. As with Ella, psychosocial symptoms are often masked by physical complaints. A multidisciplinary approach allows for physical as well as emotional assessments. The availability of other professionals within the school, as well as the family, allows the team to develop a more comprehensive assessment of the student's needs.

Even though the students are encouraged to use the health center, the social worker establishes some boundaries as part of the working alliance, which help to alleviate problems that occur when students demand to be seen daily. The social worker has to maintain an environment that is conducive to solving problems. As Ella began to deteriorate following her discharge from the hospital, the social worker saw her daily and gradually decreased the sessions as her level of functioning improved.

Outside Resources

School-Based Health Centers are strategically located in schools where there are large numbers of students at risk for social and emotional problems. The needs of a student population of over 2,000 far exceed the capacity of the SBHC staff. Therefore, outside resources become crucial to complement the school-based services. These resources may be in the form of extended family, friends, or community agencies.

In dealing with an issue such as depression, the social worker helps the family to provide the support the student may need at home. Also, for issues that require long-term treatment, the SBHC social worker becomes the link to community agencies with culturally sensitive, age-appropriate services. Ella's complex needs illustrate the requirement for links with many community agencies. Each agency involved was crucial to her improvement. For example, the inpatient evaluation provided valuable insight into Ella's psychological and emotional status. This information led to the formation of a treatment plan that depended upon the successful work of several agencies. Figure 5.1 is an ecomap that diagrams Ella's current interactions.

Reassessment and Transfer or Termination

Given the ever-changing needs of the adolescent, reassessment is an important tool in the treatment offered in the SBHC. As students feel

FIGURE 5.1. Ecomap for Ella Bogarden

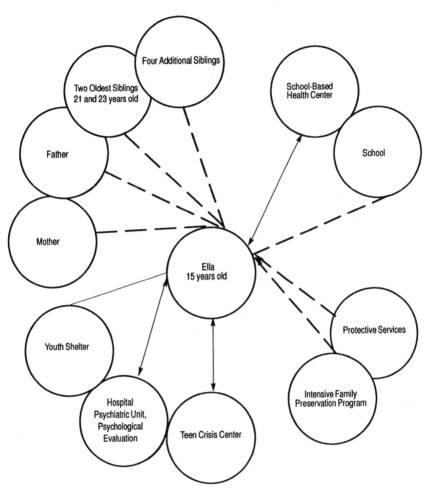

comfortable in seeking services, their needs continually change. They may initially request help with a particular issue, such as relationships with peers. Once that issue is resolved, another often emerges. This multiplicity of needs is no surprise, given the social and emotional growth that occurs during adolescence. There is also a tendency to become dependent on the social worker when faced with minor problems to solve. It is important to teach the students appropriate coping skills and then encourage them to use these skills independent of the social worker. Termination of treatment from the health center occurs at graduation or relocation to another school. If a student such as Ella is also being treated at a community agency or by a private practitioner, the health center staff will continue to work with these providers offering support and intervention as needed.

Case Conclusion

Ella's functioning has remained stable for several months. She currently attends weekly outpatient counseling sessions at the Teen Crisis Center and has remained on Prozac to treat her depression. Gaining insight into factors that trigger her depressed mood, Ella has begun to focus on her issues and develop strategies to cope with them. Academically, she continues to do well, although she still has difficulty developing friendships. Ella successfully completed the course of preventive treatment for tuberculosis. The Intensive Family Preservation Program, using a short-term model of intervention, terminated when the family reached their goals.

The social worker in the health center continues to monitor Ella's progress closely and is now helping her to develop school friendships. Most recently, Ella brought a new friend to the health center to meet the social worker. Ella's improvement is slow but stable, and she has recently begun to focus on the more normative issues of adolescence.

Differential Diagnosis

Adolescents with needs as complex as Ella's prove to be a challenge for the social worker in an SBHC. The use of clinical supervision becomes a key to the success of the treatment plan. All too often, the demands of a case with this intensity, combined with a large student population, can cause the social worker to become drained. Supervision combined with a multidisciplinary team approach led to Ella's stabilization and ultimate improvement. There are several areas, however, where alternate interventions may have been used to optimize the treatment plan.

A clearer sense of the cultural issues within this family would have been helpful in the earlier stages of involvement with Ella. Working with a community program designed to meet the needs of West Indian families might have helped to more positively engage Ella's family. In helping to understand the cultural issues as well as the family dynamics, more work should have been done with Ella's sister, who attends the same school.

This sister functions at a much higher level than Ella and might have offered additional insight to the health center staff.

Finally, team and interagency intervention could have been more proactive rather than reactive. A meeting of representatives of involved agencies was not convened until Ella was hospitalized, and should have been brought together following the referral to Child Protective Services. This would have clarified the role of each team member earlier in her care and may have prevented the extent of her deterioration. Ideally, the Child Protective Services worker should have assumed the role of case coordinator, but an extremely large caseload in that system led to the ultimate selection of the SBHC social worker for this role. If this decision had been made before the hospital discharge, Ella's subsequent decompensation might have been prevented. When working with clients whose complex needs require the involvement of multiple systems, the School-Based Health Center social worker must advocate for the student while actively working with agencies involved in the treatment plan.

REFERENCES

Adelman, H. S. and Taylor L. (1993). School-based mental health: Toward a comprehensive approach. *Journal of Mental Health Administration, 20*(1), 32-45.

Balassone M. L., Bell M., and Peterfreund N. (1991). School-based clinics: An update for the social worker. *Social Work Education, 13*(3), 162-175.

Barker L. A. and Adelman H. (1994). Mental health and help-seeking among ethnic minority adolescents. *Journal of Adolescent Health, 17*(3), 251-263.

Brice, J. (1982). West Indian families. In M. McGoldrick, J. K. Pearce, and J. Giordano (Eds.), *Ethnicity and family therapy.* New York: Guilford Press, pp. 123-133.

Department of Children and Families Hartford (Winter 1995). School-based health centers. *Primarily Prevention, 6*(2), 4-6.

Ellis, P. (1986). (Ed.). *Women of the Carribean.* London: Zed Books Ltd.

English, A. (1995, May/June). Consent and confidentiality: Important elements in adolescents' access to HIV care. *Youth Law News*, 3-6

Goldstein, E. G. (1984). *Ego psychology and social work practice.* New York: The Free Press.

Harold, R. D. and Harold, N. B. (1993). School-based clinics: A response to the physical and mental health needs of adolescents. *Health and Social Work, 18*(1), 65-74.

Harold, N. B. and Harold, R. D. (1991). School-based health clinics: A vehicle for social work intervention. *Social Work Education, 13* (3), 185-194.

Holman, A. M. (1988). *Family assessment: Tools for understanding and intervention.* Beverly Hills, CA: Sage Publications, Inc.

Irigon, F. F., Sarno, M., Sera, J., and Westgard, R. (1981). Child development centers program: An effective school based mental health service. *Child Welfare, 60*(8), 569-577.

Levy, A. J. and Land, H. (1994). School-based interventions with depressed minority adolescents. *Child Adolescent Social Work Journal, 11*, (1), 21-35.

National Association of Social Workers (1990). *Code of ethics,* Washington, DC: NASW Press.

Newton-Logsdon, G. and Armstrong, M. I. (1993). School-based mental health services. *Social Work Education, 15*(3), 187-191.

Pacheco, M., Adelsheim, S., Davis, L., Mancha, V., Aime, L., Nelson, P., Derkson, D., and Kaufman, A. (1991). Innovation, peer teaching, and multidisciplinary collaboration: Outreach from a school-based clinic. *Journal of School Health, 61*(8), 367-369.

Polster, N., Dryfoos, J., and Lear, J. (1995). School center's growth won't wither in inclement political climate. *Adolescent Medicine, 20*(10), 1-2.

Reamer, G. (1988). AIDS and ethics: The agenda for social workers. *Social Work, 33*(4), 460-463.

Rienzo, B. A. and Button, J. W. (1993). The politics of school-based clinics: A community-level analysis. *Journal of School Health, 63*(6), 266-272.

Robert Wood Johnson Foundation (Fall 1993). Building an effective team: Collaboration is the key. *Access,* Washington, DC.

Robert Wood Johnson Foundation (Winter 1995). States lead the way for school-based health centers. *Access.* Washington, DC: The George Washington University Publishers.

Robert Wood Johnson Report (1993). *The school-based adolescent health care program report.* Washington, DC.

Schlitt, J., Rickett, K., Montgomery, L., and Lear, J. (November 1994). State initiatives to support school-based health centers. *A making the grade report, November.* Washington, DC: Robert Wood Johnson Foundation.

Shulman, L. (1979). *The skills of helping individuals and groups.* Itaska, IL: Peacock Publishers, Inc.

Weist, M. D., Proescher, E. J., Freedman, A. H., Paskewitz, D. A., and Flaherty, L. (1995). School-based health services for urban adolescents: Psychosocial characteristics of clinic users versus non users. *Journal of Youth Adolescents, 24*(2), 251-264.

Zastrow, C. and Kirst-Ashman, K. (1997). *Understanding human behavior and the social environment.* Chicago, IL: Nelson-Hall Publisher.

Chapter 6

Epilepsy in Childhood:
Pediatric Neurology Clinic

Carol Appolone Ford

CONTEXT

Description of the Setting

The Pediatric Neurology Clinic is an outpatient clinic at North Carolina Baptist Hospital, the teaching hospital for the Bowman Gray School of Medicine. This medical complex is a referral center for the western third of North Carolina as well as parts of Virginia and Tennessee; some patients drive up to three hours to reach it. The clinic is held one morning a week, with approximately 25 children scheduled, most of whom have epilepsy. Two social workers attend the clinic regularly and interview families to gather psychosocial data and to assess the families' understanding of the disorder. If problems are identified, the family may be referred to an agency within their community or be scheduled for follow-up interviews with the clinic social worker, depending on the family's distance from the medical center and the nature of the problem. A packet of information on epilepsy is given to each family when the diagnosis of epilepsy is made. The families are seen briefly on follow-up visits to check the status of the child and the family's adjustment.

All patients must be referred to this clinic by a physician or by their county public health department. Many patients come from rural North Carolina, and all are low income. For these families, medical care is provided by Medicaid or by the Children's Special Health Services, a state program for children with chronic health problems, who are from low income families. All clinic visits, medications, and tests pertaining to the epilepsy are paid for by these programs. The patient population is racially mixed with the majority being white, and the patients range in age from infancy to 21 years. The frequency of clinic visits depends upon the child's degree of seizure control. Those completely controlled by medication are seen annually; those still having seizures may be seen every few weeks or months for medication adjustments.

Childhood epilepsy often causes more psychosocial problems than the medical condition would warrant. The majority of children are seizure-free when on medication, and most will eventually come off the medication and have no further problems with seizures (Aicardi, 1994; Middleton, Attwell, and Walsh, 1981). However, the family's reaction to the disorder has the potential to greatly hamper the child's psychosocial development (Hoare and Kerley, 1991; Ford, Gibson, and Dreifuss, 1983; Gardner, 1968). Underexpectation by parents and teachers may cause academic underachievement (Holdsworth and Whitmore, 1974). Many parents are fearful and anxious after witnessing a seizure, and this anxiety permeates their interaction with the child. The parental overprotection that often accompanies such anxiety can stifle a child's natural drive toward independence. Too often we see young adults whose spirits have been squelched by years of parental admonishment (Lerman, 1977). Parental guilt seems to be ever present even when there is no family history of epilepsy and no known cause for the child's seizures. This may contribute to dysfunctional parenting patterns (Voeller and Rothenberg, 1973).

It is important to intervene at the outset to educate parents about all aspects of epilepsy so that much of this can be avoided (Appolone, 1978). Children with epilepsy have been found to have a compromised quality of life when compared with normal children or to children suffering from a similar disorder (Austin, 1994). The family's perception of the epilepsy and their attitude toward it are important in the child's adjustment. Exploring the family's feelings, perceptions, and knowledge about this disorder is essential. Truly, an ounce of prevention is worth a pound of cure.

Policy

Since this is a teaching hospital, patients coming to the outpatient clinics are examined by residents and medical students who, in consultation with the attending physician, make the diagnostic and treatment decisions. The nature of medical education is such that these student doctors rotate between services, and patients usually see a different one each time they come. This results in less than optimal continuity of care. We do make an attempt to have the same attending physician see the patient each time. However, patients often do not know who to contact if problems arise between visits. In the Pediatric Neurology Clinic, the social worker provides a sense of continuity of care and serves as a person to contact if problems, medical or otherwise, arise (Caroff and Mailick, 1985).

The toll-free, statewide Epilepsy Information Service is a component of the Department of Neurology at Bowman Gray School of Medicine. Its purpose is to answer questions about all aspects of epilepsy, which patients, professionals, or the general public may have. It operates daily during business hours and is staffed by trained professionals. Patients in the clinic are advised of the availability of this resource. Not only may they use it for general information about epilepsy, but also to get in touch with the clinic doctor if problems should arise. These clinic patients often cannot afford a long distance call, frequently do not recall the name of the doctor they saw, and do not know how to locate their doctor in the medical center. Some patients do not have home phones and call from pay phones or relatives' homes. When a patient's family calls the toll-free number, a social worker who has access to the social work notes and the neurology chart, handles the call. He or she contacts the attending physician who may talk directly to the family or have the social worker convey his or her treatment decision. In this manner, clinic patients can receive much better access to medical care between visits than would otherwise be available.

Technology

Epilepsy is a collective term for a group of disorders caused by abnormal brain cell electrical activity. Each disorder of the group involves some sort of seizure associated with either loss or disturbance of consciousness, an abnormal psychic experience or behavior, or abnormal motor or sensory phenomena. Epilepsy may involve convulsive movements of the body. Sometimes it involves a blank stare, a dazed state, and/or repetitive movements with the patient having no memory of what occurred. In fact, epilepsy is not a disease but a set of symptoms (Kerson and Kerson, 1985; Schneider and Conrad, 1983).

The primary medical treatment for epilepsy is drug therapy. Complete seizure control is achieved in over half the patients (Aicardi, 1994). More than a dozen medicines are currently available, and research continues to investigate new drugs. Blood level tests are used to determine exactly how much medication is in the blood. This test involves drawing blood from the patient, a task that is particularly difficult with children.

The electroencephalogram (EEG) is the main diagnostic test for epilepsy. It measures electrical activity in the brain through electrodes placed on the scalp. Since this electrical activity may be normal between seizures, a normal EEG does not rule out epilepsy. However, an abnormal EEG may confirm the diagnosis and give the doctor important diagnostic information on the type of seizures and the drugs to be used. Another test sometimes used is a computerized tomography (CT) scan. In this procedure, X-ray beams image cross sections of the brain, allowing the doctor to diagnose structural brain abnormalities that might otherwise not be detectable. Nuclear magnetic resonance imaging is also used to detect structural abnormalities by the use of magnetic fields.

Organization

The Pediatric Neurology Clinic is staffed by three pediatric neurologists, a nurse, two social workers, and a pool of residents and medical students who may be as few as one or as many as six. Two receptionists check in patients and file forms for medical coverage. They also gather financial information, as the family stands in the entryway where, unfortunately, one's private affairs are made public. This is 1 of 13 pediatric specialty clinics operated by North Carolina Baptist Hospital. Two other pediatric clinics that are concerned with hemophilia and child abuse have social work services available for patients.

Epilepsy is historically misunderstood (Caveness and Gallup, 1980; Temkin, 1994). Parents are often frightened and confused about this diagnosis. In this fast-paced clinic, the doctor is responsive to questions the family may have, but he or she does not probe for areas of concern. Often the family is so overwhelmed by the diagnosis that they do not know what to ask. The social worker spends time with these families to cover common problem areas (Pomerantz, 1984). There is actually no funding to pay for social work services provided to the Pediatric Neurology Clinic. A research grant to design a program of comprehensive care for epilepsy patients provided funding initially, but this money ran out over a decade ago. Small grants and some state money have continued to support various aspects of the Epilepsy Information Service, which employs the social workers who attend this clinic. The hospital might be expected to provide social work services to the Pediatric Neurology Clinic, since it is one of their outpatient clinics and they do have a social work department. However, their staff of 42 social workers covers an 806-bed inpatient facility, and they do not routinely service outpatient medical clinics.

Community agencies, especially the Public Health Centers, are frequently involved in follow-up for medical as well as social and educational aspects of the treatment plan. Many patients have no phone and have chronic transportation problems, so assistance by community agencies is often our only means of determining how the patients are getting along between visits, or of contacting them when they fail to keep appointments.

Although the hospital associated with our medical school has a social work department, the medical school itself does not. Many departments employ social workers, but each answers to the department chairman, section head, or program director. Most are supported by federal grants. There is currently no effort made by these social workers to keep in touch with one another or with the social workers in the hospital network. It is the unfortunate but inevitable consequence of having no department of social work in the medical school.

DECISIONS ABOUT PRACTICE

Client Description

Jeffrey Stone is an 11-year-old boy who began having generalized tonic-clonic seizures (grand mal) eight months ago. After having unexpected difficulty in getting good seizure control, Jeffrey's pediatrician referred him to the pediatric neurologist who then hospitalized Jeffrey for further tests. Routine blood level tests found no trace of the prescribed seizure medicine in his blood. This indicated that the mother was probably not giving Jeffrey the medicine. The doctor found her to be defensive, but she offered no explanation for not complying with treatment. She was referred for social work evaluation (Heisler and Friedman, 1981).

Jeffrey is the younger of two children in a white, middle-class, urban home. His sister is 14 years old and in good health. His mother is a 36-year-old homemaker who seems to enjoy that role. His father, 38, manages a hardware store, works long hours, but spends his free time with his family. Both parents are in good health. Jeffrey's maternal grandmother lives a few hours away and has frequent contact with the family.

The initial social work contact occurred while Jeffrey was still hospitalized. Mrs. Stone was interviewed in my office. She was defensive and reticent, although no mention had been made of the medication or the compliance problem. I took a patient education approach, saying that most patients know nothing about epilepsy and that I would like to explain some things about it. Although tense throughout the interview, Mrs. Stone appeared to relax somewhat as she listened. In simple terms, I explained what occurs physiologically during a seizure, the appropriate first aid, and the role of medication. Mrs. Stone had a few questions and I praised each one saying that many parents had asked that very same question. Because parents' accounts of their children's physical problems are usually quite useful in assessing their emotional reactions to it, I asked

Mrs. Stone to tell me about Jeffrey's seizure history. By the end of the interview, Mrs. Stone had warmed up noticeably. After giving her pamphlets about epilepsy, I scheduled another interview with her, this time in Jeffrey's room later that afternoon.

At this point, there were several possible causes for Mrs. Stone's noncompliance. It was possible that she had her own ideas about the cause or nature of these seizures and that medicine did not fit into her understanding of what was going on. This is a common problem in situations of noncompliance (Voeller and Rothenberg, 1973; Tavriger, 1966). Another possibility was that the grandmother had been feeding misinformation to her daughter about this disorder and that Mrs. Stone was following her mother's dictates rather than the physician's. The influence of the grandparents on these situations cannot be overestimated. Still another possibility was that the mother had fears about giving daily medication, fears that it would have long-term side effects or lead to drug addiction. Mrs. Stone seemed neither hostile nor rejecting toward the child, nor was she a negligent mother in any other aspect of her care. There was no indication of major psychiatric problems. I had no doubt that she understood the instructions on how to give the medicine.

The purpose of this next interview was to determine why medication was not being given. Rapport had been established during the initial interview and it seemed important to follow up quickly on this. Jeffrey was out having tests when I met with Mrs. Stone in his hospital room. I opened the interview by asking whether the pamphlets had been helpful. They had. She brought up some concerns about Jeffrey becoming dependent on seizure medicine. Mrs. Stone's concern seemed mild and was obviously not the main problem. Other issues discussed were people's reactions to those with epilepsy, their misconceptions and how to handle them, and the stigma associated with epilepsy (Taylor, 1987). After about thirty minutes, Mrs. Stone seemed to feel relaxed, and I posed the question, "I know you have thought a lot about these seizures and you must have some idea about what causes them. What do you think it is?" Mrs. Stone responded in a confidential manner and seemed embarrassed at times as she explained: "I do. You see he has been watching reruns of this old TV show called *The Incredible Hulk*, and sometimes he gets to imitating the Hulk turning into that monster. Do you know how the Hulk does when he gets angry? He gets big and turns green, and it's scary. I think he got to doing that and could not stop, and it just went into one of those seizures. I did not let him watch *The Incredible Hulk* for weeks, but he begged and begged, so I finally gave in one Friday night. And do you know, he had a seizure the very next day?" Now it was understandable why medicine was forgotten so often. Medicine made little sense in the context of her unique understanding of Jeffrey's epilepsy.

Next, I focused on how frightening the seizures are, and for the first time, Mrs. Stone was able to verbalize the terror she felt when they occurred. She discussed the first seizure in detail, her thoughts, fears, and actions. She was tearful as she revealed that she thought he was dying each time he had a seizure. She was embarrassed that she had gotten so hysterical during the first seizure. I encouraged her to express her sense of helplessness and lack of control during these episodes. The goal of this interview was to uncover all of the fears that this mother kept hidden. Some information and reassurance were given about major misconceptions. I explained that behavior could not induce a seizure, that if a child voluntarily shook or jerked it could not cause him or her to go into a seizure. I again explained in simple terms the physiological phenomena and the role that medicine played. I reiterated that adequate blood levels of seizure medication should reduce the frequency of the seizures.

It was important to find out about the grandmother's and the father's reactions to Jeffrey's condition. What kinds of things did they say about it? By Mrs. Stone's account, both were concerned, but neither seemed to be contributing to Mrs. Stone's fears and misinformation. The father had not seen a seizure and was rather matter-of-fact about the whole thing. At this point, I felt confident that there were no other major issues and brought the interview to a close, making an appointment to talk with Mrs. Stone again in the morning before Jeffrey was discharged.

Later I talked with the doctor about the case, and subsequently he was able to communicate much better with Mrs. Stone. He reinforced much of what I had said, stressing the good prognosis for Jeffrey's epilepsy with the use of seizure medication. Mrs. Stone's parenting techniques and Jeffrey's school situation needed to be discussed with the mother because there was some indication that she had become quite permissive and overprotective following the onset of seizures (Ferrari, 1989). I also wanted to discuss drug treatment to make sure that Mrs. Stone was committed to following through with it.

The next morning, Mrs. Stone came to my office. When I asked about the school situation, she said that Jeffrey's teacher was fairly nervous about his condition. He had one seizure in school and that had caused an uproar. She gave permission for me to contact the school. I discussed with Mrs. Stone the importance of treating Jeffrey like a normal child and continuing with the expectations and discipline she had always imposed. Mrs. Stone realized that she set few limits now because she feared that making Jeffrey angry would cause him to have a seizure. I explained that anger did not cause Jeffrey's seizures and that it was important to treat him just as before. I warned Mrs. Stone that behavioral problems that resulted from pampering these children were difficult to correct and could create serious adjustment problems later. Although she admitted she was still fearful, Mrs. Stone agreed that she needed to be stricter with Jeffrey. I asked whether she felt comfortable about the prospect of giving medicine to Jeffrey every day for the next several years. She replied that if it would prevent seizures, she would do anything. I again explained blood levels and the importance of keeping his in the necessary range, and gave her a pill organizer to help her remember. She was instructed what to do if she should forget a dose. I explained that blood levels would be checked when Jeffrey returned to the clinic in two weeks and that I would see her again then. I gave her my phone number in case problems or questions arose. Once more, we reviewed first aid procedures. I said I would contact the school and talk with Mrs. Stone about that at the clinic visit (Fraser and Clemmons, 1989; Beniak, 1982). Mrs. Stone seemed genuinely grateful as she thanked me for my help.

Jeffrey's teacher was indeed nervous about his condition. His seizure in school had panicked everyone, especially her. She had no previous contact with epilepsy and knew nothing about it. She now watched him closely because she worried he would have another seizure. His peers were a little stand-offish immediately after the seizure, but after two months had passed, things had returned to normal. I elicited questions about the disorder and talked about first aid. I also offered to send pamphlets on epilepsy, and the teacher gratefully accepted that. She agreed to call me after reading the material. Approximately one week later, she did call and said she had enjoyed the information and had shared it with another teacher who also had a student with epilepsy. She asked whether I could present a brief talk about epilepsy at the next teacher's meeting, and I arranged to do so.

When Jeffrey and his mother returned to the clinic after two weeks, she reported that he had done well, having had no seizures and no problems. She seemed fairly relaxed and said that she trusted the medicine. She said that she was better at setting limits but still hesitated at times. I praised her efforts and encouraged her to keep it up. She had shared the written information with her husband and her mother. Her mother found it particularly helpful. I told Mrs. Stone that the school contact had gone so well that all the teachers wanted more information about epilepsy. I also told her that there were other children in the school with this disorder. The mother seemed pleased. Jeffrey was present throughout this interview. I decided to talk alone with him, and the mother stepped outside. I asked Jeffrey whether he had any questions about his epilepsy; he said not really. I asked whether he knew anyone else who had seizures. He knew such a boy in school, and he wondered whether it was true that one could catch epilepsy. I responded that one could not, and elaborated on that. He was quiet. I asked whether seizures scared him when he thought about them. He said that they scared his mother, that he had stopped breathing once and almost died. I explained that his mother had been so frightened that she misunderstood the situation. He had not nearly died. Seizures were not as dangerous as they looked. I said that I had told his mother what to do during a seizure and that she seemed to feel more relaxed now. I asked whether seizures had made any difference in school. He said that his teacher looked at him more now; he sensed her nervousness. I told him that his teacher had not known anything about epilepsy and that was why she had been nervous. Now that she was better informed, she might be more relaxed. I then told Jeffrey about a popular athlete from his state who had epilepsy, took medication, and was doing fine. Jeffrey looked pleased. I gave him my number in the event he should have any questions or problems about his epilepsy in the future.

A return appointment was scheduled in three months, and I told Jeffrey and his mother that unless problems arose, I would not need to talk with the family before then. The blood level results showed his medication to be in the therapeutic range, and both Mrs. Stone and I were pleased with that. I did tell her what the range was (10 to 20) and that Jeffrey's level was 14. Such concrete information can be reassuring and allows the family to feel more control over the situation. Mrs. Stone called me one time before the next appointment to ask whether it would be harmful to Jeffrey if she took a part-time job. She wanted to sell Avon products but needed assurance that it would not jeopardize his good progress. I encouraged her to pursue this.

When Jeffrey and his mother returned to the clinic after three months, he was doing quite well. He had had no seizures. The mother was smiling and relaxed and looked unusually stylish and well groomed. She was pleased with her job, which allowed her to meet many people as well as to have her own spending money. She was not preoccupied with his seizures any longer. In fact, she did not think of them very often. He no longer got special treatment, and things had "settled back to normal." He wanted to go to summer camp, and she wondered whether that would be all right. I asked her what she would tell the camp officials about his condition, and Mrs. Stone gave a very good explanation of his disorder and his treatment. The doctor filled out the camp medical form she had brought and gave his consent for Jeffrey to go. Jeffrey was scheduled to be seen again in a year.

Definition of the Client

The primary client in this case was Jeffrey's mother. It was necessary to assess the reason for her noncompliance and to treat those problems before

Jeffrey could come under good medical control. Jeffrey's poor seizure control created secondary problems in school. His peers had shunned him for a while after the seizure, his teacher was apprehensive and overly attentive, and he was aware of this. Jeffrey's teacher was therefore also a client. Her anxiety and lack of information needed to be addressed. The other teachers in Jeffrey's school were clients. Through in-service training, they became better prepared to deal with his problem and with other children in the school who had epilepsy. This may prevent future problems. Of course, Jeffrey was also a client. Attention needed to be given to his perception of the situation and to the problems that he identified. His awareness of the feelings of those around him is typical. Parental fears about the child's condition are usually incorporated by the patient. When parents understand and accept this disorder, the child generally does likewise (Middleton, Attwell, and Walsh, 1981; Ziegler, 1982).

Several potential clients in this case never actually became clients. The grandmother and the father might have been clients if Mrs. Stone's information had indicated problems with either of them. Jeffrey's sister was also a potential client. Sibling reactions can be very important to the patient's adjustment (Goldin and Margolin, 1975). Jeffrey's classmates might have become clients if they had continued to isolate or stigmatize him. In that case, an educational program in the classroom could be helpful.

Goals

The goals of this social work intervention were that Jeffrey achieve the best possible seizure control through medication, that his mother understand and accept his disorder, and that the emotional climate of the home and the school return to normal. Jeffrey's compliance was measured through the blood level testing. His mother's understanding and acceptance of the disorder were reflected in her willingness to give medication as well as in her openness in discussing his condition. She was cognizant of her overprotection and recognized when she began to improve and return to normal. It was relatively easy to evaluate the school situation because the teacher was cooperative and honest about feelings. Besides the social worker/client relationship, achievement of these goals depended in part on Jeffrey's physician. He was aware of what was transpiring between the mother and the social worker and was cooperative in reinforcing social work efforts rather than being overbearing or judgmental with Mrs. Stone.

Use of Contract

Although the social worker/client contract was never clearly outlined, my initial statement that I wanted to help the mother understand her child's disorder was an honest basis for all that ensued. It was not necessary to verbalize that one of the main goals was to have the mother cooperate with medical treatment. Doing so might further have alienated this mother who was already feeling threatened. It is not always best to discuss all aspects of the contract. It is important that the client have a basic understanding of why he or she is seeing a worker although the worker may have a hidden agenda.

Meeting Place

The meeting place was of some importance in this particular case. The initial meeting should have taken place in the child's room at a time when he was not there rather than in my office. This would have been a less threatening setting since it was Mrs. Stone's turf. Parents on the pediatric ward spend their nights and days in the child's room, so it becomes a temporary home for them. Bringing the mother down to my office might have seemed to her a bit more like coming to the principal's office for a scolding, considering the circumstances. I sat behind a desk in a somewhat authoritarian arrangement. When we met later in the hospital room, we sat in identical chairs facing one another in a more equal and relaxed atmosphere. However, the ideal situation cannot always be arranged, and one must work with what one has.

Use of Time

Although this client will be followed periodically over a long period of time, the social work contact was essentially short-term. The exact number of interviews with the mother could not be predetermined, but I expected to have no more than six, provided all went well. If the mother had continued to be resistant, the father would have been brought into the situation and probably the grandmother too. The time frame for each interview was not preplanned. Each lasted one and one-half hours. An interview longer than that would be too fatiguing. There were goals for each interview, and I remained cognizant of them as time elapsed.

Interventions and Use of Outside Resources

In this case, the treatment modality was crisis intervention. The crisis precipitating social work intervention was the discovery that Jeffrey's mother was not compliant with treatment for a fairly serious medical disorder. The crisis that had overwhelmed Mrs. Stone was the onset of

Jeffrey's seizures, which were terrifying and seemed life-threatening to her. The focus was on the immediate problem, and little in-depth attention was given to the social background. No attempt was made to explore or deal with problems the mother might have about specific issues, such as her need to control her anger, or her husband's long hours away from the family. No attempt was made to interpret the symbolic nature of her Incredible Hulk fantasy. In the initial interview with Mrs. Stone, I found no psychiatric problems and felt that the family's functioning before the onset of the seizures seemed fairly normal. The treatment was limited to restoring that level of functioning. (I also provided educational pamphlets and a pill organizer to the family. Educational materials were given to the school as well. No other concrete services were needed.)

Stance of the Social Worker

Because of the short-term nature of this intervention, I was direct, focusing on the immediate problem area and actively directing the course of the interviews. Initially, I took a teaching approach, carefully avoided confrontation, and supported the few concerns Mrs. Stone expressed. During the second interview, I wanted to draw Mrs. Stone out and did so with leading questions. It was important to listen during this interview, to express understanding and support for the mother's ordeal, and to universalize her feelings. Often, parents of epileptic children feel isolated and think that no one can understand their fears and experiences. It can be helpful to let them know that the worker has talked with many parents of children with epilepsy and that their fears are universally shared. This must be done carefully so as not to discount the parent's feelings but rather to lend a base of support. There was some teaching during the second interview, but I was careful not to dominate with that since the main goal was to allow the mother to express her feelings (Fraser, 1983).

The third interview consisted of much confrontation and giving of advice. Giving advice is generally shunned as a social work task, but it is a valid task at times. Mrs. Stone needed to know that if she did not change her parenting pattern, trouble lay ahead. When Mrs. Stone protested that she was scared to be firm, I confronted her. Did she want a spoiled child who was a problem in the classroom, could not get along with peers, and was impossible to live with at home? What kind of adult would such a boy grow up to be? Confrontation at this point was essential to change behavior so that problems could be prevented.

In the fourth interview, I used praise for Mrs. Stone, who was coping much better. Her efforts needed to be rewarded. I further reinforced important points covered in previous interviews. By expressing confidence in Mrs. Stone's ability to continue to handle the situation, I attempted to bolster her self-esteem. By reminding her that I was available if further problems arose, I offered her a sense of continued support. Giving permission to the mother to behave in certain ways provided the support she needed in the face of self-doubt. She needed the doctor's and my permission to treat Jeffrey normally. She also needed permission to pursue her job interest.

Reassessment and Termination

This case was reassessed each time the patient returned to the clinic, which was once a year after the first few visits. The physician and I agreed that Jeffrey and his mother continued to do well. She never had a need to contact us between scheduled appointments, but that always remained an option. Active social work intervention terminated naturally at the time of the fourth interview. By that time, the crisis was resolved. Mrs. Stone was giving the medication. Jeffrey's blood level was therapeutic and he was seizure free. The household was returning to a more normal state. The school had responded well to a minimum of intervention. I continued to check on this family, but there were no problems that required reopening the case.

Case Conclusion

Jeffrey remained on medication for four years. Since he had been seizure-free for that period of time and since his EEG was normal, the physician decided to gradually discontinue the medication. Mrs. Stone was anxious but agreed to try this. He has had no further seizures. He seems to be a normal adolescent, and Mrs. Stone continues to parent in an appropriate manner. Occasionally, her concern about his seizure history does surface, as when he went to apply for a drivers license (Krumholz, 1994; Silber, 1983). However, she is able to quell her fears, and allows him to function normally.

Differential Discussion

It might have been a good idea to bring the father in for an interview to assess his response to Jeffrey's epilepsy. However, this might have presented problems. More than likely, he was unaware that his wife was not administering the medication, and he might have been angry or accusing over that. It is possible that problems between the parents may have surfaced. There were indications that Mrs. Stone did not like her husband's long work hours and felt neglected and alone in handling the children's problems. A referral for marital counseling may have resulted. Instead, Mrs. Stone was left to cope with the seizure problem alone, and she did quite well. The successful mastering of a crisis situation can leave the person stronger than before. Mrs. Stone subsequently became more independent of her family by getting a part-time job, which afforded her an occupation outside the home and an income of her own.

The importance of parents being open with their children about epilepsy has been stressed in the literature (Schneider and Conrad, 1983). If I were to treat this family today, I would have discussed this with Mrs. Stone at the time of the final interview. I would make sure she used the terms seizures and epilepsy instead of "those" and "it," as if the condition were too horrible to call by name. While it is important not to dwell on Jeffrey's epilepsy, this topic should not be avoided if there is a need to discuss it with him or as a family.

PRACTICE IN CONTEXT

The nature of epilepsy dictates that a variety of interventions be utilized in the psychosocial treatment of epilepsy patients. Epilepsy can be a chronic, poorly-controlled seizure disorder in which the social worker provides long-term emotional support, guidance to resources, and a thread of continuity in the midst of ever-changing medical personnel involved in the treatment. Epilepsy may result in the occurrence of several seizures that are easily controlled by medication, but leave the family in a state of confusion, emotionally overwhelmed and helpless. Crisis intervention can restore the family to a state of equilibrium, as in Jeffrey's case. Although epilepsy is a chronic disorder, patients are usually normal and healthy between seizures. Social work intervention may enable the parents and patients to deal with this dichotomy and to establish appropriate expectations, limits, and goals (Lechtenberg, 1984).

Poor seizure control makes good social adjustment more difficult. Especially over the past few decades, technology has been important in the psychosocial treatment of epilepsy by making better seizure control possible. Tests that indicate the level of anticonvulsant medication in the blood are important for accurate adjustment. These can also make noncompliance evident, as in Jeffrey's case. Without blood level tests, doctors would have engaged in lengthy and fruitless efforts to adjust Jeffrey's drugs without realizing that the problem was with the mother, not with the medicine. Technology has also provided improved diagnostic tests, further refining the diagnostic process so that treatable causes for epilepsy will not go undetected. However, even if technology achieved complete seizure control for all patients, this would not eliminate the psychosocial problems that sometimes accompany epilepsy. This disorder has been associated with shame, misunderstanding, and fear for so long that many families cannot accept it simply as a medical problem. Since outpatient clinics are not routinely included in the hospital's social work network, Jeffrey was fortunate that this service was available to patients with his disorder. If Jeffrey had come in with orthopedic problems, for example, no medical social work services would have been available to help with his family problems.

In Jeffrey's case, technology was the key to further exploration of his family situation. It is ironic that the results of a chemical test were cause for social work referral. The policy of using a team approach in the Pediatric Neurology Clinic made this referral a natural consequence of the compliance problem. In cases such as Jeffrey's, social work intervention itself may be fairly straightforward. Identification of the problem and referral for social work help are crucial to achieving good medical and social adjustment.

REFERENCES

Aicardi, J. (1994). *Epilepsy in children*. New York: Raven Press.

Appolone, C.A. (1978). Preventive social work intervention with families of children with epilepsy. *Social Work in Health Care, 4*, 139-148.

Austin, J. K. (1994). Childhood epilepsy and asthma: Comparison of quality of life. *Epilepsia, 35*, 608-615.

Beniak, J. (1982). Patient education in epilepsy. *Journal of Neurological Nursing, 14*(1), 19-22.

Caroff, P. and Mailick, M. D. (1985). The patient has a family: Reaffirming social work's domain. *Social Work in Health Care, 10*(4), 17-34.

Caveness, W. F. and Gallup, G., Jr. (1980). A survey of public opinion toward epilepsy in 1979 with an indication of trends over the past 30 years. *Epilepsia, 21*, 509-518.

Ferrari, M. (1989). Epilepsy and its effects on the family. In B. P. Herman and M. Seidenberg (Eds.), *Childhood epilepsies: Neuropsychological, psychosocial, and intervention aspects*. New York: John Wiley & Sons.

Ford, C. A., Gibson, P., and Dreifuss, F. E. (1983). Psychosocial considerations in childhood epilepsy. In F. E. Dreifuss (Ed.), *Pediatric epileptology*. Boston, Bristol, and London: John Wright.

Fraser, R. T. (1983). A needs review in epilepsy rehabilitation: Toward solutions in the '80s. *Rehabilitation Literature, 44*(9/10), 264-269.

Fraser, R. T. and Clemmons, D. C. (1989). Vocational and psychosocial interventions for youths with seizure disorders. In B. P. Herman and M. Seidenburg

(Eds.), *Childhood epilepsies: Neuropsychological, psychosocial, and intervention aspects.* New York: John Wiley & Sons.

Gardner, R. A. (1968). Psychogenic problems of brain-injured children. *Journal of the American Academy of Child Psychiatry, 7,* 471-491.

Goldin, G. and Margolin, R. (1975). The psychosocial aspects of epilepsy. In G. N. Wright (Ed.), *Epilepsy rehabilitation.* Boston: Little, Brown & Co.

Heisler, A. B. and Friedman, B. (1981). Social and psychological considerations in chronic disease: With particular reference to the management of seizure disorders. *Journal of Pediatric Psychology, 6*(3), 239-250.

Hoare, P. and Kerley, S. (1991). Psychosocial adjustment of children with chronic epilepsy and their families. *Developmental Medicine and Child Neurology, 33,* 201-215.

Holdsworth, L., and Whitmore, K. (1974). A study of children with epilepsy attending ordinary schools, II: Information and attitudes held by their teachers. *Developmental Medicine and Child Neurology, 16,* 759-765.

Kerson, T. S. with Kerson, L. A. (1985). The epilepsies. In *Understanding chronic illness.* NY: Free Press, pp. 126-148.

Krumholz, A. (1994). Driving and epilepsy: a historical perspective and review of current regulations. *Epilepsia, 35,* 668-674.

Lechtenberg, R. (1984). *Epilepsy and the family.* Cambridge, Massachusetts and London, England: Harvard University Press.

Lerman, P. (1977). The concept of preventive rehabilitation in childhood epilepsy: A plea against overprotection and overindulgence. In J.K. Penry (Ed.), *Epilepsy: The eighth international symposium.* NY: Raven Press.

Middleton, A. H., Attwell, A. A., and Walsh, G. O. (1981). *Epilepsy: A handbook for patients, parents, families, teachers, health and social workers.* Boston and Toronto: Little, Brown & Company.

Pomerantz, B. R. (1984). Collaborative interviewing: A family-centered approach to pediatric care. *Health and Social Work, 9*(1), 66-73.

Schneider, J. R. and Conrad, P. (1983). *Having epilepsy: The experience and control of illness.* Philadelphia: Temple University Press.

Silber, T. J. (1983). Chronic illness in adolescents: A sociological perspective. *Adolescence, 18*(7), 675-677.

Tavriger, R. (1966). Some parental theories about the causes of epilepsy. *Epilepsia, 7,* 339-343.

Taylor, D. C. (1987). Epilepsy and prejudice. Archives of Diseases. *Child, 62*(2), 209-211.

Temkin, Q. (1994). *The falling sickness: A history of epilepsy from the Greeks to the beginnings of modern neurology.* Baltimore and London: Johns Hopkins Press.

Voeller, K. and Rothenberg, M. (1973). Psychosocial aspects of the management of seizures in children. *Pediatrics, 51,* 1072-1082.

Ziegler, R. G. (1982). Epilepsy: Individual illness, human predicament, and family dilemma. *Family Relations, 7,* 435-444.

Chapter 7

Family-Centered Care: Life Span Issues in a Spina Bifida Specialty Care Program

Wendy Schmid

CONTEXT

Description of the Setting

Medical social work plays a vital role in the delivery of family-centered care in major pediatric hospitals across the United States. This chapter describes the role social work has played in the multidisciplinary spina bifida program at The Children's Hospital of Philadelphia (CHOP) for over 30 years. The Children's Hospital of Philadelphia is a 300-bed, nonprofit, tertiary-care facility located near the center of its metropolitan area. It is a teaching hospital, adjacent to the University of Pennsylvania. Students from the nursing school, the medical school, and the graduate school of social work train at CHOP. It is also affiliated with The Philadelphia Child Guidance Center, The Children's Seashore House (for rehabilitation), and community pediatric programs.

The Spina Bifida Specialty Care Program was founded by Mary Ames, MD, in 1963. The late Dr. Ames was a pediatrician with the vision to establish a multidisciplinary program for the treatment of spina bifida. Her program was the first of its kind in the country and served as a model for other institutions because it offers the best care for patients and families. From its inception, it included social work as a key discipline. The clinic currently offers medical services to nearly 350 children and their families from diverse geographical and socioeconomic backgrounds. The population ranges in age from newborns to adults. It includes urban, suburban, and rural families. Most areas of the United States now have

health care programs for spina bifida that include all the medical specialists and colleagues in psychology and social work to provide the help that
these children and their families need (Charney, 1990).

The Spina Bifida Program sees well patients in its clinic on a regularly
scheduled basis, and the hospital offers inpatient care to those in crisis.
Clinic is held weekly, and visits are organized so that doctors and other
health professionals see these patients on the same day. X rays and other
required tests are often arranged on that same day to maximize efficiency
both for the family and the medical staff.

Policy

Until the early 1950s, babies born with spina bifida rarely survived
infancy. Major medical advances in neurosurgery and urology have
changed that. Today the majority of infants born with spina bifida can be
expected to live into adulthood and need complex and expensive specialty
care. Parents hold the primary legal and financial responsibility for their
children. In the United States, federal, state, and local health authorities
also share financial responsibility for services to these children by funding maternal and child health programs. Public and private hospitals also
provide some of the dollars for spina bifida programs.

Health Policies

The health delivery and funding system is complex and confusing to
those it supports. The federal government first became involved with
child health in 1912 by creating the U.S. Children's Bureau to investigate
and report on the welfare of children throughout the United States. The
Maternal and Infancy Act of 1921 (Sheppard-Towner Act), administered
by the Children's Bureau, was the first grant-in-aid program in the health
field. It laid the groundwork for national maternal and child health programs administered by the states and set precedents for later federal-state
relationships.

In 1935, the Social Security Act created the maternal and child health
program and the Crippled Children's program. Grants-in-aid were administered for both programs by the Children's Bureau until 1969, when the
Maternal and Child Health Service in the Public Health Service took
control. In 1989, amendments to the Title V Maternal and Child Health
Grant Program defined a national agenda for meeting the needs of children with special health care needs and their families. This agenda envi-
sions a system of services for children (and their families) with special

health care needs such as spina bifida, which is comprehensive, community-based, coordinated, family-centered, and culturally competent.

Program funding in Pennsylvania now falls under the State Department of Health, Community-Based Systems, and the Division of Children's Special Health Care Needs. The Spina Bifida Program at CHOP has received funding through this program from its inception. It must meet state requirements and reapply for funding every two years. CHOP supplements the funding of specialty care for children with spina bifida from its general operating budget.

The Pennsylvania Department of Health also provides direct patient funding. Patients can apply to the state Spina Bifida Program for supplemental coverage of medical costs. The Pennsylvania Department of Health is the payer of last resort, and all other insurance funding must be used prior to billing the state. Patients can be enrolled in the program if they meet financial requirements, are U.S. Citizens, and are Pennsylvania residents. There is no age requirement. The Department of Health no longer provides funds for services that are provided to children who have Pennsylvania Medical Assistance. There are similar programs in the states of New Jersey and Delaware, but the focus here will be on Pennsylvania.

Private medical insurance still provides most of the direct patient-care funding to the spina bifida program at CHOP. Before 1992, most of the families living in Pennsylvania applied to the state Department of Health for supplemental coverage. In October of 1992, a newsletter for Pennsylvanians with disabilities (published by the Pennsylvania Health Law Project) distributed information about a little-known regulation. This provision provided a way for more families to receive Pennsylvania Medical Assistance. The Department of Welfare decided not to look at parents' income when determining eligibility for disabled children, but to look only at the child's income. Their intent was not to cover all children, but rather to cover those children who needed medical insurance but were not eligible for Social Security Disability (SSI). The Pennsylvania Health Law Project insisted that the state apply the same rules to all applicants. Since October 1992, the Spina Bifida Program social worker has encouraged all families to apply for coverage, because it provided more comprehensive coverage than did the state spina bifida program. It remains to be seen whether families will eventually be dropped from this program or grandfathered into the program, or whether, doubtful as it seems, the program will be expanded to cover all disabled children. The State of Delaware provides medical assistance to all its disabled children. New Jersey assists some of its families with a state-supported medical assistance program.

Public and private insurance programs now dictate much of what a comprehensive specialty care program like the CHOP Spina Bifida Program can do for patients. Managed care providers authorize as much or as little care at CHOP as they consider appropriate. Primary care providers usually refer children with spina bifida to medical specialty programs, but they may require diagnostic testing and some hospitalizations to remain at local facilities. Rather than family-centered, managed care for spina bifida is often more insurance-centered. Families need to obtain referrals from their primary care providers for each visit, and there is little recourse if a request is not approved. It is crucial for specialty-care programs to help providers recognize the cost-effectiveness of treatment by professionals who know the most about the children with spina bifida. Specialty clinics need to negotiate with health care providers. Specialty teams must provide necessary teaching so that community care is safe.

Education Policies

Education as well as health care policies affect children with spina bifida because these children all have special educational needs (Lollar, 1994) Several laws have made education and employment readily accessible to the disabled. Parents and professionals involved in the education of a student with spina bifida need to learn about existing laws that guarantee educational and employment rights. The two most influential federal laws that assist students with spina bifida are at present PL 101-476, the Individuals with Disabilities Education Act (IDEA), and Section 504 of the 1973 Rehabilitation Act (PL 93-112). Each state has its own statutes and regulations governing education for children with disabilities, but these state laws may not contradict, violate, or limit the mandates of the federal laws.

The most important federal law in the area of special education is the Education of the Handicapped Act (EHA). This law, enacted in 1975, as PL 94-142 has been amended several times and is now referred to as the Individuals with Disabilities Education Act (IDEA). States that receive federal funds under part B of the IDEA must make free and appropriate public education available to all children from age 3 through 21 years of age.

Antidiscrimination Policies

Section 504 of the Rehabilitation Act of 1973, 29 U.S.C. Section 794, prohibits discrimination against children and adults with disabilities, including those with spina bifida. Section 504 recognizes that to provide a student who has disabilities with "equal access" to public education, different or additional services from those provided nondisabled students is often necessary. Both of these laws have assisted families in securing appropriate education for their children through age 21, when necessary (Rowley-Kelly and Reigel, 1993).

The Americans with Disabilities Act (ADA) enacted by Congress in July 1990, prohibits discrimination on the basis of disability in the public and private sectors in the areas of employment, public accommodations, public service, transportation, and telecommunications. The ADA expands the Rehabilitation Act of 1973 by explicitly including both public and private sectors in its coverage. In the act, a disabled person is defined in the same manner as that of section 504 of the Rehabilitation Act of 1973; that is, a disabled person is any person who (1) has a physical or mental impairment that substantially limits one or more of such a person's major life activities, (2) has a record of such an impairment, or (3) is regarded as having such an impairment. Modeled after Titles VI and VII of the Civil Rights Act of 1964, the ADA provides clear, strong, consistent, enforceable standards that address discrimination against individuals with disabilities, and it ensures that the federal government plays a central role in enforcing the standards established in this act on behalf of the 43,000,000 Americans with physical and mental disabilities (Ginsburg, 1990).

Technology

Spina Bifida is a complex birth defect. Today, it is the second most common birth defect. It occurs in approximately 0.7 to 1.0 per 1,000 live births in the United States (Charney, 1990). It is not a new disease. Archaeological discoveries have identified characteristic spinal deformities in 7,000-year-old skeletons (Gool and Good, 1986). Spina bifida affects motor, sensory, psychological, emotional, and cognitive development. The central nervous system of the developing baby fails to form at some point along its length. The location at which the defect occurs, determines the extent of the disability. This may include paralysis, hydrocephalus, mental retardation, bladder/bowel dysfunction, and musculoskeletal deformity.

Spina bifida ("split-spine") is one of a number of conditions called "neural tube defects." When the brain itself is not completely developed, the condition is called "anencephaly." Spina bifida occulta the most common and innocent form of spina bifida, occurs in 10 to 15 percent of the general population. Only the bones of the spinal column will be incompletely developed, and the nervous tissue beneath will be normal. It usually occurs at the lower end of the spine and rarely causes medical problems (The Spina Bifida Program, 1995). Meningocele is another abnormality, identified by a mass that contains cerebrospinal fluid and does not affect the spinal cord and nerves. Myelomeningocele, the most severe form of spina bifida, appears at birth as an open cyst or mass, usually located in the thoracic or lumbar area. Myelomeningocele involves the incompletely developed lining of the spinal cord and nerves, and children born with this form of spina bifida have varying amounts of physical disability. Over 90 percent have some degree of weakness of their legs, inability to control voluntarily the bowel or bladder, and a variety of orthopedic deformities. After birth, almost all babies with myelomeningocele are treated with an operation to cover the opening of the spine, which does not restore function of the abnormal nerve tissue. Once the back has been closed, hydrocephalus (accumulation of serous fluid within the cranium) then may be evaluated through head circumference measurements, brain ultra sound, or computed tomography. Management of the hydrocephalus usually involves a shunting procedure whereby cerebrospinal fluid is internally diverted to another place in the body for better absorption. The shunt was developed in 1955 by an engineer who was the father of a baby born with spina bifida.

The cause of spina bifida is still not entirely known. It occurs during the first 28 days of pregnancy, while the spine is developing. In the late 1980s researchers around the world discovered that supplements of folic acid, a common B vitamin, can reduce the statistical risk of having a baby with a neural tube defect. Specific recommendations for supplements are prescribed by doctors. Women who take folic acid daily for at least one month before becoming pregnant and who continue to take it daily during the first three to four months of pregnancy will reduce their chances of having a baby with spina bifida (The Spina Bifida Program, 1995). At present, a blood test during early pregnancy can establish risk, ultrasound can detect spina bifida, and a test called amniocentesis can establish the presence of spina bifida. Women can decide then whether to abort the pregnancy or carry it to term. In the future, we may learn how to eliminate completely this complex birth defect, but for the moment, children born with spina bifida and their families must rely on medical and social services provided by the health care system.

Organization

The Children's Hospital of Philadelphia is a large, nonprofit, teaching hospital affiliated with the University of Pennsylvania. It trains physicians, nurses, social workers, and other health care professionals. CHOP is governed by a board of directors, and managed by a chief executive officer and chief operating officer. Most recently, the hospital incorporated as a physician hospital organization to ensure its financial viability.

CHOP has expanded its services by opening several primary care sites and specialty sites in the tri-county areas. These sites provide the best community-based, family-centered care and act as feeders to the pediatric specialty and surgical departments at the main hospital.

At CHOP, the mission statement sets the tone for all programs, including spina bifida:

> "The Children's Hospital of Philadelphia, the oldest hospital in the United States dedicated exclusively to pediatrics, strives to be the world leader in the advancement of health care for children by integrating excellent patient care, innovative research, and quality professional education into all of its programs" (Administrative Policy Manual, 1995).

Family-centered care is reflected in many CHOP policies; families are viewed as part of the treatment team and are included in patient care meetings. CHOP has dedicated space and funds to a Family Resource Center, which provides families with educational materials, access to phones and fax machines for management of personal business, and private bedrooms, where parents can directly learn home care before children are discharged.

The social work department at CHOP offers services to all families who enter its doors. There are presently 32 master's level social workers, two clerical staff, two clergy, two nurses who provide support services to families waiting for children having surgery, four managers, an assistant director, and a director. The position of director was recently expanded to include 20 percent teaching, research, and grant writing funded by the University of Pennsylvania Graduate School of Social Work, with 80 percent administrative responsibility funded by CHOP.

Social workers are currently assigned either to a specialty medical service or to a specific unit, such as the emergency room or intensive care unit. Funding for social work positions varies. The majority of positions are funded through the social work department's budget. Some are grant-funded by special medical services. Funding sources can be federal, state, local, or private, and long-term or short-term. All social workers are clinically supervised by the social work department, and all participate in the on-call and on-site, weekend emergency service program. The social work department provides on-site social service to patients and families from 7:30 a.m. to 11:00 p.m. Monday through Friday, weekends from 9:30 a.m. to 6:00 p.m. On-call service by beeper is available the remainder of the time to families, physicians, and other support staff at the hospital.

The Spina Bifida Program at CHOP is directed by a pediatrician, is coordinated by a nurse clinician, and includes an orthopedist, physical therapist, part-time social worker, and part-time secretary. There is consultation from urology; neurosurgery; radiology; orthotics at Seashore House, a neighboring and related institution; and other services. Administratively, the program is part of the Department of Pediatrics at CHOP. Funding is provided by CHOP, direct patient care billing, and Pennsylvania's Maternal and Child Health Care Program.

Client Description

Bob Kelly, a 22-year-old adult, is one of the 350 patients followed from birth to early adulthood by the CHOP Spina Bifida Program. His case illustrates the long-term role of social work in one of many programs at CHOP focused on the care of chronically ill children.

Bob was born with myelomeningocele. His spinal cord lesion is at the lumbar (L3-4) vertebrae, which allows him some flexion of the knee. Even with this movement, he needed metal, long-leg braces with a pelvic band and thoracic upright appliance in order to stand and learn to walk (Gaul, 1993). The shunt that he has to prevent intracranial pressure has needed repair or replacement several times over the years. Bob was born with no control over his bowel and bladder and is seen regularly by a urologist. Today, after bladder augmentation in 1987 to increase his ability to store urine and after learning self-catheterization, he can keep himself dry and no longer needs to wear diapers. He is free of bowel accidents with timed emptying and the use of suppositories. He has had several kidney stones removed, and one kidney contributes only 15 percent to his overall renal function. Compliance with periodic urologic evaluation and follow-through on medical recommendations is essential for Bob to remain a healthy adult.

Intellectual ability is critical in determining how well a child with spina bifida can approach normal functioning. Intelligence quotients (IQs) vary greatly, but most children with spina bifida have IQs that fall in the low normal range. Most have learning disabilities that interfere with their education, so they require special education (Rowley-Kelly and Reigel, 1993). Bob was tested repeatedly over the years and found to have an IQ of 95 with evidence of visual perceptual problems. This made it difficult for him to write and made homework more tedious than usual. Bob attended Widener Memorial, a Philadelphia public school for physically disabled children from kindergarten through high school and graduated at age 21. The school is fully accessible and offers physical, occupational, speech, and other therapies and counseling to all its students. Absence from school during long hospitalizations made learning difficult for Bob. His father died of heart disease when Bob was in the ninth grade; he did poorly that year and had to repeat the grade.

The Kelly family, which was supported by the late Mr. Kelly's employment, is now financially maintained by entitlement payments to Bob, his younger sister Lisa, and Mrs. Kelly from Social Security Survivors' Benefits and by supplemental assistance to Bob from Social Security Disability. Medical costs are covered by Pennsylvania Medical Assistance. A managed care provider has contracted with Pennsylvania Medical Assistance to cover the family's medical needs. The Kellys are assigned to a primary care physician at a local Philadelphia health clinic only two blocks from their home. Dental care is available at the University of Pennsylvania dental clinic. Bob is referred by his primary care physician to CHOP for specialty care.

The Kellys live in a modest home in South Philadelphia, which is far from the most adequate, accessible dwelling one might hope for, but they make it work. A wooden ramp leads to the front door and allows Bob to come and go with relative independence. Mrs. Kelly and the CHOP social worker applied to a local fund-raising organization for assistance in building the ramp. After receiving approval and funding, the family waited until carpenters were available and it took two years from date of application to completion.

Bob recently started working in a Pennsylvania Department of Transportation Photo Identification Center (Hagner and Dileo, 1993). He earns $5.50 an hour and works 25 hours per week. He would like to work even more hours, so long as he does not lose the medical coverage that comes with his social security benefits (Social Security Administration Office of Disability, 1994). Medical insurance is not offered by the state at his place of employment. Bob continues to live at home with his mother and sister (Klein and Schleifer, 1993; Powell and Ahrenhold-Gallagher, 1993).

Goals, Objectives, and/or Outcome Measures

The spina bifida team at CHOP faces challenges that vary with each child and family. Our long-term goal is to provide comprehensive, multidisciplinary care for each child from birth to adulthood. The provision of immediate, comprehensive care for a newborn enables parents to bond with their baby. Our goal of helping each child reach its maximal developmental potential allows families to restore some of their dreams for a rewarding life for their disabled children. The specific short-term goals for the social worker on this team vary with each family situation. It is the social worker's role to help the family solve problems, as child and family face medical and social crises over time (Thompson, 1986; McCollum, 1975). Medical and social treatment of children with myelomeningocele needs to be individualized according to the needs of both the child and the family. Needs differ with the different developmental stages of each child. The short-term goals of the social worker for patient and family also change as the child grows from newborn to infant, preschooler, school-aged child, adolescent, and adult.

Family History and Impact on the Definition of Goals

The CHOP social worker's first goal in meeting a family faced with a baby who has spina bifida is to acknowledge the loss that they feel, support the feelings of love that they show for this child, and let them know they can draw upon outside support to help them meet this life challenge. Bob was the first child born to Ann and Rob Kelly. Ann was 22 years old and Rob was 33 when they married. Both had been married previously. Ann was one of 12 children born and raised in Philadelphia. Her dad worked as a bank janitor and was an alcoholic; her mother never drank, but experienced mental problems for which she was hospitalized at a public mental hospital many times. The children were cared for by their father and aunts. Between the ages of one and three, Ann lived in a Catholic home for girls. At age 16, knowing nothing about sex and longing for the love that her boyfriend offered, Ann married and had two children. She divorced her first husband after four years. Two years later, Ann met Rob, who had grown up in Chicago, one of two children. His father worked for the Board of Health and his mother was an alcoholic. Rob joined the Navy at 16 and first married at 17. He and his first wife had five children and divorced after 10 years. On retirement from the Navy, Rob took a job as manager of a night club. When he moved to Philadelphia, he became manager of a topless night club. He and Ann married after a month of acquaintance.

Bob was born at a community hospital and was transferred immediately to CHOP. Ann described her pregnancy as normal, except for the bleeding she experienced during her first trimester. Yet, she confided to the social worker that she felt there was something wrong all through this third pregnancy and, as a consequence, refused to paint the room or to get a crib. After Bob was born, Rob faced medical treatment decisions alone, and he and the obstetrician told Ann about her baby's disability after his first surgery was complete. Ann remembers that they told her Bob would be paralyzed to some degree and that they would have to watch for hydrocephalus. Ann confided that she blamed the doctors, remembering that they had told her not to push. She thought that they had dropped her baby and caused his imperfection. Despite all of this, both parents fell in love with Bob and saw him as a beautiful baby. Child care was left to Ann. Rob removed himself from the everyday care and even from medical appointments. The social worker intervened here to involve the father in appointments and care. The Kellys were introduced to the Delaware Valley Parents' Association, a support group for families who have children with spina bifida. Ann said that initially she went to a couple of meetings but did not find the members friendly.

The social worker assisted the Kellys to apply for state Medical Assistance to cover the cost of medical care not covered by Rob's job-related, union insurance. She also met with the parents when they came to the clinic to enable them to talk about their concerns and formulate questions for the medical team. Often parents are afraid to ask the questions that gnaw at them. For example, most parents worry that their children will be mentally retarded, but typically they are afraid to ask.

In that first year of life, parents of children with spina bifida face emotional devastation as well as financial worries. Rob and Ann, with few social supports, turned to alcohol. Rob drank with his friends after work. Ann drank alone at home from morning to night, sometimes as much as 24 beers a day; yet, she gave Bob the best care she could. On their hospital visits, Bob appeared well nourished, and Ann seemed fragile and nervous. Ann ignored the team's pleas that she get help for herself; finally, her pediatrician confronted her more boldly and arranged for her to be admitted to another hospital for a month of detoxification and support. The social worker assisted in the child care plans, and Bob was cared for by a maternal aunt. After discharge, Ann joined Alcoholics Anonymous, attended meetings regularly for a year, and continues in recovery. She separated from Rob for the first two years of her recovery. They later reunited, and Rob drank less and assisted with parenting Bob and daughter, Lisa, who was born six years after Bob. The social worker's goals for the family included drug treatment for both parents. These goals could be met only when they were owned by the clients. Until then, the social worker focused on Bob's safety and medical compliance. Offers of assistance and encouragement for Rob to seek assistance continued.

Goals During Preschool Years

During the preschool years, the medical goals for a child with spina bifida include independence in mobility, attempts at bowel and urinary continence, and assessment and therapy for a child's motor, language, and psychological development. Most children with spina bifida are braced between the ages of one and two years. At birth, Pennsylvania children with spina bifida who show gross motor delays are registered with the Pennsylvania Mental Health and Mental Retardation Early Intervention Program. Infant stimulation and all appropriate therapies are offered to the child and family in their own home until the age of 3, after which the local school district in Pennsylvania is responsible for providing education for that child until age 21.

It is the CHOP social worker's responsibility to ensure that families are made aware of these resources and are connected appropriately. The goals that the social worker sets with the family usually relate to financial, social, and emotional needs. For example, if equipment needs are not covered by insurance, other sources for funding must be sought. If families have limited income, the social worker helps them to learn about and apply for assistance through the federal Social Security Disability Program. Hospital support groups can help parents learn more about spina bifida and introduce them to other families who face similar problems.

At the age of one year, Bob Kelly was braced so that he could learn to walk. Funding for braces was secured through the Variety Clubs (an organization that operates nationwide to help children with these kinds of needs), after Rob's union insurance plan refused payment. Next, the social worker helped the Kellys to apply for Medical Assistance. Bob attended weekly physical therapy sessions at CHOP, and Ann joined the mothers support group led by the social worker. It met while the children were in therapy. Participation in this group was difficult for Ann, and she would rarely come. At the age of two years, Bob began attending the Easter Seal Society for therapy and preschool education five days a week (Williamson, 1987). This helped relieve some of the stress that Ann felt in parenting Bob by herself. Bob loved school and was described as outgoing by his teachers. By age four, he walked with a swing-through gait, using his crutches to propel himself forward. Bob continued as a good walker until the age of 15, when he gained weight and found it too slow to move about in his braces. There were times during those preschool years that were difficult for Bob. When he was upset watching the neighborhood children riding their bikes, the social worker helped him get a bike of his own, funded by the local Variety Club. As much as possible, the social worker supported the family and applauded their efforts as Ann successfully sought help for her alcohol addiction, separated from her husband, and then reunited with him.

Goals of the School-Age Child

Goals for the school-age child with spina bifida stress independence and learning. The medical team helps as many children as possible to overcome bowel and bladder incontinence so that they can be socially accepted by their peers. Psychological testing helps parents and their local school system plan appropriately for each child. Some of the children with spina bifida followed at CHOP are in full-time learning support classes; fewer are in regular classes with resource room help; some attend small, private schools where allowances are made for the learning needs of each child; and some, like Bob, attend public schools for the physically challenged. The CHOP team encourages parents to take one year at a time and work toward a positive relationship with their school districts. Most schools want to give each child the best they can offer. Each family is encouraged to attend the individual education planning (IEP) sessions during the year with school staff and to make sure that everything they agree on is documented in the IEP. Positive relationships with the school nurse and counselor are also essential.

Twice a year, the CHOP social worker offers an educational group session titled "Teaching the Student with Spina Bifida," which is open to parents and teachers. Videotapes are shown and followed by a group discussion. In addition, copies of the videotapes are available for parents to use at home and share with teachers. This is an example of community-based teaching used in the department.

Additionally, it is very important for each child to develop his or her interests outside of school. Children are encouraged to join groups such as the Brownies, Cub Scouts, choirs or instrumental groups, or Special Olympics or Challenger's Baseball to help them develop their talents. Also, the social worker and parents talk about the need for the assignment of chores at home in order to help the children develop independence and a sense of individual responsibility.

Bob Kelly entered the Widener School for kindergarten. His IQ was in the normal range, but he showed evidence of visual motor impairment. Mrs. Kelly could have sent him to a local school with resource-room help for his learning disabilities, but she decided instead to enroll him at Widener, where all the therapies would be available to him under one roof and where all the teachers are trained in special education. Bob studied with peers, all of whom had physical and intellectual challenges. After school and on weekends, he played with neighborhood children, most of whom were not physically challenged. If Bob Kelly were entering kindergarten in 1995, he would have the same choices because he lives in Philadelphia and Widener is still available, but the push for inclusion is stronger today.

Bob's attendance record showed many missed school days and a lot of incomplete homework assignments. This slowed the pace of his learning.

His home situation was fairly stable during those years. His father returned home, stayed employed, and supported the family. His mother provided neighborhood families with day care and was at home for Bob and Lisa. The family managed the emotional ups and downs of hospitalization with the support of extended family and the CHOP spina bifida team. The Sunshine Foundation funded a day trip to Disney World for the students at Widener. Bob and his mother went on that trip. All considered, Bob's elementary school years were stable.

Goals During Adolescence and Early Adult Years

Adolescence is a transition period. It is tumultuous for most young people even without the challenges of disability (Batshaw and Perret, 1992). For adolescents with spina bifida, it is a time of realization and recognition of their chronic problems that will require ongoing treatment and affect their life goals. For many parents, it is a time of recognition that some dependency will continue into adult years and some dreams may never be realized. Many adolescents with spina bifida experience declining physical activity, rapid weight gain, and increasing social isolation. They often choose to use a wheel chair for mobility in order to attempt to match the increasing speed and intensity of activity of their peers. As peers without disabilities become increasingly independent of their parents and move away from home, adolescents with spina bifida remain dependent on their parents and often choose to isolate themselves from peers.

It is important for the social worker to encourage as much independence as possible for these young people and to offer much support to parents. The social workers at CHOP offer a six-week course to adolescents with physical disabilities between the ages of 13 and 15 years, titled "Meeting the Challenge." The class, offered twice a year, meets weekly and focuses on self-awareness and social assertiveness. At the end of the course, each participant is given a certificate of participation (printed by the Public Relations Department at CHOP) as well as a $15.00 gift certificate donated by The GAP as an award for their participation.

Bob Kelly continued at Widener School and graduated when he was 21 years old (Wehman, 1992). During his high school years, he lifted weights and played wheelchair basketball. He and three other students formed a vocal quartet they called "Harmony Personified." They sang for a talent show at school and provided entertainment at an adolescent conference sponsored by and held at CHOP. Bob learned how to access Paratransit, a Pennsylvania public transportation system for the disabled. This allowed him some independence in travel. He used Paratransit to visit friends at their homes. After high school graduation, Bob stayed at home until he secured employment. He applied and interviewed for many jobs. His persistence resulted in a part-time job at a Philadelphia Photo Identification Center where several disabled young people are employed.

The role of the medical social worker during these years was to assist Bob with the transitions he faced. The social worker shared her knowledge of resources and assisted with job applications. Mrs. Kelly also needed help from the social worker. She found it frustrating to have Bob at home full-time. She used the social worker's support to help her think of ways to resolve conflicts at home. She also sought the help of social work in learning the rules of Social Security as they apply to employment. Answers to questions were found. Bob can keep his Pennsylvania Medical Assistance for three years even if he works full-time. If there is no accessible insurance program at that time, Medical Assistance can continue beyond the three years. Continuation of Medical Assistance is the most important issue for young people with disabilities who want to work. They often decide to stay at home rather than risk losing medical insurance.

Use of Contract

The term contract is defined here as an agreement between social worker and client as a means to achieve goals. Goals are defined jointly by the patient, the social worker, and by the patient's family. These goals need to be compatible with the goals of the spina bifida program and with the overall hospital philosophy. A contract is made when the family initially chooses to bring their child to the CHOP Spina Bifida Program. The philosophy of that clinic is explained to the family at the first meeting. The family can then choose either to contract for specialty care services with that program or not. In the past, families had the freedom to choose any doctor or hospital they wanted for themselves and their children. In the 1990s, however, it is managed care insurance programs that increasingly define the parameters and at times limit the choices available. The contract we set with the family needs to be in agreement with the contract of care set by the family's insurance company.

The social worker on the spina bifida specialty care team is introduced to the family either during the first hospital admission or at the first clinic visit. The parameters of the relationship are then defined by the social worker and explained to the family. In this case, the social work role is defined as that of advocate for the child and family in the hospital and in the community. The social worker is available to help the family cope with their emotional, social, and financial circumstances. It is the role of the social worker to locate community resources and then to assist the families in utilizing them. The overall contract between social worker and family exists from that first meeting to the patient's discharge from care at CHOP. More specific contracts are made with families as needs arise. They are usually time-limited and focused on a specific need, such as identifying financial support programs, thinking about options for education, or working through medical or psychosocial crises.

Meeting Place

The meeting place of the medical social worker, patient, and family varies. Most often at CHOP, the family of a hospitalized, newly diagnosed baby is seen at the patient's bedside. Families bringing their children for specialty medical checkups are seen in one of the orthopedic clinic rooms where the clinic is held. The family stays in one room, and professionals come in as space allows. From 10 to 20 patients and their families are seen on a typical clinic day. Most of the work done by medical social workers with families is done at the hospital.

As caseloads increase and cost cutting continues, it is increasingly difficult to allocate social work time for home or school visits. Although it would be ideal for each family to have a home visit, time does not allow for that. Instead, CHOP social workers use home care agencies and children and youth agencies to do this task. No other means compares to home visits for assessing the life of a client or family, but it is possible for today's medical social worker to visit homes or schools only infrequently. When that happens, a social worker gains a far broader perspective of life for the patient and family visited.

Social workers utilize the telephone in their work on a daily basis. It is the most efficient way to network with other agencies and to keep in touch with families who come to clinic infrequently. Conference calls between teacher or school counselor, parent, and medical social worker often are a sufficient means to resolve problems or at least to agree on a plan of action. Contacts with agencies and follow-up communication are most often done via telephone.

Use of Time

The use of time for medical social workers at CHOP is determined by caseload size and by funding. Current funding allows only for one part-time social work position for the Spina Bifida Program. The social worker uses that time to work with 350 patients and families who are seen routinely in clinic and during hospitalizations. Support groups offer a cost-effective means of educating and supporting parents and patients.

Newsletters and educational materials like the "Guide to Parents" booklet developed at CHOP offer time-conserving, cost-efficient means of communication to patients and families. In this time of "right sizing," it is increasingly important for medical social workers to keep abreast of the community resources available to families and to help families connect with those resources. Intensive counseling cannot be done by one hospital social worker serving 250 families. Often the families live far away from CHOP. It is a far better plan to locate skilled local counselors and, if necessary, to educate them on the effects of spina bifida and chronic illness on families, so that they are aware of the special circumstances. By coordinating services through community agencies, medical social workers save precious time to work with families in crisis.

Interventions

The choice of treatment modalities for the spina bifida social worker at CHOP is determined in part by the individual family, in part by the child's age and the extent of the child's disability, and in part by the constraints of time and funding. A well-educated, intact family with good extended family supports and financial means may be served best by the social worker with time-limited crisis intervention, education, and advocacy, on an as-needed basis. The single parent with a substance abuse problem, five children, and limited finances, may be served best through case management. The role of the social worker in that situation would be to locate appropriate family and community resources such as in-patient and out-patient drug programs. The social worker could help that parent get Social Security Disability for the disabled child and thus secure minimal financial stability for the family.

It is also the social worker's responsibility to ensure that each disabled child receives the proper medical care and the parenting he or she needs. The social worker spends time in monitoring medical appointments and networking with community agencies to ensure the safety of the child. A direct, authoritative approach communicates concern and establishes an action plan so that all involved players know their responsibilities and the consequences of not following through.

The spina bifida social worker at CHOP often works individually with the older patients themselves to develop independence and a social life apart from their families. If the child is severely learning disabled or mentally retarded, then much more effort is put into work with the family and community supports. The course we offer to young adolescents, "Meeting the Challenge," can be utilized only by those adolescents with the cognitive ability to think about their behaviors and social skills. These young people benefit greatly from this educational approach, which includes role plays and social interaction. In the situation where the child is cognitively limited and will remain dependent on parents or other caretakers for a lifetime, the focus of the social worker needs to remain on the family and on available community supports for things like weekend respite for parents, summer programs, home care, estate planning, and continued support of the family for a job well done.

Caseload size and funding also impact on a social worker's choice of treatment modality. There are a few social workers at CHOP with small caseloads, who provide intensive services to families at the hospital and in their own homes. Most social workers at CHOP, however, are responsible for large caseloads or a combination of administrative and clinical work, which limits the intensity of intervention they can offer families. Diagnostic interviews and family conferences can be offered, resulting in referrals to community agencies for other services. Establishing a trusting relationship with the family at an early stage of intervention allows the medical social worker on a chronic illness team to step in and out of focus as warranted by the ups and downs of life with a disabled child.

Stance of the Social Worker

The use of self in a relationship can either happen as a result of who we are and how we feel on a particular day or it can be planned to effect change. Social workers enter the profession with unique personalities and life experiences. Some are directive by nature and others are more reflective and more passive in relationships. Some know themselves well; others are less self-aware. For a medical social worker on a team, other professionals with their own approaches to life and work play a significant part in treatment decisions. In order to work successfully as a team, individuals must know not only themselves but also their teammates. This can be a plus, in that one team member can take on the role of comforter and another the role of educator or director. The nurse and social worker on the CHOP spina bifida team often cross disciplinary boundaries. Both are comfortable with this. Each is clear about specific roles on the team, but at times, the social worker can offer medical information to the family and at times the nurse offers emotional support and referrals to community resources. Because we are comfortable with this at CHOP, it works for us. There are also families that trigger countertransferential reactions in professionals. If these reactions get in the way, the CHOP spina bifida team members purposefully may decide that one or another team member take on the primary interactions with the family. The team works in whatever necessary way toward the goal of helping the patient and family.

Use of Outside Resources

The role of the CHOP spina bifida social worker as diagnostician, as supporter of child and family, as advocate, and as educator is limited by time, by caseload size, and by access to families. Outside agencies provide many services, so that together we can offer the best family-centered care. Families routinely are referred to agencies that assist with finances, education, psychosocial needs, and community-based medical care. The medical social worker serves generally as case manager to ensure that each family is aware of needed resources and actually accesses the services that are available. The CHOP booklet "Guide to Spina Bifida" provides families with access to articles on spina bifida, lists of resources, and information on educational programs. Some families manage most things on their own; other families need support and encouragement, with a dose of assertiveness training; and yet others need to be walked through the process. Occasionally, a child protective agency referral is needed to ensure that a child living in a dysfunctional family gets the necessary services to protect its health and development. Figure 7.1 is an ecomap of Bob's support structure.

Reassessment

Each time a patient and family come to CHOP, either in clinic or during hospitalization, there is a reassessment of both child and family. At clinic appointments, the doctor, the nurse, the orthopedic surgeon, the physical therapist, and the social worker offer individual assessments of the family's progress and compare evaluations at the team meeting. Recommendations are made and discussed, and a plan is agreed upon. A clinic visit summary is sent to the family and to their local physician to keep lines of communication open. Social worker, nurse, and physical therapist provide follow-up with family and community agencies as needed.

Transfer or Termination

The relationship between the CHOP social worker and the spina bifida patient and family is terminated when the child reaches adulthood and transfers care to an adult facility. Sadly, there is an occasional death, which terminates the relationship earlier, and at times, families choose to use another medical care facility or move to another state.

FIGURE 7.1. Ecomap for Bob Kelly

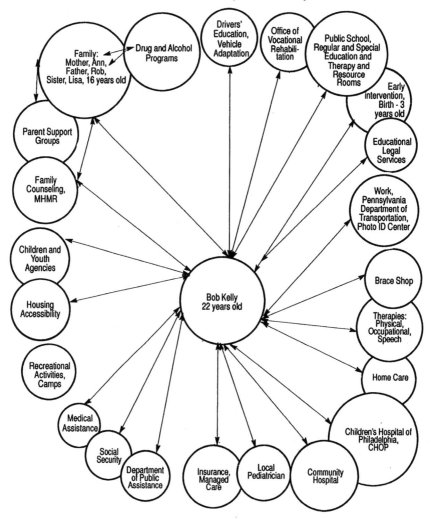

Although Bob is 22 years old, he continues to be followed at CHOP for spina bifida. The policies of the hospital are loose enough to permit young adults the option of remaining at CHOP. Adult facilities that offer a team approach to care specializing in spina bifida are few and far between. The financial incentive for doctors to develop comprehensive practices is nonexistent, because nearly all of our patients are covered by medical assistance in adulthood, and grant support is rare. Bob uses his local physician for some of his care. He comes to CHOP for annual clinic visits, as well as for orthopedic, urologic, or neurosurgical crises. He and his mother are comfortable with that arrangement. At some point, it will be necessary to transfer all of his care to an adult facility.

To measure outcome in the CHOP program we look at overall health, educational success, independence, employability, and emotional stability of the spina bifida patient and family. Patient outcomes in our clinic are compared with those of clinics across the state and the nation. Cognitive limitations and learning disabilities that accompany spina bifida interfere with goals of adult independence and employability. There is a desperate need for supported living situations and supported employment, so that as many disabled adults as possible can be productive people.

Case Conclusion

Bob Kelly is working a part-time job and loving it. He would like to work full-time. His mother is concerned about losing the Social Security payment she receives for Bob, which pays the rent, if Bob increases his employment to full-time. She is also concerned about medical insurance, which is not offered by the state in its role as Bob's employer. The job of the CHOP spina bifida social worker with this family is not complete. Eventual transition to an adult specialty care facility will change the cast of professionals assigned to Bob, but in the meanwhile social work assistance to this young adult and his family must continue. His family and a health care team will continue to assist Bob when medical, social, emotional, and financial crises occur.

Differential Discussion

The treatment of children with spina bifida by a specialty team at CHOP will continue as long as there are children who need this help and as long as there is funding for this important job. In the 1990s, the team will advocate for the benefits of this comprehensive specialty team approach with managed care programs so that their support and referrals will help to maintain the program. Family-centered and community-based care have always been the goal of the team. Communication with pediatricians, local community hospitals, and service agencies continues in the 1990s as it has for the program's first three decades, and linkage to community resources remains as an important task of the team social worker.

Rights of and resources for the disabled have improved in American society in the past ten years. Access to appropriate educational programs is easier now than it used to be. The Americans with Disabilities Act prevents the most blatant discrimination against the disabled in regard to employment. Disabled adults, like Bob, can find accessible housing in the City of Philadelphia. They can live independently, if they can manage cognitively and emotionally on their own. Yet, the need for supportive living arrangements continues. At present, there seem to be more employment programs for the mentally ill and drug-addicted adults than for the physically and learning disabled. Universal access to medical insurance is no longer a vibrant political issue, but it needs to be. Bob and others like him should not have to limit employment in order to keep state-provided medical insurance benefits.

A variety of social work interventions is utilized by the CHOP team in the psychosocial treatment of the family and the child with spina bifida. The extent of a patient's disability, the family's geographical location, and the educational and financial situation dictate how much or how little the CHOP social worker will intervene in any given case. Bob and his family did much for themselves over the years. Social work contributed to their knowledge of resources and the encouragement to use them.

Changes in health care funding will continue to affect service delivery. Managed-care insurance programs are here to stay. Negotiation and advocacy on behalf of patients and families remain important jobs of the CHOP social worker. Specialty care for serious, long-term health problems like spina bifida is best provided in tertiary-care facilities where staff are knowledgeable of both medical treatment and psychosocial resources. Primary care is best provided in the community. Communication between all the health care providers and professionals of all involved disciplines is essential to providing the best possible family-centered care.

REFERENCES

Administrative Policy Manual. The Children's Hospital of Philadelphia. 1995.

Batshaw, M. L. and Perret, Y. M. (1992). *Children with disabilities*. Baltimore, MD: Paul H. Brookes Publishing Co.

Charney, E. B. (1990). Myelomeningocele. In M. W. Schwartz, E. B. Charney, T. A. Curry, and S. Ludwig (Eds.), *Pediatric primary care: Problem-oriented approach*. Chicago, IL: Year Book Medical Publishers.

Gaul, G. M. (1993). *Giant steps: The story of one boy's struggle to walk*. New York: St. Martin's Press.

Ginsburg, H. M. (1990). The legal perspective: The Americans with disabilities act of 1990. *Pediatric AIDS and HIV Infection: Fetus to Adolescent 1*(14), 53-53.

Gool, J. B. and Good, J. D. (1986). *A short history of spina bifida*. Netherlands: Society for Research into Hydrocephalus and Spina Bifida.

Hagner, D. and Dileo, D. (1993). *Working together: Workplace culture, supported employment, & persons with disabilities.* Cambridge, MA: Brookline Books.

Klein, S. D. and Schleifer, M. J. (Eds.). (1993). *It isn't fair: Siblings of children with disabilities.* Westport, CN: Bergin & Garvey.

Lollar, D. J. (1994). Educational issues among children with spina bifida. Health and Rehabilitation Psychologists of Atlanta, Shepherd Spinal Center. Atlanta, GA.

McCollum, A. (1975). *The chronically ill child: A guide for parents and professionals.* New Haven, CN: Yale University Press.

Powell, T. H. and Ahrenhold-Gallagher, P. (1993). *Brothers and sisters–A special part of exceptional families.* Baltimore, MD: Paul H. Brookes Publishing Co.

Rowley-Kelly, F. L. and D. H. Reigel. (1993). *Teaching the student with spina bifida.* Baltimore, MD: Paul H. Brookes Publishing Co.

Social Security Administration Office of Disability. (1994). *Red book on work incentives: A summary guide to social security and supplemental security income work incentives for people with disabilities,* SSA Pub. No. 64-030 ICN 436900. Washington, DC.

The Spina Bifida Program. (1995). *Answering your questions about spina bifida,* Department of General Pediatrics, Children's National Medical Center. Washington, DC.

Thompson, C. E. (1986). *Raising a handicapped child: A helpful guide for parents of the physically disabled.* New York: William Morrow and Company.

Wehman, P. (1992). *Life beyond the classroom: Transition strategies for young people with disabilities.* Baltimore, MD: Paul H. Brookes Publishing Co.

Williamson, G. G. (1987). *Children with spina bifida: Early intervention and preschool programming.* Baltimore, MD: Paul H. Brookes Publishing Co.

Chapter 8

Family House/Womanspace:
A Residential Treatment Program
for Women and Their Children

Randee Morose Gallo

CONTEXT

Description of the Setting

The Family House/Womanspace Program is a division of Resources for Human Development, a private nonprofit corporation. Five separate programs are located in four Pennsylvania sites and one site in Louisiana. The Family House Program in Harvey, Louisiana is a six-month residential treatment program for chemically dependent women and their children. Ten women and no more than 20 children reside in the program. Family House/Womanspace sites are residential settings that have a number of therapeutic elements. The range and depth of the elements suggest the complexities of a comprehensive approach to treating mothers and children together in the presence of substance abuse problems or a recent history of drug abuse (Morris and Schinke, 1990). A multidiscipinary team consists of a primary therapist, a family therapist, life skills counselors, a prevention specialist, and a parenting specialist. Social workers at each site provide individual, group, and milieu therapy in the capacity of one of the aforementioned positions. At the Family House sites, the children also receive services. All children, from birth to five years old, receive a developmental assessment from which an educational plan is constructed. While school-age children attend local schools and receive on-site tutoring, all other children attend an on-site preschool intervention/prevention program. The children participate in self-esteem building and reading readiness activities while learning coping and decision-making skills

(Odim-Winn and Dunagan, 1991). Verbal children attend group and individual play therapy. (Johnston, 1991).

Substance abuse is seen and treated in this setting not only as a disease but as a family illness (Balis, 1989; Hanna, 1989). The challenges and rewards of Family House/Womanspace and other community-based services for substance-abusing mothers and their children are summarized by Pearlman, West, and Dalton (1982):

> The rewards of working in such a program are many and varied. In the daily contacts with mother and child, small successes are readily noticed. As mothers and children become more able to enjoy and appreciate each other, not only are the lives of the women enriched, but prospects for their children's future are enhanced. (p. 558)

In Louisiana, Family House is funded by the state and serves all areas of the state. Funds are distributed to and the program monitored by the parish in which it is located. Clients entering treatment must be eligible for medical, food, and financial assistance.

Policy

Female Chemical Addiction

Public attitudes toward the use and abuse of alcohol and other drugs affect social policy, the laws governing alcohol use, and the nature of treatment (Balis, 1989). The large number of chemically dependent women and their children require attention from society. More than 375,000 babies are born each year in the United States with traces of illegal drugs (Viadero, 1992). After their first year, approximately 80 percent of infants born with drugs in their systems are living in foster care rather than with their biological families (Macura, 1989). The United States spends over $2 billion annually to pay for the expensive neonatal care required by low birthweight babies, often caused by their mother's drug or alcohol addiction. (See Walther, Mason, and Preisinger, this volume).

Female chemical addiction crosses all cultural and socioeconomic lines. The problem is not confined to urban areas. Michael Dorris' book, *The Broken Cord,* addresses the crisis Native Americans are facing in their battle against alcoholism; approximately one-half of the adult Native American population is chemically dependent to some degree and an alarming number of babies are born with Fetal Alcohol Syndrome (FAS) or Fetal Alcohol Effect (FAE) (Dorris, 1989). Nationally, FAS is the third leading known cause for mental retardation in the United States, with an estimated 1,800 to 3,000 babies affected each year. Approximately 36,000 infants each year exhibit FAE, a less severe manifestation of FAS (Smith et al., 1987).

Historically, treatment facilities have not met the specialized needs of women adequately. Changing roles have further burdened women who must cope with single parenthood, poor housing, inadequate income, or affordable day-care, lack of education, and emotional problems (Coleman and Cressy, 1987). Present-day social conditions have led to the tremendous increase in use, and maternal substance abuse is known to be one of the critical factors in child abuse, neglect, and abandonment (Hanna, 1989). The rise of female addiction was strongly related to the appearance of crack cocaine. With the arrival of crack cocaine, the number of women seeking treatment has increased. Few treatment facilities allow women to enter treatment with their children. To choose treatment and leave children has been a great problem for women. In 1988, only ten treatment facilities in the nation allowed women to enter treatment with their children, and Family House, Norristown was one. All of the above have had a profound effect on the way women approach treatment and react to treatment (Regan, Ehrlich, and Finnegan, 1987).

The Anti-Drug Abuse Act of 1988, which funded President Bush's "War on Drugs," did not include alcoholism. This omission was not accidental. According to federal estimates, 13 percent of the nation's adult population will have alcohol abuse problems compared to 6 percent who will abuse illicit drugs; however, alcohol consumption is legal and socially acceptable, and the liquor industry is extremely powerful. Despite drunken-driving-related deaths, fetal alcohol syndrome, and the other devastating results of alcoholism, the memory of Prohibition as one of the country's greatest legislative failures makes the government proceed cautiously when it comes to restricting alcohol.

Policies in some states are leaning toward punishment rather than treatment. In California, the call for outreach to and treatment of addicted pregnant and postpartum women and their children was combined with criminal penalties for mothers who gave birth to babies prenatally exposed to drugs (National Center for Prevention of Child Abuse Newsletter, 1989). Mandatory reporting of drug use by pregnant women to child protective services is already in effect in several states. (Macura, 1989). However, problems with tranquilizers and painkillers most often prescribed to middle- and upper middle-class women are ignored while crack and heroin used by poor women are condemned. (Eitzen and Zinn, 1989). Middle- and upper-class women go to private physicians and hospitals, who are less likely to test or label their patients as drug addicts. Consequently, the women most targeted are poor.

In 1989, President Bush allocated $321 million in drug treatment and prevention programs in the schools. Some of the money was earmarked for treatment of women, and Family House/Womanspace was able to expand through this allocation. Still, the need exceeds program capacity. Future funding is not secure and cost-of-living allowances are not built into these grants. Recently, Womanspace was told not to accept any new clients because there were no available funds for residential treatment for uninsured people. Several weeks later, emergency allocation of funds to programs that provide residential treatment to uninsured people was made available with no guarantee for the next fiscal year. This population has been deemed potentially dangerous if not treated. It was reported that an additional strain on the system would be seen in street crime and incarceration expenses if funds were not available for treatment.

Laws Related to Confidentiality and Suspected Child Abuse and Neglect

In addition to funding, the Family House/Womanspace Program is affected by laws related to confidentiality and suspected child abuse and neglect. Federal and state laws require a written policy and procedure, which safeguards the residents' identities and records. Only with written permission from a resident or a "just-cause" court order may any information be divulged. Child Protective Services Laws in Pennsylvania and Louisiana mandate that employees in agencies such as Family House/ Womanspace report any suspicion of a child (aged 17 and under) being abused and/or neglected. A toll-free hotline is available at all times (Fujimoto and Kerson, 1989). Many of the residents have been identified as abusive or neglectful parents and are referred to Family House/Womanspace by Child Protective Services. In such cases, periodic meetings between Child Protective Services, Family House/Womanspace, and the resident are held to discuss any concerns of the parties involved as well as the progress of the resident in the area of parenting.

Technology

The Family House/Womanspace Program is affected by technology in various ways. In recent years, an increased number of clients have been diagnosed with concurrent mental health illness, primarily depression and anxiety disorders, and chemical dependency. Antidepressants such as Prozac and Zoloft have been used to treat the psychiatric problem, allowing the woman to stay in treatment for her substance abuse problem. Clients are referred to psychiatrists in the community. Drugs are prescribed on an individualized, case-by-case basis, and are seen as useful adjuncts to other forms of treatment (Balis, 1989). However, it has been increasingly difficult in some areas to find psychiatrists who will accept clients on Medical Assistance. When a psychiatrist has been identified, it takes six weeks or more to get an appointment for a Medicaid patient. Only when a woman is a danger to herself or others is there a chance to circumvent that long wait. The number of clients testing positive for HIV has also increased in the last five years. By taking drugs such as AZT, clients are able to stay healthy and fully participate in treatment. Clients who are HIV positive are referred to support agencies and local doctors who monitor their blood count and medication. The women are encouraged to rely on the program staff and their peers as well.

Computer technology has helped link the various sites to each other as well as to the corporate office. The use of fax machines allows for swift correspondence, which may be critical in securing funding, as a result cutting the waiting time for the client to be admitted. Computers are also used by the clients. At Womanspace, for example, clients may use the computer general equivalency degree (GED) program to help them prepare for the GED test (Schottenfeld, Pascale, and Sokolowski, 1992). In the Family House sites, children use computer programs that help prepare them for reading. The acquisition of computer skills, regardless how basic, helps build the self-esteem of the women and children.

Organization

Resources for Human Development has a decentralized organizational structure within which individual service units have day-to-day responsibility and are given maximum opportunity to develop personal autonomy and individual responsibility for their programs. The executive director delegates authority to corporate staff members who in turn manage, supervise, and support individual programs. Financial management is centralized. The central office maintains a separate account for each program thus assuring individual fiscal responsibility.

The Family House/Womanspace Program is unique to the corporate structure in that two program directors monitor and supervise all sites, and are also involved in program development and replication of the model. Each site has a project director who is responsible for the day-to-day operation. Program and project directors meet regularly as part of a method of continuous quality improvement (Lynch and Werner, 1992). Using feedback from staff and clients, they evaluate, correct, and improve the system.

At each site a multidisciplinary treatment team meets weekly to coordinate individual client work and to discuss treatment planning, clinical review, and discharge/aftercare planning. Site staff support each other and work with the staff from other sites. Family House/Womanspace Program retreats are planned periodically to share ideas within affinity groups, clarify program and individual goals and explore long-term program planning.

DECISIONS ABOUT PRACTICE

Client Description

Ethel is a 31-year-old, single, African-American woman who entered Family House, Louisiana with two daughters, Roshana, age four, and Tyesha, age two. At her request, Ethel was referred to the facility for treatment of addiction to crack cocaine by New Orleans General Hospital, where she had just completed 28 days of treatment.

Born in New Orleans and raised in Mississippi, Ethel was the third child in a family of six. She talked of being molested as a child, described herself as the "black sheep," and reported her abusive mother often told her she was no good, just like her alcoholic father. Ethel was rejected by all but one of her siblings. During Ethel's stay at Family House, the only family member to visit was her brother. When contacted by the family therapist, her mother and father verbalized support but refused to visit.

Ethel began to drink heavily at age 16, and her drinking increased steadily. She dropped out of school in tenth grade, maintained a job at a fast food restaurant for four years, and at age 26 began using cocaine. As her cocaine use escalated, her life began to spin out of control; she reported living on the street and eating out of garbage cans. Ethel entered Family House guarded, isolated from her peers, and very angry. Initially, she worked in individual sessions and was receptive to cognitive treatment approaches (Greene and Ephross, 1991). Later response to her peer group and work on a feeling level allowed for behavioral changes. After completing the treatment phase of the program, Ethel decided she needed the added time and support of the transitional housing component (Hepworth and Larsen, 1986).

Ethel's daughter, Roshana, lived with her mother on the street. Ethel reported that Roshana had been terrified when, staying with a friend who sold drugs, she witnessed a man entering the premises and shooting at the occupants. Although Roshana was nearly four years old when her family entered treatment, she barely spoke and had flat affect. At Family House,

Roshana was nurtured and encouraged to identify her feelings, and her expression of anger was considered a sign of progress. She developed language skills and learned to interact playfully with other children. Ethel's younger daughter Tyesha, who is two years old, lived with Ethel's parents, who were reluctant to relinquish custody of Tyesha but did so when Ethel threatened to go to court and agreed to enter treatment with her children. Although Tyesha had some language delays, they were not severe and she was a happy toddler.

Definition of the Client

The client is defined as the mother and her resident children. Because the Family House/Womanspace Program views addiction as a family concern, to treat an identified client alone would assume her addiction had no impact on others or others did not affect her addiction. The definition of a client, therefore, expands to include other significant persons within the client's environment (Ford, 1989). Treatment plans were written for Ethel, Roshana, and Tyesha. An effort was made to include Ethel's family of origin, but they were unwilling to participate. Ethel was unable to identify anyone other than her children as significant.

Goals

Family House/Womanspace has the following goals: (1) to increase and maintain periods of sobriety, (2) to provide a supportive environment that meets the needs of each woman as perceived by each woman, (3) to develop effective parenting skills, (4) to demonstrate an ability to live independently in the community, and (5) to provide opportunities that promote their greatest developmental growth of each child. Each goal has outcome measures. One measure, the four-level system, is task oriented; measurable tasks must be completed before advancing through the program. The four levels are orientation/stabilization, education, integration, and re-entry/completion. Each level has three areas of concentration–addiction/recovery, parenting, and life skills–and each area is monitored by a designated staff person within the discipline most related to it.

Individual goals and tasks designed to meet those goals are formulated with the adult client each month. Goal formulation is a part of the treatment process (Balis, 1989). The client meets with a life skills counselor to formulate goals in areas such as budgeting, health, hygiene, time-management, and socialization/recreation. Ethel focused primarily on budgeting and socialization/recreation (Morris and Schinke, 1990). The client also meets with the parenting specialist to develop a plan in addressing areas of concern regarding her children (Nelson-Zlupko, Kauffman, and Dore, 1995). There was staff concern regarding Ethel's lack of age-appropriate expectations, which often resulted in her becoming verbally abusive to her children. Ethel would become enraged if Roshana and Tyesha would soil their clothes or get their hands and faces dirty. She would shout at them and promptly bathe them and change their clothing. Because Ethel was sober and no longer homeless, she did not want her children's appearance and behavior to hint at the life she was trying to leave behind. It was difficult for Ethel to understand that it was important that Roshana and Tyesha participate in play rather than simply observe. Ethel agreed that this was an area she wanted to address. In order to maintain her sobriety, Ethel also met monthly with a primary therapist to discuss goals that would help her better understand her addiction and relapse triggers. Ethel focused on identifying and appropriately addressing her feelings, and she met twice weekly with her primary therapist to discuss them. Although Ethel's goals remained fairly consistent in all three areas, her tasks changed each month, allowing her to first make behavioral changes and later to gain insight.

Roshana and Tyesha each had a treatment plan and individual education plan formulated within the first month of treatment. Although plans are formally reviewed at 90 days, they may be updated when progress is made or new problems arise. A developmental assessment helped formulate the individual education plan. In addition to both girls' language delay, Roshana was also very timid and often appeared frightened when placed in new surroundings or with people with whom she was unfamiliar. Working with Ethel and the children, the parenting and prevention specialists developed goals addressing the language delay and Roshana's fear of new people and places.

Use of Contract

A preliminary treatment plan is completed 7 days after admission; an initial treatment plan is completed 14 days later; and every 30 days after the initial treatment plan, an updated treatment plan is developed. Plans are developed with the client and each member of the interdisciplinary team. A multidiscipinary team meeting is held each week to discuss updated treatment planning for designated clients. The entire family is presented, and the goals and tasks agreed upon with the client are presented. Every 90 days, clients' progress is discussed in a formal clinical case consultation. The client also presents her long- and short-term goals and plan for achieving them. The children are informally reassessed on an ongoing basis and their individual education plan is updated and modified as goals are accomplished. The children's progress is also assessed at the 90-day clinical case consultation, and their treatment may be revised. Finally, clients are reassessed dvelopmentally prior to discharge.

Family House/Womanspace also utilize behavioral contracts (Compton and Galaway, 1994). Often used when a client is in jeopardy of being discharged from the program, such contracts identify concrete behaviors that are to be changed, as well as new behaviors to adopt. Contracts are written by the team and presented in a clinical setting with team members present so that problems can be identified and discussed. The client and a representative of the team sign the contract. Most contracts are for no more than two weeks in duration. At the end of the time designated in the contract, each contract is reviewed by the team and client and disposition is considered. As a result of the review, the contract may be amended, discontinued, or the client may be discharged. In signing the contract, the client agrees to make the changes stated; by not doing so, she is choosing to leave treatment. Clients are encouraged to use their peers in the program for support.

Ethel was involved in several behavioral contracts. One concerned inappropriate behavior regarding her children, and another concerned her inappropriately taking food from the program (Henry, 1989). Ethel had become increasingly verbally abusive to her daughters. The contract was a result of Ethel's reaction to her children playing outdoors after it had rained, the culmination of many such incidents. All of the children were in play clothes and were making "mud pies" with the help of the prevention specialist. Ethel screamed at them, telling them they were nothing more than pigs playing in the mud and should be treated like animals. Chaos erupted with children crying and mothers arguing. Ethel's contract included educational assignments and concrete behavioral changes. Readings and tasks helped her to learn and practice alternative interactions as well as understand age-appropriate behavior and alternative parenting approaches (Dinkmeyer and McKay, 1982; Plasse, 1995). For example, when she became upset with her children's appearance, she was to walk away, find a peer, and discuss what it meant to her to see them unkempt. She was also given an audiotape to review, which discussed the importance of play in child development. Ethel's contract regarding her taking food from the program was also based on behavioral changes as well as cognitive tasks to help her gain insight into why she was taking the food. Writing about her past experiences allowed her to see the connection between her being homeless and hungry and her present behavior. Concrete tasks, such as listing mealtimes and creating a snack time schedule for her children and herself, gave her control of her family's eating patterns and eliminated the fear of going hungry. Both contracts were completed, therefore discontinued.

Meeting Place

I met with Ethel in the individual counseling room, a comfortable space with several love seats and chairs. We also met frequently in work situations, particularly when her house chore was cooking and she was in the kitchen. Sometimes, Ethel and I met in her apartment following her treatment at Family House and her participation in our transitional housing program. As the program director of the Family House/Womanspace Program, I am based in Pennsylvania and travel to Louisiana every two or three months. Therefore, Ethel and I also used the telephone to maintain contact. A designated time would be assigned and Ethel would call. This arrangement may not be ideal but it allowed for ongoing contact.

Use of Time

Family House, Louisiana has a six-month residential component and an optional six-month transitional housing component. The first 30 days of treatment are used for orientation, assessment, and stabilization of the families; the next 60 are used to focus on education in the areas of addiction, life skills, and parenting; and the following 60 are used to help the client integrate all she has learned. The last 30 are used to re-enter the community. Each level has goals, tasks, and outcomes. For those families entering the transitional housing component, the goals focus on independent living, work/education/vocational training, and mentorship to the families currently in treatment. Therefore, residents attend educational or vocational training, secure employment, volunteer two hours a week at Family House, and develop a community support system.

Interventions

Trust and support are established through listening, nurturing, availability and flexibility, setting mutual goals, establishing limits in a caring manner, and being supportive of the client's strength (Morris and Schinke, 1990). Treatment modalities such as psychoeducation groups; psychotherapy groups; individual, family, and milieu therapies; and self-help groups are utilized to achieve trust and provide support. The clients participate in many group activities that provide a cooperative climate for growth (Napier and Gershenfeld, 1985).

Because of the evidence linking childhood sexual abuse and addiction, groups also address these special needs of women (Tsai and Wagner, 1978). In spite of the growing evidence, not many treatment programs offer services for sexual abuse survivors. Evidence suggests that short-term group therapy is effective in ameliorating the guilt and offering hope for childhood sexual survivors (Bollerud, 1990; Yandow, 1989). Ethel revealed she had been sexually abused by her uncle as a child, and that at age 26 she was raped and left nude on the side of a highway. At Family House, a time-limited group addressing childhood sexual abuse helped her to address her anger, guilt, and shame.

In addition, she participated in two individual therapy sessions, two psychotherapy groups, and groups or seminars on addiction education, nutrition, life skills, parenting, abuse/neglect prevention, and a minimum of three 12-step meetings each week. While living in the transitional housing program, she attended an outpatient group at the Jefferson Parish West Bank Drug and Alcohol Clinic each week, the Family House Relapse Prevention Support Group, three 12-step meetings, and a transitional housing community meeting weekly.

Roshana and Tyesha attended the on-site Preschool Prevention/Intervention Program, and Roshana also participated in individual and group play therapy. Following treatment, the children participated in the weekly Children's Aftercare Support Group.

Stance of the Social Worker

My first meeting with Ethel took place two weeks after she entered treatment. I meet with identified clients each time I travel to Louisiana as well as attend a weekly community meeting. Ethel initially appeared angry, intimidating, and resistant. My second meeting with Ethel was two months later during a clinical case consultation in which she was called in for stealing food and feeding her two-year-old daughter a bottle at night when instructed not to do so, as Tyesha was already evidencing problems with her teeth. The staff was also concerned with Ethel's obsession with regards to her children's cleanliness. It was apparent that the staff was frustrated with Ethel's behavior and with the fact that Ethel was not willing to change it. I realized that Ethel's ways of thinking, reasoning, and interpreting reality sharply contrasted with the staff's, and neither understood the other (Goldstein, 1986). When children are mistreated, it is not unusual for the staff to assume this posture. The staff was ready to discharge Ethel. My role in that meeting and subsequent meetings became one of interpreter and advocate for Ethel. The staff saw Ethel as harsh, critical, and demanding, and interpreted her behavior as defiant. They believed Ethel was unwilling and unable to follow the guidelines of the program. Each confrontation became a power struggle.

On the other hand, I saw Ethel making an effort to parent her children differently than she had been parented. She wanted to assure they would be well-fed and well-dressed. I began by asking Ethel what not giving her daughter a bottle would mean. Ethel became upset and spoke of her homelessness and inability to feed her children. She stated she would never let them be hungry again. As we explored the issue further, it was apparent that Ethel's homelessness was the root of her stealing food and her need for her children not to look like they lived on the street. Ethel began to sob as I appreciated her struggle and validated her effort to be a good mother. She said no one understood how important it was for her to be a good mother. As we were able to explore the connections between her homelessness and her resistance to following the nutritional eating and play guidelines, Ethel was able to understand and change her behavior. The staff was also able to understand that Ethel's stealing of food and rigidity around her children's cleanliness and behavior were symbolic and not oppositional. As Ethel struggled through treatment, the staff learned to identify the intent of her behavior. The staff validated her efforts and supported her with new ideas, which allowed mutual trust to develop. The power struggle gave way to a partnership.

Ethel and her primary therapist asked that I be actively involved with Ethel's treatment. Both felt it would give Ethel the added support she needed. My acting as her advocate was a new experience for Ethel (Nelson-Zlupko, Kauffman, and Dore, 1995). She said she was first suspicious as to why I would want to get to know her and then afraid that when I did get to know her I would abandon her. She had never felt important or had anyone advocate for her before our meeting. At times, Ethel acted like an adolescent testing the limits by using my position and our relationship to bend the rules. This was an opportunity for me to confront that behavior and set limits (Hepworth and Larsen, 1986). It was new for Ethel to have someone care for her enough to set limits while still supporting her. Ultimately, Ethel was able to advocate for herself.

Use of Outside Resources

With the support of their life-skills counselor, clients take responsibility to negotiate obtaining cash, food stamps, Medical Assistance, and WIC as soon as they are admitted to Family House/Womanspace. Medical appointments are requested by the client but made by the unit assistant. Outside supports, which help with medication and housing, are utilized for clients with HIV-related illnesses. Support services such as

Planned Parenthood, community housing programs, outpatient drug and alcohol clinics, 12-step sponsors, and local schools and churches are used during and after treatment. An ecomap (Figure 8.1) was used in helping Ethel identify her resources, support systems, and stressors.

FIGURE 8.1. Ecomap for Ethel

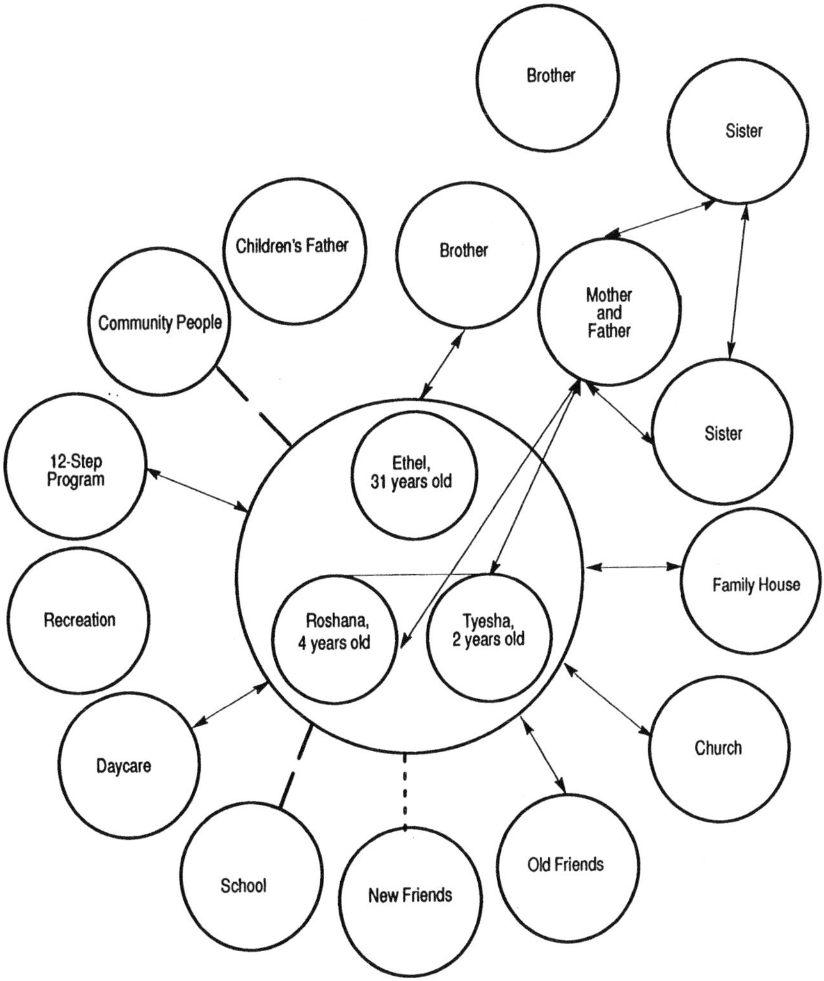

Transfer or Termination

Ethel and her daughters completed the Family House treatment program and continued in the Family House transitional housing program. Graduation was very exciting for Ethel, as it was the first time she finished any kind of educational or treatment program. She was encouraged to invite her family and friends. During the graduation ceremony, the staff shared their history of Ethel's stay in the program. Ethel wept as she shared that she was now a responsible, disciplined woman who had learned to listen and was now able to feel, love, cry, and be proud of who she was. Her presentation was followed by a candle-lighting ceremony, a tribute from her peers, induction into the alumni group, and recognition of the work that had been done by Roshana and Tyesha.

Case Conclusion

Initially, treatment focused on identifying problems in addiction. Ethel participated in group, educational, and individual counseling; used a journal to become more aware of her behaviors and emotions; and was receptive to cognitive learning. Initially, she was more responsive to individual counseling than group counseling. Ethel's destructive behavior was addressed in writing in the form of a written behavioral contract to which she was able to respond favorably. As treatment continued, issues of childhood sexual abuse and inappropriate expression of anger surfaced. During treatment, Ethel developed the ability to communicate with others, she sought support from the recovering community, and became an active member in her church and a mentor for the current clients who often seek her support. Ethel enrolled and is participating in a GED program and works part-time. A housing program helped her find affordable housing when she completed the transitional housing phase of treatment. She has been sober for two years.

During the early phase of treatment, Ethel appeared harsh and demanding of her daughters. Interactions included loud orders that often resulted in her children's withdrawing or crying. Ethel has become more aware of positive discipline methods and age-appropriate expectations. She is attentive and her positive interactions with her children have a positive influence. Both children have become more verbal and appear to laugh and smile more often. Roshana is less fearful in new situations. Prior to leaving Family House, Roshana was enrolled in a Head Start program and Tyesha in day care. Both children continue to develop their language and socialization skills.

Differential Discussion

Although some attempt was made to include Ethel's parents in family therapy, it may have been beneficial to have tried even harder. Their occasional visits with the children may have been an opportunity for an informal family meeting. Ethel's brother was supportive of her throughout her treatment, and it may have been helpful to have him participate in family therapy even when all others refused. Ethel's relationship with her family remains tenuous and stressful.

Ethel's legal problems might also have been addressed. She had been arrested several times for shoplifting, mentioned she had fines to pay, but did little to address the issue. The life skills counselor encouraged Ethel to call the courts and work out a payment schedule, but when Ethel refused, the matter was dropped. Following treatment, Ethel was summoned to court and temporarily lost her job for ignoring her fines. She could have been incarcerated for this, but instead the fines were lifted when she completed one year of treatment at Family House. Since the program's experience with Ethel, arrangements to pay all debts, including court fines, must be made in order to complete treatment.

Finally, since I am the program director, my personal involvement in Ethel's treatment intimidated some of the staff. My goal was to assist the clinical team in gaining a better understanding of Ethel's underlying behavior and alleviate some of their frustration. The staff, knowing I was an advocate for Ethel, allowed her to deviate from the some of the program guidelines as they assumed I would approve of all she did. Although my involvement was clinical, some of the staff perceived my involvement as personal. It may have been helpful to formally state my position in a staff meeting and reinforce the need for Ethel to follow the program guidelines. An educational approach in the form of an in-service training may have assisted the staff in understanding the difference between advocacy and being indulgent or enabling.

REFERENCES

Balis, S. A. (1989). Rehabilitation center for multi-faceted treatment of alcoholism. In T. S. Kerson and Associates (Eds.), *Social work in health settings: Practice in context*. Binghamton, NY: The Haworth Press, pp. 353-369.

Bollerud, K. (1990). A model for the treatment of trauma-related syndromes among chemically dependent inpatient women. *Journal of Substance Abuse Treatment, 7*, 83-87.

Coleman, J. W., and Cressy, D. R. (1987). *Social problems*. New York: Harper & Row.

Compton, B. R., and Galaway, B. (1994). *Social work processes.* Pacific Grove, CA: Brooks/Cole Publishing Co.

Dinkmeyer, D., and McKay, G. D. (1982). *The parents handbook.* Circle Pines, MN: American Guidance Service.

Dorris, M. (1989). *The broken cord.* New York: Harper & Row.

Eitzen, D. S. and Zinn, M. B. (1989). *Social problems.* Boston, MA: Allyn & Bacon.

Ford, C. A. (1989). Epilepsy in childhood: pediatric neurology clinic. In T. S. Kerson and Associates (Eds.), *Social work in health settings: Practice in context.* Binghamton, NY: The Haworth Press, pp. 137-156.

Fujimoto, M., and Kerson, T. S. (1989). Emergency room: Help for a family with an abused child. In T. S. Kerson and Associates (Eds.), *Social work in health settings: Practice in context.* Binghamton, New York: The Haworth Press, pp. 47-66.

Goldstein, H. (1986). A cognitive-humanistic approach to the hard-to-reach client. *Social Casework, 67*(1), 27-36.

Greene, R. R., and Ephross, P. H. (1991). *Human behavior theory and social work practice.* Binghamton, NY: Aldine de Gruyter.

Hanna, M. (Ed.). (1989). ODAP creates task force to address maternal addiction problem. *Addictions Association of Pennsylvania Journal, 1*, 40.

Henry, R. (1989). The importance of assessment for women entering treatment. *Addictions Association of Pennsylvania Journal, 1*, 40.

Hepworth, D. H., and Larsen, J. A. (1986). *Direct social work practice: Theories and skills.* Chicago, IL: The Dorsey Press.

Johnston, M. E. (1991). Multiple losses in children of chemically dependent families. In N. B. Webb (Ed). *Play therapy with children in crisis.* New York: Guilford Press, pp. 276-292.

Lynch, R. F., and Werner, T. J. (1992). *Continuous improvement: Teams and tools.* Atlanta, GA: Qual Team, Inc.

Macura, R. M. (Ed.). (1989). Crack. *Juvenile and Family Court Newsletter, 6*, 8.

Morris, S. K. and Schinke, S. P. (1990). Treatment needs and services for mothers with dual diagnosis: Substance abuse and mental illness. *Journal of Offender Counseling, 15*(1), 64-84.

Napier, R. W., and Gershenfeld, M. K. (1985). *Groups.* Boston: Houghton Mifflin Co.

National Center For Prevention of Child Abuse Newsletter. (1989). 1(2), 1.

Nelson-Zlupko, L., Kauffman, E., and Dore, M. M. (1995). Gender differences in drug addiction and treatment: Implications for social work intervention with substance-abusing women. *Social Work, 40*(1), 45-54.

Odim-Winn, D., and Dungan, D. E. (1991). *Prenatally exposed kids in school.* Freeport, NY: Educational Activities, Inc.

Pearlman, P., West, M., and Dalton, J. (1982). Mothers and children together: parenting in a substance abuse program. In B. Reed, G. Beschner, and J. Mondaro (Eds.), *Treatment services for drug dependent women.* Washington, DC: U. S. Government Printing Office.

Plasse, B. R. (1995). Parenting groups for recovering addicts in a day treatment center. *Social Work, 40*(1), 65-74.

Regan, D. O., Ehrlich, S. M., and Finnegan, L. (1987). Infants and drug addicts: at risk for child abuse, neglect, and placement in foster care. *Neurotoxicology and Teratology, 9*, 315-319.

Schottenfeld, R. S., Pascale, R., and Sokolowski, S. (1992). Matching services to needs: Vocational services for substance abusers. *Journal of Substance Abuse Treatment, 9*, 3-8.

Tsai, M., and Wagner, N. (1978). Therapy groups for women sexually abused as children. *Archives for Sexual Behavior, 7*(5), 417-427.

Viadero, D. (1992, January 29). New research finds little lasting harm for 'crack' children. *Education Week, 1*, 10-11.

Yandow, V. (1989). Alcoholism in women. *Psychiatric Annals, 19*, 243-247.

Chapter 9

Residential Care Facility: Treatment of a Child with Severe Disabilities

Mary O'Neill

CONTEXT

Description of the Setting

St. Edmond's Home for Children is a 40-bed, private, not-for-profit intermediate care facility for the mentally retarded (ICF/MR). The facility is licensed to provide 24-hour residential care for severely and profoundly involved children ranging in age from 2 to 21. Children are evaluated and admitted to the facility based on their ability to benefit physically and cognitively from the services offered. In addition, the emotional, physical, and financial needs of the child's natural family are considered when determining eligibility for placement at St. Edmond's. Once a child has been placed in the facility, he or she usually resides there until reaching age 21, unless advanced physical or mental development necessitates discharge to a less restrictive environment. For example, if a child begins to ambulate independently, St. Edmond's small physical structure would inhibit that child from reaching his or her full potential; therefore, he or she would be referred for discharge to a larger facility. In a similar sense, if a child begins to develop advanced expressive and receptive communication skills, St. Edmond's may have difficulty providing that child with a socially stimulating peer group, since the majority of residents are nonverbal. Consequently, the child would be referred for discharge to a facility that could provide that particular opportunity for growth and development.

In 1987, St. Edmond's was licensed as an ICF/MR. Prior to that conversion, the majority of residents were diagnosed with physical involvements, and a few were diagnosed as functioning within the mild range of mental retardation. However, as the funding for in-home services and respite care grew, these children who were considered "higher functioning" were increasingly able to reside at home. Therefore, children who were considered "lower functioning"–those who were more physically involved and functioned in the severe or profound range of mental retardation–were considered more appropriate for residential placement. In response to the growing societal need for this type of facility, St. Edmond's (under the supervision of the State Departments of Public Welfare and Health) began converting beds to ICF/MR funding in 1987 and were instructed to have all children without a diagnosis of mental retardation discharged within one year. Since that time, the majority of children residing at St. Edmond's have diagnoses of severe cerebral palsy and severe to profound mental retardation. Most residents are wheelchair-bound and are nonverbal. The neurological and physical disabilities of the children may be attributed to a number of causes ranging from genetic disorders and birth defects to birth trauma and failure to thrive. It is the objective of the interdisciplinary team of professionals to assist each child in achieving his or her potential and in living a quality life, which is particular to each child. St. Edmond's exists to offer its residents a broad spectrum of services and to help them function at their greatest capacity, both physically and mentally.

The Social Service Department has always been a vital part of the interdisciplinary team at St. Edmond's. The department consists of one director of social service and one family caseworker. The director of social service is responsible for all admissions and discharges to the facility; monitoring all residents' school placements; communicating with state, regional, and county offices of mental retardation, and departments of human service and other community agencies; individual, family and group counseling of residents and their families; investigating allegations of abuse or neglect; and other tasks deemed necessary by the administrator. The family caseworker is responsible for coordinating services and concerns of all 40 residents' families. He or she serves as the liaison between the residents and their families, advocates on behalf of the families at all team meetings, and offers supportive counseling to families when necessary. The Social Service Department is also involved in the reporting of incidents that occur at the facility and in most administrative decisions.

Policy

Internal policies originate from the director of Catholic Social Services/ Archdiocese of Philadelphia, the Board of Directors, and St. Edmond's

Home Administration. These policies typically affect services offered, organizational structure and mission, and general facility procedures. External policies that affect the continuum of care originate from a variety of sources. Since St. Edmond's is licensed as an ICF/MR, we are mandated to abide by ICF/MR regulations. Funding is provided by the federal government through Medical Assistance according to the Social Security Act (Long-Term Care Division). Federal funds are distributed to the Pennsylvania Department of Public Welfare (DPW), and that body mandates a per diem rate for each resident living at St. Edmond's. In addition, DPW contracts with the Pennsylvania Department of Health to conduct an annual survey to ensure that the facility is in compliance with federal ICF/MR regulations. DPW also conducts its own annual Inspection of Care Survey to ensure that each individual resident is receiving the appropriate level of care at St. Edmond's. In addition, St. Edmond's must abide by all federal, state, and local laws and ordinances, which include but are not limited to health and welfare safety codes; federal labor laws; life safety codes; OBRA (Omnibus Budget Reconciliation Act) standards; Federal Social Security laws; state public welfare codes; nurse practice regulations; Medical Assistance regulations (Title 55, Chapter 6210, Public Welfare code); and Public Law 94-142, which mandates educational services for all residents.

A system of managed care could affect the delivery of service to St. Edmond's residents in a variety of ways. Managed care would bring a medical, model-oriented case manager into the forefront, who may decide that St. Edmond's is too expensive or too intense a program for a given child, and who may advocate for that child to receive services in the family home, which would result in a decrease in the census for the facility and a possible decrease in quality of care for the child. The case manager would add another level of "gatekeeper" to an already complex system of funding streams and services, but this person could serve as a single source of accurate information on a given resident. If people are theoretically allotted a certain number of doctor visits per year, it is uncertain whether the children residing at St. Edmond's would be allotted a sufficient number of visits to meet their extreme medical needs. In addition, if referrals to a specialist are necessary in a managed care system, the speed with which the residents receive sometimes life-saving treatment would be crucial.

Technology

Advances in medical technology have increased the life expectancy of children with severe physical and mental disabilities. Since children with this type of diagnosis now live longer, there is an increase in the need for residential facilities, like St. Edmond's, that are equipped to care for them. In recent years, great progress has been made in developing various types of equipment that enable even the most physically involved child to function independently. This specialized equipment often provides the children with the opportunity to utilize minute body movements in an effort to control their surroundings. Some of the children residing at St. Edmond's who function at a higher cognitive level use technology such as environmental control systems to turn appliances on and off (such as lights, television, and radio); computerized voice machines to speak (with an appropriate switch for access); and power wheelchairs that they can move using a headswitch or joystick (Romanski et al., 1994). Children who function at a lower cognitive level are also able to use adapted switches to operate simple toys, tape recorders, and the like. Other types of technology employed at St. Edmond's include hydraulic lifts, both in the bathrooms and in facility vehicles; specialized bathtubs with a whirl-pool function; and multisensory equipment (aromatherapy machines; visual, auditory, and tactile stimulation machines; voice-activated picture projec-tors). These particular technological advancements assist staff in caring for and providing programming for the residents.

St. Edmond's is part of a statewide database that includes all of the children residing in the facility and the benefits (for example, Social Security Disability Insurance and Medical Assistance) that they are receiving. The information is provided through tracking the census of residents and billing for leave days, hospital days, and facility days. In addition, all admissions and discharges are immediately reported to the state database in order to maintain accurate records.

Organization

St. Edmond's is governed by the director of Catholic Social Services/ Archdiocese of Philadelphia and by a Board of Directors. Although the primary decision-making power rests with the administrator, the interdis-ciplinary team (program coordinators, therapists, nurses, residential supervi-sors, and social service representatives) advises on matters concerning health and programming. Since St. Edmond's is a relatively small facility, the director of social service reports directly to the administrator and is con-sulted frequently regarding administrative issues. The facility is staffed by approximately 120 full- and part-time employees who provide the 24-hour care of the residents.

Part of St. Edmond's mission is to provide as "homelike" an atmo-sphere for its residents as possible. Consequently, the atmosphere is informal and family-like. Administrative and supervisory staffs are visible and often assist with the daily care and program of the children. Staff communication tends to be easy on all levels, and planning takes place in both formal and informal settings.

St. Edmond's is part of a large network, and the director of social service often acts as a case manager in order to coordinate all appropriate services. Within such a complex system of services, a social worker needs to know which agency to contact when, and exactly how to approach individuals within that agency to secure necessary services and resources for each resident (Epstein et al., 1994). For example, each county's Department of Human Services retains guardianship of a number of residents and needs to give consent for various therapeutic and programmatic interventions (Downes, 1992). Also, the social worker must be aware of the particular philosophical views of other agencies in a resident's network, because these views can effect the way in which that agency meets the resident's needs. Although St. Edmond's is mandated to work closely with the state, regional, and county offices of mental retardation, those agencies tend to be philosophically opposed to residential placement and, therefore, will advocate for children with special needs to remain in the family home (Birenbaum and Cohen, 1993).

DECISIONS ABOUT PRACTICE

Description of the Client

Linda is an 18-year-old African-American client who was born at Temple University Hospital, at which time she was found to be meconium stained as a result of fetal distress. Meconium stained means that as a result of stress, often during the birth process, fecal matter is expelled, which temporarily colors the skin of the child. Linda was kept in the Intensive Care Unit for one month. At approximately six months of age, it was noted that she was extremely microcephalic and markedly developmentally delayed. By nine months of age, Linda evidenced severe spastic quadriparesis with generalized spasticity.

After being discharged from Temple University Hospital, Linda was cared for by her mother, who shared an apartment with a friend. Linda's mother subsequently abandoned her and moved to New Jersey. Linda's mother's friend brought Linda to the Department of Public Welfare where she was temporarily committed. Linda was admitted to Childrens' Rehabilitation Hospital at one year of age, until long-term arrangements could be made for her. Her mother abducted her from the hospital three days later, and abandoned her again three days after the abduction. Linda was subsequently returned to the hospital for protective custody and supportive care.

Linda was admitted to St. Edmond's Home at the age of one- and one-half-years of age and has resided there ever since. Her mother visited a few times immediately following admission, but she has not had contact with Linda since 1982, and her whereabouts are unknown. At present, Linda is adjudicated dependent and court committed to the Philadelphia County Department of Human Services.

Linda is a pleasant, social, young woman whose diagnosis continues to be severe mental retardation (IQ score between 40-55) with spastic quadriplegic cerebral palsy, microcephaly, and a seizure disorder. She is nonverbal, but she has functional communication skills through the use of an augmentative device with voice output and a language picture board, paired with gestures and vocalizations (Romanski, Sevcik, and Wilkinson, 1994). Linda is able to use her power wheelchair independently within St. Edmond's with good motor planning. She attends a community-based special education program at the local high school, under the auspices of the Delaware County Intermediate Unit.

Several volunteers have interacted with Linda throughout her years living at St. Edmond's. One consistent volunteer, Debbie, was assigned to her case in 1988 through Citizen Advocates, which is a local organization that coordinates volunteer advocates. Linda looked forward to Debbie's biweekly visits, and Debbie had been incorporated into much of Linda's programming. Debbie's visits ended abruptly in 1991, with no prior warning. Attempts were made to contact Debbie in order to bring the relationship to a close, but were never successful. Linda had a relationship with another volunteer, Tina, for approximately one year, and a volunteer from Linda's school also visited with her periodically.

Linda was referred to the director of social service for two types of intervention. At age 15, Linda was referred for counseling due to inappropriate behavior toward staff at both St. Edmond's and at school. She was periodically kicking, biting, and hitting staff—sometimes trying to run them over with her power wheelchair. She would also forcefully extend her body and scream to the point where staff were unable to attend to her personal needs. Her inappropriate behavior escalated to the point that staff at both agencies needed to be taken to the emergency room on several occasions for treatment due to her biting. She also began trying to push other children over in their wheelchairs, she punched another child in the face, and she broke her school teacher's toe by running over her foot with her wheelchair.

At age 16, Linda was referred to the director of social service for discharge planning. St. Edmond's interdisciplinary team determined that Linda had made all of the therapeutic and social gains she would make at the facility and was in need of a less restrictive environment. The team also felt that many of Linda's behavioral difficulties could be attributed to her having "outgrown" St. Edmond's (Meins, 1995).

Definition of the Client

The primary client as defined by a residential care facility is the individual resident. He or she is the person who is in need of residential placement and, therefore, is the primary target of all therapeutic, programmatic, and medical services. Although the Social Service Department considers the individual resident the primary target of treatment, from a social service perspective, the definition of a client expands to include significant others within the client's environment. Significant others can include family members, a favorite staff person, a volunteer, or a staff person from the resident's school program or from an outside agency (Baker and Blacher, 1993). The people termed significant others changes over time according to the individual resident's needs.

Linda's significant others changed many times during the course of treatment. Initially, her Citizen's Advocate volunteer, Debbie, was most significant due to her intense and meaningful relationship with Linda. When Debbie's involvement ended, other volunteers and friends from school were defined as key people during treatment. Staff people at St. Edmond's and at Linda's school program were also considered part of the client group at different times, according to their involvement in her life and how she responded to them (Halgren and Clarizio, 1993). Throughout treatment, Linda's social workers from the Department of Human Service and county Office of Mental Retardation were significant because they were actively involved in planning Linda's discharge from St. Edmond's.

Goals, Objectives, and Outcome Measures

There are three levels of goals implemented at St. Edmond's. The overarching goal set by social worker and resident at St. Edmond's is for the resident to participate fully and as independently as possible in all aspects of care. The resident must also be encouraged to be as active as possible in setting goals within the social work relationship, given his or her cognitive level of functioning (Soto, Toro-Zambrana, and Belfiore, 1994).

Program goals usually involve activities of daily living (ADL's), switch activation, sensory responses, and the like. In higher-functioning children, switch activation provides instruction in cause and effect, for example, teaching a child that operating a certain switch will activate a tape recorder or television. In some lower functioning children, sensory response goals might be worded, "demonstrate a response to a massage program" or "demonstrate a response to an oral stimulation program before dinner." A response can be anything from opening the eyes, to making some kind of vocalization, to increasing body movement. These types of goals are most often set by the interdisciplinary team, with some input from the resident if he or she is cognitively able to participate (Giangreco et al., 1994). Progress on each goal is monitered by program aides and evaluated quarterly by program specialists. Other goals are set and monitored within each discipline represented on the team. For example, physical therapy may have a walking goal for a certain resident; occupational therapy may have a hand function goal; and social work goals are usually measured in terms of changes in the resident's behavior, feelings about him or herself, and the residential program at St. Edmond's. Progress concerning this type of goal is monitored quarterly by program specialists within each discipline (Siperstein, Wolraich, and Reed, 1994).

In Linda's case, the goal of decreasing incidents of aggressive behavior was set by the interdisciplinary team. Documentation concerning frequency of incidents was maintained by program aides, and documentation regarding Linda's counseling sessions was kept by the director of social service (Belfiore, Browder, and Lin, 1993). Another goal of the Social Service Department was to commence discharge planning for Linda, since the interdisciplinary team referred her for alternate placement (Pandiani, Maynard, and Schacht, 1994). This goal was primarily the responsibility of the director of social service, with assistance from the county Office of Mental Retardation to refer Linda to other facilities.

Use of Contract and Meeting Place

In a residential setting, the need for intense intervention changes according to how the resident adjusts to his or her daily environment. Consequently, the resident/social worker relationship varies greatly at different times during treatment. For this reason and due to the low level of cognitive functioning of most residents, written contracts are rarely utilized. Linda and I established an oral contract that described the details of her behavior plan.

A variety of meeting places are available to social worker and resident. Some choices include the Social Service Department, Linda's bedroom or programming room, therapy areas, the dining room, the play yard, or an outside location. During the initial meetings with a resident, it is helpful to allow them to choose the meeting place. This opportunity not only creates a less threatening atmosphere, but also gives the resident a feeling of control within the relationship. When meetings with Linda began, she chose to meet either in her bedroom or in her program room, places that would be considered "her turf." When those options were not available, she was given the choice of meeting in a neutral location, such as a therapy area or the play yard. The office of the director of social service is usually the option of last resort due to its formal nature.

Social workers frequently meet with the residents in the community. By accompanying a resident on an outing to the mall, movies, the park, or another like place, the social worker is given the opportunity to further his or her relationship with the resident through shared experiences. Being away from the facility also sometimes enables the social worker to explore feelings with the resident more easily.

When working with residents with low levels of cognitive functioning, it is important to gradually introduce them to more threatening, intimidating, or unfamiliar meeting places, such as the Social Service Department, because they may need to meet with the social worker in these areas during treatment. For example, asking the resident to participate in a "job" that would require him or her to enter the meeting place on a regular basis helps create comfort with the particular setting. In Linda's case, meetings immediately following aggressive outbursts were held in the office of the director of social service because of its more formal nature. Prior to these meetings, Linda was asked to assist the director with bringing mail into the office each afternoon. This simple task enabled Linda to become sufficiently desensitized to meet in the office when necessary, with little or no apprehension.

Use of Time

Since St. Edmond's is a long-term care facility, time is controlled mainly by the resident's level of need and social worker's other responsibilities within the facility. The average resident's length of stay is measured in years; therefore, therapeutic interventions take place over a long period of time. The frequency and duration of planned interviews can be set by social worker and resident, and tend to vary according to the resident's needs. Unplanned interventions, like those during or immediately following an incident, tend to vary according to the availability of the social worker. The timing of the meetings depends on the resident's needs at a certain time, his or her ability to adjust to the environment, and his or her participation in treatment and in life inside and outside St. Edmond's.

Interventions

When working with children at a low level of cognitive functioning, it is crucial that the social worker act in a supportive and patient manner. Although the child with special needs experiences many stresses throughout therapeutic intervention, he or she also experiences joys and brings his or her own strengths to the process (McCallion and Toseland, 1993). The initial use of supportive techniques during treatment creates a stable, effective working relationship with a resident. Cognitive impairments, including learning disability, traumatic brain injury, and minimal brain dysfunction have characteristics that include impulsiveness, communication skill deficits, difficulties with reasoning and problem-solving, and impaired self-concept. Without appropriate intervention, these problems are likely to lead to marginal social acceptance, low levels of self-esteem, and further impaired development (Sigler and Mackelprang, 1993). In many situations, the resident's inappropriate behavior has alienated people, and the social worker needs to form an alliance with the resident to assist him or her with examining the targeted behavior (Huguenin, 1993).

When a child continues to exhibit severe and challenging behavior, however, the social worker may have to employ more confrontational techniques to facilitate the resident taking on responsibility for his or her actions (Norgate, 1994). The social worker may also need to develop positive, nonaversive behavioral support plans that would comprise multiple components such as alternative skill training or antecedent interventions. Positive support plans offer a comprehensive, proactive approach to the reduction and prevention of difficult problem behaviors (Bambara, Mitchell-Kvacky, and Iacobelli, 1994).

I formed a strong relationship with Linda initially by attending community outings with her and discussing things of interest to her. Although communication was often a barrier because she is nonverbal and uses an augmentative communication device that is limited in its function, I was able to gain insight into what frustrates her and why she acts out by asking pointed, specific questions and progressing extremely slowly (Routh, 1994). When working with a person having Linda's special needs, it is often difficult to utilize traditional therapeutic interventions. A social worker needs also to advocate and mediate for the client and educate significant others about relating to him or her (Maisto and Hughes, 1995).

The program Linda and I agreed upon consisted of positive rewards that she specified, which were given at specific times of the day if she did not act out (Repp and Karsh, 1994). Rewards included age-appropriate stickers and cards she could put on her wheelchair, special phone privileges, and private time with favorite staff people. If Linda acted out during the day, the staff was instructed not to reprimand her but to tell her that she would not be receiving her reward for the day (Prasad et al., 1992). Linda remained on this program successfully until her discharge. There was a significant decrease in her incidents of inappropriate behavior with periodic reassessment and change of motivators (Iwata et al., 1994).

Another issue we talked about in our sessions was how much Linda liked to socialize with adults and her desire to do things independently. Consequently, we decided on some "jobs" she could do at St. Edmond's and at school, which would provide the interaction and independence she desired (Newton and Horner, 1993). The jobs she enjoyed most were delivering attendance sheets to classrooms at school, taking messages to the kitchen at St. Edmond's, and delivering communication notebooks from the school bus drivers to my office each afternoon. All the jobs enabled Linda to move about independently, feel useful, and interact with people in new ways (Staub and Hunt, 1993).

One aspect of Linda's personality that she wanted to focus on was making transitions from one activity to another. Linda recognized that she had trouble and would act out when activities she enjoyed ended, and she let me know that she needed more time to prepare herself emotionally. We worked out a system of transition time whereby the staff was instructed to set a timer, which was attached to her wheelchair tray with Velcro, for ten minutes before an activity would end so Linda would have time to prepare herself for the transition to another activity (McIlvane et al., 1995). I trained the staff both at St. Edmond's and at Linda's school to implement the reward system and the transition time plan, since she spent a great deal of time in both places (Rasnake et al., 1993).

Although Linda does not have any family involvement, she has a large, extended support system of people at St. Edmond's, at school, through volunteer programs, etc.–all of whom are invested in her success and well-being. Linda is a pleasant and social person who was consistently motivated to participate in our sessions. She seemed to enjoy and benefit from our relationship and saw me as someone who understood her and could assist her with communicating thoughts she may have been unable to express on her own. I also initiated extensive staff training regarding all programs throughout treatment to facilitate more appropriate and healthy communication between Linda and significant others in her environment (Fleming and Reile, 1993).

The residents at St. Edmond's are entitled to a variety of services, and the social worker also functions as liaison, advocate, and case manager to ensure that each resident receives those services in a timely and appropriate manner (Epstein et al., 1994). Methods of advocacy might include staff training and development, representing the resident during court hearings, or initiating contact with community volunteer organizations. Advanced case management skills are required due to the size and complexity of the mental retardation system.

Stance of the Social Worker

My stance as a social worker stems mainly from my beliefs about the rights of children with special needs and their families. My first belief is in the basic human right of these children to have as much control over their environment as possible. When a child acts in a disruptive fashion, that child is trying to communicate something that he or she cannot communicate verbally (McLean and McLean, 1993). Each resident also has the right to be as independent as possible within the environment, and it is the job of the social worker to act on that child's behalf—to be the advocate, liaison, messenger, or voice to communicate to others what he or she cannot (Heal and Rusch, 1994).

A second strong belief of mine is that parents who have residentially placed a child with special needs should be treated with the same respect and dignity as those who have not placed their child (Wasow and Wikler, 1983). Society, in general, views a family who has residentially placed their child as "giving the child up" or "institutionalizing" him or her, and the families tend to be stigmatized. The social worker needs to work toward educating both staff and the general society about the difficulties of caring for a child with special needs in the family home, and the need for residential placement in many cases (Black et al., 1985).

Use of Outside Resources

Given the level of functioning of most residents at St. Edmond's and the complexity of the system of services available to them (See Figure 9.1), it is ultimately the social worker's responsibility to coordinate, monitor, and secure all concrete services. Although some residents may eventually learn to be independent in activities of daily living, mobility, or use of a communication device, many are not cognitively aware enough to advocate for or obtain their own services. The social worker must ensure that needed services are available within St. Edmond's prior to a resident's admission and are available within another facility in the event of a resident's discharge (McDonald, Owen, and McDonald, 1993).

Reassessment

In a residential care setting, reassessment does not occur at specific times during treatment but occurs as the social worker/resident relation-

FIGURE 9.1. Ecomap for Linda

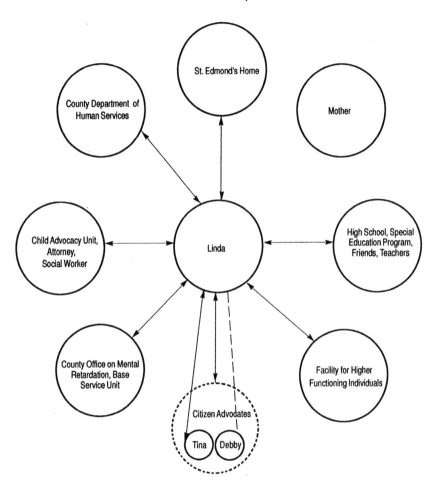

ship progresses. Reassessment can be initiated by either party at any time during treatment and occurs continually throughout treatment. During Linda's treatment, reassessment concerning her behavior was initiated on a formal level by the interdisciplinary team who met monthly regarding her case. Informal reassessment between her and the director of social service took place according to their relationship and goals. In addition, when planning for Linda's discharge, reassessment occurred repeatedly with Linda, St. Edmond's interdisciplinary team, and the facilities considering her for admission.

Termination or Transfer

Termination of the social worker's therapeutic intervention is determined by program specialists, the behavior management consultant, and the social worker, based on a substantial decrease in the number of disruptive outbursts. However, termination is very often temporary. Given the level of cognitive functioning and the retention rate of the residents, a case is always terminated with the understanding that treatment can be resumed at any time for any reason. Planned transfer to another facility is usually initiated by the interdisciplinary team or necessitated by reason of the resident's age. In either case, the director of social service commences discharge planning and oversees the transfer to an alternate placement. Once a resident is transferred to another facility, he or she is not readmitted to St. Edmond's; consequently, the transfer of all information concerning the resident's care is vital. The director of social service also makes appropriate referrals for therapeutic intervention when necessary and does not continue meeting with a child once he or she is residing elsewhere.

Linda and I addressed issues surrounding her discharge to another facility. After having lived at St. Edmond's for many years, Linda was apprehensive about moving into alternate placement. While she was anxious and realized that she would miss St. Edmond's terribly, she also knew that she did not have a peer group there for socialization and relationships. Most of the residents function at a lower cognitive level than Linda, and she has always craved an appropriate peer group.

Case Conclusion

Linda resided at St. Edmond's until July 1995, when she was transferred to another facility that offered her greater community experience and opportunities for interaction with peers. Linda was discharged to a facility like St. Edmond's whose residents are higher-functioning. Some of the residents at the new facility were familiar to Linda as they had lived at St. Edmond's when they were younger. I trained the staff at the new facility regarding Linda's programs and made sure all necessary information was passed on to them (Ittenbach et al., 1993). Linda adjusted smoothly to her new residence and relates well to a peer group of friends, spends a substantial amount of time in the community, and has made several visits back to St. Edmond's to see people who have been significant in her life for many years.

Differential Discussion

Overall, I found my work with Linda to be a positive experience for both of us. I feel that if I had advocated for a more sophisticated augmentative communication device, we would have been able to discuss her issues around anger and frustration more in depth. However, funding difficulty and time required to order a new device would have likely interfered with that plan. Another avenue I believe I could have pursued more vigorously would have been to involve more of Linda's significant others in our work. Our work was fairly confined to the staff at St. Edmond's and at her school program. Perhaps if I employed a volunteer visitor, Linda would have had even more opportunity for social interaction (Soto, Toro-Zambrana, and Belfiore, 1994). Although I made several unsuccessful attempts to involve Linda's Department of Human Services social worker in the process, it would have been helpful for him to learn about her behavior since he would be following her case after her discharge from St. Edmond's (Downes, 1992). Due to funding concerns, our behavior management consultant was only available on a limited basis, but she could have been involved more with the ongoing monitoring of Linda's behavior plan. I also think that Linda was appropriate for discharge from the facility far sooner than she was actually transferred. If I could have secured alternate placement for her a few years earlier, she may have been given opportunities for socialization to offset some of her behavioral outbursts. However, given the availability of appropriate placements for children like Linda I realize that earlier discharge would have not been possible.

PRACTICE IN CONTEXT

The availability of appropriate placements not only affected Linda's quality of life, but is an issue of great importance concerning all the residents at St. Edmond's and their families. As medical technology advances, children like Linda are living longer. When Linda was born, she was given a very short life expectancy, but due to the available technology and excellent care, she has far outlived anyone's expectations. It follows then that if children with special needs are living longer, more residential placements must be made available for them. However, policy makers have been slow to recognize the overwhelming need for residential facilities because they feel that such facilities cost too much and devalue notions of family preservation. Consequently, the existing facilities operate at full capacity and rarely have openings, often leaving families with children like Linda living at home in desperate situations and people like Linda with few options for placement after St. Edmond's. Families that are able to mobilize themselves and advocate for residential placement in the face of adversity are unusual. Policy makers have yet to fully understand that in some cases, children with special needs can be physically, emotionally, and/or financially draining for a family, and residential placement is the best option for all involved. Until this is realized, many special children and their families will be living with uncertainty, frustration, and numerous questions about their future. In these situations, social workers must advocate for the creation of new facilities while they continue to support the children and families trying to survive in a system that is less than sympathetic to their needs.

REFERENCES

Baker, B. and Blacher, J. (1993). Out-of-home placement for children with mental retardation: Dimensions of family involvement. *American Journal on Mental Retardation, 98*(3), 368-377.

Bambara, L., Mitchell-Kvacky, N., and Iacobelli, S. (1994). Positive behavioral support for students with severe disabilities: An emerging multicomponent approach for addressing challenging behaviors. *School Psychology Review, 23*(2), 263-278.

Belfiore, P., Browder, D., and Lin, C. (1993). Using descriptive and experimental analysis in the treatment of self-injurious behavior. *Education and Training in Mental Retardation, 28*(1), 57-65.

Birenbaum, A. and Cohen, H. (1993). On the importance of helping families: Policy implications from a national study. *Mental Retardation, 31*(2), 67-74.

Black, M., Cohn, J., Smull, M., and Scrites, L. (1985). Individual and family factors associated with risk of institutionalization of mentally retarded adults. *American Journal of Mental Deficiency, 90*(3), 271-276.

Downes, B. (1992). Guardianship for people with severe mental retardation: Consent for urgently needed treatment. *Health and Social Work, 17*(1), 13-15.

Epstein, M., Cullinan, D., Quinn, K., and Cumblad, C. (1994). Characteristics of children with emotional and behavioral disorders in community-based programs designed to prevent placement in residential facilities. *Journal of Emotional and Behavioral Disorders, 2*(1), 51-57.

Fleming, R. and Reile, P. (1993). A descriptive analysis of client outcomes associated with staff interventions in developmental disabilities. *Behavioral Residential Treatment, 8*(1), 29-43.

Giangreco, M., Dennis, R., Edelman, S., and Cloninger, C. (1994). Dressing your IEPs for the general education climate: Analysis of IEP goals and objectives for students with multiple disabilities. *RASE: Remedial and Special Education, 15*(5), 288-296.

Halgren, D. and Clarizio, H. (1993). Categorical and programming changes in special education services. *Exceptional Children, 59*(6), 547-555.

Heal, L. and Rusch, F. (1994). Prediction of residential independence of special education high school students. *Research in Developmental Disabilities, 15*(3), 223-243.

Huguenin, N. (1993). Reducing chronic noncompliance in an individual with severe mental retardation to facilitate community integration. *Mental Retardation, 31*(5), 332-339.

Ittenbach, R., Chayer, D., Bruininks, R., Thurlow, M., and Beirn-Smith, M. (1993). Adjustment of young adults with mental retardation in community settings: Comparison of parametric and nonparametric statistical techniques. *American Journal on Mental Retardation, 97*(6), 607-615.

Iwata, B., Pace, G., Cowdery, G., and Miltenberger, R. (1994). What makes extinction work: An analysis of procedural form and function. *Journal of Applied Behavior Analysis, 27*(1), 131-144.

Maisto, A. and Hughes, E. (1995). Adaptation to group home living for adults with mental retardation as a function of previous residential placement. *Journal of Intellectual Disability Research, 39*(1), 15-18.

McCallion, P. and Toseland, R. (1993). Empowering families of adolescents and adults with developmental disabilities. *Families in Society: The Journal of Contemporary Human Services, 74*(10), 579-589.

McDonald, L., Owen, M., and McDonald, S. (1993). Quality care in residential placement for children and youth with developmental disabilities. *Behavioral Residential Treatment, 8*(3), 187-202.

McIlvane, W., Kledaras, J., Iennaco, F., McDonald, S., and Stoddard, L. T. (1995). Some possible limits on errorless discrimination reversals in individuals with severe mental retardation. *American Journal on Mental Retardation, 99*(4), 430-436.

McLean, L. and McLean, J. (1993). Communication intervention for adults with severe mental retardation. *Topics in Language Disorders, 13*(3), 47-60.

Meins, W. (1995). Symptoms of major depression in mentally retarded adults. *Journal of Intellectual Disability Research, 39*(1), 41-45.

Newton, J. and Horner, R. (1993). Using a social guide to improve social relationships of people with severe disabilities. *Journal of the Association for Persons with Severe Handicaps, 18*(1), 36-45.

Norgate, R. (1994). Responding to the challenge: Planning for the needs of children with severe learning difficulties who present behavior difficulties. *Educational Psychology in Practice, 9*(4), 201-206.

Pandiani, J., Maynard, A., and Schacht, L. (1994). Mathematical modeling of movement between residential placements: A systems analytic approach to understanding systems of care. *Journal of Child and Family Studies, 3*(91), 41-53.

Prasad, M., Sitholey, P., Dutt, K., and Srivastava, R. (1992). ADL (activity of daily living) training and treatment of temper tantrums in a severely retarded aphasic child. *Indian Journal of Clinical Psychology, 19*(1), 37-39.

Rasnake, L., Martin, J., Tarnowski, K., and Mulick, J. (1993). Acceptability of behavioral treatments: Influence of knowledge of behavioral principles. *Mental Retardation, 31*(4), 247-251.

Repp, A., and Karsh, K. (1994). Hypothesis-based interventions for tantrum behaviors of persons with developmental disabilties in school settings. *Journal of Applied Behavior Analysis, 27*(1), 21-31.

Romanski, M., Sevcik, R., Robinson, B., and Bakeman, R. (1994). Adult-directed communications of youth with mental retardation using the system for augmenting language. *Journal of Speech and Hearing Research, 37*(3), 617-628.

Romanski, M., Sevcik, R., and Wilkinson, K. (1994). Peer-directed communicative interactions of augmented language learners with mental retardation. *American Journal on Mental Retardation, 98*(4), 527-538.

Routh, D. (1994). Commentary: Facilitated communication as unwitting ventriloquism. *Journal of Pediatric Psychology, 19*(6), 673-675.

Sigler, G. and Mackelprang, R. (1993). Cognitive impairments: Psychosocial and sexual implications and strategies for social work intervention. *Journal of Social Work and Human Sexuality, 8*(2), 89-106.

Siperstein, G., Wolraich, M., and Reed, D. (1994). Professionals' prognosis for individuals with mental retardation: Search for consensus within interdisciplinary settings. *American Journal on Mental Retardation, 98*(4), 519-526.

Soto, G., Toro-Zambrana, W., and Belfiore, P. (1994). Comparison of two instructional strategies on social skills acquisition and generalization among individuals with moderate and severe mental retardation working in vocational setting: A meta-analytical review. *Education and Training in Mental Retardation and Developmental Disabilities, 29*(4), 307-320.

Staub, D. and Hunt, P. (1993). The effects of social interaction training on high school peer tutors of schoolmates with severe disabilities. *Exceptional Children, 60*(1), 41-57.

Wasow, M. and Wikler, L. (1983). Reflections on professionals' attitudes toward the severely mentally retarded and the chronically mentally ill: Implications for parents. *Family Therapy, 10*(3), 299-308.

PART II:
ACUTE AND HIGH-TECHNOLOGY CARE

Chapter 10

Discharge Planning
in a Community Hospital:
A Patient Whose Symptoms
the System Could Not Manage

Danielle L. Hammer
Toba Schwaber Kerson

CONTEXT

Description of the Setting

Montgomery Hospital is a private, nonprofit, 240-bed community facility first established as the county hospital in 1889. The hospital provides a comprehensive range of medical services, including specialty programs in cardiology, oncology, psychiatry, surgery, rehabilitation, skilled nursing, and home care. It is located 30 miles west of Philadelphia in Norristown, Pennsylvania–Montgomery County's seat of government. Once a busy area for heavy industry, Norristown has experienced urban blight but is surrounded by burgeoning white-collar business and residential communities. In the last few years, the town itself has created several initiatives for internal economic development. The population surrounding the hospital is ethnically, racially, socially, and economically diverse. Traditionally, the hospital's patients have lived or worked within a 10 to 15 mile radius of the institution; however, the hospital is now extending its service area in order to increase its patient base.

Policy

Montgomery Hospital meets the standards determined by its prime accrediting body, the Joint Commission on the Accreditation of Hospital

Organizations (JCAHO). In addition, most of the policies that affect discharge planning at Montgomery Hospital relate to reimbursement for hospital charges and the measures that government, business, and the insurance industry have taken to curtail the escalating cost of medical care. A series of such measures have been instituted since the early 1970s. Of greatest importance to discharge planning are prospective payment, utilization review, and managed care. In 1983, the federal government altered the reimbursement system for Medicare recipients from one in which hospitals determined the cost of care to prospective payment in which reimbursement is based on the severity and kind of diagnosis or diagnostic-related groups (DRGs) (Muller, 1993; Dobrof, 1991). This system of reimbursement plus the concerns of other third-party payers make it necessary for the hospital to monitor hospital use through a system called utilization review. Utilization review tracks services and, as part of its mission, prevents patients from being hospitalized unnecessarily (Penchansky and Macnee, 1993; Wickizer, 1991). Utilization review has become an important function for social workers in many acute care hospitals. It is one way for hospitals to gauge the appropriateness of admissions, length of hospital stay, and use of resources. All of this information helps hospitals to contract more clearly and effectively with insurers. If a patient meets the acute care criteria set by his or her insurance company, the hospital will receive the precontracted rate of pay per day. If the patient does not meet the criteria for acute care, the hospital is either paid at a lower contracted rate of subacute or skilled care if the patient meets the insurance company's criteria for that level of care or it is denied payment. The hospital can appeal the denial of payment; however, denial usually occurs after the patient has left the hospital and the hospital is left with an unpaid bill for services rendered.

In 1986, the Social Security Act (Public Law 99-509, Oct. 21, 1986) stated that every hospital must have in place a process of planning discharge that, early in each hospitalization, identifies patients who without such planning would be likely to experience adverse health consequences. The plan is to be included in the medical record and discussed with the patient and/or his or her representative. This law was designed to avoid discharge delay (Sharpe, 1991).

Managed care is a concept used by health maintenance organizations as well as many forms of health insurance, including the Blues, private insurance companies, and Medicaid and Medicare, who use this process to control access to and the cost of health care. An additional federal policy that affects discharge planning is the Patient Self-Determination Act, which mandates that hospitals and other health care institutions discuss with patients their advance directives, that is, their wishes for medical intervention in case they are not competent to make decisions (Soskis and Kerson, 1992). Patients are advised about making a living will as well as granting a trusted relative or friend Durable Power of Attorney.

Technology

Advances in medical technology have contributed substantially to the cost of health care; however, many high-cost technologies such as IV infusion, ventilator care, wound management, and apnea monitoring can now be managed in subacute, skilled nursing, or home settings. Thus, in some ways, advances have placed greater responsibility on the discharge planner to help to move the patient to a subacute or skilled level of care as quickly as possible and to ensure that the patient will be safe and well cared for after discharge.

An important tool in facilitating the discharge planning process is the creation and development of clinical pathways (also called caremaps or critical pathways)–efforts to coordinate and standardize clinical care by making hospital stays more predictable. Clinical pathways are a guide to the expected care to be delivered to a patient during and after hospitalization (Clare et al., 1995; Clark, 1995; Morgan, Hofmann, and Butler, 1995; Lord, 1994; Milne and Pelletier, 1994). Here, a hospital stay is divided into individual days of service. For example, a patient admitted for a total hip replacement may receive care from a physical therapist, social worker, nurse, internist, and orthopedic surgeon and be expected to stay in the hospital for four days. The clinical pathway illustrates the activities these and other disciplines would carry out with the patient. If the patient has no medical complications, progresses therapeutically as predicted, and has an established discharge plan, discharge should occur on the expected day to control and maximize resource use and deliver successful care at a predictable cost (Walsh and Coldiron, 1993). Although insurers and the hospital wish to see medical care function in this rational manner on a day-to-day basis, physicians argue that it cannot be so (Davis et al., 1995; Feather, 1993). Often, the patient's social situation is less predictable than this rational model supposes, and the burden falls on the social worker as discharge planner to move extremely quickly to respond to the cadence set by the caremap.

For example, patients admitted to the hospital for total joint replacement are prescreened and either interviewed by phone or in person by the social worker during prehospital testing. Prehospital testing usually includes blood work, X rays, anesthesia assessment, and registration of insurance information. Such prehospital discharge planning allows the social worker and patient to anticipate the needs upon discharge from the hospital. As payers increasingly incorporate daily review of patients and capitated reimbursement into their payment structure, the social worker must work quickly to identify the patients' needs and plan for their aftercare. Often, these posthospital needs, such as equipment and the services of a visiting nurse and physical therapist, must be confirmed by the third-party payer as well. Patients are often ignorant of their benefits, and the social worker must be knowledgeable in order to advocate for the patient, especially in terms of obtaining postdischarge services to which the patient is entitled. These timely interventions will facilitate the patient's safe and appropriate discharge from the hospital.

While larger hospitals rely on either laptop computers or social work computer software to compile service statistics and productivity measurements, our department gathers this information by hand and enters it into a Word Perfect software file (Mutshler, 1990). The department uses the hospital's patient data system to collect financial, demographic, and medical test results information (Booth, Ludke, and Fisher, 1994; Rosenstein, 1994). All social workers have an approved access code for retrieval of this confidential information.

Organization

Historically, discharge planning has been the primary role of social workers at Montgomery Hospital and serves as the defining factor for the social worker's relationship with patients and family members (Kadushin and Kulys, 1994; Soskolne and Auslander, 1993; Abramson, 1990; Blumenfield and Rosenberg, 1988; Report on the Task Force, 1987). Social work maintains this overarching function because of our training in psychosocial assessment, as well as our knowledge of and close working relationship with community resources. The American Hospital Association (AHA) states that discharge planning is an interdisciplinary process that should be guided by the following essential elements:

1. early identification of patients likely to need complex posthospital care;
2. indication of patient preferences for posthospital care;
3. patient and family education;
4. patient/family assessment and counseling;
5. planning, development, coordination, and implementation, which includes health and other community resources needed to assure continuity after discharge; and
6. postdischarge follow-up to ensure services and plan outcome (American Hospital Association, 1984).

At Montgomery Hospital, the Social Work and Utilization Review Departments have combined to form the Department of Case Management, which is staffed in-house, seven days a week (Brennan and Kaplan, 1993). Here, the social workers and nurse utilization coordinators are teamed to identify patient needs and plan aftercare. The department consists of two full-time master's-level social workers, one of whom is the director; three full-time and one part-time bachelor's-level social workers; and four full-time and one part-time nurses. Home care coordinators, who are registered nurses, arrange homecare and equipment but do not screen admitted patients. Social workers are assigned to specific units such as psychiatry, surgery, and cardiac care and rotate at least semiannually. This rotation offers the social workers the opportunity to practice with various populations and to relate to a wide range of professionals, staff, and community resources. Montgomery offers a continuum of services including a short-stay surgery center, a skilled nursing unit, and home care; thus, a patient's discharge can be planned with those services in mind (Rock et al., 1995; Schwartz, Blumenfield, and Simon, 1990). These increased options allow the social worker and patient to develop a long-term service plan from the acute hospital, to skilled nursing to home care and finally to visits to physicians' offices.

Daily clinical team patient reviews assist social workers in early identification of patients requiring discharge planning, and social workers review all new admissions daily to identify patients needing such services. High-risk indicators include the following: (1) clinical pathway patients with total joint replacements or pneumonia; (2) patients over 70 years old with complicated medical illnesses such as significant cardiac, respiratory, renal, or orthopedic problems or stroke (Berkman et al., 1990); (3) the presence of substance abuse or psychiatric diagnoses (Allen and Phillips, 1993); (4) patients admitted with changes in mental status (Travis, Moore, and McAuley, 1991); (5) patients readmitted within 15 days of prior discharge, (6) nursing home residents; and (7) children admitted with failure to thrive, orthopedic problems, or potential diagnoses resulting from abusive situations (Lockery et al., 1994; Oktay et al., 1992; Proctor and Morrow-Howell, 1990).

PRACTICE DECISIONS

Description of Client

Mr. Johnson is a 40-year-old, single, white, male, who was admitted to the Critical Care Unit after having "passed out." He has a past history of alcohol abuse, seizures, esophageal ulcers, cirrhosis, electrolyte abnormalities, assaultive behavior, and incarceration. The diagnosis of alcoholic anoxic encephalopathy–lack of oxygen to the brain as a result of alcohol intoxication–resulted in Mr. Johnson's arriving in the hospital alert and awake, but disoriented and confused. Mr. Johnson did not recall his drinking, falling, or passing out on the bed at home where his grandmother found him. He did not know where he was or what day it was but recognized his mother and grandmother.

Mr. Johnson was considered high-risk for discharge planning as a result of substance abuse and was referred to social work the day after he was admitted (Holden et al., 1995). He was not able to hold a conversation beyond initial courtesy introductions and spent the day watching television. Attempts to engage Mr. Johnson in therapeutic activities met with little success due to his poor concentration and mentation. He could perform repetitive tasks such as separating paperwork in two easily discernible stacks or pushing a courtesy cart with a volunteer supervisor. A psychiatric evaluation determined that the patient would remain impulsive, totally dependent, helpless, and disoriented. The psychiatrist indicated that an involuntary commitment to the County Mental Health Crisis Center was appropriate for treatment of Mr. Johnson's assaultive behaviors, which included impulsivity, verbal explosions, and sexually inappropriate behaviors exhibited during his hospital stay. The attending medical physician was in agreement with the psychiatrist's recommendation and confirmed that Mrs. Johnson could not manage her son in her home with her 87-year-old mother present as long as Mr. Johnson was confused, disoriented to time and place, assaultive, and impulsive. His options for discharge were severely limited by his behaviors and age.

Prior to admission, he lived with his mother and grandmother. Mr. Johnson had a long history of alcohol abuse, and a brother had recently died due to complications from alcohol abuse. Mr. Johnson had been released from prison approximately six months prior to admission. He also has a young son with whom he has no contact (Brown, 1995; Daley and Raskin, 1990).

Definition of the Client

Although Mr. Johnson was the primary client, the limitations on his ability to make decisions for himself or care for himself made it necessary for me to work, primarily, with his mother. Mrs. Johnson had received Durable Power of Attorney from her son when he was incarcerated, and Mr. Johnson had not revoked this agreement prior to his hospital admission. Because the Durable Power of Attorney allowed Mrs. Johnson to make decisions regarding Mr. Johnson's health and finances, guardianship was not pursued during his hospitalization. Selected information was shared with Mr. Johnson; however, he gave no evidence of understanding his situation.

Mrs. Johnson, in her early 60s, worked full-time as a bookkeeper for a local company, as she had for all of her adult life. A very determined, heavyset woman, she looked younger than her years. She was long divorced from Mr. Johnson's alcoholic father. We worked well together because Mrs. Johnson was so willing to advocate for her son and was not going to allow strangers to decide what would happen to him. This was her only living child; while she could not care for him directly, she could make sure that he received proper care. She began immediately to educate herself about the system and continues to do so. Although at times Mrs. Johnson has been depressed over her son's state, because of her need to remain her son's advocate she has never become immobilized. Late in Mr. Johnson's hospitalization, Mrs. Johnson increasingly infantilized him, even checking to see if he had soiled himself. I helped her to understand that she was reacting in that way because of the level of her son's dependence. Mrs. Johnson and I also discussed the need for her to eventually seek legal guardianship (Keith and Wacker, 1994). The power of attorney granted to her when her son went to prison may not hold, and guardianship is a more permanent solution to what is a permanent problem.

Goals and Contract

I met with Mrs. Johnson to review her understanding of Mr. Johnson's current status and discuss discharge options. Contracting with Mrs. Johnson was not difficult because she was prepared to plan for her son's needs. We agreed to share responsibility for contacting potential long–term care facilities. We explored the possibility of Mr. Johnson's living in a facility that would provide supervision 24 hours a day or his returning home with community day programs such as adult day care and/or attendant care to meet his personal care needs. Mrs. Johnson felt that while returning home might be the long-term goal, the immediate need was for 24-hour supervised care in a safe environment other than home. Possibilities included placement in a psychiatric facility or an extended care facility; however, it soon became clear that Mr. Johnson would not be accepted into the mental health system because his behaviors and outbursts were a result of permanent neurological damage. Therefore, his symptoms were not amenable to change through psychiatric treatment or hospitalization.

Meeting Place

At the hospital, Mrs. Johnson and I met either in my office or in the family lounge on the patient's medical floor. We also worked through telephone calls when face-to-face visits were not possible due to time or weather constraints. The Social Work Department is centrally located floors away from the unit where Mr. Johnson was being treated, so it was not possible to meet with Mr. Johnson in the department office. The patient was in a semiprivate, two-bed room. Although he was medicated with Ativan and Haldol to decrease his outbursts, he was easily agitated by information that he was unable to process. Thus, the usual issues of confidentiality in a nonprivate space were compounded by Mr. Johnson's inability to manage any significant information. While I assured Mr. Johnson that I was locating a place in which he could continue to be cared for, I could not include him in discussions of finances, which addressed his eligibility for placement under Medical Assistance rules and the federal Omnibus Reconciliation Act (OBRA), both of which require that applicants to nursing homes be screened for any preexisting mental health or mental retardation diagnoses. Upon placement, Mr. Johnson was not found to have a targeted psychiatric diagnosis that under OBRA would have required the State Office of Mental Health to approve his placement.

Treatment Modality

Primary modalities were task-centered and problem-solving. Crisis intervention is also commonly used in discharge planning, but in Mr. Johnson's situation, it was only appropriate for the earliest stages of the work. Because Mr. Johnson was unable to help himself and because the systems with which we had to deal were so large, powerful, bureacratized, and complex, much of my work involved advocacy techniques. My work was constrained by the various systems I had to confront on the patient's behalf. The chosen modalities best allowed me to help Mrs. Johnson plan for her son's short- and long-term needs because she was ultimately responsible for her son after his hospitalization and she wanted to understand and be able to cope with his needs for the long term. After Mrs. Johnson and the medical staff at the hospital understood that Mr. Johnson required 24-hour supervision and that his return home would be unsafe, we began to plan together for an extended care facility placement. It was an overwhelming process, which I helped Mrs. Johnson to divide into specific tasks and then establish priorities. Problem solving became my primary treatment modality as I waded through the myriad systems with which I had to deal to plan for Mr. Johnson. It was extraordinarily unusual for Mr. Johnson to remain in the hospital for the duration of time he was hospitalized; however, a safe discharge home was not feasible.

After approximately four months of psychiatric evaluation for placement at the County Psychiatric Service and State Hospital, the patient was officially refused placement because he had had no preexisting psychiatric diagnosis. Even though he had exhibited behaviors such as physical and sexual aggressiveness, and noisiness and eloping, these facilities and the State Office of Mental Health determined that he was organically affected with an alcoholic dementia due to his alcohol-induced anoxic encephalopathy. In addition to pressing for and monitering Mr. Johnson's psychiatric evaluations, I continually searched for and referred him to extended care facilities. Engaging Mrs. Johnson in these tasks allowed her to cope with and feel as if she had some control over her son's situation.

Due to Mr. Johnson's age, behaviors, and the potential for life-long placement, it was extremely difficult to find an appropriate living arrangement for him. The County Office on Aging determined that he was appropriate for long-term institutional nursing care; however, more than 60 nursing facilities, including the County Nursing Home, refused to admit him, citing his age and behaviors that were beyond their ability to manage. Finding this experience frustrating and bewildering, I assumed the stance that nursing home placement had been determined clinically appropriate. I worked with Mrs. Johnson on contacting local, state, and federal representatives and helped her to file a complaint against one of the facilities with the Office of Civil Rights for discrimination based on age (Report on the Task Force, 1987). The case is currently under investigation.

Finally, Mr. Johnson was placed at a facility that had an opening for younger patients with a psychiatric diagnosis and/or dementia. This facility was 60 minutes away from his home and outside of his county of residence. Taking the steps necessary to evaluate this location for her son and making the decision for placement was a very emotional process for Mrs. Johnson. However, given our relationship and joint efforts at case planning and responsibility for Mr. Johnson, Mrs. Johnson was able to mobilize herself, and agree to and accept her son's placement (Showers et al., 1995).

Outside Resources

The Office on Aging played a critical part in the evaluation of the patient for nursing home placement via the options process. This is the process through which the County Office on Aging evaluates the medical appropriateness of a patient for short- and long-term nursing home care paid for by Medical Assistance. Once the Office on Aging makes that determination, the information is sent to the County Assistance Office, which determines financial eligibility. Once financial and medical eligibility are established, the individual will receive a Medical Assistance grant for nursing home placement. Their original determination that Mr. Johnson did not require psychiatric placement reinforced Mrs. Johnson's and my goal of placement in a long-term, extended-care facility. It was also necessary to work with the county and state Offices of Mental Health to clarify the psychiatric component of the situation. Finally, the Office of Civil Rights was valuable in determining whether Mr. Johnson's rights had been violated because of his age. Figure 10.1 is an ecomap for Mr. Johnson, which outlines the many resources at work.

Reassessment

Mrs. Johnson and I reassessed our discharge plan at three critical points in Mr. Johnson's care. First, after the initial assessment, it became necessary to think of a living situation for Mr. Johnson other than his home; second, it became necessary when Mr. Johnson was found to be inappropriate for psychiatric placement; and third, it was necessary when supported by the county's options process. When we had secured a place at an extended care facility that specialized in younger adults with dementia, we reassessed our options and what help Mrs. Johnson would need from me to follow through with the hospital discharge and nursing home admission. Mrs. Johnson's and my assessment of each other's successes and failures continued to strengthen our resolve on behalf of Mr. Johnson.

Termination

Traditionally in hospitals, relationships between the patient, family members, and the social worker end when the patient is discharged from the hospital. For the most part, this is true for the Johnsons and myself; however, because a civil rights claim had been filed on behalf of Mr. Johnson against one of the nursing facilities from which he was refused admission, Mrs. Johnson and I remain in touch regarding the progress of the case. In that regard, I have been interviewed by the Civil Rights Office and have obtained written consent from Mrs. Johnson to release information in order to respond to case inquiries on Mr. Johnson's behalf. If Mr. Johnson were readmitted to our facility, the department would follow him for postcare planning.

FIGURE 10.1. Ecomap for Edward Johnson

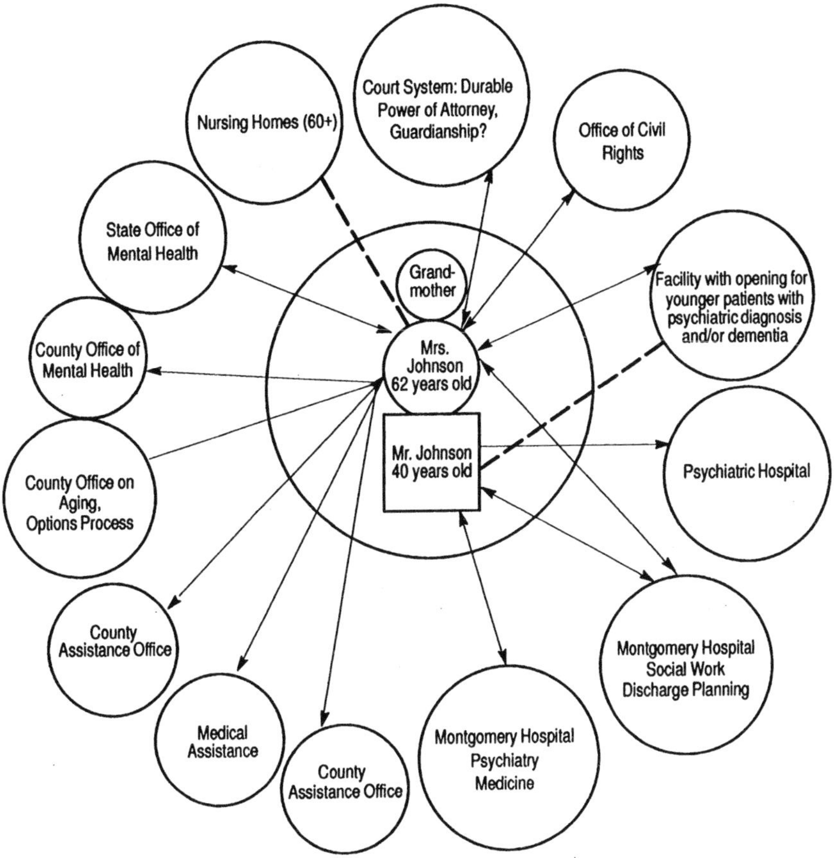

Case Conclusion

Mr. Johnson has remained in the nursing facility since his discharge from the hospital more than a year ago. His level of care has not changed; however, long-term confinement continues to be difficult for him. He requires extensive supervised activities and continued psychiatric medication to control outbursts and aggressive behavior. He has been hospitalized twice in a psychiatric facility for over 30 days for continued aggressive behaviors. Returning Mr. Johnson to a community environment with less than 24-hour supervision is highly unlikely; however, it is always a possibility. Facilities will continue to use chemical and behavioral techniques that will enable them to discharge him to the community. Because Mr. Johnson will agree with that goal, it is critical that his mother be granted guardianship in order to protect her son.

Differential Discussion

Mr. Johnson's placement could have progressed more quickly if additional referrals had been made earlier and to facilities in a wider geographic area. Originally, placements were purused only in Mr. Johnson's county of residence so that his mother would be able to visit him more easily; but eventually, he was referred to facilities in a five county area. In addition, consultation with the Office of Mental Health earlier in the process could have eliminated the psychiatric stigma and made Mr. Johnson's placement in an extended care facility less of a challenge. Also, because Mr. Johnson did not have a previous psychiatric diagnosis or hospitalization, he could not be referred to any community mental health or halfway house programs. It would have been helpful if the psychiatrist had not identified that the patient should be psychiatrically institutionalized the same day the county home was evaluating him for long-term placement. It would also have been beneficial to the placement process if the psychiatrist had discussed the patient's diagnosis with the Office of Mental Health to assist the psychiatrist in determining whether psychiatric placement was feasible and/or appropriate. Finally, Mr. Johnson's hospital stay was prolonged because I thought it was unsafe for him to wait at home for a community facility opening. Although I hope that payers will continue to respond to such concerns, managed competition and the bottom line may press payers to press the hospital to discharge without sufficient regard for safety. Although the social worker will continue to advocate for patients such as the Johnson's, advocacy will be an uphill battle.

PRACTICE IN CONTEXT

Due to the hospital's legal obligation to provide evidence of reasonable efforts at establishing the patient's discharge to a safe environment, the constraints on making a discharge to home, and the lack of community supports and facilities to meet his needs, Mr. Johnson's length of stay exceeded four months. Different levels of government declared his reimbursible length of stay and appropriate utilization of services in this acute care facility; several county and state agencies had to "certify" or "not certify" diagnosis and treatment. From the outset, it was clear that Mr. Johnson's options were limited by the payer (Medical Assistance), degree of medical complexity (alcoholic anoxic encephalopathy), disagreement about the presence of a psychiatric diagnosis, and lack of access to community resources (mental health community services, psychiatric placement, and extended nursing facility care). Mrs. Johnson, the mother of the patient and the one who acted as his guardian, understood the limits of the hospital services with respect to length of stay, level of care, 24-hour supervision, and the activity level of the patient. Clearly, the health system is severely limited in its ability to appropriately and efficiently provide for the long-term care needs of a 40-year-old man with an alcohol dementia.

PROFESSION IN CONTEXT

Social workers' skills, values, and resources make them able to act as discharge planners because they advocate for clients; understand policy constraints and organizational ethics; ensure continuity of care through knowledge of relationship building, organizational dynamics, and community resources; and monitor the costs and duplication of services within their respective health care institutions. This unique combination of knowledge, values, and skills has never been as important as it is now in the managed care environment. Social workers remain necessary to the provision of efficient and high-quality patient care in acute-care hospitals as they are to the entire range of facilities in the U.S. health care system.

REFERENCES

Abramson, J. S. (1990). Enhancing patient participation: Clinical strategies in the discharge planning process. *Social Work in Health Care, 14*(4), 53-71.

Allen, M. G. and Phillips, K. L. (1993). Utilization review of treatment for chemical dependence. *Hospital and Community Psychiatry, 44*(8), 752-756.

American Hospital Association. (1984). *Discharge planning guidelines*. Chicago, IL: American Hospital Association.

Berkman, B., Miller, S., Holmes, W., and Bonander, E. (1990). Screening elder cardiac patients to identify need for social work services. *Health and Social Work, 15*(1), 64-72.

Blumenfield, S. and Rosenberg, G. (1988). Towards a network of social health services: Redefining discharge planning and expanding the social work domain. *Social Work in Health Care, 13*(4), 31-48.

Booth, B. M., Ludke, R. I., and Fisher, E. M. (1994). Reliability of a utilization review instrument in a large field study. *American Journal of Medical Quality, 9*(2), 68-73.

Brennan, J. P. and Kaplan, C. (1993). Setting new standards for social work case management. *Hospital and Community Psychiatry, 44*(3), 219-222.

Brown, S. (1995). (Ed.). *Treating alcoholism.* San Francisco, CA: Jossey-Bass.

Clare, M., Sargent, D., Moxley, R., and Forthman, T. (1995). Reducing health care delivery costs using clinical paths: A case study on improving hospital profitability. *Journal of Health Care Finance, 21*(3), 48-58.

Clark, R. E. (1995). The STS Cardiac Surgery National Database: An update. *Annals of Thoracic Surgery, 59*(6), 1376-1380.

Daley, D. C. and Raskin, M. S. (Eds.) (1990). *Treating the chemically dependent and their families.* Newbury Park, CA: Sage.

Davis, J. T., Allen, H. D., Felver, K., Rummell, I. M., Powers, J. D., and Cohen, D. M. (1995). Clinical pathways can be based on acuity, not diagnosis. *Annals of Thoracic Surgery, 59*(5), 1074-1078.

Dobrof, J. (1991). DRGs and the social worker's role in discharge planning. *Social Work in Health Care, 16*(2), 37-54.

Feather, J. (1993). Factors in perceived hospital discharge planning effectiveness. *Social Work in Health Care, 19*(1), 1-14.

Holden, G., Cuzzi, L. F., Grob, G., and Bazer, C. (1995). Decisions regarding the order of opening multiple high-risk cases: A pilot study in an urban hospital. *Social Work in Health Care, 22*(1), 37-55.

Kadushin, G. and Kulys, R. (1994). Patient and family involvement in discharge planning. *Journal of Gerontological Social Work, 22*(3/4), 171-199.

Keith, P. and Wacker, R. (1994). *Older wards and their guardians.* Westport, CT: Praeger.

Lockery, S. A., Dunkle, R. E., Kart, C. S., and Coulton, C. J. (1994). Factors contributing to the early rehospitalization of elderly people. *Health and Social Work, 19*(3), 182-191.

Lord, J. T. (1994). Architects of care: How we build support for clinical pathways. *Hospital Health Network, 68*(6), 20-21.

Milne, C. T. and Pelletier, L. C. (1994). Enhancing staff skill: Developing critical pathways at a community hospital. *Journal of Nursing Staff Development, 10*(2), 160-162.

Morgan, J. W., Hofmann, P., and Butler, R. (1995). Simple pneumonia: A critical pathway approach to care. *Inside Case Management, 2*(8), 4-6.

Muller, A. (1993). Medicare prospective payment reforms and hospital utilization: Temporary or lasting effects? *Medical Care, 31*(4), 296-308.

Mutshler, E. (1990). Computerized information systems for social workers in health care. *Health and Social Work, 15*(3),191-196. ·

Oktay, J. S., Steinwachs, D. M., Mason, J., Bone, L. R., and Fahey, M. (1992). Evaluating social work discharge planning services for elder people: Access, complexity and outcome. *Health and Social Work, 17*(4), 290-298.

Penchansky, R. and Macnee, C. L. (1993). Ensuring excellence: Reconceptualizing quality assurance, risk management and utilization review. *Quality Review Bulletin, 19*(6),1 82-189.

Proctor, E. K. and Morrow-Howell, N. (1990). Complications in discharge planning with Medicare patients. *Health and Social Work, 15*(1), 45-54.

Report on the Task Force on Legal Issues in Discharge Planning (1987). Discharging hospital patients, legal complications for institutional providers and health care professionals. Chicago: American Hospital Association.

Rock, B. D., Beckerman, A., Auerbach, C., Cohen, C., Goldstein, M., and Quitkin, E. (1995). Management of alternate level of care patients using a computerized database. *Health and Social Work, 20*(2), 133-139.

Rosenstein, A. H. (1994). Cost-effective health care: Tools for improvement. *Health Care Management Review, 19*(2), 53-61.

Schwartz, P., Blumenfield, S., and Simon, E. P. (1990). The interim homecare program: An innovative discharge planning alternative. *Health and Social Work, 15*(2), 152-160.

Sharpe, L. (1991). Discharge planning: Before the fact. *Society for Hospital Social Work Directors of the American Hospital Association Discharge Planning Update, 11*(3).

Showers, N., Simon, E. P., Blumenfield, S., and Holden, G. (1995). Predictors of patient and proxy satisfaction with discharge plans, *Social Work in Health Care, 22*(1), 19-35.

Soskis, C. W. and Kerson, T. S. (1992). The patient self-determination act: Opportunity knocks again. *Social Work in Health Care, 16*, 1-18.

Soskolne, V., and Auslander, G. (1993). Follow-up evaluation of discharge planning by social workers in an acute-care medical center in Israel. *Social Work in Health Care, 18*(2), 23-48.

Travis, S. S., Moore, S. R., and McAuley, W. J. (1991). A comparison of hospitalization experiences for demented and nondemented elders: Findings of a retrospective chart review. *Journal of Gerontological Social Work. 17*(1/2), 35-46.

Walsh, C. M. and Coldiron, J. S. (1993). Enhanced length of stay management through monitoring of discharge planning parameters. *American Journal of Medical Quality, 8*(3), 128-133.

Wickizer, T. M. (1991). Effect of hospital utilization review on medical expenditures in selected diagnostic areas: An exploratory study. *American Journal of Public Health, 81*(4), 482-484.

Chapter 11

Psychological Recovery from Burn Injury: Regional Burn Center

Betsy C. Blades

CONTEXT

Description of the Setting

The Baltimore Regional Burn Center is a tertiary-care facility of the Maryland Emergency Medical System for the treatment of seriously burned patients. It is one of a small number of facilities in the nation to be designated a burn center and is the only one in the state of Maryland. Approximately 250 to 300 patients are admitted annually.

Policy

Organizational and Operating Policy

Maryland has a highly sophisticated emergency medical system. The Maryland Institute for Emergency Medical Services Systems (MIEMSS), is responsible for planning, implementing, and coordinating the system. The system includes such tertiary facilities as a shock trauma center, neonatal units, a hand center, and a spinal cord center. The Burn Center is designated by MIEMSS as the facility to receive patients from throughout the state with major burns. The American Burn Association (ABA) has established criteria for burn-care facilities, and "burn center" is the designation reserved for those facilities that maintain the highest level of ser-

The author would like to acknowledge Dr. Andrew Munster for his assistance in updating this chapter.

vices, equipment, teaching, and research. The ABA guidelines specify the need for a social worker and recommend some of the social work responsibilities as well (American Burn Association, 1990). Certification of burn-care facilities has recently been undertaken by the ABA and will eventually be a requirement for reimbursement. MIEMSS policy establishes criteria for burn-center admission, which is consistent with the ABA recommended guidelines.

Reimbursement Policy

Reimbursement policy is an essential part of any discussion of inpatient hospital care, and both state and federal policies influence tertiary care. Prospective payment systems that provide reimbursement according to Diagnostic Related Groups (DRGs) are in current use in most states under Medicare and in many states under Medicaid. DRGs were initially viewed as a particular threat to burn-care facilities and consequently a threat to access for patients in need of such care because of the high cost of burn care and the large number of outliers in specialty centers. However, with considerable documentation by members of the ABA and the efforts of the National Coalition of Burn Care Hospitals, burn DRGs have been modified to provide more appropriate reimbursement to specialized centers. The ABA currently maintains a national registry that allows, among other things, the ability to track cost data.

Maryland is one of a small number of states with a Medicare waiver so that hospitals are reimbursed by all payers according to the same methodology rather than by the prospective payment formula. Rates for each hospital are set by the state hospital's Cost Review Commission, and the cost of a hospital's uncompensated care is included in its rates. This method results in higher rates for teaching hospitals and for those that serve a disproportionate number of the uninsured. A recently approved plan will distribute the cost of charity care over all hospitals in the state. This will lower charges for hospitals serving large, uninsured populations and raise rates for the others. Thus, the threat of limiting access to currently high-cost specialty facilities, a concern for patients insured through HMOs and other managed care plans, will be reduced.

Medicaid reimbursement policies for inpatient hospitalization vary by state, and reimbursement rates are often very low. In states without a strong emergency medical system, there is an incentive for nondesignated hospitals to transfer patients with potential for low reimbursement to specialized facilities while keeping those with potential for higher reimbursement. Such conditions pose a threat to access for some patients with the need for specialized care.

Another Medicaid policy that varies among states is participation in optional programs such as Medicaid for the Medically Needy and Medicaid for Two-Parent Families. When states participate in both programs, the uninsured or inadequately insured family with low income or wage earner who has no income once he or she becomes ill can easily "spend down" to the level of eligibility by accumulating a hospital bill that relieves them of responsibility for all charges above that level. Because the cost of burn care is so high, a family with a modest income may also be eligible for Medicaid through the "spend down" provision. A state's participation in such optional programs will have an important impact on both the family and on the facility providing treatment for those without insurance or with inadequate coverage. In Maryland, these programs apply only to families with children, as the state does not provide Medicaid coverage for single persons. Single persons can obtain Medicaid only if they qualify for Social Security Supplemental Income (SSI), which requires an anticipated 12-month disability; SSI recipients are eligible for Medicaid from the onset of disability. The typical burn patient, however, is ready to return to work in less than 12 months (Bowden, Tompson, and Prasad, 1989). For those who have been declared disabled for the purposes of obtaining SSI and Medicaid, there may be a disincentive to returning to work particularly for those who have low education and few job skills (Wrigley et al., 1995). Other programs that vary by state include programs for catastrophic illness, state insurance pools, and other programs to cover the cost of uncompensated care.

In many states, including Maryland, patients must be admitted into the emergency medical system based on the need for treatment without prior inquiry as to ability to pay. The now-terminated federal Emergency Medical Services Systems Program, which promoted development of emergency medical systems (EMS), set this as a condition of receiving federal grants, and many states have included this in their EMS laws (Emergency Medical Services Systems Act, 1973). In Maryland, there is also a requirement with a basis in the former federal EMS program that individuals have access to facilities in neighboring states when appropriate and necessary. Patients from Pennsylvania are admitted to the burn center in Maryland, and patients from some areas in Maryland are routinely admitted to the center in Washington, DC, because these are the closest appropriate facilities. In many states, there are problems collecting reimbursement from state programs across state lines. There are also reimbursement problems for out-of-state patients when the home state has differing Medicaid policies, such as a limit on days of reimbursement or eligibility of two-parent families. These situations have the potential to limit access of the injured person to the most appropriate facility for his or her need. Hospitals, for example, may respond to the threat of lost revenue by denying access to out-of-state residents. In states without comprehensive EMS laws, cooperation in an EMS system is voluntary, and hospitals may decide to restrict access to patients from outside their usual catchment area in order to limit potential loss.

Increasingly, patients are insured through health maintenance organizations (HMO) or other managed care plans that require approval for admission and monitor ongoing treatment. Although tertiary care cannot be preapproved, authorization for ongoing care is not usually a problem as specialized burn care has been shown to be cost effective (Munster, 1994). Managed care plans can be creative and may arrange for items not otherwise covered in order to reduce length of hospital stay. Managed care programs through Workman's Compensation insurers place a priority on enabling the patient to return to work and be very creative in assisting the patient to meet this goal. The creative insurer can be very helpful to the social worker who must often seek assistance through scarce resources. Other managed care plans may also seek to limit the number of days of acute care, but may do so without creativity. For example, when Medicaid is the sole payer, patients may be enrolled in an HMO. Although the HMO may press to reduce the inpatient stay, some subacute and rehabilitation facilities will not accept Medicaid as the primary payer; some Medicaid HMOs have such a poor reputation that no facility will accept their patients.

One alternative that permits early discharge while allowing for continuity is home care, which has grown tremendously in response to the pressure to shorten lengths of stay. Home care programs can provide skilled nursing, physical and occupational therapy, social work and dietary consultation, and personal care services. The home care agency that is a member of the particular health system that includes the burn center is obviously familiar with burn care. It provides services to all patients within a reasonable distance from the city and has a network of services prepared to provide for long-distance patients. This agency will provide services for patients without insurance coverage when such provision will help to reduce hospital loss. Home care is another resource that eases the posthospital planning responsibility of social work.

Families with inadequate insurance coverage, such as policies that have a low dollar cap on reimbursement, may sustain substantial loss of savings and other financial resources even if they can "spend down" to Medicaid eligibility levels. Beyond costs associated with acute care, other unmet expenses may include the cost of nonprescription supplies for outpatients, which can be substantial; the cost to families for lodging away from home; and the loss of income during the recovery period.

Income Insurance Policy

Programs such as SSI and Social Security Disability Insurance (SSDI) require an anticipated period of disability of at least 12 months. In the case of SSDI, payments do not begin for at least six months. However, if eligibility can be established, both programs provide support during a trial work period, which can allow for gradual reentry to employment.

Policy Discussion

While policy provides for access of the patient to the most appropriate treatment facility, this may be a considerable distance from home, which can affect the degree of family involvement and the frequency of follow-up by the social worker after discharge. Work with the patient may be complicated by serious financial issues that, at the extreme, may include the need to move to more affordable housing. Reimbursement policies can affect the amount of acute care time that is available to work with the patient and can affect options for rehabilitation. However, creative insurers can assist the social worker with posthospital planning. Income insurance policies can provide support for return to work, but they can also provide a disincentive to those who are marginally employed.

Technology

Overview of Burn Injury

Because a burn injury affects all functions of the body, treatment technology involved is very complex. A burn most obviously affects the skin, the largest organ of the body, which acts as the first line of defense against infection, controls temperature, and serves to contain fluid. The severity of a burn is determined by its depth and the percentage of the body surface involved. A full thickness or third-degree burn is the deepest and involves all layers of the skin. Nerves, hair follicles, and sweat glands are all destroyed. The capacity to regenerate skin is lost; skin must be grafted. A second-degree burn is a partial-thickness burn, and nerve endings are exposed. With no complications, the skin will regenerate within several weeks. First-degree burns are similar to sunburns; because they do not cause systemic damage, they are not considered in calculating burn size.

One factor affecting the depth of a burn is the source of the injury. Typical sources are flame, electricity, chemicals, scalds, and contact with hot objects. Burns may involve muscles, tendons, and other underlying structures in very deep injuries, such as electrical burns. Burn size, burn depth, and the age of the patient are significant factors in determining mortality, as are other general physiological conditions.

A partial thickness or second-degree burn is very painful, as nerves are partially damaged and the endings are exposed. All of us have experienced partial thickness skin loss when the skin is scraped, for example, a skinned knee or a brush burn, or when burned by a grease splatter, an oven pan, or a hot iron. The seriousness of the burn increases with the size of the surface involved.

Because it destroys the nerves, a third-degree or full-thickness burn is not painful. However, there are usually patches of second-degree burns within and around third-degree areas. Donor areas from which partial thicknesses of skin have been removed for grafts are the equivalent of second-degree injuries.

Treatment Technology

When a patient is admitted, he or she is brought directly to the burn center, where the burn size and depth are estimated. The patient is placed in a tub of water, washed, and dead skin is removed. The burned areas are covered with an antibiotic cream and wrapped in gauze dressings. The patient is then x-rayed, and catheters and needles are inserted to monitor all body functions. Depending on the circumstances of the injury, the patient may require an endotracheal tube to assist breathing, in which case he or she will be unable to talk. Burned extremities are elevated in slings, and rigid splints are required to maintain proper position. A heat-radiating shield may be placed above the bed to help compensate for the diminished ability to control body temperature. For patients with burns on the back or buttocks or for those patients with potential for skin loss from pressure, an air-fluidized support system may be used. This is essentially a bed on which the patient "floats" so that no pressure is exerted on the body. While the bed prevents further skin loss and permits healing, the experience is unique and can exacerbate disorientation particularly for elderly patients.

The appearance of the burn patient may change markedly. Vascular changes cause the patient to swell massively; if the face is burned, the patient may be unable to open his or her eyes and will be largely unrecognizable to friends and family during the initial period. Patients are usually quite lucid at this time and are often talkative; however, few if any are able to comprehend the seriousness of their injuries.

Dressings and creams are changed at least twice each day during the acute phase of treatment. The patient is usually "tubbed" once daily. This procedure involves several staff members washing the patient to remove creams and dead skin. Physical and occupational therapy are instituted daily to exercise joints to aid in the prevention of contractures, which result from the tightening of healing skin. All of these necessary procedures cause additional pain for the patient. Many feel the tub water burns. Wounds are covered with cream before they are wrapped, and washing or wiping the creams off is very painful for the patient, some preferring to do this themselves. There is also pain associated with positioning and with maintaining a position for a period of several days while grafts heal. Healing burns itch and often continue to itch for months. Some patients feel that this experience is more stressful than the pain.

Pain varies from individual to individual. Patients who are relaxed, for example, find exercising far less painful than those who are tense, because anxiety, fear of pain, and visual stimuli compound the feeling of pain. Patients often cry, moan, or swear, but despite the seriousness of the injuries and discomfort of the treatment, burn centers are not filled with constant expressions of pain.

While healing, patients need massive amounts of calories to maintain normal body temperature and to promote healing. This requires that those patients with large calculated calorie requirements be fed high-calorie substances continuously through nasogastric tubes or intravenous lines. Those who can must eat as much as possible.

Patients with full-thickness injuries require skin grafting. This procedure, performed with anesthesia, involves the excision or removal of devitalized skin from the burned area and its replacement with a partial thickness layer of skin from an unburned area. The first of often multiple grafting procedures is usually done within a few days following admission. Following grafting, the patient must remain immobile without pressure to grafted areas until a blood supply has formed to the grafted skin. Dressings over grafts are not changed but must be kept wet with antibiotic solutions. Once the graft takes, tubbings and exercises resume until the next grafting procedure. In recent years, the practice has been for surgeons to perform early excision and grafting with a relatively short time between subsequent procedures. This has led to improved survival as well as a coincident decrease in length of hospital stay (Munster, 1994).

Throughout the time the patient has areas of unhealed burn, infection is a constant threat. Although this can be minimized by various medications and procedures, organisms that normally exist within and on the healthy human almost inevitably infect the burn wound. If the infection reaches to blood stream, the patient may become quite ill and may die.

With the available technological arsenal, even the fatally injured patient can be supported for quite some time, in some cases more than a month, during which time he or she is often quite alert and oriented. The course of treatment for those not fatally injured is often, at best, marked by ups and downs. Pain, periods of immobility, therapeutic exercises, physical isolation, and interrupted cycles are all necessary parts of the treatment process. Psychological defenses, which are all mobilized initially, are often depleted over time, and this can result in reduced ability to tolerate further treatment. There are also personality and psychological factors that contribute to the variability of pain tolerance (Thurston et al., 1995; Blumenfield and Schoeps, 1993). Medications are often used to dull the pain, to control infection, to aid sleep and promote relaxation, and to minimize itching in healing areas. There are also alternative techniques for providing relief such as hypnosis and relaxation techniques (Blumenfield and Schoeps, 1993).

Once the wounds are covered or healed, the patient is fitted with custom-made pressure garments to minimize scarring. These garments are worn over affected areas during the time when scarring is most likely to occur. Splints may be necessary to prevent contractures. Plastic surgery may also be required after discharge for reconstruction of burned areas or for release of contracted scars over joints.

Social work involvement with the patient, as well as with the family, must begin immediately with an assessment of the circumstances of the injury, the preinjury functioning of the patient and family, and their initial responses to the injury. Early involvement is extremely important as recollection of the preinjury situation is often distorted with time.

Organization

Physical Organization

The burn center is located in a 300-bed teaching hospital, which has been a part of the Johns Hopkins Medical System since 1984. The hospital recently opened a new acute-care wing, which includes a very modern and attractive space for the burn center. The center is organized as a ten-bed intensive care unit for critically injured adults and children with a contiguous ten-bed intermediate care unit that serves as a stepdown unit for recovering adults and as the site of care for those with less serious injuries. There is also a physical and occupational therapy suite, serving both inpatients and outpatients, and an adjoining operating room. Burned patients who do not require admission are also treated in the unit.

Treatment Team Organization

Leadership is provided by a general surgeon and a plastic surgeon who are codirectors holding medical school faculty appointments. The house staff physicians are part of the Johns Hopkins Surgical Training Program and are assigned for periods ranging from one to six months, depending on their level of training. One nursing staff serves both the critical care and the step-down units. The nurses are also cross-trained to work in the adjoining Surgical Intensive Care Unit (SICU), so that they can respond to changes in census. Thus, SICU patients can fill burn center beds or vice versa if there is an overflow on one side or the other. Likewise, when the combined census is low, patients can be confined to a single nursing care unit. This type of flexibility is important both to retain highly skilled burn nurses and to respond to the fluctuating incidence of burn injury in a cost-effective manner. Other members of the team include a nurse practitioner, a nurse clinician, occupational and physical therapists, and a clinical psychologist. A full-time social worker is assigned to the burn center and the plastic surgery service. Consultants who are available include psychiatrists and a cosmetologist. Virtually all of the patients are followed in the burn clinic after discharge. Patients requiring reconstruction are usually transferred to the burn reconstruction clinic after approximately three months. The burn center social worker has responsibility for both clinics.

The hospital social work department has 15 FTEs (full time equivalents), and social workers are assigned by the department's director on a nonrotating basis to medical services and units. The social workers assigned to the burn center have had considerable stability with only three different social workers over the past 20 years. The treatment program is organized on a team model with a clear commitment that the whole patient must be treated. The expectation is that all team members will become involved with the patient within three days of admission. Weekly rounds in which each patient is discussed in a comprehensive manner are well-attended by team members as well as by representatives of outside resource programs. Individual patient care conferences are held as needed. The center's codirectors are accessible to patients, staff, and families, and families are encouraged to approach staff members with questions and concerns.

The demands of caring for burn patients can be quite stressful to the staff. Burn nurses often regard their work as more demanding and requiring more comprehensive knowledge than other critical care areas. When nursing shortages do occur, the demands of wound care continue, and there is less emphasis on total patient and family care. A high level of professionalism for all team members is encouraged, which can turn a feeling of isolation into an attitude of exclusiveness or specialness. Many burn team members teach in the hospital and in the community. Students from most disciplines, including social work, receive training at the center. Professional association memberships, professional meeting attendance, and research are encouraged for all team members. Logo patches, t-shirts, baseball caps, and social events also serve to promote team identity.

Anxiety about burns on the part of many people in the hospital and community can create problems in obtaining resources for patients. It is difficult, for example, to arrange for certain services when the interviewer does not visit, is afraid to visit, or is bothered by burns. For example, it is frequently difficult to arrange vocational rehabilitation and substance abuse services.

Patients and staff generally address each other by first names. Former patients frequently visit and correspond with the staff, sometimes for several years. There is a support group for former patients but attendance is inconsistent when there is no dynamic patient participation. Staff members are sometimes able to utilize the continued interest of former patients by having them visit the newly burned.

DECISIONS ABOUT PRACTICE

Client Description

The Client's Injury

Paul was a 32-year-old male admitted to the Burn Center with a flame burn over 40 percent of his body surface. He was injured when his car caught fire and ignited his clothing. He suffered full- and partial-thickness burns on his head, face, chest, arms, and neck; very deep burns on his hands; and a severe injury to his lungs from the inhalation of smoke, superheated air, and toxic fumes from the burning car's upholstery. He was admitted via helicopter transport from the scene, approximately 50 miles from the center. His condition was critical; he required a lengthy period of respirator support and was unable to talk for the first ten days. In terms of his age and burn size, his survival estimate was 85 percent, but this estimate was significantly lowered due to his lung injury.

Paul's face and head were burned, and what remained of his beard and hair in the burned areas had been shaved. On the day following his admission, which is when I first saw him, his face was extremely swollen. Although he is a small-framed man, he appeared to be very large, almost massive. His eyes looked like slits because of the swelling of the lids and surrounding areas. His lips and lower face were so swollen that the lower lip stuck out and the inside surface was exposed. His head and face were covered with white cream, and his hands and arms, which also appeared very large, were wrapped in dressings and suspended in slings.

Social Work Assessment

Initial assessment information was obtained primarily from Paul's wife, Marsha, on the day following his admission. Paul lived with Marsha, to whom he had been married for five years; they had one four-year-old daughter. He had a nine-year-old son from a previous marriage, who lived with his first wife and with whom he had limited contact. His mother lived about 50 miles from the hospital in the opposite direction from the patient. Paul's parents divorced when he was 14, and he has had no subsequent contact with his father. Two older sisters lived outside the state; he and Marsha lived in the same community as Marsha's parents and sister. While they each had friends through work and other activities, Paul and Marsha did not have close friends with whom they socialized as a couple. The entire family, including their parents, enjoyed water-related activities. Paul kept a boat docked near his mother's home, and this was their main source of recreation.

Paul worked as a mechanic specializing in diesel engines. He had worked with the same firm for eight years and was a supervisor. Marsha had a job as a department administrator in an office where she had started as a secretary. Insurance was provided by a federal employee group health plan with comprehensive coverage for inpatient and outpatient services; the direct cost of medical care was not an issue for the family.

Paul was described by both his wife and mother as a quiet person who tended to keep his concerns to himself and to withdraw under stress. His wife described him as a heavy drinker. This had been a source of discord between them; she had threatened to leave him if he did not seek help. He had attended several meetings of Alcoholics Anonymous, but his wife felt he never acknowledged that he was an alcoholic. This was later confirmed by the patient. They had not been involved in any other counseling or therapy. Before he was burned, Paul had wanted to buy a house in the waterfront community where his mother lived. He thought a change and the opportunity to pursue their water-related interests would solve their marital problems. They had recently contracted to purchase such a house and were awaiting final financial approval for possession. Marsha saw herself as the stronger of the two and the decision-maker of the family. She felt she had a close relationship with her family and a positive relationship with Paul's mother. Paul's mother was very protective of him, and she denied that there were any preexisting problems in his life.

The circumstances of the injury were somewhat obscure. Paul had been drinking with friends while they were working on a car that they were restoring. The friends had left him to close up the garage after they had finished their work for the evening. He was next seen several hours later running from the scene with his clothes in flames. While he maintained that the car exploded when he turned on the ignition switch, he had no recall of the event, and he could not account for the lapse in time. Based on the severity of his lung injury, it is speculated that he had been sitting in the car while the upholstery smoldered, the result of a fire probably caused by a lit cigarette.

Several significant facts were learned from the initial assessment. Paul's injuries were potentially lethal, and, at best, would result in physical limitations to his hands. An obscure account such as the one he gave is often associated with substance abuse. Of those who were drinking at the time of injury, a large majority are alcoholics (Jones et al., 1991). Paul had experienced considerable stress from the demands of his job as well as from his marital problems and a planned major financial commitment. His stress was complicated by his use of alcohol, which I interpreted, at least in part, as an attempt to cope with stress. Preinjury stress is recognized both as an antecedent as well as a complicating factor for recovery from burn injury (Cobb, Maxwell, and Silverstein, 1991). His difficulty verbalizing his concerns and his search for magical solutions (in which his wife collaborated to some extent) were significant in light of the task he faced of reconciling himself to his losses. In addition, Marsha was quite angry with him; she blamed him not only for injuring himself but also for disrupting their lives and plans. Positive factors were his supportive family system, his history of employment stability and success, and his apparent desire to maintain his marriage.

Definition of the Client

A traumatic event such as a severe burn injury constitutes a crisis for the entire patient-family system; each part of the system is affected in different ways and each part must be addressed (Bernstein, 1976; Bowden, 1979). Team efforts are primarily directed toward the patient's physical, psychological, and social recovery, not only because of his or her physical injury but also because his or her available emotional resources become the most depleted. However, the patient can not be separated from his or her family, and intervention takes place along a continuum of client definitions, ranging from only the patient at one end to the whole family only at the other end. The degree of social work involvement along this continuum changes over the course of time, depending upon the urgency of the need and the accessibility of family members and patient.

Paul's psychosocial recovery was my primary concern from the time of his admission; however, he was unable to talk because of the need for respirator support. Because of the burns, his face was quite swollen initially, he was unable to open his eyes, and he could not make himself clearly understood by moving his lips. His hands were in splints and elevated in slings, so he could not write, and he had a limited ability to gesture. During this time, he was, therefore, not directly accessible to me.

Marsha was overwhelmed by a sense of helplessness. She was able to visit and was aware that he could hear her, but she could not understand his attempts to communicate, and she could not anticipate his concerns. He became agitated when she visited. She was accessible to me and was expressing a need. By helping her, I could also provide for some of Paul's needs. If Marsha could reduce her anxiety and regain a sense of control, she could be supportive to him and in turn help reduce his anxiety. When Marsha gained control over her anxiety, it became obvious that she was angry with Paul. She had been trying to force him to make financial decisions when he was barely able to communicate. My accepting her feelings as legitimate and encouraging her to express herself, allowed Marsha to recognize that she wanted to punish him when his suffering was already great, and she was able to stop trying to increase his burden. Also, helping Marsha to focus her anger early, made it less likely for her to express it in a more detrimental manner later toward Paul, his family, or the center's staff.

Marsha did become much more comfortable visiting Paul and also resumed her responsibilities at home and work. Paul, on the other hand, felt very frustrated and helpless. He required high levels of pain medication, ate poorly, and was withdrawn. I decided that Paul's stress might be eased with an opportunity to verbalize his concerns, a task which had been difficult for him in the past. He now became the primary focus, and Marsha's process of adaptation was merely monitored.

These decisions represented different points of intervention along the patient-family continuum. There are many times when the most accessible point of intervention or the need in the client-family system is more difficult to define. For example, in another case, I became involved with a grief-stricken and guilt-ridden husband whose critically injured wife had requested that he not be permitted to visit. They had separated on the day of her injury. Because of her condition, she was not accessible to me, and he was requesting help. He could not see her, and although he was experiencing the loss of separation, he could not comprehend the effect of her severe injuries. By becoming involved with the patient's husband, I lost the opportunity to develop a relationship of trust with the patient at a later point.

Goals, Objectives, and Outcome Measures

The team has general goals for every patient. Whether these become the goals for the patient/social worker relationship depends on how well the patient is able to negotiate the tasks involved without intervention and on the decisions made by the patient and the social worker. The most general goal for the treatment program is to help the patient and family achieve the best possible level of functioning. Functioning is defined in terms of physical, social, and psychological goals; primary among them is the ability to pursue one's usual work and to be independent. This general goal includes an important recognition that the physical survival of the patient is not the exclusive focus of treatment. While life-saving efforts are priorities, intervention in psychological, social, and physical functioning must begin even before survival is assured.

To achieve these goals, the patient and family must undergo a process of adjustment (Goodstein, 1985). They must first recognize that something terrible has happened. The next step is to try to explain the injury and to place it into a rational framework. Patients ask questions such as "What did I do to deserve this?"; "Why am I being punished?"; or "Why have I been chosen?" They must understand that they do not deserve their injuries and that there is no rational explanation of this sort for why they have been injured. Patients must accept that the injury is unrelated to punishment or divine wrath before they can fully participate in their own rehabilitation. Then they can consider how their lives have been changed and how they will need to adjust their lives for the future. These steps are not discrete and may be reached at different rates. The adjustment process is marked by periods of great anxiety, depression, and regression. The social worker's goal is to help the patient negotiate this process. A related goal is to assure continuity of care with posthospital planning.

Burn patients define their goals predominantly in physical terms. Patients and families generally feel that once the patient leaves the hospital, all their past, present, and future problems will be solved. Intervention often begins without clearly defined mutual goals, but the patient is helped to comprehend his or her situation more realistically and to participate in defining goals for psychosocial adjustment.

Paul initially thought only of surviving the pain, discomfort, and frustration of physical recovery. He often could see no further into the future than the time for his next pain medication. When he first thought about leaving the hospital, he thought about operating his boat. As he began to think about actual hospital discharge, however, he began to think more realistically about what postinjury life would be like for him. At this point, we were able to begin to define mutual goals for our work.

One outcome measure for inpatient social work is length of stay or, in particular, days of denied payment for stays beyond those which are medically necessary. The goal of course is zero, but even when the delay is caused by the failure of a physician to complete a form in a timely manner or when an insurer has such a poor record of payment that no other facility will accept the patient, delay days initially reflect on the social worker.

The Burn Specific Health Scale is an instrument that was developed several years ago in an effort to quantify quality of life in surviving adult patients (Blades, Mellis, and Munster, 1982; Munster, Harwitz, and Tudhal, 1987). While it was anticipated that it could be used longitudinally to track changes in progress, it is still being used only in conjunction with more standardized instruments in research protocols (Pryzinsky et al., 1992). Thus, to this point the only outcome measures beyond survival and discharge indicators are clinical impressions.

Use of Contract

Contracts with patients are usually broad in the beginning, unless there is a particular immediate need. They are almost always oral and flexible to accommodate the treatment process and the physical and emotional fluctuations that frequently arise between interviews. Patients and families have rarely had another experience with which to compare a burn injury, and their knowledge of social work is often limited. For my initial assessment, I ask clients for information about themselves, particularly about how the patient and family respond to stress. When family members know their information is important to the patient's care, they begin to be involved in his or her treatment. I explain that the patient's recovery process will be difficult for everyone, but that I can assist them by answering questions, explaining the process, and providing support. I often see family members daily for the first few days.

My introduction to the patient is often limited to asking him or her about the circumstances of the injury. Reviewing the experience helps the patient incorporate the reality of what has happened. The first loss the patient experiences is his or her preinjury sense of invulnerability. After verbalizing thoughts about the experience and the loss, the patient is surprised by the relief felt through talking. This recognition of the importance of talk helps me explain my role. As the patient progresses physically, social and psychological goals are better defined. Patients are usually so attuned to the present that planning far into the future is not realistic. If we do establish a contract, it is to remind us of the tasks on which we have agreed.

Paul could not recall the circumstances of his injury or the first ten days of his hospitalization. His increasing awareness that he had "lost" ten days of his life was very alarming to him, and this awareness needed to be incorporated into his recovery process and our discussion. He was also concerned that his limited hand function would make it hard for him to be a father to his daughter. He presented a long list of things he could not do with her. I agreed that it might be difficult for him to do these things but suggested that there were other things he could do with her—things we could figure out together. I told him that I could help him think of options he had never considered. We agreed to focus on what he really needed to be able to do and on what he could do. For his part of the contract, Paul agreed to work on tasks that used his hands, such as holding a glass, between our sessions.

Clearly, one does not need hands to be a good father, but Paul was focusing on his preinjury situation and present experience exclusively in those terms, and he could learn to think in other ways. In establishing a contract to focus on his hands, tasks, needs, and realistic abilities, Paul was to commit himself to this relearning and thinking process. His desire to be a good father helped me motivate him to cooperate in his physical therapy and to begin to deal realistically with his rehabilitation.

Meeting Place

Both the injury and the treatment process frequently dictate where the meetings can take place. For example, a patient interview could take place in the patient's room when he or she is in bed in the morning. However, this may be a time when the patient is anticipating tubbing and dressing changes. In the afternoon, the patient may be up in a lounge chair or out in the hallway, feeling less anxious and therefore better able to participate in the process.

Privacy is more often a concern for me than for the patient. There are few private moments in the patient's treatment process, and the patient frequently loses his or her sense of need for privacy through exhaustion, regression, or adaptation. Families are less likely to have lost their need for privacy, and office meetings may be arranged for them. During the first few days following the patient's admission, families are often reluctant to leave the visitors' waiting area. Early meetings may take place there if there is an opportunity and if there is no need for more privacy.

Use of Time

The length of hospitalization is an important issue for burn patients. When patients ask how long this will last, they are also expressing their concerns about their ability to endure the physical process. At this point, they do not anticipate emotional difficulties beyond enduring the pain and discomfort of physical recovery or any problems beyond the end of hospitalization. Patients are told that they will be changed by this experience and that their physical, emotional, and social functioning can improve for a year or longer. No matter how much they talk about going home, patients and families experience very high anxiety at this time and frequently attempt delaying tactics. Altering the discharge date for any reason reinforces their fear that the patient is not ready. It is necessary for the social worker and other staff to work with physicians to determine the discharge date so that there is adequate time to carry out necessary tasks without having to postpone the date.

In other aspects of time, I again favor a flexible approach. In Paul's case, I knew that if he survived, his hospitalization would be a lengthy one, which would allow for a longer period of intervention. Depending on our task and his physical state, we could meet as often as several times a week. At other times, it would only be possible to maintain contact for very brief periods of time. Patients are also given permission to not talk with me if they don't feel up to it. Once given this permission, I have found that patients rarely use it. However, if they do not wish to talk, it is important to assess whether this is a healthy exercise of control or an avoidance tactic that needs to be addressed.

Interventions

Like other social work decisions, interventions can vary depending on the client of the moment, the vicissitudes of recovery and treatment, or the needs of the institution. Intervention may be in the form of support for the family or the patient, information and referral, or identification of options for the patient to assure continuity of care in the posthospital period. Intervention may also involve education or arranging for a conference to provide clarification for the patient or family. It may also be necessary to intervene with an employer on behalf of a patient. While other professions may define a narrow focus for their work, it is often consistent with the nature of social work that decisions about intervention be flexible.

When working with a patient, I most often use a problem-solving approach. Although the patient must complete a lengthy process of adjusting to his or her losses, he or she accomplishes this process by solving a series of problems experienced individually and on a day-to-day basis. This approach meets the patient's need for short-term goals and solutions, and solving problems helps reduce anxiety and provides a sense of control. This modality can also be expanded from a brief crisis intervention model to a longer problem-solving model. I used a long-range, problem-solving approach when Paul expressed his concern about fulfilling his role as a father to his daughter. He was recovering and was better able to tolerate working toward a longer-range goal. This approach allowed him to think about what he wanted to do as a father. He was already losing contact with his son, as his own father had lost contact with him; Paul did not want to repeat this with his daughter.

When considering the choice of modalities, the social worker needs to recognize the enormous effects of the burn. The patient relates everything to the burn itself, and it takes a long time before the patient and his or her family are able to recognize that preinjury problems will recur. So much has changed for the patient that he or she feels everything has changed. Paul imagined that his marital conflicts had ended and that he would never want to drink again. Modalities such as family therapy are not often useful until much later in the recovery process.

Stance of the Social Worker

When I began working with Paul, I encouraged him to talk about his experience. I gave him minimal direction, listening instead. I knew he needed to incorporate what had happened to him. Verbalization assists this process, helps to relieve some of the patient's anxiety, and reduces the frequency of dreams or nightmares of the injury event, which are often indistinguishable from reality. I took a rather passive stand with Paul because that was all he needed in order to carry out the task.

I was more active with the family, encouraging them to express their feelings, because they required reassurance that their feelings were legitimate. I also had to interject notes of reality, which are important to counter feelings of overoptimism and guilt about feeling pain. I helped the family regain their sense of control by passively listening to their descriptions of how they learned about Paul's injury and by being attentive to the individual experiences they were describing. I was active in teaching them about the burn center and the ways in which Paul could be helped. They had many questions about treatment and the physical process. Although staff members had previously explained the situation and answered questions, the family's anxiety had blocked their ability to process some of this information, which would have helped them to feel somewhat more in control of this experience. My understanding of the treatment and recovery process enabled me to answer questions that simplified or clarified what they had heard. My initial stance, therefore, may be active, passive, or a combination of both. Techniques of teaching, clarification, listening, and support are frequently all that are needed to help the patient and family negotiate the early stages of the treatment process.

I was at times more directive and confrontational with Paul when he was having difficulty negotiating a step. At one point in his recovery, he became obsessively concerned about his loss of hair. Without minimizing the importance of this change for Paul, I knew that the loss of hair was in the configuration of natural baldness and was clearly not his major loss. He talked about it incessantly as it related to his worry that his daughter would not recognize him. At the same time, he regarded his hands with detached interest. He looked at them and tried to use them, but he did not talk about his losses in terms of either appearance or function. The reality of the situation was that his hands did not work very well and would not work well in the near future. He could wear a hat in public, but people would stare at his hands. By confronting Paul with his avoidance, I enabled him to move to the next step of his adjustment process.

Use of Outside Resources

Decisions about concrete services are based on whether or not patient and family involvement is necessary and whether their involvement would increase their sense of competency. A worker can help the family become involved in the recovery process by assisting them with various tasks. Marsha, a capable person striving to regain control, needed some assistance to make a list of tasks she could implement. She was then able to arrange for Paul's sick and insurance benefits, obtaining the necessary information from doctors without any further assistance.

Paul did not require any appliances for exercising or function. He did have a hand splint to maintain position and to apply pressure to his palm. Patients rarely require any special equipment at home as they either leave the hospital with maximal function, which they must work to maintain, or they are transferred to a rehabilitation or subacute facility where therapy will continue. Wheel chairs and other assistive devices could potentially contribute to loss of function as scarring and contractures develop. In many cases, outpatient therapy is required primarily to maintain function that may be lost as healing (scarring and contracting) continues. Arrangements were made for Paul to receive physical therapy at a hospital near his home. They negotiated a schedule, and Marsha arranged the necessary transportation. Marsha's needs and abilities were determining factors in my not offering assistance in making these arrangements.

Reassessment

Reassessment may be formal, informal, comprehensive, or problem-specific. Decisions about reassessment relate to when it should and should not take place. Paul experienced periods of depression and regression that are typical in the recovery process. Attempts to help the patient recognize progress through reassessment at times like these may result in the patient viewing the worker's attempts at reassessment as false reassurance. In timing reassessment with the patient, I take into account his or her preinjury style of coping, the duration of regression and depression periods, and his or her awareness of the recovery process.

A formal reassessment took place at regular intervals following Paul's discharge. Originally instituted as part of a research protocol, the assessment involved discussing his preinjury functioning with him and assessing change in relation to that level. This comprehensive assessment included work, independence, physical functioning, family and social relationships, psychological functioning, and subjective concerns. The patient and social worker together identified problems and growth areas.

The benefit of this type of comprehensive reassessment approach can be seen in Paul's case. He was focusing on his diminished hand function as an indicator of his lack of progress. He had not considered the fact that he was not drinking and that his relationship with his family had improved. When he did, he was able to view his progress in a new light, and it helped to increase his sense of efficacy. We identified his inability to work as a problem but not one accessible to intervention at that point.

Transfer or Termination

After Paul left the hospital, he and Marsha were seen regularly each time he returned to the clinic or for further surgery. After the typical high anxiety they experienced at the time of his discharge, Paul found the home environment to be quite supportive. He avoided some of the problems that patients often face when returning home to friends and acquaintances because they moved to their new home and were far from former associates. If a need had been identified for family counseling or therapy, Paul and Marsha would have been referred to an agency near their home because of the distance and decreasing frequency of their hospital visits. However, a large number of patients fail to follow up with outside referrals for psychosocial services (Blumenfield and Schoeps, 1993).

As Paul became more independent, Marsha stopped accompanying him, so there was no formal ending with her. Paul and I reviewed his progress for the last time one year after discharge. He had exceeded or achieved his preinjury levels of functioning in most areas. He was still not employed, but he regarded employment as a future goal and not a problem that was causing him distress at that time. Significantly, he was able to admit that apart from the possibility that he might not ever be able to do the type of work he had been doing, he had found the work stressful and had not really enjoyed it. In his decision to consider a more satisfying type of work in the future, he had made a positive step. We agreed that he could and would contact me if he required assistance in this or other areas in the future.

Case Conclusion

Several years have elapsed since Paul's burn injury. The injuries to his hands were severe and required several reconstructive surgical procedures to achieve the maximum degree of function. At this point, Paul's only physical limitations involve his right hand where all of the digits are partially absent. Although he has developed a grip with his palm, he is limited in the size of objects he can pick up with that hand. The left hand is now dominant, but functions that require bilateral fine movements are limited.

When Paul left the hospital, his hair had grown back on the sides of his head. His nose was red—the color of actively healing skin. He wore a hat and long-sleeved shirt to avoid exposure to the sun and a custom-made glove on his left hand to apply pressure to minimize scarring. His right hand was very dark red and somewhat swollen. The skin on his arm was also red. Although I do not know what Paul looked like before his injury, he described his hair as thinning. He is now bald on top of his head and deep over the crown. He has some scarring on his nose that would not be remarkable except that the contour of his nose is somewhat changed (the end is larger and slightly lumpy). He has some flat scars on his chest and left arm. The grafted areas of his arm have a meshed appearance. His right hand is as described, with thumb and fingers completely or partially absent. His skin is tanned now, and he has a full beard.

Paul talks more with Marsha now and recognizes when things ought to be discussed. These discussions are still not easy for him, and he often must rehearse before he begins. Paul at first felt sexually awkward, but as he became more comfortable with himself and accepting of his limitations, he and Marsha were able to resume a satisfactory sexual relationship.

Paul did not return to his former job. Upon his discharge, he quickly assumed responsibility for the care of his daughter while Marsha worked. He received Social Security Disability Insurance payments for two and a half years, which provided income necessary to contribute to family expenses while allowing him time to explore employment options. Although he did not solicit contact with his son, his former wife returned him to live with him. He welcomed this opportunity to be a father to his son as well as to his daughter.

Paul also found a new drive for mastery. He quickly learned to drive his car and to operate his boat. He developed an interest in woodwork, which he was able to sustain, even though it took him several hours to do what most individuals could do in an hour. Eventually, he was able to develop a new career that built on his interest in boating. He did not require any special training program. He was able to figure out how to do the work by persistent trial and error, and he devised the necessary adaptive equipment himself. Paul's adjustment to his losses is considered good, both in terms of the measures he has taken to help himself and in terms of his ability to reassess his situation. He has not resumed drinking, and he and Marsha both describe their relationship in positive terms. It is fortunate that they had been able to continue with their planned move. If they had not been able to fulfill this dream due to Paul's injury, feelings of guilt and blame could well have contributed to a different outcome.

Differential Discussion

The impact of the burn injury is such that most of the patient's energy is directed toward coping with the present. Paul and Marsha had difficulties prior to the injury, but their marriage had not collapsed. As in many such cases, they felt their preinjury difficulties would not recur. For this reason, problems such as Paul's drinking, chronic communication difficulties, and problems assuming responsibility were not focused on directly. However, these are all issues that might have warranted a referral to outside resources if problems had persisted because of distance and the decreasing frequency of patient contact. Unfortunately, a patient's injury can be so overwhelming to community resource professionals that it is difficult for them to focus on the underlying problems. If a patient's preinjury functioning was chronically chaotic and now results in intensification of preexisting problems, I intervene only in major crises that interfere with his or her ability to participate in the treatment program. In these cases, I help the patient do some problem-solving, but I know he or she will probably still have major areas of dysfunction when he or she leaves the hospital.

When an individual has difficulty negotiating the steps of adjustment, the process may halt at any point. Because Paul was expected to have physical limitations that would require his dependence on others to carry out basic functions initially, regression was a likely complication. When he did regress, it might have been possible to introduce behavior modification or other directive techniques, but I chose to stay with my original problem-solving approach. Paul's early involvement in the problem-solving process increased his sense of competence during a very stressful period and possibly helped him to avoid persistent regression.

A major role for social workers is early and ongoing psychosocial assessment of the patient and family. Through comprehensive assessment, preinjury problems that are often associated with hospital adjustment and long-term adjustment may be identified (Blumenfield and Schoeps, 1993; Bowden, 1979). This assessment can be used to guide planning of multiple team interventions to address both immediate needs and as a basis for posthospital planning. By meeting with family members on the day after Paul's admission, their immediate needs for education were assessed and arrangements were made to meet those needs with the assistance of several team members. Marsha's need to be more in control of her anxiety and to focus her anger were identified and addressed. Communicating with the staff that Marsha was angry enabled them to look for indications that she may be using her anger in a detrimental way; there was no evidence of this reported after the first few days. A great deal was learned about Paul and his usual methods of coping, which staff members were able to use to guide their communication with him even before he could tell us about himself. Knowing that Paul enjoyed water sports and found boating relaxing enabled the staff to evoke relaxing memories for him when he became agitated.

Paul, in many respects, was unusual in that his injuries were more disabling than most. The long-term loss of function is often less of a problem for the patient than disfigurement. While patients can have difficulties such as traumatic stress disorder (Patterson, et al., 1990) and sexual dysfunction (Whitehead, 1993), the long-term emotional outcome for most patients is good. The most important factor associated with good long-term outcome is perceived social support, which can mediate the long-term effects of both burn size and visible disfigurement (Blalock, Bunker, and DeVillis, 1994). In Paul's case, the initial assessment indicated that his family had a strong potential for providing social support although his nonfamily support system did not appear to be strong. The task was to bolster this support system by meeting their immediate needs and to monitor their ongoing response to avoid overprotectiveness or other behavior that would interfere with his engaging in his treatment in his own behalf. Because the family unit remained supportive, minimal intervention was required with them after the initial period, although other families require more extensive intervention (Reddish and Blumenfield, 1986). In Paul's case, the only direct psychosocial intervention focus was provided by the social worker, although this would vary with the patient and the setting, depending on policy and available resources. Paul was not evaluated by an alcoholism counselor or other professional. This decision was based on a knowledge of available resources and on the belief that he was not amenable to intervention during hospitalization. Although he did not resume his drinking after hospitalization, patients usually do return to former behaviors, and it is often possible and desirable for intervention to be planned during hospitalization (Powers et al., 1994).

Although I favor a flexible approach, other approaches have been found to be effective (Blumenfield and Schoeps, 1993; Gilboa, Friedman, and Tsur; 1994). Possibly a more structured approach to goals, contract, meeting times, and other practice considerations might provide a greater sense of security for the patient. That I feel a more flexible approach is less stressful to the patient may reflect my own need, which is also a factor in decision making.

PRACTICE IN CONTEXT

The Burn Center's context is most obviously shaped by its technology. Although patients now leave the hospital after shorter lengths of stay than a even a few years ago, the treatment remains long, painful, and emotionally draining for the patient and his or her family (Thurston et al., 1995). The center's multidisciplinary team organization not only saves lives and promotes healing but also works to achieve a high quality of life for survivors. The social worker's involvement from the beginning helps to anticipate and prevent problems that may develop in the patient's adaptation process.

Because the Burn Center is required to maintain the highest level of technology and expertise, the patient's initial prognosis was improved by his speedy admission to the center where the expertise and experience of treating similar injuries was available. Although Paul's injuries were particularly handicapping, the treatment team at the center included therapists and other staff who were familiar in working with these unusual injuries. At the time of discharge, he had maximal function, and his present function is excellent in light of the potential disability. Tertiary care facilities do have the disadvantage of removing the patient from friends and family, and it can be difficult to ease the transition to outpatient care when the person is from another part of the state; however, the advantages outweigh the disadvantages. Policies that affect the organization and delivery of emergency medical services vary by state and will affect access.

Changes in financial policies of various insurers provide challenges for treatment centers and for social workers. Although some of the policies that affect burn care are national in scope, many vary with the state and can affect both the insured and the uninsured directly and indirectly. Changes in financial policies, in general, are contributing to the need to develop measures to reduce the length of stay, and the need to identify and develop resources constitutes a challenge that involves social work. While Paul was hospitalized for a considerable length of time, a shorter length of stay would have altered some of the decisions about practice.

In this case, the organization of the center was supportive of the social worker's role. While support from the director of the center was probably most important in beginning to establish a role in this setting, ongoing support and cooperation from the entire staff are important for further development of roles for intervention. While this case involved only social work intervention, there can be difficulties planning intervention with and through other professionals such as psychologists and others who work on a fee-for-service basis to support their positions.

The problem-solving approach proved effective in reducing Paul's anxiety and providing him with a feeling of competence. By beginning my work with Paul early in his hospitalization, I was able to help him establish a pattern of problem solving early in his recovery and adaptation process. My understanding of the Burn Center's technology and resources and my knowledge of the process of adaptation to burn injuries helped me define problems and realistic goals. Paul was able to utilize what he had learned about problem solving to define problems and to establish goals, thus continuing his psychosocial recovery postdischarge.

REFERENCES

American Burn Association (1990). Hospital and prehospital resources for optimal care of patients with burn injury: Guidelines for development and operation of burn centers. *Journal of Burn Care and Rehabilitation, 11,* 97-104.

Bernstein, N. R. (1976). *Emotional care of the facially burned and disfigured.* Boston, MA: Little, Brown & Co.

Blades, B. C., Mellis, N., and Munster, A. M. (1982). A burn specific health scale. *Journal of Trauma, 22,* 872-875.

Blalock, S. J., Bunker, B. J., and DeVillis, R. F. (1994). Psychological distress among survivors of burn injury: The role of outcome expectations and perceptions of importance. *Journal of Burn Care and Rehabilitation, 15,* 421-427.

Blumenfield, M. and Schoeps, M. (1993). Psychological care of the burn and trauma patient. Baltimore, MD: Williams & Wilkens.

Bowden, M. L. (1979). *Psychosocial aspects of a severe burn.* Ann Arbor, MI: National Institute of Burn Medicine.

Bowden, M. L., Tompson, P. D., and Prasad, J. K. (1989). Factors influencing return to employment after burn injury. *Archives of Physical Medicine and Rehabilitation, 70,* 772-774.

Cobb, N., Maxwell, G., and Silverstein, P. (1991). The relationship of patient stress to burn injury. *Journal of Burn Care and Rehabilitation, 12,* 334-338.

Emergency Medical Services Systems Act of 1973. Public Law No. 93-154, 87 Stat. 594 (1973) (Repealed 1981).

Gilboa, D., Friedman, M., and Tsur, H. (1994). The burn as a continual traumatic stress: Implications for emotional treatment during hospitalization. *Journal of Burn Care and Rehabilitation, 15,* 86-94.

Goodstein, R. K. (1985). Burns: An overview of clinical consequences affecting patient, staff, and family. *Comprehensive Psychiatry, 26,* 43-57.

Jones, J. D., Barber, B., Engrav, L., and Heimbach, D. (1991). Alcohol use and burn injury. *Journal of Burn Care and Rehabilitation, 12,* 148-152.

Munster, A. M. (1994). The effect of early surgical intervention on mortality and cost-effectiveness in burn care, 1978-1991. *Burns, 20,* 61-64.

Munster, A. M., Horowitz, G., and Tudhal, L. (1987). Abbreviated burn specific health scale. *Journal of Trauma, 27,* 425-428.

Patterson, D. R., Carrigan, L., Questad, K. A., and Robinson, R. (1990). Posttraumatic stress disorder in hospitalized patients with burn injuries. *Journal of Burn Care and Rehabilitation, 11,* 181-184.

Powers, P., Stevens, B., Arias, F., Cruse, C. W., Krizek, T., and Daniels, S. (1994). Alcohol disorders among patients with burns: Crisis and opportunity. *Journal of Burn Care and Rehabilitation, 15,* 386-391.

Pryzinsky, T., Rice, L., Himel, H., Morgan, R., and Edlich, R. (1992). Psychometric assessment of psychological factors influencing adult burn rehabilitation. *Journal of Burn Care and Rehabilitation, 13,* 79-88.

Reddish, P. and Blumenfield, M. (1986). A typology of spousal response to the crisis of severe burn. *Journal of Burn Care and Rehabilitation, 7,* 328-330.

Thurston, M., Reilly, S., Hanson, J., Hrenewich, B., and Sleith, J. (1995). Emotional responses of hospitalized patients with burns to debridement during the acute phase. *Journal of Burn Care and Rehabilitation, 16,* 269-275.

Whitehead, T. L. (1993). Sexual health promotion of the patient with burns. *Journal of Burn Care and Rehabilitation, 14,* 221-226.

Wrigley, M., Trotman, K., Dimick, A., and Fine, P. R. (1995). Factors relating to return to work after burn injury. *Journal of Burn Care and Rehabilitation,* 444-449.

Chapter 12

Confronting a Life-Threatening Disease: Renal Dialysis and Transplant Programs

Margo Regan Bare

CONTEXT

Description of the Setting

The Hospital of the University of Pennsylvania (HUP) is a 600-bed teaching hospital affiliated with the university. The Renal Dialysis Unit at HUP was created in 1952 for the treatment of patients with acute renal failure. In 1963, a three-bed unit for chronic dialysis and research was established. There is now an eight-bed, hospital-based hemodialysis unit for inpatients and patients whose medical problems preclude being dialyzed in the Outpatient Dialysis Unit. In 1977, HUP initiated a home training program for peritoneal dialysis. Initially, a three-bed unit was located in the inpatient unit, where patients were trained for continuous ambulatory peritoneal dialysis (CAPD) and intermittent peritoneal dialysis. Because of the increasing number of patients diagnosed with end-stage renal disease (ESRD), a freestanding hemodialysis unit affiliated with HUP was opened in 1979, and all medically stable patients who were dialyzed in the inpatient program were transferred to the outpatient unit. In 1984, the CAPD Program was moved to the outpatient unit.

One of the major functions of the Inpatient Dialysis Unit is to provide dialysis treatment to both pre- and postrenal transplant patients. The first renal transplant at HUP was performed in 1966; that year, four transplants were completed. Since that time, the program has grown substantially; the number of transplants completed in 1995 was 150. Approximately 45 percent of the recipients had living related donors, with the remaining 55 percent receiving kidneys from cadaveric donors.

All patients being considered for maintenance hemodialysis, home peritoneal dialysis, or transplant are referred to the social worker for a full psychosocial evaluation to assess the appropriateness of a given treatment alternative. Factors that are important in determining appropriateness include the emotional stability of patients and their families, a patient's ability to cope with the stress that accompanies a given treatment modality, and available support systems. As the renal social worker at HUP, I also participated in a number of multidisciplinary meetings in both the dialysis and transplant units and, in this way, facilitated communication between members of the treatment team.

Policy

Before 1972, a person in need of chronic dialysis who lacked substantial personal resources or insurance coverage was compelled to forgo the treatment, with physical deterioration and death the inevitable result. Because of limited funding and equipment, the opportunity for dialysis was severely limited. Decisions regarding which particular patients would receive dialysis were made by admissions/uremia committees, which are multidisciplinary groups composed of medical, legal, religious, and lay representatives who assessed a candidate's value to society and determined whether dialysis would help the individual remain a productive member of society (Fox and Swazey, 1974). The decisions of these so-called "death committees" had an adverse impact upon disenfranchised racial and economic groups and patients suffering with systemic diseases such as diabetes and lupus who were likely to continue to have serious medical complications despite dialysis.

In 1972, however, the need for such life and death decision-making was largely eliminated by the enactment of Public Law 92-603, Section 2991 (known as HR 1), which amended the Social Security Act to provide Medicare coverage for persons with ESRD (Adams, 1978). The legislation provided funding for in-center hemodialysis after the first three months, coverage for transplant surgery, kidney donor costs, and one year's postoperative coverage. In the ensuing years, technological advances made home peritoneal dialysis a viable, lower-cost treatment alternative for many renal patients. In 1978, Congress amended HR 1, extending Medicare coverage to include peritoneal dialysis (with no waiting period if the patient dialyzes at home) and three years of post-transplant coverage. Medicare coverage for the ESRD program has been expanded to include immunosuppressive therapy to kidney transplant recipients for up to three years, and erythropoietin therapy for dialysis. Medicare insures 92 percent of dialysis patients and 90 percent of kidney transplant recipients (Held et al., 1995). Many of the gaps in the Medicare program's insurance coverage have also been filled by the Pennsylvania State Renal Program, which is based on income eligibility and provides funds for renal-related medications and the initial three-month period of hemodialysis not covered by Medicare.

These legislative changes reflected a shift in social policy, which led legislators to conclude that no person suffering from renal disease should be denied treatment because of prohibitive costs or limited resources (Rettig, 1996). Broadened public funding is a major factor in allowing HUP's dialysis and transplant units to exist and offer a panoply of treatments and services. It is interesting to note that HR 1 represents a rare singling out by Congress of a particular disease for such funding assistance. Congress has targeted only ESRD for such extensive insurance coverage of their treatments (Friedman, 1996; Rettig, 1996; Iglehart, 1993). Important to social work is the fact that in 1976 the federal regulations titled "Implementation of Coverage of Suppliers of End Stage Renal Diseases" mandated the availability of social work services to patients with ESRD (Fortner-Frazier, 1981). Probably, this mandate enhances the importance of the social worker on the team.

Although managed care has had a significant impact on other areas of health care, it has had a minimal effect on the treatment of patients with ESRD, who are specifically exempted from prospective payment regulations. One important example of the power of managed care in the realm of ESRD treatment occurs when a patient's coverage for the first year of treatment is provided by an HMO, which is permitted to dictate where a patient will be dialyzed and/or transplanted.

Technology

There are four alternatives available for the patient suffering from ESRD: hemodialysis, peritoneal dialysis, transplantation, and no treatment (which will eventually result in death). Dialysis acts as a substitute for impaired or lost kidney function; it does not restore kidney function. Dialysis is designed to compensate for two of the functions the damaged kidney is failing to perform: (1) the removal of waste substances produced by normal body activities and (2) the removal of fluid (salt and water) from the body. Dialysis cannot perform either of these functions as well as a healthy kidney. It is therefore necessary to supplement dialysis with additional measures, such as medication and dietary restrictions (Fortner-Frazier, 1981).

During hemodialysis, which may be performed in the hospital, dialysis center, or home, blood flows through tubing attached to the patient's body into a machine that filters out accumulated waste products. Before beginning hemodialysis, the patient must undergo a surgical procedure to create an access route, that is, to make his or her circulatory system accessible to the machine tubing. The cleansed blood is then returned to the patient through another line of tubing. This continuous circulatory cleansing process lasts between three and five hours and is done three times a week, 52 weeks a year (Czaczkes and Kaplan-DeNour, 1978).

The other form of dialysis is peritoneal dialysis, which prior to 1968 was done only in acute cases. In 1968, the advent of the Tenchkoff Catheter, a permanent plastic catheter that can be placed in the patient's abdomen, made peritoneal dialysis a treatment alternative for chronic renal failure and one that could be performed in the hospital or at home. In this treatment, tubing is attached to the permanent catheter and the diffusion of excess waste occurs through the peritoneum, which is the sac surrounding the intestines. This waste filtration does not require removal of any blood from the body (Brey and Jarvis, 1983).

There are three forms of peritoneal dialysis: intermittent peritoneal dialysis (IPD), which is done on an inpatient basis; continuous ambulatory peritoneal dialysis (CAPD), developed in 1976; and continuous cyclic peritoneal dialysis (CCPD). Only the first two forms of dialysis are performed at HUP. In IPD, concentrate is introduced through the tubing into the abdomen, where it bathes the peritoneal membrane. Patients are admitted to the hospital for this procedure, which takes approximately 48 hours, usually once a week. IPD is used temporarily until the individual is transplanted or begins a chronic hemodialysis or CAPD training program. CAPD does not involve any machinery, and the patient is essentially continuously dialyzing. The patient has a permanent catheter with tubing attached to a two-liter bag of concentrate, which empties into the abdomen through the tubing and remains there for approximately four hours, drawing off wastes from the body. The patient then replaces the bag with a fresh bag of concentrate, performing four such exchanges a day. It requires approximately three to seven days to train an individual to handle CAPD independently. Once trained in CAPD, an individual returns to the hospital only once a month for clinic visits, where he or she is seen by the entire dialysis team, including the nurse, social worker, dietitian, physician, and administrator.

The third alternative is transplantation, which involves surgically placing a new kidney in the patient's pelvic area. Whenever possible, it is preferable to procure the new kidney from a living, related donor, in which case the kidney survival rate at one year is 92 percent, as opposed to a cadaveric donor, in which case the kidney survival rate is 84 percent;

(Creecy, Wright, and Berg, 1992; Held et al., 1995). The major threat in transplantation is rejection, which may be temporary or permanent and may occur at any time. Rejection occurs when the body's natural defense mechanisms against foreign bodies attack and attempt to destroy the transplanted kidney. In some cases, rejection can be reversed with massive doses of immunosuppressants. Cyclosporine, an immunosuppressant developed in 1987, has essentially revolutionized organ transplant. The success rate for both living-related and cadaveric kidney transplants has increased dramatically with this drug. In cases where immunosuppressants are unsuccessful in reversing rejection, the transplanted kidney must be removed and the patient be forced to return to chronic dialysis. He or she may or may not choose to attempt transplant again. When the transplant is successful, the patient is able to resume a relatively normal lifestyle. The patient receiving a transplant is hospitalized an average of nine days to three weeks and must take immunosuppressant drugs for the life of the transplanted kidney (Dhooper, 1994).

Both dialysis and transplant have serious, though different, physiological and psychological ramifications for the patient. Dialysis is merely a maintenance treatment and not a cure for renal failure. Unless the patient undergoes successful transplant surgery, dialysis will be necessary for the remainder of the patient's life. Transplantation, on the other hand, is the nearest available thing to a cure for renal failure. The dialysis patient faces a wide range of chronic and periodic medical problems, including, but not limited to weakness, fatigue due in part to anemia, bone disease, clotting of access routes, and sexual dysfunction arising from both physiological and psychological reasons. The patient on dialysis is also placed on a restrictive diet that limits both fluid intake and many foods high in potassium and sodium. Additionally, patients must take medications to supplement certain functions the diseased kidney no longer performs (Frazier, 1981).

Transplant patients also encounter medical problems, although they are not generally as severe as those confronting dialysis patients. Most of these problems result from the continuous use of immunosuppressants. Side effects may include fat deposits in the cheeks, abdomen, and back of the neck; increased susceptibility to opportunistic infections; steroid-induced diabetes mellitus; acne; elevated blood pressure; increased appetite; excessive hair growth or loss of hair; gastric irritation; and altered mental states such as lability, irritability, and nervousness (Fortner-Frazier, 1981). Cyclosporine can be nephrotoxic (toxic to the kidney), and consequently the levels of the drug must be closely monitored.

With either transplant or dialysis, the threat of death is omnipresent. Among dialysis patients there is a mortality rate of approximately 25 percent each year. Transplant patients have a one to five percent mortality rate, depending on whether they have living related donor transplants or cadaveric transplants. Those receiving transplants from living related donors have a lower mortality rate. (Held et al., 1995).

Organization

The Renal Dialysis Unit falls within HUP's Department of Medicine, and the transplant program falls under the aegis of the Department of Surgery. Somewhat uniquely in this instance, both renal patients and the renal social worker move between the two services. For instance, although dialysis is considered a medical procedure, it contains a surgical component in that a surgeon is required to place an access route to facilitate dialysis. Conversely, following transplantation the patient is closely followed by a nephrologist, who is a member of the Department of Medicine, to monitor the functioning of the new kidney. Although the hospital and university may attempt to segregate medical and surgical functions for administrative purposes, these lines are not nearly as obvious to the patients, particularly those who move from dialysis to transplant and, in some instances, back again. Different personnel may comprise the dialysis and transplant teams, but a common denominator is the social worker, who assists the patient in identifying the team member best able to address a question or concern. These formal organizational lines are also blurred for staff, due to the collaborative approach to treatment and decision making that prevails in the dialysis and transplant programs. The multidisciplinary teams in the dialysis and transplant programs work together in formulating and implementing treatment plans and aftercare planning for all renal patients. Social work has a primary responsibility for aftercare planning, both in dialysis and transplant.

Kidney One, the regional organ procurement agency, is an organization in the HUP network of services that affects transplant patients. At any given time, there are about 30,000 people waiting for kidney transplants (Held, 1995). Patients awaiting transplantation must endure the stress and uncertainty waiting for a suitable kidney. While Kidney One's primary function is to provide organs for transplantation, a major function of the renal social worker is to help the patient cope with the pressures associated with waiting for a kidney, by providing information, as well as supportive counseling and education related to transplantation.

DECISIONS ABOUT PRACTICE

Client Description

Robert Jones, an intelligent, sensitive, handsome, muscular, 24-year-old African-American man, presented himself as self-assured and in control, but was actually quite anxious and depressed. He began dialysis in 1978 and was being hemodialyzed three times a week at the inpatient unit at HUP. Partly because of his manipulative behavior, Mr. Jones made a less than satisfactory initial adjustment to hemodialysis. Before the onset of his illness, he had maintained a high level of activity and had never been seriously ill or hospitalized. The onset of his renal disease was quite sudden and accompanied by multiple complications. When his condition finally stabilized, he was unable to cope with the limitations imposed by chronic hemodialysis, and he responded by being demanding with the staff.

Mr. Jones was aware that renal transplant was a treatment alternative for him. During the initial stages of his illness, his entire family was tissue-typed to determine whether any member would be a suitable donor candidate. However, because of medical and personal problems, none of them volunteered to donate, so Mr. Jones was placed on the list of those waiting for a cadaveric donor. Mr. Jones had undergone multiple surgeries as a result of his renal disease. He did not cope well with the stress of hospitalization and often became quite nervous, exhibited regressive behavior, and acted out his emotions. Additionally, he had never been able to deal with any sort of pain, most notably pain caused by the needles used for hemodialysis. The staff had attempted several methods to alleviate his pain but achieved only moderate success. Mr. Jones admitted to taking none of his medications, justifying his behavior by asserting that he did not perceive any appreciable difference in his condition when he took the medications. He also felt that taking medications reminded him of his illness, which, when not on dialysis, he denied.

Mr. Jones lived alone in an apartment in Philadelphia, having separated from his wife, who maintained custody of their eight-year-old son. A high school graduate, Mr. Jones was unemployed at the time of our initial interview. He had a series of odd jobs, but although he professed a desire to work, he rarely followed through with referrals that might have led to employment. Mr. Jones was the eldest of four children. His parents were divorced and both had remarried. His siblings, a brother and two sisters, all in their late twenties, lived independently, and he saw them occasionally. Mr. Jones reported to have been raised by his paternal grandmother; consequently, his closest relationship was with her, and she tended to dote on him. Despite their closeness, however, Mr. Jones resented the continual advice she gave him. He was not particularly close to his mother, toward whom he harbored a great deal of anger for her neglect of him when he was young. Mr. Jones had, however, recently become close to his father.

Before the onset of his illness, most of Mr. Jones' interests and energies were channeled into physical activity. He was an accomplished athlete and held a black belt in karate. He expressed that his appearance had always been very important to him. It was difficult for him to settle into a more sedentary lifestyle and he was unable to cope with the multiple stresses of chronic illness, including loss of his independence and, most important, changes in his body image. His multiple surgical scars had altered his body image and diminished his self-concept. Mr. Jones was markedly depressed and in intense emotional pain. He denied this, however, and his psychic pain manifested itself in physical pain. At that point, demands for pain medication were the only way Mr. Jones could cope with his depression. This accounted for his repeated requests for pain medication and analgesic abuse.

Definition of the Client

In every case, the primary focus in terms of client population is the patient. As a renal social worker, it is the patient with whom I have the closest continuous contact. However, renal disease by its nature affects the patient's family, and so the family is also usually included in the definition of the client (Gorman and Anderson, 1982). In Mr. Jones' case, as with many others, several family members were part of the client system. Actually, the definition of the client was fluid, depending on which members of his family were active in his case at any given point. For instance, when Mr. Jones was first diagnosed, all the members of his family expressed concern and the possibility of donation for transplant was discussed. Although several members of his family, including his mother, were indicated by tissue-typing to be suitable matches, no one volunteered to donate. At that point, his mother's involvement in Mr. Jones' case virtually ceased, as did her inclusion in the client group. Later, however, when Mr. Jones suffered a cardiac arrest and nearly died, his mother rallied around him, so to speak, and for a time became more involved with her son, thereby becoming part of the client system again. This phenomenon of family members dropping in and out of the patient's case and the client's system, depending on the patient's medical condition, is commonplace. As a patient stabilizes and adjusts to renal disease and its treatment, some nonpatient members of the client system tend to distance themselves from the patients and get on with their own lives.

Goals, Objectives, and/or Outcome Measures

My role as a social worker was to assist Mr. Jones in redefining his life goals in light of the limitations imposed by hemodialysis. Most goals and objectives were ongoing because they involved actions that were continuous and repetitive. Although these were some more specific goals, such as obtaining a resource, most of our work together involved ongoing goals (Hepworth and Larsen, 1993). In my work with Mr. Jones, the target areas involved intrapersonal subsystems as well as Mr. Jones' interaction with his social and physical environment, such as the dialysis unit and the hospital. We set the goals together, always understanding the place of his medical situation. Goals included changes in his cognitive thinking, such as helping him to understand the reasons for his noncompliance and reframing compliance so it was consistent with his understanding of his illness; altering his emotional thinking; helping him to feel less depressed about changes in his life caused by his renal disease; and helping him to make behavior changes such as reducing his demand for analgesics and his manipulative behavior (Hepworth and Larsen, 1993).

The first goal after addressing emotional needs arising from the diagnosis of renal disease is to ensure that the client is educated in all the treatment alternatives. Since Mr. Jones was immediately placed on dialysis, I helped him to understand hemodialysis. Once his medical condition stabilized, we discussed other treatment alternatives and their ramifications. Like many patients, Mr. Jones viewed a transplant as a panacea, an opportunity to regain his independence, return to his previous lifestyle, and forget he had ever been afflicted with renal disease. My task was to help him understand the risks and complications that accompany transplantation (Carosella, 1984). Most clients view transplant as a salvation from the negative aspects of dialysis, consequently tuning out its drawbacks. Nevertheless, I attempt to prepare the patient for the stresses which accompany the process of and life with renal transplantation.

Another early goal was to help Mr. Jones adjust to life on dialysis. Although dialysis was keeping him alive, Mr. Jones found it a decidedly mixed blessing. Dialysis imposes very stringent limitations on the patient's lifestyle because it involves time commitments; travel restrictions; and frustration of basic drives such as food, water, and sex (Fortner-Frazier, 1981). Like most patients, Mr. Jones deeply resented the restrictions and impositions that dialysis entails. Specifically, it is critical for the patient on dialysis to comply with medical and dietary regimens. Thus, Mr. Jones had to assume an active role in his treatment and rehabilitation. Because he needed to deny his illness and his dependence on the machine, Mr. Jones did not take care of himself (Kaplan-DeNours and

Czaczkes, 1972). Since such behavior was maladaptive and interfered with his treatment, I helped Mr. Jones recognize the reasons for his noncompliance and to channel his denial and need for control into more positive directions, including employment and handling as much of his own medical care as possible. As part of this work, I helped Mr. Jones' family to adjust to his being on dialysis and to redefine their roles within the family. Since Mr. Jones's grandmother tended to want to keep her grandson dependent, I helped her to understand and reinforce with Mr. Jones the importance of his looking after himself.

In Mr. Jones' case, evaluation of outcomes involved assessing the results achieved based on our jointly agreed upon goals. The type of evaluation we used was goal attainment scaling, which allows for degrees of achievement. A goal can be fully achieved, mostly achieved, moderately achieved, somewhat achieved, or no progress might be made. Given Mr. Jones' baseline personality and the number of setbacks he experienced, it was necessary to articulate goals that indicated progress and accomplishment in gradations of completion. This approach afforded both of us a sense of accomplishment and reframed Mr. Jones' attainment in a more positive light.

Use of Contract

In the early stages of our working together, I left the terms of my relationship with Mr. Jones fairly open-ended and undefined. I initially let him know that I would be available and would meet with him weekly to discuss problems and issues of concern for which we would jointly formulate goals and strategies. It soon became apparent, however, that such a broad definition was insufficient. Instead, I decided he would benefit more from an explicit, task-oriented contract outlining our respective roles and goals. Although the initial contract was verbal, we renegotiated the contract after a medical crisis and jointly agreed that we would employ a written contract. The rationale for this change was to reinforce the commitment to follow through on agreed goals and to minimize misunderstandings about either of our roles and responsibilities. The contract included goals ranked according to priority; responsibilities of Mr. Jones, myself, and other parties; interactions and/or techniques to be used; the time frame; and how progress would be monitored (Hepworth and Larsen, 1993).

The medical condition of the patient ultimately governs most considerations. If, for example, the patient has agreed to complete a job resume within three weeks, but a cadaver kidney becomes available for a transplant, the agreement deadline is discarded in favor of attending to the client's more immediate needs. Because of the uncertainty of Mr. Jones' medical condition, the contract had to be altered to accommodate his changing circumstances. Renegotiation occurred frequently to address Mr. Jones' evolving situation. We formulated a contract that identified specific tasks to work on and set a time frame within which we hoped to accomplish these tasks. Mr. Jones tended to be overwhelmed when faced with broad, nonspecific objectives, so we divided these general goals and plans into more defined, achievable components. We found utilizing such a step-by-step approach gave Mr. Jones a sense of accomplishment that provided him with the motivation to work on other identified goals. As specific tasks such as composing a job resume within three weeks were completed in accordance with our agreement, Mr. Jones and I would formulate additional specific tasks and goals. Hence, we were continually recontracting with varying terms within the same general format.

Meeting Place

Meetings between Mr. Jones and myself occurred in several different settings. During the periods of his hospitalization, we met in his hospital room. If he was physically able, I would encourage Mr. Jones to get out of bed and sit in a chair during our meetings in order to minimize his feelings of illness and to make our interviews as normal as possible. On other occasions, I met with Mr. Jones while he was dialyzing. Physically, this entailed my sitting next to his bed. I preferred to avoid, if possible, meeting with clients in the dialysis unit because the patient's connection to the machine tends to reinforce his or her feelings of powerlessness and negatively highlights the differences between the social worker and client. In a real sense, the client is a captive audience in that he or she lacks the option simply to get up and leave.

The negative aspects of the dialysis setting may be ameliorated somewhat by, for example, drawing curtains around the patient's station for privacy; however, the most desirable setting for patient meetings is a small, private conference room located off the dialysis unit. The room is furnished with several chairs, but there is no desk or table to create any barrier between the worker and patient. In this setting, the meeting may be carried on in as normal and as private a setting as possible, and the worker and patient can relate to each other more as equals. In any of these settings, there are possibilities for physical contact, if appropriate, between worker and client. This contact generally takes the form of holding the client's hand or putting a hand on the patient's shoulder when he or she is experiencing physical or emotional pain.

Use of Time

As a general rule, the social worker/client relationship continues in one form or another for as long as the patient remains in the Renal Dialysis Unit at HUP. Since neither dialysis nor transplant patients are ever discharged, in the sense that they no longer need medical treatment, I as the social worker remain available to them. The intensity of the relationship, of course, varies with the psychosocial factors, medical condition, and treatment phase of the patient and family. I saw Mr. Jones and his family quite frequently when the diagnosis of ESRD was made and he was having considerable difficulty adjusting to dialysis. In most cases, the frequency of contacts declines as the patient stabilizes and adjusts to dialysis or transplant. Mr. Jones, however, experienced many emotional and medical crises, such as loss of self-esteem that resulted from changes in body image and learning his family would not act as donors for his transplant, followed by cadaver transplant, rejection of the transplanted kidney, readjustment to dialysis, and a cardiac arrest, which led to debilitation that required extensive rehabilitation services. The number of crises and losses Mr. Jones suffered necessitated more frequent and intensive intervention.

The duration of each meeting with him was dictated by his psychological and/or medical condition. When he was doing poorly, our meetings tended to last longer, as they did when he was hospitalized for transplant and when he faced losing the transplanted kidney. During this time, I helped Mr. Jones deal with disappointment and feelings of hopelessness in losing the kidney and returning to dialysis.

Interventions

Crisis intervention was a frequently utilized treatment modality in Mr. Jones' case since many crises developed during the course of his illness, which caused disequilibrium and interference with his emotional functioning. The first crisis, of course, was the sudden onset of his renal disease and his need for dialysis treatments. The goals of social work crisis intervention at the initial stage matched those of the dialysis staff: relief of symptoms and restoration to the fullest extent possible of pre-crisis functioning. Utilizing anticipatory guidance, I helped Mr. Jones to foresee future crises that might develop and to plan effective coping strategies based on problem-solving skills learned during preceding crises. The most relevant strategies were analyzing sources of distress, accrediting successful efforts in coping with past crisis situations, anticipating needs, identifying and utilizing support systems, and formulating and implementing tasks (Hepworth and Larsen, 1993). When each succeeding crisis occurred, I utilized the same treatment approach to help Mr. Jones achieve a maximum level of functioning.

Another modality of treatment was education. Renal patients are usually frightened of the prospect of dialysis. On the theory that gaining knowledge about something hitherto unknown may reduce anxiety, I immediately attempted to expand Mr. Jones' understanding of his illness and his treatment alternatives. As mentioned before, much of the information imparted at the outset of treatment is not successfully integrated, because at that stage the client is overwhelmed physically and emotionally by his or her disease and tends to deny the long-term need for treatment. Therefore, this educational process continues throughout the course of my relationship with a client (Gorman and Anderson, 1982).

Furthermore, since by definition renal disease affects all members of the family, the Jones family was seen several times in an effort to determine the nature of their emotional involvement and the degree of stress Mr. Jones' disease caused. I attempted to identify dysfunctional interactional patterns and replace them with more facilitative ways of relating to one another. Mr. Jones needed positive feedback from his family. This was particularly important after he learned that he would not have a family donor for transplant. The involvement of his grandmother, parents, and siblings provided Mr. Jones with reassurance and encouragement. The family sessions seemed particularly to enhance the relationship between Mr. Jones and his father.

While he was aware intellectually that medication and dietary compliance are critical to successful treatment, Mr. Jones nevertheless refused to adhere to medication and dietary requirements because of his high level of denial regarding his illness. Above all else, he desired a transplant. Through extensive counseling, he identified his reason for noncompliance and realized he could only be eligible for a transplant if he demonstrated that he was able to manage his medical, dietary, and other regimens.

Case management was used when Mr. Jones suffered a heart attack. It became my responsibility to plan and orchestrate the service delivery in a systematic and timely manner. Mr. Jones' coping style was manipulative behavior through which he could "divide and conquer" those involved in his care and treatment. Functioning as his case manager allowed me to develop a unified strategy so that the various services were not working at cross purposes (Hepworth and Larsen, 1993). In this role, it was necessary to advocate on behalf of Mr. Jones with the visiting nurses, the volunteer transportation service, the Office of Vocational Rehabilitation, as well as the transplant department. The majority of my advocacy would be termed case advocacy because it was work on behalf of Mr. Jones and his family. A goal of my advocacy for Mr. Jones was to encourage him to advocate for himself. This was demonstrated when Mr. Jones contacted the hospital Office of Vocational Rehabilitation counselor to follow up when she did not get back to him with information she agreed to provide by a specific date. He followed through with her and her supervisor until he got the needed information.

Another technique utilized successfully with Mr. Jones was task-oriented counseling. In order to enhance his self-esteem, his motivation, and ability to deal with his medical and emotional problems, Mr. Jones and I concentrated on setting those successively attainable goals discussed earlier. Finally, I used supportive therapy on several occasions during Mr. Jones' treatment. Different forms of support were offered to meet Mr. Jones' needs, including protection, acceptance, validation, and education (Nelson, 1980). I found this therapy tool particularly useful in helping him adjust to dialysis initially and cope with returning to dialysis after his transplanted kidney was rejected.

Stance of the Social Worker

My stance in relation to Mr. Jones was necessarily variable. I adopted different roles depending upon, for instance, whether he was in crisis or stabilized medically and emotionally, or whether he was making progress toward his goals or was stymied. The onset of Mr. Jones' renal disease left him so overwhelmed by his medical problems and introduction to dialysis that it would have been futile to try to get him to participate actively in a social worker/client relationship. At that stage, it was necessary for me to adopt a directive, active stance with Mr. Jones. I "took him by the hand" in almost a literal sense, trying to impress upon him the meaning and ramifications of dialysis and treatment options. Once Mr. Jones had achieved a fairly complete, rational understanding of what lay ahead for him, I was able to reduce the directive aspect of my role and relate to Mr. Jones as more of a partner as we discussed and mapped out both medical and life goals for him.

Choices such as support or confrontation were also largely determined by Mr. Jones' emotional and medical condition at a given time. For instance, when Mr. Jones rejected his transplanted kidney, he was at first so devastated that it was most effective to provide Mr. Jones a shoulder to lean on and a friendly ear to hear his concerns, fears, bitterness, and hopelessness. I had to be wary, however, of taking the supportive stance too far and reinforcing Mr. Jones' dependence and self-pity. He tended to adopt a passive role, manipulating others, including me, in an attempt to get them to handle his problems and achieve his goals for him. Such manipulative behavior signaled to me a need to prod Mr. Jones, using confrontational tactics if necessary, to take more control of his life and participate fully in treatment and life decisions.

I also found a direct approach to be most effective with Mr. Jones. Since he often denied his illness, it was difficult to get him to arrive at conclusions about appropriate courses of action in an inductive manner. We made considerably more progress when we discussed the problems he faced and reviewed potential options that might increase coping and problem-solving skills. We would then make concrete plans and divide the steps necessary to achieve his goals.

Use of Outside Resources

In three instances, I helped Mr. Jones with other resources. As elsewhere, my overriding concern here was to maximize Mr. Jones' participation in his own care. The first instance occurred when Mr. Jones and I agreed that it he should try to obtain a job. Toward that end, I made the initial contact with the Pennsylvania Office of Vocational Rehabilitation and conferred with the counselor assigned to the hospital, explaining Mr. Jones' medical condition and his desire for counseling that might lead to employment. From that point on, I gave him the counselor's name and telephone number so he could set up an appointment. Later in the process, I gave Mr. Jones an article detailing preparation of a resume. After we discussed the format and what points to emphasize, he prepared a rough draft, which we then refined for typing and submission. Throughout the process, I supported Mr. Jones' progress by providing positive reinforcement for tasks he performed.

The second instance was after Mr. Jones suffered a cardiac arrest that resulted in brain damage, making it impossible for him to return to his previous independent lifestyle. Although his brain damage was felt to be reversible, home care services were necessary until he fully recovered. Because of Mr. Jones' serious, albeit temporary, physical and mental disabilities, it was necessary for me to take an active role in arranging for necessary services, including home physical therapy, visiting nurses, and home health aides. Additionally, a family meeting was convened to review Mr. Jones' emotional and physical needs, discuss family concerns, and make arrangements for family members to assist with Mr. Jones' care, since he could not be left alone during the period immediately following his discharge.

The third instance involved arranging for Mr. Jones' transportation to dialysis following his discharge from the hospital after his unsuccessful transplant. When Mr. Jones was physically able, he traveled to dialysis by public transportation. However, when his physical condition precluded this, I made arrangements for a volunteer organization to transport him. When he improved to the point where the special transportation arrangements were no longer necessary, he nevertheless attempted to persuade me to continue them. Recognizing that cooperating with Mr. Jones' manipulative behavior would only reinforce his dependent sick role, as well as abuse the volunteer system, I resumed working with him toward the goal of reassuming responsibility for his own transportation arrangements. Figure 12.1 outlines Robert's various available outside resources.

Reassessment

Reassessment occurred regularly on two levels. First, each month his condition, progress, health care needs, and treatment plans were discussed at the patient-care conference. At these conferences, the entire treatment team, including doctors, nurses, technicians, social worker, dietitian, and pharmacist discussed the full range of issues affecting Mr. Jones and his care. They included his analgesic abuse, demanding behavior, rehabilitation potential, high fluid gains between treatments, and medication noncompliance. At each meeting, I identified and discussed issues and problems I was confronted with at the time. Soliciting the suggestions of the other members of the treatment team, I was able to think through alternative strategies that might be helpful. These multidisciplinary conferences also offered valuable opportunities for me to update the other members of the team regarding the treatment plan I had formulated for Mr. Jones. As Kress states, "The goal of the treatment plan is to offer care in a way the patient can tolerate and to provide a regimen within the context of the client's personality structure and family life" (1975, p. 43). The second type of reassessment, between the client and me, took the form of a periodic contract renegotiation concerning Mr. Jones' goals and tasks.

Transfer or Termination

Only death or the social worker's leaving absolutely terminates the relationship between the social worker and the renal patient. In some cases, the patient may be adjusted and stabilized to the point that the relationship will be reactivated only if a specific problem that requires additional social work intervention arises. The only other instance would be the transfer of the client to another dialysis unit. This occurs, for example, when a patient unsuccessfully transplanted at HUP is transferred back to

FIGURE 12.1. Ecomap for Robert Jones

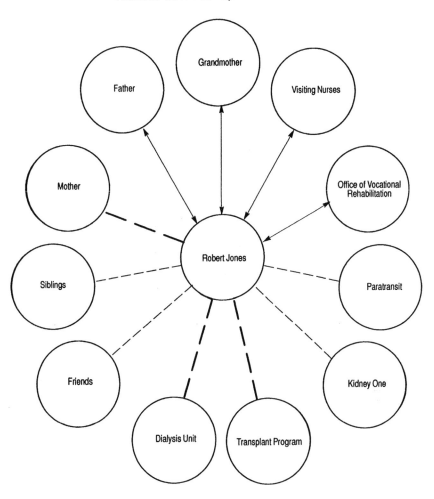

the referring dialysis unit for continued treatment. In these cases, it is essential to maintain contact with the social worker at the referring unit so that he or she is able to prepare for the client's return. In Mr. Jones' case, a similar type of transfer occurred. HUP established an outpatient hemodialysis unit several blocks from the hospital. The renal program transferred patients who could participate in their own care to this outpatient unit, reserving the inpatient unit for medically unstable patients and pre- and post-transplant patients. Mr. Jones viewed his impending transfer with trepidation. The prospect of facing a new facility and entirely new staff (with the exception of the physicians) created feelings of anxiety in Mr. Jones. Like many patients, he had a substantial emotional investment in the people and surroundings that had sustained him through a crisis-ridden period in his life. It was my task to make Mr. Jones' transition to the outpatient unit as smooth and free of problems as possible, and this included establishing a relationship between him and the new social worker.

In completing Mr. Jones' transfer, I was able to evaluate the degree to which goals were accomplished. Together we found a "mixed bag," with goals either moderately or somewhat achieved. Although the overriding goals may not have been completely fulfilled, specific objectives were fully achieved, leading to a sense of accomplishment and mastery for Mr. Jones and myself. The goals that we had not fully achieved became part of Mr. Jones' contract with the social worker in the outpatient unit. To facilitate this transfer, I scheduled a series of conferences for Mr. Jones, the new social worker, and myself to familiarize Mr. Jones and the new worker with each other, to review his progress and remaining goals, and to orient him to the new unit. In an effort to reduce his anxiety over his transfer, I attempted to impress upon Mr. Jones that the move represented significant progress in his overall adjustment to dialysis. I believed that helping Mr. Jones positively view his transfer, through which he would take a more active role in his dialysis treatment by performing limited self-care, would boost his self-esteem and feelings of independence. At that point, although Mr. Jones might have been referred to me if the outpatient worker was unavailable, our relationship ended.

Case Conclusion

Mr. Jones was transferred to the outpatient dialysis unit. As anticipated, he experienced significant anxiety that manifested itself in manipulative behavior with the staff, increased requests for pain medication, and regression in goal attainment. As he began to settle into the routine of the outpatient dialysis unit and developed relationships with fellow patients and staff, his demanding behavior decreased, as did his requests for pain medication. Mr. Jones is currently hemodialyzed three times weekly on the evening shift. His main problem continues to be noncompliance with the medication regimen and periodic high fluid gains between treatments. While in some respects his noncompliance allows him to maintain a fairly high level of functioning, the dysfunctional element of the noncompliance will likely become apparent over the long term as Mr. Jones develops complications such as bone disease associated with long-term medication noncompliance.

Despite an initial setback in goal attainment upon transfer to the outpatient unit, Mr. Jones developed a good relationship with the social worker there. Prior to his transfer, Mr. Jones and I agreed that it might be beneficial for him to do volunteer work in an effort to prepare himself for other types of employment. He began volunteering at a local pediatric hospital and his experience not only increased his self-esteem but helped Mr. Jones become more responsible, which was an essential element of obtaining employment. Mr. Jones has since gone on to a series of jobs, including security guard and taxi driver. Most recently, he went into business with his father.

When Mr. Jones realized he would require dialysis on a long-term basis he felt anxious about his ability to form and sustain a relationship with a woman because of the limitations imposed by his disease. However, as he began to accomplish goals that boosted his self-esteem, he became more willing to engage in relationships. After his transfer to the outpatient unit, Mr. Jones became involved with the local church and began dating a young woman. They are now married and Mr. Jones helps raise his wife's daughter from a previous relationship. He is quite devoted to the daughter; he thinks of her as his daughter and assists with her care since his wife works.

Mr. Jones has demonstrated a significant amount of growth. He has become increasingly responsible, as evidenced by his employment, his commitment to his marital relationship, and the responsibility he has assumed for his wife's daughter. Despite his recurrent noncompliance, he has greatly improved from the time he began dialysis, when he refused to take any medications, demanded analgesics prior to needle sticks, and had excessive weight gains between every treatment. Mr. Jones' noncompliance is not surprising in light of his desire to deny his illness when he is not in the unit. In the past, he saw the cause and effect of his noncompliant behavior and modified it appropriately. Now, however, given the absence of immediate impact of his failure to follow his prescribed regimen, he does not perceive any problems associated with his noncompliance and is thus less motivated to modify his behavior. Given Mr. Jones' personality, his current behavior is to be expected.

Differential Discussion

In general, I feel the relationship between myself and Mr. Jones was a positive one. Many of the goals we established were accomplished and Mr. Jones was able to utilize problem-solving skills successfully in subsequent crises. There were times when I became very frustrated with his noncompliance and manipulative behavior, and I know this interfered with my effectiveness in the therapeutic relationship. Furthermore, since Mr. Jones often alienated the staff with his demanding behavior, I sometimes allowed the staff's opinion to influence my assessment and evaluation of him. Obviously, this led to incorrect assumptions on occasion, and I had to redefine the assessment to ensure relevant interventions. Additionally, I had to guard against focusing on the pathology or negative aspects of Mr. Jones' behavior. Unfortunately, this pathology approach is part of the medical model and was often the focus in team meetings. Consequently, I found it necessary to emphasize the positive and functional aspects of Mr. Jones' personality and behavior, not only to enhance his self-esteem and motivation but to help the staff to see the incremental improvements in a positive light.

Although there were several family sessions, in retrospect it would probably have been more beneficial for Mr. Jones if I had been more aggressive about consistently including his family in the treatment program. I tended to push for family involvement during periods of crisis, and allowed them to disengage once the disequilibrium had resolved. Perhaps their consistent involvement would have further eased Mr. Jones' adjustment to chronic dialysis and minimized some of the problems he experienced.

PRACTICE IN CONTEXT

The treatment of patients in dialysis and transplant programs is profoundly affected by social policy and technology. The targeting of renal disease for special legislative attention and appropriations has obviated the need for the sort of life and death decisions that were common 20 to 25 years ago. Twenty-five years ago, Robert Jones would very likely have succumbed to his illness within a few weeks of reaching end-stage renal disease; considering his socioeconomic situation and multiple medical problems, he may well not have been selected by the admissions/uremia committee to receive treatment. Today, however, virtually any patient suffering from chronic renal failure can be treated, regardless of socioeconomic or medical considerations. In the future, finite resources and other pressures may restrict the ability to treat all individuals with ESRD and the quality of care provided.

Hand-in-hand with policy issues go the technological advances that have so affected the treatment of renal disease. The increased number of treatment options available in recent years not only gives the staff a greater variety of medical alternatives but also creates many more opportunities and challenges for social work intervention. For instance, the choice and success of a given treatment (the decision made largely by the patient and family with staff advice) dictate whether the patient will spend a great deal or relatively little time in the unit; whether his or her family will actively participate or merely provide emotional support in the treatment; and whether the patient will lead a relatively normal or severely restricted life. These and similar issues provide fertile ground for assistance by the social worker.

Perhaps the most perplexing aspect for the individual who is on dialysis or who has received a transplant is the notion that he or she should not focus on being ill and should get on with his or her life. This is often difficult when the patient is receiving mixed messages from the staff. Because of the physical location of the dialysis and transplant unit, the patient must come to the hospital for treatment. He or she may be an outpatient, but he or she is aware that a hospital is a place where people go when they are sick and where other people do everything for them. However, the philosophy of both the dialysis and transplant programs is to expect the patient to participate fully in his or her care and to perform tasks independently. We encourage patients to return to their pre-illness lifestyles and to function as independently as their condition allows. On the other hand, we reinforce dependency needs and the concept of illness by having patients come to the hospital, where they are constantly reminded of their illness by medications, the care given them, and by dietary restrictions (Landsman, 1975). This almost schizophrenic existence tends to confuse the patient and often makes social work intervention frustrating. In Mr. Jones' case, he became quite comfortable with the sick role and was reluctant to perform tasks independently. Conceptualizing the individual as part of several systems allows me to define my role and work with the patient toward goals that are realistic and achievable.

Most important to remember about social work practice in a renal program is that patients and their families are confronting a life-threatening disease. There is no escaping that fact, although patients and their families often deny it in order to return to some semblance of a normal lifestyle. The role of the social worker is to educate the patient and family in the treatment alternatives available for renal failure and to help the people affected by the disease make a positive adjustment, redefine their life goals in terms of the limitations imposed, and rehabilitate themselves to their fullest potential. Legislative aid, improving technology, and a supportive staff all contribute in a meaningful way to that social work effort.

REFERENCES

Adams, L. (1978). Medicare coverage for chronic renal disease: Policy and implications. *Health and Social Work, 3*(4), 41-53.

Brey, H. and Jarvis, J. (1983). Life change: Adjusting to continuous ambulatory peritoneal dialysis. *Health and Social Work, 8*(3), 203-209.

Carosella, J. (1984). Picking up the pieces: The unsuccessful kidney transplant. *Health and Social Work, 9*(2), 142-152.

Creecy, R. F., Wright, R., and Berg, W. E. (1992). Discriminators of willingness to consider cadaveric kidney donation among black Americans. *Social Work in Health Care, 18*(1), 93-105.

Czaczkes, J. W. and Kaplan-DeNour, A. (1978). *Chronic hemodialysis as a way of life.* New York: Brunner/Mazel.

Dhooper, S. S. (1994). *Social work and transplantation of human organs.* Westport, CT: Praeger.

Fortner-Frazier, C. (1981). *Social work and dialysis: The medical and psychosocial aspects of kidney disease.* Berkeley, CA: University of California Press.

Fox, R. and Swazey, J. (1974). *The courage to fail.* Chicago, IL: University of Chicago Press.

Frazier, C. (1981). Renal disease. *Health and Social Work, 6* (Supplement), 755-825.

Friedman, E. A. (1996). End-stage renal disease therapy: An American success story. *Journal of the American Medical Association, 275*(14), 1118-1122.

Gorman, D. and Anderson, J. (1982). Initial shock: Impact of a life-threatening disease and ways to deal with it. *Social Work in Health Care, 7*(3), 37-46.

Held, P. J., Port, F. K., Webb, R. L., Wolfe, R. A., Bloemberger, W. E., Turenne, M. N., Holzman, E., Ojo, A. O., Young, E. W., and Mauger, E. A. (1995). U.S. Renal Data Systems, USRDS 1995 Annual Data Report, *American Journal of Kidney Diseases, 26*(4), (Supplement # 2), 1-186.

Hepworth, D. and Larsen, J. (1993). *Direct social work practice theory and skills.* Chicago, IL: Dorsey Press.

Iglehart, J. K. (1993). The end-stage renal disease program, *The New England Journal of Medicine, 328*(5), 366-371.

Kaplan-DeNour, A. and Czaczkes, J. (1972). Personality factors in chronic hemodialysis patients causing noncompliance with medical regimen. *Psychosomatic Medicine, 34*(4), 333-344.

Kress, H. (1975). Adaptation to chronic dialysis: A two-way street. *Social Work in Health Care, 1*(1), 41-46.

Landsman, M. (1975). The patient with chronic renal failure: A marginal man. *Annals of Internal Medicine, 82*, 268-270.

Rettig, R. A. (1996). The social contract and the treatment of permanent kidney failure. *Journal of the Americal Medical Association, 275*(14), 1123-1126.

Chapter 13

Beyond Survival by Machine: Reflections of a Spouse

Elisabeth Doolan

THE BEGINNING

In 1964, a few months before our wedding day, my husband-to-be, Tom, was told that he had very little renal function left and would probably have only a few years to live. In the early 1960s, hemodialysis was not offered as a treatment option to patients suffering from chronic renal failure, and kidney transplantation was just in its infancy. Tom therefore was instructed to follow a very stringent diet in order to postpone total kidney failure until a program of chronic hemodialysis could be established at the hospital where his physician was practicing.

Tom was the director of the export section of a small family business. Before his illness, he traveled extensively, but as he weakened he had to confine himself to desk work. During the following two years, he lost a substantial amount of weight and muscle tone, felt nauseated most of the time, and gradually gave up all interest in life. He spent the year of 1967 in and out of the hospital undergoing surgery and several types of dialysis, some quite crude and experimental. At the end of that year, Tom was unable to stand, walk, or concentrate enough to sustain a conversation.

During this time, I read extensively about kidney disease and began to familiarize myself with various hemodialysis treatment approaches. One program at the University of Washington Hospital in Seattle had begun to train patients for home dialysis using a machine that, compared to other machines, required more hours of treatment but was less taxing to the patient. The Seattle group was reported to be remarkably supportive of patients and families and committed to emotional as well as physical rehabilitation. When Tom failed to improve after several months of thrice-weekly hemodialysis, I asked his nephrologist to let us go to Seattle to try the Kiil artificial kidney and be enrolled in the home training program. He agreed, and two weeks later, we were on our way to Seattle.

At the end of one week of treatments in Seattle, Tom's mood and thinking had already improved greatly. His blood studies were much better than they had been in months. He was less irritable, more cooperative, could follow and participate in conversations for a longer time, and seemed to regain some of his zest for life. It finally looked as if we were going to have a chance at a better life. After one month in the hospital, Tom was enrolled in the home dialysis training program. The Seattle philosophy was to teach the patient first so that he or she would assume responsibility for his or her own life. The patient, in turn, under a nurse's supervision, was to teach a mate or helper. Then, patient and helper were to function as a team, with the patient as captain or leader. For us, however, the plan did not work very well. Tom's mind still seemed quite foggy at times, and he was slow to comprehend new ideas. Because of his physical and mental handicaps, it was difficult for him to learn new skills. Lack of adequate dialysis in the early stage of his illness had caused extremely high blood pressure and numerous seizures. In addition, the nerve damage to his feet and hands prevented him from standing up or manipulating medical instruments or supplies with dexterity. Since he could not realistically be expected to be the leader of our team, the medical staff agreed to let me assume that role, with the condition that we would share responsibilities more as Tom improved and returned to work.

I welcomed this decision. Home dialysis was our only chance of having a near-normal life, and I saw in the procedure of dialysis a true challenge: it was an opportunity to learn new skills, a test of my competence, a way of proving my love for Tom, and a means of regaining some control of our lives. After two months of training, Tom felt much better and everyone agreed we were ready to go home. I flew back to Philadelphia to set up the kidney machine and organize the medical supplies, and Tom joined me a few days later. Surprisingly, I was not apprehensive or anxious. On the contrary, I remember experiencing a sense of elation. I was actually eager to go ahead with our first dialysis and embark on this new way of life.

Despite various crises, Tom made a remarkable recovery, gradually regaining strength and the ability to walk and return to work full-time. He loved his work, which constantly provided him with challenges, mental stimulation, and enhanced his self-worth. After a fairly smooth first year, dialysis became an integral part of our lives. Having chosen for our training an institution and a particular group of nephrologists who were located 2,000 miles away, however, was not without problems. It meant that we accepted the policies and technological solutions of that institution and often had to fight to have the center and physicians responsible for Tom's care accept our methods. Repercussions of that decision would be felt in our having to be more self-reliant and later retaining technological solutions that many considered outdated.

As Tom's health improved, we wanted to be a more complete family and decided to have a child. We were elated when I became pregnant and gave birth to a healthy boy we named Gregory. For many years, despite the crises that most dialysis patients face, Tom felt fairly well; he worked every day, thrived on the challenges of his business, enjoyed family life, and did not mind his thrice-weekly dialysis schedule. After some years, I regarded dialysis as fairly routine–a necessary drudgery, perhaps–but quite manageable most of the time. When our son entered first grade, I determined that I would benefit from resuming professional interests, and I entered graduate school in social work. Our life had become almost "normal."

OUR DIALYSIS PROCEDURE

Initially, because we lived in a small apartment, the kidney machine was in our bedroom. We took off the carpeting, installed a linoleum floor and ran a few hoses to the bathroom for water supply and drainage. It was not the most romantic setting, but we managed this way for four years. Eventually, we built a house with a "kidney room" that adjoined our bedroom and was closed off when not in use. We dialyzed three nights a week for an average of eight hours. Because we did not use a blood pump, the blood flow through the dialyzer was slow and therefore treatment sessions needed to be longer.

We were often asked why we continued dialyzing for so many hours when the trend was to shorten each treatment. Tom found daytime dialysis difficult, no matter how short the time period, and he claimed that if he had to dialyze during the day, he would soon develop serious psychological problems. With our method, he could relax watching television in the first few hours of the treatment and eventually go to sleep. We both slept during dialysis, although not quite so well as on other nights.

Operating our first dialyzer was time-consuming and frustrating. Sometimes, hours were spent building and rebuilding the Kiil kidney before it finally tested properly. One particular hot summer Sunday comes to mind: Tom was out of town attending a funeral and was to return home in time to be dialyzed. After Gregory, then an infant, was settled, I proceeded to take the Kiil kidney apart to clean and rebuild it. Eight hours later, I realized I had spent the entire day taking the dialyzer apart and putting it together without success. The technicians at the training center were unavailable and the staff at our hospital were not familiar with the Kiil system. To make matters worse, Greg had cried off and on all day. Exhausted and disgusted, I was angry with Tom for leaving me with a crying baby and a recalcitrant kidney. On the whole, however, things were usually not that bad. I became adept at rapidly rebuilding the kidney and enjoyed the challenge of increasing my speed and solving problems. Preparing the machine became part of my household chores.

In the early 1970s, dialysis centers began to use artificial kidneys that were smaller, presterilized, partly disposable, and easier to handle. Despite this advance, we persisted with our old method for 11 years; we rationalized that we were successful with the old procedure and that it was too complicated to return to a center on the other side of the country to be retrained in the use of a different dialyzer and machine. We were finally forced into making this change because supplies for the Kiil artificial kidney and parts for our machine were increasingly hard to find. In retrospect, I see that change was difficult for me. Familiarity with the old method gave me a sense of security and control.

TRANSPLANTATION

Invariably people ask why Tom never had a kidney transplant. Before the advent of immunosuppressant drugs, people in need of renal transplantation were dependent on a good tissue match of a close relative. Since Tom's only close relative, his brother, did not seem willing to be considered as a donor, transplantation was not a possibility in the earlier stages of Tom's disease. Since then, of course, improved organ preservation, tissue typing, and constant progress in immunosuppressant therapy have made the transplantation of cadaveric organs highly successful.

Our reasons for not choosing transplantation were probably more emotional than logical. Tom remembered how close to death he had been before dialysis and was afraid to be in a similar condition again. He had seen friends reject a graft and subsequently become very ill. The transplantation statistics were not good enough for him until he became too debilitated and ill to have a transplant. Although his life might not have appeared so good to others, Tom thoroughly enjoyed every day of it. He believed that it would be foolish to "upset the apple cart" after almost two decades of doing well.

Initially, I shared this view. As years went by, however, I could see the likelihood of a successful kidney transplant. I knew that if I had been the person with kidney disease, I would have chosen transplantation because I would have found the dependency on a machine and other people's goodwill for my care and survival too difficult to tolerate. Despite the risks, I would have wanted a chance to feel totally healthy and normal again. Yet I recognized that this was a very personal decision. Only Tom could make this decision.

THE LAST YEARS

In the summer of 1983, two months after Tom had decided to retire, he fractured his right hip. The next year and a half were to be the most difficult of our lives. There were multiple prolonged hospitalizations. Tom underwent hip surgery three times. No sooner would he begin to recover than he would face a new fracture and more internal bleeding. After each hospitalization, he would try very hard to make a comeback, working with a physical therapist several times a week, forcing himself to go out with his walker or his wheelchair, but there were constant setbacks. We were both getting tired of the struggle. Although we did not talk about the future, we both felt that nothing would ever be good again.

During one of Tom's admissions to the hospital where I worked, he had an episode of internal bleeding. With great courage and sensitivity, the nephrologist on whose service I was a social worker explained to me that Tom was suffering from esophageal varices caused by liver damage. He told me that in all likelihood these varices would some day hemorrhage and cause Tom's death, though nothing could be done to prevent it from happening. Tom was told about the varices but not about the possible prognosis. He chose not to ask any questions; I chose not to tell him any more than he wanted to know. He was always good at protecting himself when he sensed that not much could be done about a problem, and he only sought information about his medical condition when there was some specific solution.

For many months, we just hobbled along. Tom kept hoping that he would never again have to be hospitalized because he was so frightened of hospitals, and I was hoping that I would have enough time to get help if the varices caused major hemorrhaging. In December of 1984, three days before Christmas, Tom woke up after dialysis feeling very weak, anxious, and irritable. His blood pressure was extremely low and I knew immediately that he must be bleeding internally. With great difficulty, I convinced him to let me take him to the emergency room, from which he was admitted to the intensive care unit for his last and most difficult hospitalization.

THE END STAGE

It was eight o'clock on Saturday morning, and the phone was ringing. My heart immediately started to pound, flooding me with anxiety. The phone always startled me when Tom was in the hospital, and this time, I was particularly weary because we had spent the preceding six weeks on a physical and emotional roller coaster. During the latest hospitalization, Tom had undergone surgery to arrest internal bleeding caused by esophageal varices. The surgery had left him disoriented, confused, anxious, agitated, and subject to hallucinations. Yet despite his confusion, he could at times appear logical and very convincing; he would forcefully demand that I be there all the time or that I convince his doctors to let him go home. He often behaved in this manner when he was in the hospital. Whenever that happened, I became confused myself and did not know what to believe or do. Now I understand better that the irritability and forceful demands were, in fact, a protective cover for his fears and confusion.

His physicians had explained to me that the disorientation was caused by severe encephalopathy that could only be controlled through medication, which in turn caused constant diarrhea. The diarrhea left him so sore that he cried whenever he was being cleaned. He had wasted away to skin and bones, and his body ached all over. His nephrologist had begun to vaguely discuss the possibility of discontinuing dialysis, but I had no sense of who would ultimately be responsible for making that decision if Tom was too confused to decide for himself. As a nephrology social worker, I had participated in team and family conferences where termination of treatment was presented as an option, and I knew I did not want to be alone responsible for making such a final decision about my own husband.

As I answered the phone that Saturday morning, I was surprised to hear Tom's voice. Instead of an agitated and confused person, I was hearing a calm and pleasant one. I could not believe that he was alert and that his mind was clear. He sounded calm, but concerned about the reason for this hospitalization: he could not understand why he had so much diarrhea and was so sore. He was not remembering any of the events of the previous weeks, but kept repeating how he hated being in the hospital and wanted to be home. I cannot recollect exactly how the conversation proceeded, but I do remember that we began to talk about the possibility of discontinuing dialysis. I hurriedly dressed and rushed over to the hospital, not quite sure what to expect. As I walked in, Tom said, "I think the time has come to stop everything. I want to go home. I want to be home in my nice sunny room."

I wondered whether his words were a function of his confusion and if he understood that giving up dialysis meant dying. I remembered how scared he had always been about dying. Memories of his dark humor and jokes about death came back to me, and I asked directly, "Do you know what this would mean?" I could tell by his answer that he clearly understood, and suddenly I felt an overwhelming sense of urgency. I sensed that Tom might again lose some clarity of thought. I wanted him to enjoy himself at home before he died, to be with us in the house he liked so much, away from the cold hospital environment where he felt isolated and assaulted.

Because it was Saturday, his physician was not there and could not be reached. I was hesitant to take Tom home without the hospital's approval. On the one hand, I thought we should wait until the following Monday when Tom would be dialyzed and we could discuss this with his nephrologist; on the other hand, my heart was telling me that there was no time to plan, no time to waste. The time had come to make a decision. Some weeks earlier, the nephrology social worker had said, "When the times comes, you will know deep down in your heart, and you will be able to make the right decision."

I asked Tom whether he wanted to go home immediately. Saying yes, he told me to call his brother so that he could tell him about his decision to discontinue dialysis treatment. After Tom spoke to his brother, a nurse located the physician on call whom I informed of our decision. Because he knew us well and was familiar with Tom's condition and prognosis, he was willing to go along with whatever plan we had. Within an hour, we were on our way home in an ambulance, accompanied by a private duty nurse.

When we arrived home, Tom was elated to be back in his familiar sunny room and to find Gregory, our son, with whom I had spoken earlier. It was like a happy reunion. All three of us acted as if we had escaped something terrible and we could now safely be together for a long time. We hugged and kissed and talked euphorically about the things we would do during the following week. Later, when Tom rested, I realized I had to make some practical arrangements. Since I wanted to be totally available to him, I called my social work colleague and asked her to take over my work responsibilities and to inform everyone that I would not be in until after my husband's death. Tom and I also decided that Gregory should not have his usual routine disrupted, but continue to go to school every day.

The first night at home was very difficult. I was up all night, holding Tom's hand, turning him, washing him, and changing his pajamas; it became clear that I would not be able to care for him by myself. In the morning, I called a friend who directed a hospice program and asked for a recommendation of good nurses with experience in terminal illness. An hour later, she called back to ask tactfully how I planned to manage alone.

She reminded me that what I needed to be was Tom's wife, not his nurse or social worker, and she suggested our using hospice care.

Hospice was an invaluable help in Tom's care during that last week. Regular attendance by a physician and nurses, as well as pain control, meant that he would not have to suffer. Hospice allowed me to devote myself totally to him, be available emotionally, hold his hand when he needed me, talk, listen, and let him rest. And the hospice team was there for all of us, giving us a sense of security.

On Sunday, Tom wanted his brother and nephew to come say goodbye to him, and they visited briefly. The following day, two of Tom's favorite physicians came to say goodbye: the internist who had diagnosed his renal disease 20 years earlier and the surgeon who had performed all of his procedures over that long period. Both men had become good friends of ours, and their approval was very important to Tom, who needed to know that by discontinuing dialysis, he was not disappointing two friends who had fought for his life for so many years. By reviewing his struggles, accomplishments, and happy times, the two physicians were able to reassure him that it was right to recognize when the time had come to let go.

It was an unreal week, sad and beautiful at the same time. Even though it was February, there were some sunny days. Tom's room faced east, and when the morning sun poured in, he talked about the warmth of the sun on his face. I sat next to him and we held hands quietly. Greg would come home from school and talk about his day. That week, Greg, who had never been an athlete, played basketball and was proud to report that he had made several baskets. He also received an acceptance from the high school that his father wanted him to attend, and Tom was delighted.

All his life Tom had been a man who made his own decisions, and now, in the last week of his life, he still behaved in the same manner. Even though he was confused at times, he was determined to do everything for himself; he needed to be in control, sitting up, eating, drinking, being washed or not washed on his terms. He reminded me to order baseball tickets so Greg and I would continue to attend the Phillies games and think of him. He also told me to make sure I would always have some champagne in the house, since I loved champagne and it would be good to have a glass whenever I was too sad. One day, he began to cry and wondered how Gregory would grow up without parents. I reminded him that I would be there for Gregory, and with a smile, he turned to me and said, "Oh, that's right. I had forgotten that you are going to stay here. You are not coming with me."

Sometimes Tom would start to fantasize about a wonderful miracle that would make him well. One day, he asked me if perhaps we could give all our money to a charity in the hope of being rewarded with a miracle. At those times, I would hold his hand and tell him that the miracle had already happened: he was home with us and not suffering, we loved him, and I would make sure that he would not be hurt any longer and would go in peace. After these conversations, he would rest again. I would look at him and be surprised that I still loved him so much despite all the changes in his body. I wanted to crawl into his bed and have him hold me and tell me that I had been a good wife, but I also remembered that he did not want to be touched and needed to detach himself. Once he asked me why I was not letting him go home. Thinking he was confused, I told him he was home, and he replied, "You know what I mean."

As the week progressed, Tom began to sleep more and more, and his periods of alertness grew shorter. While he was alert, however, we had wonderful conversations and I felt very close to him. I do not think that I quite realized that after that week he would never be with us again. At the time, I needed to isolate my feelings to be available to him and to protect myself from suffering. The night before his death, I left the house for the first time that week to get suppositories at the hospital in case Tom could not longer swallow pain medication. Gregory walked over with me, and we talked about Tom's imminent death. We talked about how sad it was to lose one's father at such an early age. Gregory reminded me that five years earlier I had come to school to tell him that Tom had been hospitalized with a possible heart attack and that he might not survive. He thought then that he would lose his father, and he felt fortunate now to have had his father for 14 years of his life. That night, I went to sleep very late. At three o'clock in the morning, I felt the nurse tapping my shoulder. When she said, "It won't be long now," I quickly went to Tom's room. His breathing was very shallow. I took his hand and waited. Ten minutes later, his breathing stopped. Everything was quiet and peaceful, sad but beautiful. I felt a great sense of relief: Tom would never again have to suffer, and I would never again have to worry about him.

REFLECTIONS: PERSONAL AND PROFESSIONAL

Friends and other professionals sometimes ask how we lived and coped with end-stage renal disease and dialysis for more than 20 years. Perhaps the best way to review our experience is to look at the dimensions of our lives that were most supportive and those that were most difficult. At the beginning of Tom's illness we were newly married, in love, very devoted to each other. Our only obligations were to each other, and his care was at the center of our lives. While we were certainly not wealthy, our financial resources allowed us to pay for his medical care at a time when only a few select people were accepted in chronic dialysis programs. In the 1960s, many kidney patients who did not have the means to pay for their treatment died; others survived only through public appeals for financial help. In 1972, after intense lobbying by patients and health professionals, Congress and President Richard Nixon signed into law a Social Security amendment that provided coverage under Medicare for all patients with kidney failure, no matter what their age. From then on, our medical costs dropped sharply at a time when Tom's earnings also increased, enabling us to afford a nice house, household help, a babysitter when needed, and eventually graduate school tuition for me. There is no doubt that our financial resources were the greatest factor in easing the adjustment to Tom's illness. We had privileges that helped compensate for some of the deprivations associated with renal dialysis.

Our personality characteristics were also helpful. Tom's strong desire to live, his discipline, and his take-control style enabled him to forget that he had physical limitations. He often appeared surprised that anyone could think his illness affected our lifestyle. He saw himself as different from most other kidney patients, more disciplined and motivated, and therefore functioning better. He took pride in the fact that he had no psychological problems. His denial protected him from painful feelings and helped him to live with very real restrictions.

I, on the other hand, fit the style of the obsessive-compulsive, somewhat parental, nurturing spouse that is described in the literature as a good dialysis partner. In the dialysis situation, I was the "mother protector" and Tom was the "dependent child." During crises, in particular, we assumed complementary roles: when the situation required fast decisions and prompt action on my part, Tom remained very calm while supporting and guiding me; when he was overly anxious or apprehensive, I was able to calm him down. Of course, other times, we lost patience with each other and fought. On the whole, though, we managed to negotiate these roles fairly well, which may have contributed to our adaptation to home dialysis.

Just as returning to work was important for Tom, renewing outside interests and resuming a professional career helped me see that life did not have to revolve around a dialysis machine only. Besides offering challenging opportunities to put my experience and knowledge in the service of others, working outside of the home provided me with a connection to the world, a different perspective on life, and much-needed emotional rewards. It allowed me to come home refreshed and more understanding of Tom; it helped me keep my sanity. After Tom's death, my professional activities enabled me to direct my attention toward others and avoid becoming deeply depressed. Had I not had a career in social work, it would have been much more difficult to find meaning in a life without my husband.

The greatest step in the direction of normalcy, however, was our decision to have a child and become a more complete family. Our son Gregory brought Tom and me great joys and he constantly taught us to take our minds off ourselves. He forced us to build into our lives moments of fun and enjoyment despite Tom's illness and the dialysis regimen. He, of course, had to live with dialysis as well. He seemed to take it in stride; he knew nothing else, of course. I remember once when he was a tiny boy, he told me that when he grew up and had a home of his own, it would have a dialysis room just like ours. We had to explain to him that not all daddies were on dialysis. Gregory was 14 years old when his father died. Throughout these fourteen years we talked freely with him and tried to keep him informed as much as possible of Tom's medical condition while at the same time attempting to give him a sense of security. Although we did not have the support of a close extended family (my family lived in Europe where I was raised, and Tom had only one brother), various self-help patient organizations and our son's school gave us the opportunity to develop a network of friends and supportive health professionals who were willing to be there for us and let me talk about my pain, my doubts, and my conflicts. Still, dependency on the medical staff and institution for survival was threatening to us. We knew that our independent, very cautious, and questioning attitude was not always welcome and often viewed as offensive by the medical staff. Independence and responsibility are not rewarded in the medical system. It was very difficult to be assertive. The fear of being abandoned, albeit irrational, was always there.

The very personality factors that served us well in dialysis also created problems with intimacy. Tom, who took so much pride in his independence and fought so hard to stay alive, tried to shun conflict at any cost. It was easier and less threatening for him to avoid knowing what I felt and to act detached and aloof. In the last year, when he was more debilitated, Tom needed all his energy just to stay alive. He began to withdraw increasingly and show less interest in anything unrelated to his body and his world. The literature abundantly describes the physical and sexual limitations of dialysis patients. These limitations are also the lot of the spouse. I often felt frustrated, deprived of emotional nurturance and unsupported, but believed (erroneously, of course) that I had no right to add to Tom's problems by expressing my needs. The frustration and deprivation caused resentment and anger followed by intense guilt. To compensate for my negative feelings toward Tom, I became more of a perfectionist, gave excessive attention to detail, worried about him, and probably frequently became controlling. A healthy intimacy is difficult to achieve in a dialysis marriage.

Isolation can be a problem in the lives of dialysis patients and their families. Because home dialysis is so time-consuming, there is little time for social activities. In addition, most people feel uncomfortable with a sick or handicapped person, and they handle their discomfort with avoidance of the person. My husband joked about the parties we were not invited to, but he was truly surprised that his presence could make some people so uncomfortable. To compensate for feelings of anxiety and deprivation, dialysis couples develop primitive urges towards psychological closeness. Spouses often use the pronoun "we" instead of referring to the dialyzed person by name. We certainly fit that description. I frequently said, "When we were on the machine last night," or "What are the results of our blood tests?" My husband sometimes asked, "Have you found out what is wrong with your machine?" This kind of closeness helps bond the couple, but also perpetuates isolation and can deprive one of individuality. The balance of caring, being cared for, and maintaining one's autonomy is not easy to achieve.

There is never any reprieve in home dialysis. In essence, the whole family is attached to the kidney machine and has to weather crises. Over the years, we had our share of crises: major surgery, episodes of internal bleeding, frightening postponements of dialysis sessions due to mechanical problems, and serious blood loss while Tom was on the machine. Crises represented setbacks; they revived all the initial pain and anxiety, which affected our functioning for many weeks. Although we coped with them, they never became routine. Every single one was frightening, because it could be the last one. Crises were a painful reminder of the precarious nature of life with dialysis.

Yet, despite the stresses, Tom and I took pride in our ability to manage home dialysis so well. We were inclined to show only our strengths and hide our frustrations and anxieties. We remembered the initial, very difficult years, when we thought there was no hope, and we were grateful that this new technology was available to make our lives as close to normal as possible. From an emotional perspective, though, the road was always more difficult for me, because Tom was more adaptable than I, and I tended to assume more responsibility for his treatment than he did. It is now more evident to me that denial helped us to survive these years. To some extent, Tom and I both believed that I would always be able to take care of him and maybe even protect him from death.

TODAY

It has been a little over 30 years since Tom's initial diagnosis and ten years since his death. As a social worker in dialysis, I thought I knew a great deal about loss and grief, but nothing prepared me for the pain caused by my husband's death. I did not know about the excruciating intensity of the pain and the loneliness. Being a mental health professional does not spare you; no amount of work or reading can prepare you for the personal experience of grief. Like everyone else, I had to make the arduous journey of experiencing the feelings and learning to find new meaning without my loved one.

After Tom's death, I worked for one more year as a renal social worker, then started a private practice with another clinical social worker, providing counseling to individuals and families who have experienced loss through illness and death. A few years ago, my colleague and I were asked to develop a bereavement program for the Organ Procurement Organization in our area: once again organ transplantation was entering my life. In addition to seeing our own clients, we now coordinate this support program for families who have donated the organs and tissues of loved ones who have died sudden, unexpected deaths. As a result of our personal experiences with illness and loss, we both know that illness and death reach far beyond the person stricken, and that the entire family is affected. Although we cannot quite walk in the shoes of our clients, their pain is not unfamiliar; we can remember how it felt when we were there. Our own experience, we believe, gives an additional dimension to our professional work.

Gregory, now 25, is a graduate student in a doctoral philosophy program. He has grown to become a fine young man, perhaps stronger for his early experiences, and he continues to bring me joys and challenges. Not infrequently, however, I wonder if my focus on his father's care and the (often unconscious) anxiety I was experiencing at the time of his growing up prevented me from being emotionally available to him and meet his needs. We are fortunate, though, that we are now able to talk about the past and be open with each other, even about painful topics. We reminisce about his father and remember his appreciation for even the smallest pleasures of life, and we are able to laugh about some of his foibles.

As I reflect on the past 30 years, I see more clearly how difficult these years sometimes were for all of us, although we did not always realize it at the time. In retrospect, however, considering our lack of sophistication about the medical system at the beginning of our "career in dialysis," and the absence of family support, I am surprised at how well we functioned. We made rather good use of whatever internal and external resources we had. Most of all, we were fortunate to live in an age when a new technology was developed in time to save my husband's life, in a country where governmental policies would insure payment for treatment, and to have the education and financial resources to avail ourselves of the help we needed to turn what could have been major problems into opportunities to live full and challenging lives.

BIBLIOGRAPHY

Adams, L. R. (1978). Medicare coverage for chronic renal disease: Policy implications. *Health and Social Work 3*(4), 41-53.

Binik, Y. M. (1983). Coping with chronic life-threatening illness: Psychological perspectives on end stage renal disease. *Canadian Journal of Behaviour Science 15*(4), 373-391.

Binik, Y. M., Chowanec, G. D., and Devins, G. M. (1990). Marital role strain, illness intrusiveness and their impact on marital and individual adjustment in end-stage renal disease. *Psychology and Health, 4*(3), 245-257.

Caplan, A. L. (1992). If I were a rich man could I buy a pancreas? Problems in the policies and criteria used to allocate organs for transplantation in the United States. In A. Caplan (Ed.), *If I were a rich man, could I buy a pancreas?: Other essays on the ethics of health care.* Bloomington and Indianapolis: Indiana University Press, pp. 158-177.

Carpenter, C. B. (1990). Immunosuppression in organ transplantation. *The New England Journal of Medicine 322*(17), 1224-1226.

Conley, J. A., Burton, H. J., DeNour, A., Kaplan, A., and Wells, G. A. (1981). Support systems for patients and spouses on home dialysis. *International Journal of Family Psychiatry, 2*(1-2), 45-54.

Devins, G. M. (1994). Psychosocial issues in end-stage renal disease: Introduction. *Advances in Renal Replacement Therapy, 1*(3), 195-197.

Devins, G. M., Mann, J., Mandin, H., Paul, L. C., Huns, R. B., Burgess, E. D., Taub, K., Schorn, S., Letourneau, P. K., and Buckie, S. (1990). Psychosocial predictors of survival in end stage renal disease. *Journal of Nervous and Mental Disease, 178*(2), 127-133.

Evans, R. W., Manninen, D. L., Garrison, L. P., Hart, L. G., Blagg, C. R., Gutman, R. A., Hull, A. R., and Lowrie, E. G. (1985). The quality of life of patients with end-stage renal disease. *The New England Journal of Medicine, 312*, 553-559.

Fortner-Frazier, C. L. *Social work and dialysis: The medical and psychological aspects of kidney disease.* Berkeley: University of California Press.

Friedlander, R. J. and Viederman, M. (1982). Children of dialysis patients. *American Journal of Psychiatry, 139*(1), 100-103.

Gilmore, B. (1979). Home dialysis: A second look. *Perspectives, The Journal of the Council of Nephrology Social Workers, 3*(1), 44.

Goldman, L., Cook, E. F., Oye, R., Desbiens, N., Reding, D., Fulberson, W., Connors, A. F., Covinsky, K. E., Lynn, J., and Phillips, R. S. (1994). The impact of serious illness on patients' families. *Journal of the American Medical Association, 272*(23),1839-1844.

Goldman, R. H., Cohn, G. L., and Longnecker, R. E. (1980). The family and home hemodialysis: Adolescents' reactions to a father on home dialysis. *International Journal of Psychiatry, 10*(3), 235-255.

Green, G. J., Pedley, J., and Littlewood, J. (1986). Coping with chronic renal failure. *British Journal of Social Work, 16*(2), 203-222.

Holden, J. O. (1980). Dialysis or death: The ethical alternatives. *Health and Social Work, 5*(2), 18-21.

Iglehart, J. K. (1993). The American health care system—the end stage renal disease program. *The New England Journal of Medicine, 328*(5), 366.

Kaye, J., Bray, S., Gracely, E. J., and Levison, S. (1989). Psychosocial adjustment to illness and family environment in dialysis patients. *Family Systems Medicine, 7*(1), 77-89.

Krakauer, H. J. (1983). The recent U.S. experience in the treatment of end stage renal disease by dialysis and transplantation. *The New England Journal of Medicine, June*, 308-317.

Landsman, M. K. (1975). The patient with chronic renal failure: A marginal man. *Annals of Internal Medicine, 82*, 268-270.

Leick, N. and Davidsen-Nielsen, M. (1991). *Healing pain: Attachment, loss and grief therapy.* London and New York: Tavistock/Routledge.

Levy, N. B. (1994). Psychological aspects of renal transplantation. *Psychosomatics, 35*(5), 427-433.

Littlewood, J., Hardiker, P., Pedley, J., and Olley, D. (1990). Coping with home dialysis. *Human Relations, 43*(2), 103-111.

Lownace, D. C., Singer, P. A., and Siegler, M. (1988). Withdrawal from dialysis: An ethical perspective. *Kidney International, 34*, 124-135.

McCue, K. (1994). *How to help children through a parent's serious illness.* New York: St. Martin's Press.

Moguilner, M. E., Bauman, A., and DeNour, A. K. (1988). The adjustment of children and parents to chronic hemodialysis. *Psychosomatics, 29*(3), 289-294.

Moskop, J. C. (1987). The moral limits to federal funding for kidney disease. *Hastings Center Report, 17*(2), 11-15.

Page, S. and Weisberg, M. B. (1991). Marital and family characteristics of home and hospital dialysis patients. *Loss, Grief and Care, 5*(1-2), 33-45.

Palmer, S. E., Canzona, L., and Wai, L. (1982). Helping families respond effectively to chronic illness: Home dialysis as a case example. *Social Work in Health Care, 8*(1), 1-14.

Palmer, S. E., Canzona, L., and Wai, L. (1985). Finances and adaptation to illness: A study of home dialysis patients. *Social Worker/Travailleur Social, 53*(2), 57-60.

Peterson, K. J. (1984). Integration of medical and psychosocial needs of the home hemodialysis patient: Implications for the nephrology social worker. *Social Work in Health Care, 9*(4), 33-44.

Peterson, K. J. (1985). Psychosocial adjustment of the family caregiver: Home hemodialysis as an example. *Social Work in Health Care, 10*(3), 15-32.

Procci, W. R. and Martin, D. J. (1985). Effect of maintenance hemodialysis on male sexual performance. *Journal of Nervous and Mental Disease, 176*(6), 366-377.

Rando, T. A. (1985). *Treatment of complicated mourning.* Champlain: Research Press Co.

Rideout, E. M. and Littlefield, C. H. (1990). Stress, social support and symptoms of depression in spouses of the medically ill. *International Journal of Psychiatry in Medicine, 20*(1), 37-48.

Roy, R. (1990/1991). Consequences of parental illness on children. A review. *Social Work and Social Sciences Review, 2*(2), 109-121.

Ruchlin, H. S. (1984). The public cost of kidney disease. *Social Work in Health Care, 9*(4), 1-9.

Sheridan, M. S. (1988). Renal disease and the social worker: An update. *Perspectives, The Journal of the Council of Nephrology Social Workers, 9*, 43-56.

Sherwood, R. J. (1983). Compliance behaviour of hemodialysis patients and the role of the family. *Family Systems Medicine, 1*(2), 60-72.

Smith, M. D., Hong, B. A., and Feldman, R. D. (1985/1986). An assessment of the social networks of patients receiving maintenance therapy for end stage renal disease. *Perspectives, 7*, 49-56.

Terasaki, P. I. (Ed.). *History of transplantation: Thirty-five recollections.* Los Angeles, CA: UCLA Tissue Typing Laboratory.

Viswanathan, R. (1991). Helping patients cope with the loss of a renal transplant. *Loss, Grief and Care, 5*(1-2), 103-113.

Wagner, K. D. and Wagner, R. E. (1985). Effect of chronic renal disease on sexuality. *Medical Aspects of Human Sexuality, 19*(1), 168-175.

Wolcott, D. L., Nissenson, A. R., and Landsverk, J. (1988). Quality of life in chronic dialysis patients: Factors unrelated to dialysis modality. *General Hospital Psychiatry, 10*, 267-277.

Worden, J. W. (1991). *Grief counseling and grief therapy.* New York: Springer Publishing Co.

Chapter 14

Adult Oncology:
Helping a Terminally Ill Woman
to Plan and Cope

Lesley Sharp Haushalter

CONTEXT

Description of the Setting

Rising up among the row homes of a racially and ethnically blended community in the heart of Trenton, New Jersey, Helene Fuld Medical Center (HFMC) is a 353-bed, acute-care teaching facility and a member of the Robert Wood Johnson University Hospital Network. The hospital's patient population is drawn mainly from Mercer County, in which it is located, as well as several contiguous New Jersey counties and nearby Bucks County, Pennsylvania. Within this region, neighborhoods run the gamut from low income to affluent, and hospital clientele reflect this variation. However, because HFMC is an inner-city facility and has a number of programs that help to meet the needs of the underprivileged, nearly one-third of its patients are covered by Medicaid or are of "self pay" status. Roughly 41 percent are privately insured and 27 percent are Medicare recipients. Forty-eight percent of the hospital's patients in 1993 were white, while 40 percent were black, and the remainder represented other ethnic groups (K. Fritsch, personal communication, August 24, 1995).

The oncology program at HFMC is still in the early phases of its development. Though oncology patients have long been treated at this century-old facility, it was not until 1992 that ten beds on one pavilion were dedicated specifically to the care of patients receiving chemotherapy and other medical treatment for cancer. This marked the establishment of the hospital's Oncology Unit, which is now slated for further development. The work of the oncologists on this unit is complemented by a multidisciplinary staff with specialized training in cancer management. The creation of the Oncology Unit has effectively centralized inpatient medical oncology in the interest of enhancing the quality of cancer care.

Surgical oncology patients are those undergoing complete excisions or radical resections of malignant tumors who may then receive adjuvant radiation or chemotherapy once they have recovered from their surgery. Cancer patients may also be admitted for palliative surgery (i.e., to reduce the size of a tumor and increase patient comfort) when a cure is not possible. These patients are admitted to the hospital's 30-bed Concentrated Surgical Care Unit (CSCU) where they are integrated with patients undergoing surgeries for disorders other than cancer.

Outpatient cancer treatment is offered at two locations. In the hospital's on-site Infusion Unit, registered nurses certified in the administration of intravenous chemotherapy provide this service as well as blood transfusions, antibiotic treatment, and other interventions. Radiation therapy is carried out at an adjunct facility approximately nine miles away from the medical center. The hospital provides free patient transportation to this facility for those who need it. It is also planning, along with another Trenton area hospital, to build and operate a radiation oncology center in the immediate area by 1996.

To facilitate cancer prevention within its community, HFMC provides a variety of free cancer screenings and educational programs during the course of each year. In 1993, while I was there, 397 patients were diagnosed with cancer. Some of these diagnoses were made via the screening process. Though the hospital provides services that touch a wider constituency through its strong programs in emergency services, nephrology, mental health, and neonatology, it also maintains a close relationship with the members of its local community who seem to embrace HFMC as their medical center. During my employment at Helene Fuld, I had the experience of counseling one neighborhood man with leukemia and learning that the woman hospitalized with lymphoma just a few rooms away was his sister-in-law. It was not unusual to know of extended families that had several members utilizing the medical center for a variety of services. This was then and is now indicative of the hospital's role within its community.

Policy

The center is fully accredited as an acute-care teaching hospital by the Joint Commission on Accreditation of Healthcare Organizations and is certified by the New Jersey Department of Health. Acute care is defined as "intense, short-term medical, nursing and related services given to patients to restore their previous state of health or to prevent their present health status from worsening" (Snook and Ruck, 1987, p. 1). Hence, an acute care hospital is a facility "that cares primarily for patients with acute diseases or conditions and whose average length of stay is less than 30 days" (O'Leary, 1994, p. 19).

If a hospitalized patient is given a terminal prognosis and it is determined by his or her attending physician that no further acute-level surgical or medical interventions will be of benefit, the patient's social worker and others who have been involved in planning the discharge help the patient prepare to move to a more appropriate care setting. Depending on the provisions of insurance coverage, the support system available, and his or her wishes, the patient may return home and receive home care or hospice services; or the patient may go to an inpatient hospice or a long-term care facility. In any case, once the patient no longer requires an acute level of care and can be kept comfortable with skilled or custodial care, he or she is not supposed to remain in an acute-care facility. Exceptions to this rule arise, of course, if there are dispositional problems (i.e., no bed is available in a long-term care facility and there is no family support at home), and patients sometimes remain in an acute-care facility because no suitable alternative is readily attainable. In arranging the discharge, the social worker makes plans with the patient and his or her family to ensure that he or she will move from the hospital into a safe environment where physical and emotional needs can be met.

There are possible consequences for failing to discharge a patient from an acute-care setting in a timely manner. One is that the patient's insurer may terminate reimbursement to the hospital for the services being provided or may reimburse the hospital at a lower rate, which could mean that the unpaid fees would fall on the shoulders of the patient. For example, for a Medicaid patient, the hospital may be reimbursed at a lesser Medicaid rate rather than the full hospital rate if Medicaid considers that there is an unwarranted extended stay. A second potential consequence is that certifying and accrediting agencies, in reviewing the hospital's practices through the examination of patient charts and other means, may find fault with the hospital unless justifiable circumstances that delayed the discharge are documented. For these and other more patient-centered reasons, the social worker's role in helping the terminally ill patient to plan for discharge from an acute-care setting is crucial (E. Calabro, personal communication, August 8, 1995).

The determination of where the patient will go following his or her hospital stay is, in large part, driven by the insurance provider. The patient who will be discussed in this chapter was enrolled in the New Jersey Medicaid Only Program for which she qualified by meeting the criteria for Aid to Families with Dependent Children (AFDC) as a low-income, single mother of two children. Eligibility means that a family may receive medical assistance covering a broad range of services but may not additionally receive cash assistance to supplement its income. This is one of the regular Medicaid programs jointly funded by both federal and state governments, authorized under Title 19 of the Social Security Act, and administered by the Division of Medical Assistance and Health Services of the New Jersey Department of Human Services (New Jersey Division of Medical Assistance and Health Services [NJDMAHS], 1992a).

If a terminally ill individual covered by New Jersey Medicaid wishes to die in the comfort of his or her own home rather than in a long-term care facility or an inpatient hospice, that individual may choose to receive either home hospice or home care services. If he or she chooses hospice, an Election of Hospice Benefits Statement must be signed and in doing so, he or she waives rights to most regular Medicaid services but will be offered palliative interventions. If the individual has an acute medical problem unrelated to the terminal illness, Medicaid will pay for the treatment of that problem. If he or she chooses to institute a "break" in hospice care he or she may do so but might, as a result, lose some of the days of care allotted under the hospice benefit. In most cases, the individual would still be able to resume hospice care following such a break in services. If the terminally ill patient decides to go home with home care services rather than hospice, Medicaid will pay for this (E. Calabro, personal communication, August 8, 1995; NJDMAHS, 1992b).

One service that is not covered for a terminally ill patient by New Jersey Medicaid, under either the hospice benefit or as part of home care services, is the administration of total parenteral nutrition (TPN). TPN entails the intravenous infusion of nutrients into the bloodstream for a patient who, for whatever reason, is unable to eat normally or has a disease that interferes with the ability to digest food. It is unusual to discuss TPN as a possible aspect of terminal care via hospice since the use of extraordinary, life-sustaining interventions runs counter to the program's philosophy. But there is sometimes a measure of flexibility in hospice policy if circumstances warrant it. The patient under discussion in this chapter was able to eat but had metastatic cancer, which prevented her intestine from digesting and absorbing nutrients. In light of this and because the patient expressed hopes that her TPN would not be withdrawn, I explored whether Medicaid would pay for the administration of TPN in conjunction with either hospice or home care.

My investigation revealed that Medicaid would pay for the actual liquid nutrients that constitute the TPN but it would not pay for the private duty nursing care, which the patient requires to receive this treatment at home. The only exception to this rule for my patient could be found in the state's Model Waiver III program. If a patient chooses to have home care services, he or she can apply for this waiver. There are only 150 Model Waiver III slots available statewide each year. But if the patient meets the criteria and a slot is available, under this waiver he or she can receive a full range of home care services, and Medicaid will also pay for the private-duty nursing care necessary for TPN administration. If a patient elects the Medicaid Hospice Benefit, however, he or she is prohibited from applying for a Model Waiver III. So, the patient may either choose to have home care services with the possibility of TPN through the Model Waiver III provision or choose to have hospice services without TPN (E. Calabro, personal communication, August 8, 1995; NJDMAHS, 1991).

Finally, it is interesting to note that it was only as recently as September 1, 1992 that the State of New Jersey authorized the provision of hospice services for its terminally ill residents enrolled in the regular Medicaid program. This benefit was also pursuant to Title 19 of the Social Security Act and the subsequent New Jersey state statute. Prior to this date, only AIDS patients enrolled in a special New Jersey Medicaid waiver program could receive hospice care. Fortunately, the woman discussed in this chapter received her terminal prognosis in the fall of 1993, after her state's law made hospice care an option for her (NJDMAHS, 1992c).

Technology

Colorectal cancer, the form of malignancy that affected my client, is one of the most commonly diagnosed cancers in both men and women in the United States. It is second only to lung cancer in both incidence and mortality and has an overall five-year survival rate of 56 percent. This survival rate improves to 92 percent and 85 percent for colon and rectal cancer, respectively, when the disease is discovered at a localized stage. The American Cancer Society estimates that 149,000 new cases were diagnosed in 1994 (Garfinkel, 1995; Steele, 1995).

Adenocarcinoma is the cancer most commonly found in the colon and rectum and is a malignancy that involves the cells lining the walls of various organs throughout the body. When colorectal cancer metastasizes, or spreads from its primary site to distant areas of the body, it often invades the liver and lungs. The process of diagnosis begins with a physical examination and complete medical history. If the physician finds reason to, he or she will then order further studies, which may include procedures such as a biopsy; a colonoscopy, which involves the use of a lighted, flexible instrument to explore the colon via the rectum; a barium enema and an air contrast examination done to facilitate X ray visualization of any growths in the colon; or a computerized tomography scan (CT scan) of the abdomen and pelvis. Further workup to determine the extent of the disease may involve a liver scan, chest X ray, or other tests (Redfield and Reilly, 1991).

Stages

Once the extent of the disease is learned, the cancer is classified in one of five stages ranging from Stage 0 to Stage IV, which represent the earliest to the most progressed forms of the disease. Stage 0 cancer has not moved beyond the inner wall of the colon, while Stage IV cancer has grown all the way through the intestinal wall and spread to the lymph nodes as well as distant parts of the body. Accurate staging of an individual's cancer is important because it assists in the selection and planning of the most appropriate treatment for either cure or palliation (American Cancer Society [ACS], 1995; Lenhard, Lawrence, and McKenna, 1995).

Treatment

The primary treatment for colorectal cancer is surgery, and when the disease is caught in its early stages, the outlook is generally positive. Radiation therapy (treatment of the affected site with high-energy radiation) may be used in addition to surgery to treat Stage II, Stage III, and Stage IV cancers. This therapy is used to reduce the size of a tumor before surgery, to destroy residual cancer cells after surgery, or to help shrink recurrent cancers to relieve symptoms. Chemotherapy (administration of powerful cancer-fighting drugs either intravenously or by mouth) was previously used to palliate advanced colorectal cancer and provide pain relief. But trials have revealed that a drug called 5-fluorouracil (5-FU), used in combination with other agents after surgery, has produced favorable results in increasing survival time for some patients (ACS, 1995).

With either radiation or chemotherapy, a patient may experience side effects. These might include mild skin irritation, nausea, diarrhea, or fatigue from radiation and hair loss, lowered resistance to infection, nausea and vomiting, diarrhea, or mouth sores from chemotherapy. New drugs being administered in conjunction with chemotherapy can help to lessen or eliminate nausea and vomiting related to that treatment. Side effects can be quite challenging for patients. This is an area in which supportive, well-informed social work intervention can shore up patient and family tolerance by encouraging a patient's focus on realistic goals and by sustaining hope. Fortunately, side effects are not experienced by all patients, and symptoms usually subside once treatment has ended (ACS, 1995).

Follow-Up

After a patient has been treated for colorectal cancer, it is important for him or her to be followed carefully by a medical team to evaluate his or her response to treatment and determine whether there has been any recurrence of the disease. One follow-up study that is routinely used is a test for the presence or amount of carcinoembryonic antigen (CEA) in the blood. CEA is a tumor marker that, when measured in a blood sample, may indicate the existence of colorectal cancer and signal the need for further treatment. It is a very effective marker for patients who have CEA-producing adenocarcinomas. However, "its limitation is the absence of curative approaches (for most patients) once recurrence is defined by serial CEA elevation" (Steele, 1995, p. 247).

Because colorectal cancer interferes with the systems by which we normally take in nutrients and eliminate waste, there are certain procedures that may be used to aid in these processes during treatment and, in some cases, for a period of time after. One of these interventions, TPN, has already been explained. Another intervention is a nasogastric tube, which is a narrow plastic tube that is inserted into the nose and passed down the esophagus into the stomach. It may be used for the delivery of nutrients or to suction out stomach contents that are not being properly digested. A gastrostomy is a surgical procedure in which an opening is made so that a feeding tube can be placed directly into the stomach from outside the body. This is known as a gastrostomy tube (G-tube) and can also be used to deliver food directly to the stomach or to drain stomach contents, if necessary. A colostomy is created when a surgeon makes an opening between the colon and the surface of the body to permit the elimination of body wastes. Though colostomies can be permanent and require considerable emotional and physical adjustment on the part of the patient, many are temporary and are later surgically reversed once the area of the tumor resection has fully healed.

HFMC is technologically equipped to provide comprehensive cancer diagnosis and treatment using the means described above as well as others. Another important area of technology is the use of hospital-wide computer systems. At HFMC and other hospitals, reports from CT scans, laboratory and pathology studies, magnetic resonance imaging, and many other tests are input into a computer system as soon as they are complete, thus making them immediately available to the health care team on site. At HFMC, these data are simultaneously faxed to outlying physician's offices as soon as they are entered into the system. For many tests, there is no longer a need to wait for hard copy reports to arrive via interdepartmental mail. The obvious advantages are that anxiety-provoking waiting periods are somewhat reduced for patients and treatment planning is expedited.

Organization

HFMC's cohesive social service department consists of 14 social workers and a secretary. The departmental director reports to one of five hospital assistant administrators. Social workers cover all areas of the hospital and are well-regarded for the perspective they bring to the medical center's multidisciplinary approach to patient and family care.

The oncology social worker is responsible for assessing the psychosocial status of newly diagnosed cancer patients as well as any cancer patient having difficulty coping with treatment, refusing treatment, or having problems with activities of daily living as the result of their illness. The social worker provides individual, family, and group counseling and facilitates linkage to outside resources. Inpatient counseling on the medical and surgical oncology units is complemented by the efforts of an excellent discharge planning social worker who is assigned to the same areas and handles the more concrete aspects of patient care. Because the number of patients being treated for cancer in the hospital warrants it and due to the often overwhelming impact that cancer can have on families, HFMC includes the counseling position on its social work staff.

Since the patient under discussion in this chapter was hospitalized in the Concentrated Surgical Care Unit (CSCU), I will focus on its organization with regard to physical space, services, and staffing. The unit consists of 15 semiprivate rooms. There are specific criteria for admission or transfer to the CSCU, but generally speaking, any surgeon can admit a patient with a surgical diagnosis to the unit. Subsequently, patients are hospitalized there for a variety of disorders that require surgery, including, in many cases, cancer. Most patients are admitted to the unit either immediately postoperatively or after a transitional stay in the intensive care unit.

The physician director of the CSCU is also the hospital's director of surgical services and an oncologic surgeon. Along with other professional accomplishments, he is known for his particular skill in gastrointestinal surgery and has developed and disseminated new techniques in this area. He is also a very warm, approachable individual who highly values the contributions that social workers make to the treatment of the whole patient. A number of other surgeons with different specialties operate on surgical oncology patients at the hospital as well.

The staff member with whom I worked most closely throughout the hospital, was the oncology clinical nurse specialist. We functioned as a team in meeting patient and family needs, keeping lines of communication open between families and staff members, and ensuring patient understanding of the course of treatment. Additionally, we cofacilitated a monthly cancer patient and family support group as well as two biweekly staff development groups designed to address the professional and emotional concerns of staff members working with oncology patients.

The nurse manager for the CSCU ran a tight but good-spirited ship and played a significant role in setting the tone on the unit. The nursing staff, social workers, dietitian, unit clerk, and other key staff members carried out their responsibilities with the utmost professionalism and a feeling of family unity. This kind of bonding, which occurs in many work settings, can be intensified in medical settings in which professionals work shoulder-to-shoulder in caring for individuals with life-threatening illnesses. At HFMC, there is considerable longevity of employment, which contributes to this feeling as well.

Two additional dimensions of the organization support and enhance the work of oncology and strengthen professional alliances. The Cancer Committee, with representatives from the administration, medical staff, and various disciplines, plans, initiates, and evaluates cancer care at the hospital. The Tumor Board provides a multidisciplinary, biweekly case conference.

PRACTICE DECISIONS

Description of the Client

Tracy Lane was a 37-year-old, divorced, white, Catholic mother of two adolescent daughters, Kimberly, aged 17, and Sarah, aged 15. She lived with her children in a low-income neighborhood just outside of Trenton in a home that had once belonged to her mother. The eldest of eight children, Tracy had come to realize the pressures of single parenting at the age of 24 when her mother died. Her father had died previously and so Tracy, already divorced with two small children of her own, effectively became the head of her original household the day she lost her mother.

Tracy took her role very seriously and, with some help from relatives, managed to keep her five sisters and two brothers together during the years that followed. Eventually, three of them moved out of the area, one brother was killed in an auto accident, and four of the sisters remained in the Trenton area. Tracy's husband, who had been repeatedly abusive toward her during their marriage, moved away after their divorce and provided her no assistance. Tracy worked at various jobs to support herself and her children and was employed as a salesclerk until her illness necessitated her resignation.

At the time of Tracy's admission, she and her daughters were sharing the family home with her 31-year-old, divorced sister, Gale, and Gale's five-year-old daughter, Ashley. Tracy's youngest sister, Kristen, was living in the home as well. The fourth locally residing sister, Sandy, lived just a few blocks away and, along with being deeply concerned for Tracy, was fighting her own battle with alcohol dependence.

Tracy's family was loving, but their intense level of preexisting anxiety tended to undermine their functioning. Terminal illness in one family member tests each member's level of emotional maturity. Though Tracy's siblings performed many loving acts toward her during her illness they could not always be counted on for consistency and reliability. Tracy's children understandably demonstrated some acting-out behaviors in response to the threat of losing their mother. Sarah, in particular, had problems with truancy.

Though Tracy also brought a fair amount of generalized anxiety into her situation, she benefited from considerable ego strengths that served to elevate her abilities above the level of her siblings. She was perceptive and had the capacity to rally and become goal-oriented in the face of her crisis. Her higher level of functioning was reflected in her role as the family elder and caretaker. She was a devoted mother who focused on her daughters' needs even as she endured great emotional and physical pain (Goldstein, 1984).

Tracy was first diagnosed at HFMC with colorectal cancer in the spring of 1992. At that time, she underwent surgery to remove an obstructing left-sided colon carcinoma, specifically diagnosed as adenocarcinoma. This was followed by several months of outpatient chemotherapy using 5-fluorouracil. During a follow-up examination and testing the following spring, Tracy was found to have a rising CEA level in her blood. A CT scan was ordered and revealed a new mass, metastasis, in the right lobe of her liver. She was immediately scheduled to have a right hepatectomy, an excision of the affected portion of her liver.

Unfortunately, intraoperatively Tracy's surgeon discovered that her cancer had metastasized not only to her liver but also to her small intestine and her left ovary. The hepatectomy was aborted, the intestinal metastasis was biopsied, and her left ovary, with a very large tumor attached, was removed. She received further chemotherapy over the months that followed under the care of her oncologist. However, "metastases from . . . intestinal cancers are less amenable to treatment and, in such cases, the outlook is not good" (Clayman, 1989, p. 234). This, then, was Tracy's situation.

In November, Tracy presented in the emergency room with complaints of abdominal distention, nausea, and vomiting, and reported having had a ten-pound weight loss in a brief period of time. Her surgeon examined her and admitted her to the hospital, suspecting a possible small bowel obstruction from her cancer. This time a CT scan revealed a huge tumor underlying Tracy's small intestine in a location that made it inoperable.

On a cold fall afternoon, Tracy's surgeon met with her in her hospital room on the CSCU, just a few doors away from the room where her mother had died of colorectal cancer 13 years before. There he gave her the kind of news that physicians are loathe to deliver; that her newest tumor was inoperable and that nothing more could be done to prevent her cancer from taking her life. Tracy's sister was there with her and the doctor spent some time with both of them to offer his support and answer any questions they might have. Tracy could not bring herself to ask how long he expected she might live, though he would have told her whatever she wanted to know. He did inform the oncology nurse specialist and me later that day that he did not expect her to live until Christmas. As he emerged from Tracy's room, I was waiting in the hallway to go in to see her. The doctor and I spoke for a moment and then I went into Tracy's room to meet her for the first time, to offer my support, and to learn what I might possibly do to help this young mother.

Definition of the Client

My client, in this case, was primarily Tracy, as she and I had the most continuous contact throughout her five-week stay at the hospital. She remained lucid and able to make her own choices about her care as well as other issues of concern to her. It is not unusual to begin working with a terminally ill patient and her family and to have the work shift entirely to the family members as the patient slips further into the illness and becomes unable to communicate. Fortunately, this did not occur with Tracy while she was hospitalized and we had time to accomplish some things before she went home.

I also worked with Tracy's family as they were deeply affected by her illness and prognosis, but I did not have the same frequency of contact with them. Because Tracy's sisters and her eldest daughter were employed during the day, they often came to visit in the early evening after I had left the hospital. I did conduct some sessions that involved only

Tracy's daughters, in order to assess their coping and provide supportive counseling. I also met with Tracy, along with various family members, on a number of occasions and spoke with her sisters by phone to make arrangements and provide support. Two nights before Tracy's discharge, we held a family meeting, which everyone attended for the purpose of preparing Tracy and her family for her return home. Thus, as is common for a social worker in an acute-care setting, I worked with a variable client unit. The nature and continuity of the work that Tracy and I engaged in, however, made her the principal client.

Goals

The earliest goals materialized within moments of our meeting and included (1) helping Tracy through the crisis of receiving a terminal prognosis, and (2) preparing Tracy to tell her children about her prognosis and supporting her through the task. This is something that Tracy told me almost immediately that she needed to do and that she expressed great fear of doing.

Consequent goals that followed included (3) linking the children with resources for bereavement counseling and (4) making arrangements for Tracy's home-based terminal care. Tracy identified the need for bereavement counseling very early. She wanted to be certain that they would have counseling available to them following her death. I suggested the children would likely benefit from immediate intervention and she agreed. The terminal care goal was both policy driven and self-determined. Though the policies of any acute-care hospital would dictate that Tracy be transferred to another setting to receive palliative care (if possible), she also had her own reasons for wanting to return home. She wanted to be in her own environment and among her family. Arranging home-based care produced two related goals: assisting Tracy through the process of choosing between having "home care services with TPN" or "home hospice without TPN," and reestablishing telephone service at Tracy's home to facilitate 24-hour, on-call nursing service and to make it possible for Tracy's out-of-state siblings to call her. Other identified goals were to (5) help Tracy to learn and complete New Jersey's legal process for transferring custody of her daughters to her sister effective at the time of her death, and to (6) help Tracy to reconnect with her parish priest per her request.

Ongoing goals included (7) assisting Tracy's family in dealing with their impending loss and in preparing to take an active role in Tracy's care, (8) empowering Tracy to make her needs known with regard to pain management and in communicating her needs to her family, (9) helping to reduce Tracy's anxiety about medical and surgical procedures and pain by providing her with support and means for control, (10) facilitating Tracy's self-determination by educating her about her choices, and (11) sustaining hope. Although this may seem to be a goal incongruous with work with the terminally ill, an individual might have goals regarding how he or she will live out the rest of his or her days and what can be accomplished in that time. Social workers can play a significant role in supporting patient efforts to identify and reach final goals, depending on the patient's level of energy. This can have the beneficial effects of revitalizing hope and facilitating a life lived fully to the end. As stated in The Dying Person's Bill of Rights (from the Southwestern Michigan Inservice Education Council quoted in Tatelbaum, 1980, p. 164), "I have the right to be treated as a living human being until I die . . . I have the right to maintain a sense of hopefulness, however changing this might be."

Use of Contract

With all of my oncology patients, contracts were verbal and flexible. Cancer and its treatment can sweep families along on the physical and emotional equivalent of a white-water rafting trip, replete with periods of calm and frenzy. Careful review of a patient's medical chart combined with a thorough initial interview help to clarify needs for social work intervention or the lack thereof. However, an oncology social worker understands that the patient who expressed no needs yesterday may suddenly develop some as the result of an unforeseen disease or treatment complication. Thus, it is necessary to maintain an awareness of the progress of all patients, through participation in multidisciplinary rounds, in the event that social work services might be needed in the future.

In Tracy's case, the need for social work intervention was immediately apparent. She was in crisis and readily expressed a desire for help, beginning with her great concern for her daughters. As the literature on crisis intervention describes, the vulnerability and disorganization experienced by an individual in such a state renders one more receptive to professional help than might otherwise be (Woods and Hollis, 1990). My meeting with Tracy's daughters on the day that they learned of her prognosis, a prompt response to her first concern, contributed much to our early process of joining. From there, we continued to explore and respond to other needs and verbally laid plans to accomplish goals that were important to her. In addition, I agreed to be there for her, to provide emotional support and safe, nonjudgmental opportunities for her to ventilate the feelings she experienced as she endured the challenges that her circumstance presented. This was the substance of our contract.

Meeting Place

Due to the extent of Tracy's tumor burden and its impact on her level of energy and mobility, she spent most of her time in her hospital bed relieved by brief periods of sitting in a nearby chair. Eventually, she had difficulty walking, and wheelchair transport was hindered by the various medical equipment attached to her. Thus, all of our meetings took place in her room with me at her bedside.

I met with most of my oncology patients in their hospital rooms simply because it was the easiest place for them to be, given their illnesses and the fact that they were often connected to IVs and sensitive monitors for chemotherapy infusion. This gave the patient the advantage of being on the small amount of hospital turf that was his or hers, but it also presented challenges with regard to privacy. The majority of the rooms at the hospital were semiprivate with just a curtain available to create a thin barrier between patients. The Oncology Unit did have a private supportive care room used to meet with the families of patients who were very ill, but with patients, the curtain existed as the fourth-wall convention.

With Tracy, I did not face the usual predicament of trying to find ways to create a sense of privacy, for even though she was staying in a semiprivate room, the second bed was never occupied. The CSCU nurses apprised the hospital admissions staff of Tracy's health status and they, in turn, managed to keep the other bed empty for the duration of her hospital stay. They would never have compromised service to another patient to provide this environment for Tracy, but the census permitted it and the staff was caring enough to make the extra effort.

As a result, my meeting place with Tracy was as ideal as possible within a hospital setting. I could close the door to her room, and we would have quiet and freedom from outside distraction. This is certainly not the norm for hospital-based social work but it was one of the benefits of working within the mores of the institution and the unit. A planned reorganization of the Oncology Unit includes private rooms for cancer patients.

One remarkable aspect of my meeting place with Tracy was its location on the same hospital unit where her mother had died. This, of course, was addressed in our work together and actually served as a vehicle for Tracy's introspection.

Use of Time

"Most of the requests for oncology social work services stem from a person who is experiencing crisis" (Stearns, Lauria, Hermann, and Fogelberg, 1993, p. 108). Given this fact, consistent access to a social worker can be very important to a patient undergoing treatment for cancer. In my work, I would usually see a patient or family at least every other day. If a patient was in crisis, I would see him or her daily and on some occasions, multiple times within the same day. Since I worked in various areas of the hospital, patients and families were told they could reach me by beeper and were encouraged to do this without hesitation.

Because of Tracy's terminal condition and her family situation, I met with her daily. Some meetings lasted an hour if she was really struggling and needed to talk. Others lasted only moments on days when she was too exhausted to deal with emotional or practical matters. However, those momentary meetings just to say, "I'm sorry you had such a rough day" or "I hope you sleep better tonight" were, in a way, as valuable as the hour-long sessions because of their effect in maintaining our rapport and lessening Tracy's anxiety.

Interventions

Crisis Intervention

Given the circumstances of my first meeting with Tracy, crisis intervention was my initial treatment modality. I continued to use crisis intervention techniques at various times throughout the five weeks in which we worked together. Tracy required extra help to get through some distressing palliative surgical procedures, and she remained in a "general" state of crisis once she was given a terminal prognosis. Woods and Hollis (1990) have noted, "If we always assume that crisis resolution must occur within a short time period, we may find ourselves pushing clients too fast and too hard" (p. 430). Most significant in Tracy's case was the reality that she still had the crisis of dying ahead of her.

Several aspects of my early crisis assessment enabled me to better understand Tracy's situation and help her to regain some sense of equilibrium. First, for her, a terminal prognosis meant that there would be unrealized dreams; that she would lose her children as well as their futures; and that she, as head of the household, would be leaving the family members who had depended on her for years. Second, her preexisting personality structure was adaptive and strong. Ironically, this was to some degree a result of her previous losses and an important factor in understanding how she was perceiving her current crisis. Between her mother's death and her own 18-month struggle with cancer, she had lost the illusion of being "invulnerable," which many people maintain and which causes them to be more overwhelmed when tragedy strikes. Though she was certainly in shock during the early part of our work together, Tracy had a realistic view of the world, which helped her to rally and begin to plan. Third, Tracy said that her mother had received wonderful care but had endured much pain and been isolated from the family due to her need to be hospitalized. Fourth, Tracy expressed concerns about her family's functioning during our first meeting, saying that she knew that her family loved her but wondered if they could be helpful to her.

As I explored these and other areas, I responded in ways that would assure her that she was being heard and that I was willing to help her manage. The clinical nurse specialist and I talked with her about the hospital's pain management team and the fact that the staff was committed to working to keep her comfortable. I informed her that there were ways that we could arrange for her to be cared for at home among her family. I gave her ample time for ventilation of her sadness and fears, which provided some relief. I validated her expressions of current and anticipated losses and of fear, thereby normalizing her response to her crisis. Finally, by helping her initially with the task of telling her daughters of her prognosis and assisting her in beginning to plan, I was able to facilitate her regaining some sense of control.

Case Management

The sum of my work with Tracy and her family, including this crisis intervention, could be characterized as case management. My professional efforts involved providing individual and family counseling concerning coping and grieving; calling on outside resources to assist us in the accomplishment of goals, and in providing the best environment and care for Tracy and her family; educating; advocating; and ultimately working to prepare both patient and family for Tracy's return home.

Clinical Interventions

In my clinical work, I drew upon the tenets of Bowen Family Systems Theory. For example, it was useful in my exploration of Tracy's family history to pay attention to multigenerational transmission processes. Getting some idea about the kinds of emotional responses that had been reinforced over the generations gave me clues about the current family's capacity for weathering this crisis (Friedman, 1985).

One of the general areas to keep in mind when evaluating the cancer patient and family, according to Kerr (1981), is the level of existing anxiety in the patient and his or her important relationship systems. Given the patterns of reactivity, which I observed among Tracy and her family, it was helpful for me to remain, as much as possible, an objective, nonanxious presence in working with them. My ability to be clearheaded and less reactive in this highly emotionally charged situation seemed to help modify the family's anxiety (Friedman, 1985).

My clinical interventions with Tracy also involved the discussion of spiritual beliefs. Referring to spirituality and religion at a conference of oncology social workers, Summerville (1993) concluded, "We have not really been seeing or working with this dimension of our client's lives in social work." In truth, this is an area of exploration often neglected in practice. Yet spirituality can be a central aspect of a client's life. As a Catholic, Tracy believed in heaven and held hopes of being reunited there with her mother and brother. Our discussions of this and other spiritual issues were a great source of comfort for Tracy and provided me with important information about her. I was glad not to have overlooked this opportunity to further enrich the work we shared.

Humor was an element of our work together as well. The inclusion of laughter in our therapeutic relationship provided periods of much-needed relief. As Friedman states, "Anxiousness and seriousness are blood brothers" (1985, p. 182). Thus, to the extent that we were able to be a little less serious on occasion and engage in a moment of playfulness, we effectively tapped some of the anxiety and contributed to Tracy's continued enjoyment of the lighter side of living.

Intervention Intersects Policy

One particular area of intervention with Tracy was directly influenced by the three policies outlined at the beginning of this chapter. Tracy's need for only palliative care made it necessary to transfer her to a setting more appropriate for her long-term supportive care needs. Knowing that Tracy would have her own feelings about where she wanted to spend the last weeks of her life, I gently began to explore the issue of her supportive care with her. She told me that she wanted to be at home with her family if possible, and so I spoke with her about the options of home care and home hospice. When she wanted to learn more about how hospice would work in her case, I called New Jersey-based Samaritan Hospice and arranged a meeting between her and a hospice social worker. I also consulted one of our home care nurses and the Medicaid district office to determine what home care and home hospice services would be available to Tracy.

It was through this series of discussions that I learned of the difficult choice that Tracy would have to make with respect to her supportive care. Due to her intestinal obstruction, hospice would allow Tracy to keep her total paremteral nutrition (TPN) as long as they could get the Medicaid reimbursement that they would need in order to provide this service. However, I then discovered, as described previously in the policy section, that New Jersey Medicaid would not pay for TPN administration under the hospice benefit. Medicaid policy dictated that Tracy could have TPN under the Model Waiver III program, but only if she chose home care services instead of hospice. At Tracy's request, I sat in on her meeting with the hospice social worker. As the discussion between the three of us progressed, it became clear that Tracy took great comfort in what she heard about the hospice program. When the conversation turned to the subject of TPN, I also realized that Tracy was unaware that this was a life-sustaining medical intervention for her and not just a temporary measure that could be withdrawn without physical consequences.

The next morning, I spoke with Tracy's surgeon and explained the policies to him. It was important that Tracy be educated about the purpose of her TPN and the effects of withdrawing it so that she could make a fully informed decision whether to elect home care with TPN or hospice without it. Her surgeon agreed and we went directly to Tracy's room to discuss this with her. For Tracy, this was almost like receiving her terminal prognosis again. It was a difficult conversation for all of us. The dilemma surrounding her TPN presented Tracy with a great emotional conflict. She had been so relieved to learn about hospice care and its provision of bereavement counseling for her children and family, but to choose this now meant giving up nourishment, necessary for survival. Making this choice forced Tracy to face her impending death even more directly and took the two of us to a deeper level in our clinical work together.

We could have essentially pieced together the services that hospice would have provided if Tracy chose home care and her family took advantage of support groups in the area; however, my own bias was in favor of hospice. In light of the family's compromised ability to provide a strong support system for Tracy, I thought the less splintered her care was, the better it would be. I believed that the family would benefit from the continuity and comprehensiveness that the hospice package would provide. I did not articulate my bias to Tracy but rather, tried to help her come to her own decision. I realize now though, that I became reactive to the policies that seemed to be preventing my client from having the best of care. I became focused on trying to find some way to get her exactly what she wanted without giving much consideration to the option of home care accompanied by other services.

Finally, in the midst of our wrestling with this issue, I said to Tracy, "You know, if you choose hospice and go home without your TPN and decide that you don't like how things are going, you can call us and we'll change your services and get the TPN back for you." It was a simple bit of common sense (the accuracy of which I verified in advance of my statement), but it provided Tracy with a safety net that freed her to make a decision she had been too fearful to make. She was able to move beyond her fears and choose to have hospice and have her TPN terminated. Once she returned home, she never did ask for TPN to be reinitiated. The availability of technology and the constraints of policy had forced her into an extremely difficult emotional struggle, but they had effectively moved her forward in dealing with her own death.

Stance of Social Worker

In working with Tracy, my stance was consistently supportive. I gave her plenty of room to make her own choices and then contributed to their realization in any ways that I could as a professional. While my supportive stance colored all of my interventions with Tracy, I moved freely between passive and active roles as the situation dictated. When she needed to ventilate grief-related emotions, I was basically passive. At other times, I was more active, exploring issues that needed to be addressed and nudging our discussion in a particular direction. Facilitating the accomplishment of certain concrete, resource-specific goals necessitated my taking a more active approach as well. I would investigate resources or procedures and then discuss with Tracy what she needed to do if, for example, securing a service required her participation. By and large, my relationship with Tracy was a partnership. She would do what she could from her bed, I would do what I could "on the move," and we would enlist the help of family members as needed.

With Tracy's family, I was supportive and directive when they were unsure how to proceed with tasks. For instance, when Tracy's sister, Gale, asked for help in the transfer of custody of Kimberly and Sarah, I called Mercer County Legal Aid and inquired what steps were necessary. I then helped Gale to complete her part of the process. At other times, I took a directive approach to encourage family members to perform responsibly. For example, once Tracy had chosen home hospice, she needed a working home telephone to have the 24-hour, on-call nursing service available. The phone had previously been disconnected because Gale had run up a bill and had failed to pay it. I advocated for Tracy with Bell Telephone, and they agreed to reinstate local phone service for the duration of Tracy's life, as long as Gale contacted them and arranged some form of payment plan. Once I had this agreement in place, I informed Gale of what she needed to do in order to make phone service available for Tracy's care. She followed through without hesitation.

An insidious challenge to my ability to remain objective and balanced in my work with Tracy and her family was the positive transference/countertransference phenomenon that may have emerged within the relationship between Tracy and myself. Tracy was just 14 months older than I and our age similarity contributed to the feelings of partnership and closeness with which we set about pursuing our goals. In retrospectively evaluating our relationship, I have come to wonder about the possibility that, for Tracy, I may have represented a longed-for, reliable sibling. For my part, I have one sibling, a sister who has always been one of the most important people in my life. We have a great love for one another and a wonderful friendship. She is two-and-a-half years older, has two children, and happens to have physical features that are similar to Tracy's.

In looking back, I have come to realize a disparity between my work with Tracy and my other oncology patients. With my other patients, I did counseling with some resource linkage. In Tracy's case, despite the fact that I worked with an excellent discharge planner, I took over. It has only been in reviewing this case that I have become aware of the degree to which I overfunctioned. It has occurred to me that the emotional impact of my countertransference may have fueled my need to take special care of Tracy. The negative impact of this, however, was that it interfered with my ability to shift more responsibility to the family and likely contributed to their feelings of powerlessness. Thus, while Tracy was in the hospital, I was inadvertently limiting their opportunity to rise to the challenge presented by her dying. To have gotten out of their way and allowed them a greater chance for growth would have probably been a more helpful intervention.

Of course, being a nonanxious presence in the midst of a family's crisis is something that can be achieved to varying degrees. My abilities to remain clearheaded, to problem solve, and to subsequently defuse some of the anxiety within this family were manifestations of my relative success. However, my countertransference-based (anxious) concern with providing Tracy with everything she needed, demonstrated by my overfunctioning, was evidence of my own limitations.

Use of Outside Resources

The resources utilized are represented in the ecomap in Figure 14.1. As stated earlier, Tracy asked me to contact her priest during our first meeting, at the height of her initial crisis. As a divorced Catholic, Tracy had been away from her church for some time, which probably contributed to her reluctance to make the contact. I spoke with her priest and he subsequently visited Tracy, which provided her with some measure of reconnection and solace.

When Tracy originally asked about securing counseling for her daughters, I contacted two local family service agencies with appropriate services. These agencies became standby resources in case Tracy decided not to choose home hospice, which had bereavement counseling as a component of its services. The American Cancer Society provided funding directly to Bell Telephone to pay the nearly $200 charge for reinstating the family's phone service. The hospital's security office had some extra phone equipment available and I was able to secure a loaner phone for the family from them.

The custody hearing regarding Tracy's children took place at Mercer County Family Court. As Tracy could not attend, she was required to write a letter, for presentation in the court, that expressed her wish for Gale to become the guardian of her children at the time of her death. This was a very difficult task for her, and she originally asked me to help her write the letter. But after several quiet talks with her children and Gale, as well as conversations that she and I had together, Tracy was eventually able to perform this last rite of motherhood on her own. One night, during the last week of her hospitalization, she wrote a beautiful letter that expressed her wishes for her children's care. We had the letter notarized in the hospital and it was presented in family court two days later.

Reassessment

Tracy and I continually assessed what we had accomplished and what was left to accomplish during her admission. We were both highly motivated by the time limits that Tracy's short life expectancy and her more immediate impending discharge from the hospital imposed upon our work. When the day arrived for Tracy to leave, we had met our goals. From a clinical standpoint, I never expected to help Tracy move to a place of acceptance in the relatively brief time we had together, nor did I ever consider this an important or likely outcome. What I did consider important was that she have a safe environment and ample opportunity for grieving, reflection, and life review. It was important too that she be emotionally supported through these processes, her many medical procedures, and the difficult tasks she had to undertake in preparing for her death. To the extent that my role within a hospital setting allowed, I believe that I helped in certain ways to provide the opportunity and the support, which Tracy required to do some of the work of dying.

FIGURE 14.1. Ecomap of Tracy's Support System

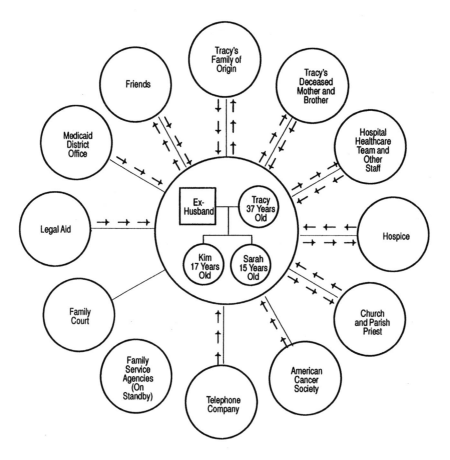

Transfer or Termination

Tracy left HFMC after 37 days. She and I spent some "quiet time" the morning of her discharge reviewing the last details of her care arrangements and our relationship. The actual termination of my relationship with Tracy came several weeks after she left. Following her discharge from the hospital, I made two home visits. The first was planned by the clinical nurse specialist and myself; however, when Tracy's surgeon and his secretary learned that we were going to see her, they asked if they could join us. Consequently, on that particular day, the physician threw his parka on over his scrubs and drove the four of us to Tracy's home. My last visit with Tracy was on the day before I myself left HFMC due to my family's relocation to another area. On this occasion, just the nurse and I visited.

Case Conclusion

Samaritan Hospice has established five levels of patient care, which correspond to family levels of functioning, the first coinciding with the most functional of families and the fifth indicating the least functional families with the greatest levels of need. According to their assessment, Tracy and her family began at the fourth level of care and remained there for the duration of the hospice intervention (C. Garber, personal communication, August 7, 1995). Nevertheless, when Tracy died, she was in her own home, surrounded by her family as she wished.

Differential Discussion

The collective impact of Tracy's youth, personality, strength, and fate was deeply felt by the staff members who cared for her on the CSCU. Just as I have described my own overfunctioning as problematic, the staff's level of attachment to Tracy, coupled with their normal caregiving roles, may have caused her family to feel somewhat shut out and even less confident in themselves as potential caregivers.

In reviewing my case notes from the week before Tracy's discharge, I noticed evidence of this dynamic. One afternoon, I mentioned to Tracy that on a couple of occasions she had alluded to being fearful of returning home. When I then asked her if she would like to have a meeting to address her and her family's fears, she became tearful and said that she would. She added that she felt her family "pulling away" from her. After assuring her that this was not indicative of a diminishing of her family's love for her, I suggested that the staff's continual efforts in actively helping her may have been exacerbating her family's feelings of helplessness. I also speculated that her ability to respond with strength in times of crisis may have been making it hard for her to understand others' different functioning in crisis situations.

A few nights before Tracy's discharge, the clinical nurse specialist and I held a meeting with Tracy, her sisters, and her children. The family fully utilized the opportunity to express both fears and sadness and to have questions answered. The meeting ended with the nurse teaching the family how to administer Tracy's pain medication through her nasogastric tube. The family member who stepped forward first to administer the medication that night was Tracy's youngest daughter, Sarah. This not only seemed to elevate the family's level of confidence, but also gave Sarah some sense of control over her situation by providing her with a way in which she could help her mother (unlike Tracy's experience with her own mother).

As Barnsteiner and Gillis-Donovan (1990) have noted, "Empowering families enables them to become increasingly competent, confident, knowledgeable, calm, and in control, rather than helpless, dependent, frightened, immobilized, and uninvolved in care and decisions" (p. 224). If I were presented with a similar case now, I hope that I would be better at recognizing when to step back and allow the family to engage in the helping process. Though I have a profound respect for the capacity of families to minister to their loved ones, this family's behavior and my feelings for Tracy both compelled me to function in a manner inconsistent with my beliefs.

Furthermore, in my role as an interdisciplinary team member, I would utilize rounds or the biweekly staff group the encourage the staff to examine their level of involvement with the patient and ways in which we might more effectively relate to both patient and family. It is not possible to predict the extent to which such a family might meet the challenge of caring for a dying loved one. But if, as helping professionals, we allow them the opportunity to intervene, they will have a greater chance to gain some degree of mastery over their own anxious responses and to develop increased emotional resources for contending with future crises.

REFERENCES

American Cancer Society. (1995). *Cancer response system: Colorectal cancer* [Computer program printout]. Atlanta, GA: Author. (Document 10007).

Barnsteiner, J. H., and Gillis-Donovan, J. (1990). Being related and separate: A standard for therapeutic relationships. *Maternal Child Nursing, 15,* 223-228.

Clayman, C. B. (Ed.). (1989). *The American Medical Association encyclopedia of medicine.* New York: Random House.

Friedman, E. H. (1985). *Generation to generation: Family process in church and synagogue.* New York: The Guilford Press.

Garfinkel, L. (1995). Cancer statistics and trends. In G. P. Murphy, W. Lawrence Jr., and R. E. Lenhard Jr. (Eds.), *American Cancer Society textbook of clinical oncology,* Second Edition. Atlanta, GA: American Cancer Society, pp. 1-9.

Goldstein, E. G. (1984). *Ego psychology and social work practice.* New York: The Free Press, Macmillan.

Kerr, M. E. (1981). Cancer and the family emotional system. In J. Goldberg (Ed.), *Psychotherapeutic treatment of cancer patients.* New York: The Free Press, Macmillan, pp. 273-315.

Lenhard Jr., R. E., Lawrence Jr., W., and McKenna Sr., R. J. (1995). General approach to the patient. In G. P. Murphy, W. Lawrence Jr., and R. E. Lenhard Jr. (Eds.), *American Cancer Society textbook of clinical oncology*, Second Edition. Atlanta, GA: American Cancer Society, pp. 64-74.

New Jersey Division of Medical Assistance and Health Services. (1991). *Home care services manual*. Trenton, NJ: Author, Chap. 60, pp. 48-52.

New Jersey Division of Medical Assistance and Health Services. (1992a). *Administration manual*. Trenton, NJ: Author, Chap. 49, pp. 1-10.

New Jersey Division of Medical Assistance and Health Services. (1992b). *Hospice services manual*. Trenton, NJ: Author, Chap. 53A, pp. 1-32.

New Jersey Division of Medical Assistance and Health Services. (1992c, September 1). To announce the coverage of hospice care for Medicaid recipients who are terminally ill. *Newsletter, 2* (57).

O'Leary, M. R. (1994). *Lexikon: Dictionary of health care terms, organizations, and acronyms for the era of reform*. Oakbrook Terrace, IL: Joint Commission on Accreditation of Healthcare Organizations.

Redfield, C. S. and Reilly, N. (1991). Colorectal cancer. In S. B. Baird, M. G. Donehower, V.L. Stalsbroten, and T. B. Ades (Eds.), *A cancer source book for nurses*. Atlanta, GA: American Cancer Society, pp. 191-199.

Snook Jr., I. D. and Ruck, K. M. (Eds.). (1987). *A guide to hospital words, terms and phrases*. Philadelphia, PA: Ephraim Publishing Company.

Stearns, N. M., Lauria, M. M., Hermann, J. F., and Fogelberg, P. R. (1993). *Oncology social work: A clinician's guide*. Atlanta, GA: American Cancer Society.

Steele Jr., G. (1995). Colorectal cancer. In G. P. Murphy, W. Lawrence Jr., and R. E. Lenhard Jr. (Eds.), *American Cancer Society textbook of clinical oncology*, Second Edition. Atlanta, GA: American Cancer Society, pp. 236-250.

Summerville, M. E. (Speaker). (1993). *Spirituality in oncology social work: A neglected dimension* (Cassette Recording No. F43). New York: National Association of Oncology Social Workers.

Tatelbaum, J. (1980). *The courage to grieve*. New York: Harper & Row.

Woods, M. E. and Hollis, F. (1990). *Casework: A psychosocial therapy*, Fourth Edition. New York: McGraw-Hill.

PART III:
REHABILITATION, LONG-TERM
INTERVENTION, AND ADVOCACY

Chapter 15

Family Therapy
with a Chronic Pain Patient:
Rehabilitation Hospital

Genevieve S. Coyle

CONTEXT

Description of the Setting

The New England Rehabilitation Hospital is a 197-bed, for-profit facility that began in 1969. Founded during a period of expansion of medical services, the hospital is adapting to the age of managed care and competition. It is now part of a corporation that provides a range of rehabilitation services in New England. In addition to rehabilitation, the corporation has expanded into home health services and assisted living for the elderly, as well as those challenged by physical disabilities. This corporation is a stark contrast to the original facility founded by a physician who began the hospital after his own personal experience with rehabilitation. Previously, the personal interest of the founder and the personality of the first administrator contributed to a small, intimate atmosphere in which staff and administration knew each other and patients frequently returned as volunteers or employees.

The hospital provides specialized rehabilitation services to people suffering from chronic pain, burns, spinal cord and brain injuries, strokes, oncological and cardiac disease, or amputations. These specialized programs have physically self-contained units with their own multidisciplinary staff tailored to the diagnosis. This inpatient facility also has an affiliated day treatment program and an outpatient program. Eighty percent of the patient population is over 65 years old. The vast majority of the staff and patients are Caucasian.

Policy

The hospital is accredited by the Joint Hospital Accreditation Commission (JHAC), and the chronic pain service meets the criteria established by the

Commission on Accreditation of Rehabilitation Facilities (CARF). As a rehabilitation hospital, the program is geared to the restoration of physical function, which means that medical diagnosis and acute treatment are usually completed before the patient arrives for rehabilitation services.

In Massachusetts, most medical care is now managed, and competition among providers for patients has had significant impact on the hospital policy, its staff, and patients. In order to survive in a competitive managed care environment, this hospital must provide excellent patient care with competitive costs and length of stay. The resultant staff fiscal conservatism has produced a streamlined staff at a time when patients with a higher acuity of illness are the norm and documentation standards are more rigid and time-consuming. Often patients find that hospital choice and timing may be restricted by their insurer. Patients usually come to New England Rehabilitation Hospital from an acute care hospital. Then after this hospitalization, they may continue with services in a chronic rehabilitation facility, outpatient clinic, or home services. Patients do remark about the difficulties of using so many providers during one episode of illness.

In the early 1990s, one of the hospital's methods of coping with managed care was to establish the Case Management Department, composed primarily of nurses. This decision led to the elimination of the Social Work Department, which dramatically reduced the psychosocial programs. Limited psychiatric consultation was available primarily to evaluate Axis I diagnosis and to provide pharmacologic treatment and some patient support groups. Widespread concern about the absence of a psychosocial program caused the only staff family therapist to propose the present Family Therapy Program, which is partially funded by Medicare. Family therapy responsibilities include individual, family, or group therapies for patients and support groups for staff. The discharge plans are made by case managers whose responsibilities include communications with the insurer regarding treatment goals, expectations of length of stay, and discharge planning. This separation of therapeutic interventions from discharge plans does free the social worker from time-consuming resource management, but may also eliminate a bridge for some patients or families stressed by illness. Those who may be reluctant to engage in a therapeutic conversation may find it easier to build a relationship around discharge planning that might include their particular needs around the stress of illness.

Managed care has also had a significant impact on chronic pain in patient treatment. Chronic pain programs began in the 1960s, a time of great medical expansion when inpatient programs proliferated and issues regarding time limitations and patient selection were not emphasized. As medical costs escalated, managed care appropriately began to evaluate services; as a consequence, present programs focus on functional restoration and monitor length of stay (Mueller, 1993; Mechanic, 1986). In addition, pain treatment advances allowed for more targeted approaches that did not always require hospitalization. This combination of new knowledge and the constraints of managed care stimulated an expansion of more targeted treatment approaches that did not rely exclusively on inpatient care. This outcome may also be responsible for the decrease in chronic pain admissions, since some of the patients who would have developed chronic pain syndrome may have benefited from earlier, effective interventions. Still, the reluctance of the managed care system to hospitalize chronic pain patients can have a deleterious effect on some chronic pain patients who need hospitalization.

The stigma attached to pain patients has not abated, and lack of a defined, medical diagnosis that has a high value in many managed care systems may hinder necessary hospitalization. Additionally, these patients may be capable of independent life even though they may be impaired in many roles; thus, the managed care system may not attach the same importance to the patients' rehabilitation needs as they do to acute care patients. The medical costs of chronic pain patients are frequent outpatient visits, referrals for consultations, and prescription drugs. These costs may not be monitored as carefully as an acute hospitalization and become more apparent over years of care. Additionally, as managed care providers merge or adopt new patient groups, the medical records of an individual patient may not be transferred to the new case manager. A patient with chronic pain may need to rebuild a medical record to get appropriate services. Finally, physicians whose pain patients are refused admissions for hospitalization may stop making referrals (Calafatis, 1995). While the numbers of pain patients are small, the costs to the individual patient can be high. Their occupational, social, and family roles may be severely restricted.

Technology

The Chronic Pain Service is the antithesis of high technology medical care. Thus, those who work with chronic pain patients frequently see the results of failed or unnecessary surgical procedures, misdiagnosis, and inappropriate use of medications, particularly narcotics. The strategic approach of this program is heavily weighted toward physical and occupational therapy and that of alternative treatments such as relaxation, meditation, and lifestyle issues that may affect pain. Occasionally, acupuncture or massage is used, but the philosophy of the program is to avoid dependence on any intervention that the patient cannot perform at home. The primary goal is restoration of physical function, and achievement of this goal should enable the patient to resume occupational and social roles.

Organization

The Chronic Pain Service is organized according to the standards set by the Committee for the Accreditation of Rehabilitation Facilities (CARF). These standards include criteria for professional staff, patient evaluation, and treatment. The staff is organized as a team and consists of a psychiatrist, who is the medical director; a physiatrist (a physician who specializes in rehabilitation medicine); nurses, physical, occupational, and family therapists; case manager; and a vocational counselor. Additional specialists may be consulted to evaluate or treat patients.

The patients who participate in this program are there for physical rehabilitation, the goal of which is restoration of physical function. Those accepted must have pain that is related to an accident or illness. The program is based on the concepts of milieu therapy used in psychiatric services (Osterweis, Kleinman, and Mechanic, 1987). Group treatment is the norm in all disciplines so that patients learn from each other and reduce the social isolation that many living with pain have experienced. Each discipline conducts individual evaluations of the patients, and these findings are discussed in team meetings in which treatment plans for each patient are formulated.

Within the hospital staff, the Chronic Pain Program is viewed as different from other programs despite similarities in staffing and approach. The differences are that patients are usually treated in groups, and instruction in stress reduction and lifestyle alterations are emphasized. These differences may account for some ways in which the program is seen by the hospital as different, but they do not account for all perceived differences. In our society, there is a stigma attached to those with chronic pain syndrome, and the hospital community reflects society's views (Kleinman, 1988). Pain patients do not escape this stigma and frequently are told that they should not complain because their pain is viewed as different from those with more visible conditions.

All disciplines including family therapy have professional departments with whom they may relate for supervision or professional collaboration. The family therapy department is composed of five part-time family therapists, and during the school year four social work interns usually participate in the hospital program.

PRACTICE DECISIONS

Definition of the Client

Sue Atkins, a 21-year-old high school graduate and recent graduate of a technical school, was admitted to the Pain Clinic because of chronic pain related to reflex sympathetic dystrophy (RSD), secondary to a sprained ankle that had occurred 18 months ago (Osterweis, Kleinman, and Mechanic, 1987). RSD, a diffuse, persistent pain, usually in an extremity, and often associated with vasomotor disturbances, trophic changes, and limitation or immobility of joints, frequently follows some local injury. Sue walked on the toes of her right foot and did not wear a shoe or sock because of pain. She experienced frequent spasms of her right leg. Sue lived at home with her parents and a brother who is two years younger.

Sue's accident was expensive on a personal, family, and societal level (Turk, Meichenbaum, and Genest, 1983). Sue had been involved in the medical system since the accident and with the Massachusetts Rehabilitation Board for over one year. The board, funded through employer contributions, insures and provides case management services to employees who have worker-related accidents and illnesses. Sue's accident was work-related in that she tripped on the second of two steps while leaving work. The initial medical diagnosis, a sprained ankle, was amended to a hair-line fracture, which the patient understood to have been improperly casted (Osterweis, Kleinman, and Mechanic, 1987) and which was later labeled reflex sympathetic dystrophy. Sue, a young, attractive, physically healthy woman had many medical interventions prior to her hospitalization. These interventions included a leg cast, 21 nerve blocks, outpatient physical therapy, psychotherapy, and a polypharmacological program that included three different narcotic pain medications, antidepressants, antianxiety drugs, and anti-inflammatory drugs. Also, she had left an inpatient pain program against medical advice.

By the time Sue was admitted to our program, pain was consuming her life and that of her family. Her mother was in psychotherapy because of stress related to Sue and on medical leave because of a back injury. She left the house with reluctance because of her anxiety about Sue. She responded to Sue's every demand out of fear that a refusal would cause more problems. Sue's father was furious with her mother for not adhering to any limits, and he withdrew to avoid arguments. The couple had no privacy as Sue invaded their bedroom at night with complaints of pain. Because of their fears and growing relationship difficulties, they had given up all social activities and plans for an early retirement in Florida.

Sue's younger brother, who was heavily involved with alcohol, was rarely home. Sue's grandfather, anxious about his favorite granddaughter, called repeatedly to castigate Sue's parents for their failure to solve his granddaughter's health problems. After Sue's hospitalization, he transferred his critical comments to the hospital administration. Prior to the accident, the family described their daughter as bright, willful, and responsible. She was a good student, and a hard worker who had ambitions to own her own business. The parents spoke with obvious pride of Sue's success before the accident and felt that they had failed as parents because of Sue's current disability and their son's ongoing alcohol abuse and recent suicide attempt. They had high hopes for their daughter whose ambition and intelligence reminded them of themselves. Their despair over their daughter had convinced them that their next step was to set up a trust fund to support her. She had no plans to return to work, and although her boyfriend remained her only companion, their relationship narrowed to that of a caregiver and patient. Their plans to live together and marry were put on hold.

At the time of admission, Sue was demanding of attention, requested that staff members sit on her leg to stop spasms, fell frequently, and wanted increased individual physical therapy time. Her thinking was confused, she had difficulty completing sentences, and was emotionally labile. When the staff set limits, it was met with resistance and threats to leave. Initial evaluation indicated that Sue was on a potentially fatal dose of narcotics and that her physical impairment appeared psychogenic in nature. A structured behavioral program began, which included attendance at all programs, a narcotic detoxification schedule, and a program to manage her falls and spasms by wheelchair transport from therapies to her room. Her pain was acknowledged, but its source was not debated with her.

As Sue's thinking was clouded by her use of narcotics, therapeutic conversations with her were limited, and her family became my primary client. The parents had become so exquisitely tuned to Sue's demands that they did not appreciate that Sue was out of control and that they were following her nonsensical direction (Lewis, 1986). After an initial meeting, the family agreed to come for weekly sessions, and in the first sessions they provided some openings that shaped future sessions. Sue's mother was distraught over the attempted suicide by her son and Sue's use of pain medications. She felt that Sue's involvement with drugs was out of control. As their son had used Sue's pills in his suicide attempt, she had been desperately trying to lock up all medications and felt this hospitalization was their last chance. She felt this was a matter of life or death. In response to my question about his understanding of the source of this pain, Sue's father hesitantly offered that as they searched for a medical answer, some physicians had suggested that Sue had psychogenic reflex sympathetic dystrophy. When asked about the strength of his belief, he remarked that he thought there was at least a 75 percent chance that this was true. I acknowledged that this was a significant consideration in the initial evaluation. With many interruptions from Sue, the family considered this possibility. This family was desperate, and the father had begun to shift his thinking from medical interventions to psychological ones.

For Sue, the overarching goal of this hospitalization was the restoration of her physical functioning. I needed her family's support to ensure that this goal was accomplished. Sue had been in charge of decision making for most of this illness, and her parents responded to her requests many times against their better judgment. For successful treatment, her parents had to resume appropriate parental roles and support treatment goals (Rolland, 1994; McDaniel, Hepworth, and Doherty, 1992).

The family was seen in four formal sessions. In the first session, high emotional tension interfered with communication. The family members were unable to observe simple social rules such as allowing one another to complete sentences or listening to each other's ideas. By the second session, the parents had cooperated with plans to continue Sue's hospitalization, visit appropriately by telephone and in person, and restrict the interference of the grandfather. As the parents' high level of emotional expression calmed, they acted together, and Sue began to respond behaviorally to their decisions even when she disagreed verbally.

By the third family session, the parents had not succeeded in getting the son to a session; they were suspicious of his behavior and were concerned that alcohol was becoming a larger part of his life. Their grief and sadness over the state of their children's lives was palpable. They felt that they had failed as parents and lost hope that their children's lives might be salvageable. Everyone was quiet, which was unusual in this family of southern-European background in which constant chatter was the norm. With the acknowledgment of sadness came some recognition of the hopes and dreams they had had for their first child. Sue's parents recalled her as a bright, adaptive child. They regretted working so much but were pleased they could send their daughter to college. Her father recalled the skillful ways in which she had debated with him. These recollections cheered the family, and the meeting closed with renewed hope and good will.

While many psychological issues surfaced in the four sessions, the primary goal of this therapy—to enable Sue's parents to resume an appropriate parental role for their daughter and support the treatment—was achieved. The parents began to act as a team and together refused to take Sue home the night she packed her bags and told them to take her. Later they refused her request for a long-distance calling card but initiated appropriate calls to her. The parents divided some tasks. For example, Sue's mother set limits with her own father who was interfering with parental roles, while Sue's father contacted her physicians and requested that they stop prescribing narcotic medications for his daughter. Sue's parents began to trust their judgment and were surprised that Sue cooperated.

Goals

The overarching goal for the chronic pain patient is restoration of a functional life in which appropriate social, occupational, and personal relationships can be attained despite pain. While it is hoped that pain will be reduced during rehabilitation, the purpose of the program is to enable patients to learn physical and mental techniques to decrease pain and related behaviors. The absence of pain is not a goal (Kabat-Zinn, 1991). Cessation of all narcotics is required. While all patients are informed of these goals and agree to them prior to admission, the implementation of these goals and their many nuances is difficult for most patients. Fear, anger, disbelief, shame, and resistance are common reactions during the initial stages of hospitalization.

Prior to admission, most patients, particularly those with complicated histories, meet with the medical director to decide if the program will be helpful and if the prospective patient is interested in the type of treatment offered. Sue had agreed to these goals; however, severe dependency on narcotic pain medications limited Sue's ability to think clearly and participate in a treatment plan. Consequently, Sue was minimally involved in the goal-setting discussion; instead the team focused their goals on behavioral modification, and her parents became my primary client. Team goals for Sue included detoxification from medications, attendance at all therapy sessions, and swift removal by wheelchair to her room to avoid any secondary gain should her leg develop spasms. Sue's parents were the key to her successful therapy, and my goals were set with them as the primary client.

Contract

While the emotional component of the chronic pain patient is acknowledged by staff, the patient's use of psychotherapy sessions is voluntary. Families are not required to attend family therapy sessions, and Sue's family could have chosen not to participate. My contract with Sue's family was verbal and included agreement about time and frequency of the meetings. Sue objected to the primacy of the contract with her parents but did not refuse to participate.

Meeting Place

In an inpatient program there are a variety of meeting places, but confidentiality can only be preserved in the therapist's office or a conference room. Less structured meetings can take place in patients' rooms, but interruptions are frequent and roommates may be present. The meetings with Sue and her parents were highly structured and took place in a formal meeting room governed by time limits that guide traditional therapy. I had one formal session with Sue, and all others were brief and in her room.

Use of Time

Time is an important framework and is set by the terms of the patient's insurance which determines length of stay on the basis of Diagnostic Related Groups. For inpatient chronic pain programs, four weeks is the norm, though it may vary with individual patients. Treatment must conform to this time allotment. At the time of admission, as the social worker on the "Chronic Pain Unit," I meet with patients individually to ascertain their understanding of their pain and its source. This understanding includes their history prior to the onset of pain, and the effect of pain on them, their relationships, and roles. Usually I make arrangements for a private session with agreed-upon time limits. If subsequent therapy occurs, it is by joint agreement. Family involvement is most often initiated with the patient's knowledge and consent. Since the team appreciates the emotional component in chronic pain, there is greater acceptance of psychologically therapeutic time being substituted for a physical therapy session than in other areas of rehabilitation. In my clinical work with Sue's family, therapy time was structured, but Sue and I met occasionally and informally. She participated in structured therapy groups but, until the third week, left early because of the interference of her symptoms.

Interventions

My interventions on the pain unit are intertwined with the interdisciplinary program on the "Chronic Pain Unit." The team interventions include an evaluation process that incorporates a weekly reassessment of progress, and a physical and occupational therapy program that includes a strong component of stress management and relaxation. My clinical interventions with chronic pain patients are informed by and benefit from the patient's experiences in the total program and the team's ongoing assessment. For example, the team assessed that Sue's physical limitations were caused by limited and inappropriate use of her foot and ankle, and that with appropriate physical therapy she could be 100 percent functional. The evaluation indicated that Sue was physically capable of complete physical restoration of her leg, her use of drugs was to be gradually stopped, and further evaluation of her emotional needs would be made as she became free of drugs. If further evaluation had indicated that she had limited use of her leg, I may have made different interventions.

Sue's case is an illustration of some of the changes that have taken place in chronic pain treatment centers over the past decade in response to the brief hospitalizations encouraged by a managed care system. The goal of Sue's medical interventions and subsequent hospitalization is the restoration of physical function. Nevertheless, as seen in her previous treatments, unless psychosocial issues are addressed, the goal of physical restoration may be compromised. She had been the recipient of many targeted treatments, the focus of which was her leg, and in her first inpatient program, the family was not involved. This may have contributed to her father's decision to facilitate her discharge against medical advice. In this hospitalization, Sue did achieve her goal in that her physical functioning was restored, but it was achieved with psychosocial interventions that included family therapy (Rolland, 1994). Most of Sue's individual psychological issues must be managed after discharge, and this creates some uncertainty about her ultimate success in resuming appropriate social and occupational roles.

In my initial evaluation, I explore experiences, observe dynamics, and create an environment that allows families to acknowledge problems, recognize their strengths, and set their goals. By broadening the concept of pain beyond the physical, to include some of the family and patient dynamics that may contribute on an emotional level, I provide new opportunities for the patient to make positive changes (Griffith, Griffith, and Slovic, 1990).

Thus, I consider many theoretical issues during treatment. The life stage of the patient and family at the time of the onset of pain is one of those issues (Carter and McGoldrick, 1980; George and Gold, 1991; Rolland, 1987). Sue was beginning to physically separate from her family and become self-supporting. Her technical training after high school opened a door to financial independence, and she had a long-term boyfriend and a circle of friends. As long as Sue was not able to walk or wear shoes and was in severe pain, appropriate developmental issues involving career choices, a sexual relationship, and physical separation from her family were put on hold. Her parents, after a youthful marriage and a hectic life of careers and childrearing, were confronting the loss of their parental roles and a troubled marriage. Sue's pain and its treatment might facilitate the avoidance of any one of these issues to concentrate on her physical problems. Finally the parents had ongoing difficulties in their relationships with their parents. Sue's father had been cut off from his family for years, and the couple's relationship to the mother's intrusive father had always been difficult (Penn, 1983). Sue's crisis may be a reflection of this family's struggle to establish a personal identity and maintain healthy ties to their families. The family's description of their experiences helped me to understand the issues that have meaning for them.

Other pertinent theoretical considerations relate to the chronic pain syndrome. In Sue's case, repercussions of an accident were out of proportion to the event. While one should not rule out a significant physical finding that cannot be definitively diagnosed, the evaluation of her physical limitations by physical therapy were not congruent with her stated injury. Thus, I considered the other components frequently found in the chronic pain paradigm, which include factors related to affective disorders, substance abuse, and traumatic life experiences (Osterweis, Kleinman, and Mechanic, 1987). Substance abuse issues played a role in the lives of Sue and some family members. Sue's involvement with pain medications was life threatening; she had not divulged her full use of medicines and began to experience withdrawal symptoms when routinely given the dose she acknowledged. As far as we knew, Sue had abstained from alcohol and illegal drugs, but her brother remained significantly involved, and her mother continued pain medications for a back injury. Chronic pain patients, particularly those involved with substance abuse issues, may also have histories of trauma that include physical, sexual, or emotional trauma (Wurtels, Kaplan, and Keairnes, 1990). Sue's previous therapist had not documented any incidents, but Sue also had had periods of anorexia and, connected with this illness, periods of compulsive exercise. She and her family had a cluster of symptoms that would indicate that this family was experiencing difficulties, and Sue's transition from adolescence to adulthood was difficult for them. The family acknowledged marital discord but suggested no relevant traumatic physical or emotional events in Sue's life (Pozatek, 1994).

The hospital chart usually contains some basic psychosocial information and history of the patient's pain syndrome, but my goal is to maintain a neutral position and listen to the patient's and family's story. Most patients have had many evaluations and years of medical care in which they have answered many questions and have been given explanations of their pain. In each first session, I gather the patient's experience of the illness and include the history of the illness in the fullest sense. I want to know each facet of the pain and the patient's account of the illnesses' intrusions on their past and present family, occupational, and social relationships. I try not to overlook the reasons that patients attribute to their suffering. Patients sometimes blame bad medical care or may believe that God is punishing them. I also ask patients to describe their future if they must live with pain. These questions open personal areas of the patients' experience. Arthur Kleinman's work, *The Illness Narratives*, is a model that I have used to conceptualize my thinking about the personal experience of illness as contrasted with medical diagnosis of disease (Kleinman, 1988). In Sue's case, pain had penetrated every aspect of her life and that of her family. Her parents were demoralized and had lost confidence in their decisions about their daughter; the repercussions of their daughter's pain had changed most aspects of their lives. They acknowledged difficulties in balancing their home and professional lives. Their marital relationship was troubled, and they wondered if it had a negative effect on their parenting. They were pessimistic about the future and believed that their daughter's remaining life might be one of total dependence.

In my work with pain patients, I have found the techniques of narrative theories to be successful (White and Epston, 1990). These techniques were not sufficient for this family as they could not observe normal social amenities that allowed one another to be heard. In addition, Sue's mother feared repercussions, so she continued to try to meet Sue's demands. Occasionally Sue's father verbally erupted at mother-daughter interactions, but usually stood by in silence and anger or carried out their wishes. Thus, with this family, structural theories and techniques were used (Umbarger, 1983). As a chalkboard eraser was available, this became the symbol that identified the speaker. The family observed the rules that they had to have the eraser to speak and should repeat the last speaker's thoughts before they began their own. The family quickly got the idea and within two sessions had mastered talking in turn. They began to act as a team weighing their daughter's requests in "life or death" terms, and Sue began to ask them rather than demand, and although she frequently objected to their decisions, she did not behaviorally disagree. Through this process, the parents gained confidence in their ability to draw a line separating behaviors that would enable Sue to regain a normal life and those that might put her at risk.

These parents needed help to structure their family and reclaim their roles as parents (Umbarger, 1983). The use of the eraser allowed the family meeting to go forward in an orderly manner so that even Sue knew she could not interrupt until she had a turn. The parents, through my repeated referral of appropriate decisions to them, acted competently. Thus, Sue's mother restrained her desire to give in to her daughter, and her father became more active. My use of the mother's statement that this was a case of "life and death" helped them to evaluate each request in terms of whether it would help Sue live or die.

As this family gained confidence that they could listen to one another, the concepts related to narrative therapy became relevant to subsequent sessions (White and Epston, 1990). Many pain patients focus on their pain and medical care and exclude other stressful or successful life events. The conceptual framework of narrative therapy helps to enlarge the patient's focus, which in turn frequently helps the patient explore untapped resources and new solutions. Narrative therapy emphasizes the patient as the authority over his or her life and respects the stories that families value about themselves. It does not gloss over problems. Thus, Sue's father and mother appreciated the opportunity to relate the full impact of her pain in their lives. The father spoke of the thoughts of Sue's pain that kept him from concentrating and led to a serious automobile accident. He was not able to attend to his business and began to think of himself as a failure. Sue's mother was overcome with a sense of responsibility for Sue and had given up all of her interests. After they had acknowledged the devastation that Sue's pain had brought into their lives, they were able to relate stories that reflected the values they cherished and their previous successes. In their family, children were treasured and all decisions were made in light of the children's interest. The evening that Sue's family shared stories about their determination and hard work resulted in a renewal of the family's pride. She glowed as her parents described their pleasure in her abilities to express her opinions, persevere, and work hard. Soon after this session, she began to talk about returning to work and future plans.

Other concepts of narrative therapy that were useful in Sue's treatment were those of unique outcomes and objectification of problems (White and Epston, 1990). Patients set in a downward spiral frequently overlook some successful efforts and, as a result, fail to gain a sense of accomplishment. Initially, Sue's family failed to note that Sue respected their decisions, and only as I brought their success to their attention were they able to regain confidence in their parental roles. In highlighting some of the patient's successes, hope may be reestablished along with maps to a more successful life.

Finally, most pain patients internalize the stance of our larger society—that lack of diagnosis means internal character deficiencies. As I help patients identify pain as an object to manage rather than as a characterological flaw, they are able to develop strategies to work with pain and its resultant behaviors. Thus, Sue's family was able to enlarge upon the impact of pain beyond Sue's leg to look at the ways it had invaded all of their lives and to establish guidelines to defeat the pain and its impact. For the first time in two years, they were able to work together, as Michael White would say, to defeat pain (White and Epston, 1990). The objectification of pain helped to reduce their immobilizing demoralization around Sue's pain.

Use of Outside Resources

While some chronic pain patients may need continued physical therapy, the inpatient goal is to restore physical functioning; thus, recommendations for health clubs, vocational counseling, substance abuse counseling, or psychotherapy are as likely as referrals for medical interventions or recommendations for ongoing physical therapy. Patients' uncertainty about the ability to carry over hospital success into daily life is common. They are particularly fearful if the discharge plan is not oriented to continued physical therapy.

Sue's discharge recommendations can serve as an example. First, a letter was sent to the prescribing physician stating that Sue's physical condition no longer required narcotic medications. Second, there was no recommendation for post-hospitalization physical or occupational therapies, which made the nonphysical nature of this problem clear to parents and patient. Third, recommendations for continued family and individual therapies were made.

Reassessment

Weekly reassessment is made by the team in collaboration with the patient, and this ongoing assessment provides a framework for the therapies of each team member. The patient's physical capacity and physical progress guide my work with families and individuals and set a frame for me to formulate goals. In retrospect, my work with Sue's family probably ensured that Sue would complete this hospitalization. Her family's compliance in attending meetings, acceptance of limits, and progress in family therapy allowed other team members to work successfully with Sue.

Transfer or Termination

While most of our patients complete the program, a small number transfer to an acute care hospital because further medical evaluation is required or suspected acute medical illness needs further evaluation. Approximately 2 percent of the patients leave because they decide that they want to continue chronic use of pain medications. Another 1 percent may leave because they do not agree with the team's assessment of their rehabilitation needs. Sue is an example of a patient who left an earlier rehabilitation program prematurely and probably stayed this time because her parents did not cooperate when she demanded to leave.

Four weeks is the average length of stay in the "Chronic Pain Unit," although some accomplish their goals in less time. A small number of our chronic pain patients have complicated physical, emotional, or substance abuse histories and may need a longer hospitalization; however, managed care companies may be reluctant to extend the time and some patients may return home prematurely. Sue's treatment shows that managed care may support a complicated patient. Her managed care program extended her length of stay by one week, which required efforts at the hospital and the managed care program above the case management level. This is an instance in which a history was not lost as she stayed with the same program throughout the entire treatment of her ankle. Finally, her situation demonstrates that managed care does not guarantee appropriate patient care as she was certainly overtreated with nerve blocks and medications in other programs.

Case Conclusion

During Sue's final week in the rehabilitation program she had completed the narcotic detoxification program and was able to engage in therapeutic experiences with staff and her fellow patients, some of whom were her age. Her thinking cleared and she did not seem depressed. She was able to attend all sessions for the last week and was involved with other patients in appropriate discussions about careers and relationships. She participated in discharge plans to participate in a health club, though she would have preferred continued physical therapy. She planned to return to her previous psychotherapist and agreed to formally terminate with the physician who had prescribed her narcotic medications.

Sue's transition to home was not smooth. Her parents were undecided about the decision for the family to continue therapy, and although they made one appointment with a family therapist, they did not continue. She attempted to see her previous therapist, but this was denied because she no longer needed physical therapy and her psychotherapist was employed by the outpatient rehabilitation program. Her managed care program through the state rehabilitation office approved individual therapy, but their approved therapists had waiting lists. Three months after discharge, Sue had not been assigned to a therapist. Sue, however, was able to remain off medications, enjoy a normal social life, hold a part-time job, and take one course. Her mother's back problems became more severe and she consulted a variety of physicians about possible treatments. Her brother continued his alcohol abuse and decreased his limited work schedule. Thus, six months after discharge, Sue continued to resume a more normal life, but the status of her mother and brother had worsened, and her mother remained in therapy. Her father remained on the periphery, and the relationship of the couple remained difficult.

Thus, six months after discharge, physical restoration–the goal of Sue and the insurance company–was maintained. She had not returned to narcotics and had no physical limitations. This hospitalization was a success. Some uncertainty remained about individual issues that could require future psychological interventions. Sue was insured through the state rehabilitation services. While it may be appropriate for the State Rehabilitation Board to restrict Sue's access to psychotherapy, she was only partially employed and her health insurance opportunities were limited. The family continued to have significant health-related problems for which they pursued medical interventions. Additional family therapy may have been successful in addressing the issues that remain within this family and may have potentially reduced their need for ongoing medical interventions.

Differential Discussion

In reviewing this case, I believe that family therapy was successful and that my involvement of Sue's parents was a critical therapeutic move. If I had not invited Sue's parents to join the treatment process or if they had refused to participate, I am convinced that she would have left this program. Sue's parents were confused by Sue's accident and bewildered by the sophisticated medical diagnoses that she had received. They wandered from one medical treatment to another and accepted without question Sue's evaluations that treatments had failed. The parents needed a therapeutic intervention that could encourage them to trust their abilities as parents. Sue needed her parents to set limits until she was able to act on her own.

I had some systemic supports that limited the parents' choices and encouraged them to put their energies and hope into the treatment at New England Rehabilitation Hospital. This family needed some boundaries and were intelligent enough to understand several realities. Sue's parents knew that her insurance company would not support another inpatient treatment program and that Sue's use of narcotic medications was at a dangerous level. Finally, her parents had spoken to enough physicians to realize there were no more treatment options.

Within the hospital, I was fortunate to have an experienced team that understood how to work with a patient whose pain exceeds the extent of the physical injury. My colleagues knew how to acknowledge pain, set limits, and provide encouragement even if the patient was heavily influenced by narcotic medications. Sue's behavior was very difficult. She may not have stayed with a less caring or less knowledgeable staff.

This family treatment demonstrates that systemic therapies can be successfully used with a targeted symptom such as Sue's chronic pain and that these therapies can be provided within a brief treatment model. Sue was so involved with narcotic medications that she had little psychic energy to explore issues related to anorexia nervosa or questions about possible traumatic life events. Sue also needed her parents to support her treatment rather than respond to her immediate pain. If I had concentrated on these individual issues, I do not believe her treatment would have succeeded.

Her family, however, continued to identify individual members who needed services and were not able to consider that involvement in a systemic family approach might foster changes. The couple did not want to continue to assess the family dynamics that may have contributed to their son's addiction, her mother's back pain, and the couple's estrangement. They preferred to continue to address targeted issues of individual members.

REFERENCES

Calafatis, S. (1995). Personal Communication.

Carter, E. A., and McGoldrick, M. (Eds.). (1980). *The family life cycle.* New York: Gardner.

George, L. and Gold, D. (1991). Life course perspective on intergenerational and generational connections. *Marriage and Family Review, 16,* 67-88.

Griffith, J., Griffith, M., and Slovic, L. (1990). Mind-body problems in family therapy: Contrasting first- and second-order cybernetics approaches. *Family Process, Inc., 29,* 219-233.

Kabat-Zinn, J. (1991). *Full catastrophe living.* New York: Delta.

Kleinman, A. (1988). *The illness narratives.* New York: Basic Books.

Lewis, J. (1986). Family structure and stress. *Family Process, Inc., 25,* 235-247.

McDaniel, S., Hepworth, J., and Doherty, W. (1992). *Medical family therapy.* New York: Basic Books.

Mechanic, D. (1986). *From advocacy to allocation.* New York: The Free Press.

Mueller, K. (1993). *Health care policy in the United States*. Lincoln, Nebraska: University of Nebraska Press.

Osterweis, M., Kleinman, A., and Mechanic, D. (Eds.) (1987). *Behavioral and public policy perspectives*. Washingtin, DC: National Academy Press.

Penn, P. (1983). Coalitions and binding interactions in families with chronic illness. *Family Systems Medicine, 1*, 16-25.

Pozatek, E. (1994). The problem of certainty: Clinical social work in the postmodern era. *Social Work, 39*, 396-403.

Rolland, J. (1987). Chronic illness and the life cycle: A conceptual framework. *Family Process, Inc., 26*, 203-221.

Rolland, J. (1994). *Families, illness, and disability*. New York: Basic Books.

Turk, D., Meichenbaum, D., and Genest, M. (1983). *Pain and behavioral medicine*. New York: Guilford Press.

Umbarger, C. (1983). *Structural family therapy*. New York: Grune & Stratton.

White, M. and Epston, D. (1990). *Narrative means to therapeutic ends*. New York: W. W. Norton.

Wurtels, S., Kaplan, G., and Keairnes, M. (1990). Childhood sexual abuse among chronic pain patients. *Clinical Journal of Pain, 6*, 110-113.

Chapter 16

Rehabilitation of a Quadriplegic Adolescent: Regional Spinal Cord Injury Center

Judith F. Hirschwald

CONTEXT

Description of the Setting

Magee Rehabilitation Hospital is a 96-bed, free-standing, not-for-profit physical rehabilitation center. Opened in March 1958, the hospital offers comprehensive inpatient, outpatient, and follow-up services to individuals with physical disability. Patients are evaluated and admitted based upon their ability to benefit physically from the services offered and on their potential to utilize these functional gains within the home and community setting. Thus, admission criteria are both medical and social. The average length of stay is approximately 27 days. The majority of patients are newly disabled and will return home with some degree of permanent disability. In addition to the inpatient services, the hospital has comprehensive outpatient and follow-up services.

In 1978, in conjunction with Thomas Jefferson University, Magee received federal designation as the Regional Spinal Cord Injury Center of Delaware Valley. This designation altered the general characteristics of the patient population and provided impetus for the development of specialty programming in spinal cord injury. Since statistically the 18 to 23-year-old male is at highest risk for spinal cord injury, the overall population became younger. In addition, a system of lifetime care was designed to provide a resource for the rehabilitation needs of this population over their lifetime. Over time, similar resources were developed for other specialty populations, particularly brain injury and stroke. Recent changes in health care have significantly reduced lengths of inpatient stay, thus increasing the need for more complex and comprehensive outpatient and follow-up services.

Throughout the history of the hospital, social workers have functioned as integral members of the rehabilitation team with the primary role of discharge planning. Discharge planning has encompassed not only the myriad of details, services, and referrals needed to accomplish a safe, quality discharge, but also the work with patient and family to cope with the lifestyle changes engendered by the disability. With the advent of managed care and changes in health care delivery, the social workers have also assumed the primary role in communication with the managed care providers and in collaboration with the physician in managing the utilization of resources and length of stay. At this writing, the social work department is in transition to a department of case management. The major functions of case management, as defined by the hospital, will be discharge planning, utilization review, and system coordination. The number of staff has been reduced to eight full-time staff and will include individuals with both social work and nursing credentials. These staff will now have full responsibility with the medical staff for the management of the rehabilitation process and rehabilitation team throughout the patients' length of stay. The extent of social work or case management integration into the outpatient and follow-up areas is yet to be defined.

These changes mirror the changes that are occurring in health care throughout the country, where perhaps the only constant theme is "change." Social work is again restructuring its contribution to patient care and defining new opportunities in a rapidly changing health care environment.

Policy

Polices affecting delivery of service in physical rehabilitation originate from both internal and external sources. Internally, the primary policies derive from the Board of Trustees and the hospital administration. Such policies affect the scope of hospital services, admission policies, and overall hospital mission. External forces that influence delivery of care include third-party payers, accrediting agencies, and general governmental and societal sanctions.

Probably no other single entity has so totally affected the health care delivery system as the rapid growth of managed care. The term "managed care" is generic, and in the absence of any national policy or structure, emerges in a myriad of models and designs. In general "managed care is an alternative to fee-for-service health care. . . . The financing and delivery of medical care are integrated through contracts with selected physicians and hospitals furnishing a comprehensive set of services to enrolled members, usually for a predetermined monthly premium" (Keigher, 1995 p. 146). The prevailing message is quality care at lower cost. The rapid growth of managed care is reorganizing the health care delivery system at both the macro and micro levels. As these changes are still in progress, it is difficult to predict the structure of health care in the twenty-first century. However, in today's world, some effects of the changes are obvious in the daily services to patients:

1. Lengths of stay are shorter in both acute care and rehabilitation.
2. Transfers to rehabilitation must be preauthorized as to both the need for rehabilitation services and also the specific rehabilitation provider.
3. All nonroutine services must be preauthorized, for example, out-of-hospital consultations, durable medical equipment, home health services, and outpatient services.
4. Choices as to providers for durable medical equipment, home health services, etc., are limited to those providers under contract with the managed care company.
5. Admission and discharge decisions are specifically impacted by the managed care provider.

While critical pathways, clinical pathways, and practice parameters are being designed to standardize treatment, they are not universally accepted nor applicable to all patients. While outcome measurement is the buzz-word of the 1990s, payers and providers are both struggling to define outcome. The cost of care is being reduced as hospitals are downsizing, rightsizing, and restructuring, as well as reevaluating the resources expended for a given diagnosis. However, the impact of these changes on quality of care and outcome is yet to be quantified. The chronically ill and/or disabled populations present a particular challenge to managed care as they are potentially high risk, high users of resources with perhaps a more difficult dilemma in measuring outcome. Consequently, the pressure to find alternative, less costly levels of care is great and impacts significantly the traditional population of an acute rehabilitation facility, both in the initial rehabilitation effort as well as in the maintenance of health in the community.

The increase in managed care is an outgrowth of the national consensus to reduce the cost of health care. However, the National Health Care Reform discussions of 1993/1994 did not produce consensus on how to effectively accomplish this goal. Therefore, powerful commercial forces are quickly transforming the U.S. health care system with far more effect than policy discourse (Keigher, 1995). Underlying this transformation is a consistent philosophical stance that enormous dollar expenditure can be justified only if the result is the restoration of the individual to normal, productive functioning. These policies have tended in the past to release funding for care of individuals who are younger, perhaps less severely disabled, and who demonstrate a potential for return to competitive employment. However, more recently there have been some significant policy shifts and new legislation affecting the lives of individuals with severe disability. Title VII of Public Law 95-102 (Amendments to the Rehabilitation Act of 1973, 1978), made provision for the development of consumer-directed independent living centers for the severely disabled. Since 1980, independent living centers have grown significantly, providing information, referral, and advocacy services for severely disabled persons. The Americans with Disability Act (ADA) signed into law in 1990 finally articulated the civil rights of individuals with disability. Even in a climate of shrinking health care dollars, some monies are being directed to quality-of-life issues in the community.

Lastly, Magee's commitment to lifetime follow-up care for individuals with catastrophic injury (specifically spinal cord injury) has been influenced at least in part by the stance of the Commission on Accreditation of Rehabilitation Facilities (CARF) and by the former Department of Health, Education, and Welfare, who originally designed and implemented the model systems concept for spinal cord injury (Standards Manual for Organizations Serving People with Disabilities, 1987). Both of these organizations place emphasis on outcome, requiring the collection of follow-up data in order to measure patient outcome. The need to collect data following discharge dictates the need for a system to track patients to determine their current status in defined parameters. Around this data-collection system evolved a commitment to a service system and consequently the design of a lifetime follow-up system.

Thus, the philosophical stance and hence the policies to address the needs of individuals with disability, from point of onset through a lifetime in the community, remain somewhat contradictory. While additional resources are being expended to allow the maintenance of an independent lifestyle in the community, more controversy arises over the expenditures in the initial months following onset as to the appropriate level of care and dollar expenditure to attain maximum level of independence.

Technology

Increased technology has had a significant influence in the field of physical rehabilitation in two primary spheres. First and foremost, increased medical technology has significantly lowered the mortality rates for many individuals with traumatic injuries and severe medical insults. The result of this new technology is that individuals with more severe residual disabilities are surviving the initial trauma and being transferred for rehabilitation services. Many of these individuals, however, require significant support, in both human resources as well as technology, to survive in the community. Only creative planning and a productive partnership with funding resources can allow for a safe discharge to the community and potential for an acceptable quality of life.

Advanced technology, particularly with increased computer sophistication, has also made available equipment that can allow even the most severely disabled individual some degree of independent functioning. These systems may be operated by verbal cues, a shoulder shrug, breath control, or a mouth stick, sometimes the only motion available to the individual. Elaborately adapted vans can make driving a reality for an individual with quadriplegia. However such advanced technology comes with a high price tag, and often this high-tech equipment, while having potential to enhance the individual's quality of life, is not justifiable to the payer as medically necessary.

Thus, the area of technology reintroduces some of the dilemmas in the health care debate. Should the most sophisticated technology be made available to every person or should health care be rationed by some criteria? If the most severely traumatized individual is to be kept alive at the scene of the accident and in acute care, to what extent are the ongoing survival needs of this individual to be supported?

Organization

Magee Rehabilitation Hospital is governed by a Board of Trustees who represent a variety of community and hospital interests. The chief executive officer is also the president and medical director, so that the ultimate decision-making power, both medical and administrative, rests in one office. In the new organizational structure, there is no director of Social Service. There is a coordinator of case management who reports to the chief operating officer. Case management will consist of eight full-time staff and appropriate support resources. For over five years, the hospital has also been organized around programs (product lines). Program directors are responsible for programmatic planning, resource identification, and profitability. This coexistent structure of program directors and department directors has dictated a matrix management structure in all clinical areas. As a relatively small institution, Magee lends itself to an informal atmosphere and to easy staff communication on all levels. Administrative staff are quite accessible, so planning occurs both formally and informally. Magee is not currently a formal partner in a network system except for the formal affiliation with the Regional Spinal Cord Injury System. Relationships with a variety of other organizations, in both health care and the larger community, facilitate transfer of patients into rehabilitation and from rehabilitation into the community.

DECISIONS ABOUT PRACTICE

Client Description

Jeffrey Bauer was admitted to Magee in September, following an automobile accident in late July. He was 19 years old, had graduated from high school the previous June, and was working as a maintenance engineer in his local school district. He was one of six passengers in a car, all friends, returning from a weekend at the shore. Jeff was the only one injured in the accident. He sustained a complete fracture of his sixth cervical vertebra that left him paralyzed below the neck. While drugs and alcohol were suspected to have been factors in the accident, Jeff was not heavily into either, prior to his injury. Following acute medical treatment at a local community hospital, Jeff was transferred to Magee for physical rehabilitation services. Although a complete bed patient on admission, he could be expected to attain mobility at a wheelchair level, learn to feed himself, transfer to and from the wheelchair, and dress himself with minimal assistance. Jeff's own goal on admission was to return to his "normal" level of physical functioning.

Although he was technically living at home prior to his injury, Jeff rarely spent any time there except to sleep. His major activity centered around his friends from high school. He was not an outstanding student in high school, although whether his low achievement was a result of lack of ability or lack of application was unknown. He had not chosen a career goal for himself, but was planning to enter the armed services to secure training in some area. Generally, his life at this time consisted of having a good time with his friends and using the money from his employment for his own enjoyment.

He was a good-looking, personable young man, but was not especially verbal except with his own peer group. He clearly valued his beginning independence from his family and, throughout the time in the general hospital, communicated with them as little as possible regarding his feelings and plans made with him for his ongoing care. His mother and father were feeling shut out by him, angry at his unwillingness to communicate with them, and guilty that they were not performing appropriately in their role as parents of a severely injured son (Wheeler, 1977).

Jeff's medical care coverage was through an HMO, which he had selected from a menu of plans offered by the local school district. As Jeff was expected to contribute toward the cost of his health coverage, he had selected a plan with a minimal out-of-pocket expense. As such, the plan did not offer full comprehensive benefits, but in Jeff's words "I was 19 years old and in perfect health. Why would I need good heath insurance?" Immediately following the accident, the insurance company assigned a case manager to monitor his care in recognition of both the catastrophic nature of the injury as well as the risk to the insurance company. Their plan was to transfer Jeff for his rehabilitation to a local center with whom they had a contract. However, Jeff's mother and father had done some research following his injury and advocated for Jeff's transfer to a Regional Spinal Cord Injury Center. Although Magee did not at the time have a negotiated contract with this HMO, they were willing to negotiate out-of-contract. Consequently, Jeff was transferred to Magee.

Definition of Client

The primary client as defined by a physical rehabilitation center is the individual patient. He or she is the key person who needs to gain an understanding of and ability to cope with his or her disability, and is therefore the primary target for all educational efforts regarding his or her care and needs. To treat the client alone, however, would be to assume that the individual will live in a vacuum. The definition of client, therefore, expands to include significant other persons within the client's environment (Crewe, Athelstan, and Krumberger, 1979; David, Gur, and Rozin, 1981; Zola, 1981).

The delineation of significant other persons often changes during the course of rehabilitation as the patient and the family or friends begin to recognize the effects of severe disability and the implications for the future. For example, at times an employer or an attendant becomes part of the definition of the client. Jeff's significant others changed over time. Initially, his parents were most significant. As he began to go out for weekends, his younger brother became important. The brother's ability to cope emotionally and physically with Jeff's care was critical. In later stages of rehabilitation, Jeff's friends became important.

For the social worker and for Jeff, the case manager from the HMO was also a significant and integral part of the client system. This individual was the link between the client, the rehabilitation process, and the payer. No decisions could be made or plans formulated without her involvement and concurrence.

Goals, Objectives, and/or Outcome Measures

The broadest goal set by the social worker and the patient is to enable the patient to participate fully in the rehabilitation program and to return home at the highest possible level of functioning. Initially, the patient's goals are usually physical–most often complete recovery–and are not realistic regarding the limits of the disability. It is the social worker's first task then to enable the patient to begin the long process of coping with the reality of the disability (Athelstan, 1978). Obviously, the sudden onset of a physical disability is an overwhelming experience. Dealing with the totality of the disability usually immobilizes the patient. Consequently, the joint setting of small, manageable goals helps the patient begin to cope. At an early stage of treatment, a shift must occur in the patient's perception of him or herself. The patient must change from viewing him or herself as a sick person who is the passive recipient of care to a disabled person who has the ability and the right to participate actively in his or her own program (Orbaan, 1986; Lane, 1975). In order to assert him or herself in this role, the patient must be given choices within the setting. For instance, the patient may not realistically have a choice of treatment, but he or she may be able to decide when it occurs.

For the most part, goals set by the social worker and client are measurable in terms of changes in the patient's behavior and feelings toward him or herself, his or her disability, and his or her rehabilitation program. As the patient begins to be able to assume more responsibility, he or she will become more active in setting goals within the social work relationship and within the program as a whole. Ideally, the patient will begin to demand what he or she wants from the social worker and assume the initiative in setting appropriate goals.

Many outside factors impinge on the kinds of goals that social worker and client can set. One obvious and consistent reality is the physical disability itself. Goals that do not account for the limitations of the disability cannot be set. Another critical factor is that the accomplishment of certain goals may be limited by the structure of the institution, the plans of another staff person, or a patient's family or significant others. The lack of resources within the community or within the institution may also alter the ability to accomplish certain goals.

In addition, the goals jointly established by the patient, rehabilitation team, and support system need to be evaluated by, and compatible with, the goals of the insurance company. In Jeff V's case, initial goals and anticipated length of stay were negotiated with the case manager the first week of admission. However, the role of the case manager was to continually monitor progress toward these goals and to continually certify the appropriateness of the level of care and length of stay.

Use of Contract

In working with Jeff, a written contract was never utilized. At Magee, written contracts have only been used in instances where behavioral issues are interfering with participation in the rehabilitation process. In these situations, contracts may be initiated to delineate expectations of both staff and patients. An oral contract was established with Jeff at the beginning of our relationship, which did define mutual expectations and goals. As the relationship progressed, our goals and expectations were redefined, but only on a verbal level.

Meeting Place

Within a physical rehabilitation setting, there are a wide range of meeting places. Choices include the social worker's office, the patient's room, therapy areas, the dining room, the patient lounge, or, at times, a place outside the institution. Each place selected by the social worker or the client reflects the intent of the meeting, the amount of control each can exert, and the opportunity available for an extended, intensive meeting. The most structured, formal, and private atmosphere is the social worker's office. Other meeting places are informal and generally unstructured. They do not promise privacy or uninterrupted time, but they do demonstrate an interest in the patient's daily activities. The informal areas tend to be regarded more as the patient's turf, and as a place where his or her control over the content and length of the interview is greater.

With Jeff, as with many of my younger patients, my style of working tends to include the very conscious use of meeting place as a dynamic in building a relationship and in sustaining certain aspects of it. In general, my feeling is that our young patients in particular are wary of a structured, formal setting in which they feel they have limited physical control. In fact, as with Jeff initially, they do have limited physical control and cannot independently remove themselves from a situation in which they do not wish to participate. Many of the younger patients also initially view a request to see a social worker or psychologist in his or her office as an indication that they now have an emotional as well as physical problem. Therefore, my initial meetings with Jeff were deliberately structured to occur on his turf and in as unthreatening an atmosphere as possible. These meetings occurred in either occupational therapy, physical therapy, or his room. Since my intention was to build a relationship with Jeff through an interest in his activities and his adaptation to the center, the meetings were frequent and deliberately brief. Little pressure was put on him to discuss his feelings. Instead, we discussed his current activities in the center, and I answered any specific questions he had regarding his program, passes from the center, etc. Once we had established a relationship, our meeting in the more formal atmosphere of my office was not threatening to him. Eventually, he reached the point where he set the meeting place. His choice was generally acceptable to me unless my goals for our meeting together differed from his. If so, we negotiated; but these negotiations were really about the purpose of our getting together at that time, and not the place itself.

If a patient has an especially difficult time forming a relationship and yet clearly has a need for it, several other alternatives are helpful in reducing the threat. Patients often participate in a structured, therapeutic, recreational program, both within and outside the center. Activities within the center may include volleyball, bingo, and parties; trips outside can be to baseball games, restaurants, concerts, etc. Accompanying a patient on such a trip is often a useful dynamic in establishing a relationship when other efforts have failed. This meeting place is the least threatening, affords patient and social worker the opportunity to share a common experience, and provides a beginning with which to explore the patient's feelings about participating in an activity from a wheelchair, perhaps for the first time.

Use of Time

In a physical rehabilitation setting, time is controlled by the relationship and by outside factors. The frequency and duration of interviews can generally be set by patient and social worker. As needs of patients tend to vary during the inpatient phase, the frequency and duration of meetings is continually renegotiated. While general points of high stress for the patient can be identified—for example, admission, discharge, first visit home, or goal-setting meetings with physician and staff—patients have their own patterns. Some do not really face their disability until after discharge, while others seem to be hit hardest upon admission. No typical pattern exists, nor does the timing of the point of greatest impact of the disability bear any real relationship to the eventual ability to cope. Therefore, the timing of interviews parallels the needs of the individual patient, his or her ability to cope, and his or her participation in treatment and in life outside the center.

The crucial factor in determining the relationship period is the patient's length of stay in the center. Discharge is determined primarily by the attainment of physical goals. This may dictate a premature ending to the relationship. Within reason, the length of stay can be extended for social or emotional causes, but certainly not for any prolonged period. The opportunity for continued patient/social worker contact after discharge is limited because of lack of transportation for the patient and lack of time to make home visits on the part of the social worker. Thus, the time period during which the relationship occurs is only minimally controllable by the patient or the social worker.

Interventions

Within the general practice framework, a social worker will assume multiple roles with patient/family, rehabilitation team, payer, and outside resources. The role definitions frequently include (1) counselor/sounding board, (2) teacher, (3) advocate, (4) consultant, (5) resource specialist, (6) arbitrator/negotiator, and (7) case manager. In practice, these roles are intertwined and an experienced social worker will fulfill multiple roles within a single encounter.

Counselor/sounding board is an obvious social work function with patient/family, but assumes equal importance at times with the rehabilitation team or insurance case manager. Particularly in working with adolescents, professional staff are frequently frustrated and concerned regarding episodes of noncompliance, acting-out behavior, reticence in revealing feelings, objectively poor choices in relation to treatment regimes or future goals, or seeming lack of motivation. In many of these critical incidents, the behaviors are simply age appropriate, particularly within the context of prior lifestyle and the struggle to cope with a life altering disability. In addition to providing an outlet for the expression of frustration, the social worker often assumes a consulting role with staff regarding the dynamics of the situation. Staff may momentarily forget that the patient is only 17, has a right to make choices, and may be only struggling to control his or her environment. Families may also need the same reassurance as adolescent sons or daughters exhibit the same behaviors that frustrated their families prior to onset.

At times within this same framework, the social worker may assume a strong advocacy role with the team in asserting the patients' rights to make certain choices, even with the realization that other responsibilities and consequences may derive from those choices. In cases of persistent or extreme acting-out behaviors, the social worker may function as the negotiator/arbitrator with the patient and team in redefining the boundaries of acceptable conduct and responsible behavior. Perhaps the staff can be more flexible, the patient more compliant. The role of advocate may also be assumed in negotiating with a managed care case manager or with a community resource in securing resources or services that do not conform to standard policies. For patient/family, staff, and insurer, the social worker is the individual who functions as the case manager, organizing the system and the resources to accomplish the defined goals and the discharge plan. The social worker is the point of contact for the coordination and synthesis of all the elements of the process. The social worker is the specialist regarding available resources and guides patient/family, and sometimes case manager, through application and approval processes. Perhaps the least articulated role of social worker is that of teacher. Continually throughout the process, the social worker imparts knowledge of the rehabilitation process, of resources, and of strategies in coping with disability. To the extent possible, the social worker teaches patient and/or family those skills necessary to ultimately function as their own advocate/case manager. In daily practice, the social worker is rarely aware of the assumption of multiple roles and moves easily within a single encounter from one role to another. However, only in the synthesis of these multiple roles does the social worker offer the full range of his or her expertise.

Stance of the Social Worker

From my experience, I have drawn three conclusions that affect my stance as a social worker. The first concerns a prominent treatment theory. Many articles in the literature adhere to a stage theory of adjustment to disability, which identifies shock, denial, depression, anger, and then acceptance as the phases of disabled patients' attitudes (Cook, 1979; Hohmann, 1975; Kerr, and Thompson, 1972; Siller, 1969). In my experience, this theory has not been a useful construct. One can rarely discover distinct sequential stages; patients do not seem to follow consistent patterns; and in fact, adjustment or acceptance, as traditionally defined, may not be a realistic or desirable goal. A given patient may definitively state that he or she will never accept his or her disability. There is no need for a total acceptance. An individual must and does learn to live in spite of or with the disability, but probably never loses the hope that one day he or she will be able to return to normalcy. Thus, the professional whose goal for the client is to hear him or her say "I know I will never walk again and I accept that as a fact" will in most cases never attain his or her treatment goal. The patient may in fact say "if I don't walk again" or "until I am able to walk," but those statements continue to imply hope that some day life will be different. In my opinion, that hope itself may be the essential thread allowing the patient to continue to go on living with or in spite of the disability. In general, the "markers" of the patient's feelings about him or herself as disabled are revealed through adaptive or nonadaptive behaviors and rarely through actual words.

A second strong belief of mine is that understanding the intrapsychic process may, for many patients, be a less important treatment goal, in the long run, than the need to maximally manipulate the environment in order to allow the disabled person to resume as much of his or her previous lifestyle as is possible. Depression may be more directly related to a patient's total physical dependence on a family member or inability to return to work and provide for family than to the actual fact of the patient's disability (Judd, Burrows, and Braun, 1986). Providing attendant care to help relieve a patient's feeling that he or she is a burden to family, and reducing architectural and attitudinal barriers within the employment market may be far more appropriate treatment goals than the intrapsychic exploration of the patient's depression.

Third, the early attitudes of the able-bodied persons with whom a newly disabled individual comes in contact are crucial (Woodrich and Patterson, 1983). For most patients, the most consistently encountered able-bodied persons are close family members and hospital and rehabilitation personnel. Their attitudes are critical in beginning to help the individual form good initial opinions about him or herself as a disabled person. The individual needs to know that with the exception of now needing physical care, he or she is the same person as before and should be treated the same way to the extent possible. The adolescent, in particular, needs to know that previously unacceptable behaviors are still unacceptable. The newly disabled person must assume responsibility for making decisions regarding his or her own life and for the consequences of those decisions.

Obviously, an individual brings to his or her disability the same problems and uses the same coping mechanisms that he or she had prior to the onset of the disability. For many, the support, understanding, acceptance, and willingness of the social worker to be with him or her and to believe in his or her continuing value and capabilities as a human being are key elements in the helping relationship. For other patients, a total behavior modification approach is needed to help them change maladaptive, destructive forms of behavior. A psychoanalytic approach may be the treatment of choice for still others. For many, a combination of modalities will be needed at different times during the rehabilitation (Trieschmann, 1978).

The ability to cope with a severe disability develops over time, and intervention strategies must be employed with an acute sensitivity to this fact. The period a patient actually spends in the inpatient phase of rehabilitation is only a small beginning in learning to live with a disability. In fact, many patients say they did not begin really to deal with their disability until after they were discharged (Richards, 1986). The key decisions about modality are made according to the goals of the relationship and the assessment of the patient's ability to assume greater responsibility. In the very early stages following the onset of disability, the social worker will usually assume a more supportive role, accept some of the responsibility for certain decisions, and tolerate an expected level of maladaptive behavior. The role of the social worker changes, however, as the patient assumes more responsibility. If needed, confrontation is used to help the patient examine behaviors and attitudes.

Peer group therapy is frequently used because the peer group is a critical source of support in a physical rehabilitation center. With formal groups, usually an integral part of the services offered, peer relationships can sometimes be influential. This is important because peer influences are ever present and may be most crucial in determining a patient's attitudes. The status of each patient in the peer group and the impact of the group values on the goals of the individual patient also provide significant information to the social worker.

An individual with a disability must develop the behavioral skills necessary to survive in a society that will be generally hostile to him or her. He or she has to learn to manipulate his or her environment constructively and assertively. For these reasons, assertiveness is taught at Magee. It is a critical component in dealing successfully with different people and systems with which the disabled individual will now be forced to interact. For example, the individual may need to develop the skills to hire, supervise, and fire, if attendant care is to be a routine part of his or her life. The individual must also know how to handle agencies such as social security and insurance companies.

Use of Outside Resources

The provision of concrete services is obviously essential in a rehabilitation setting, as there are a myriad of services that need to be in place prior to a patient's discharge. In general, who assumes responsibility for obtaining needed services is determined by the goals of the relationship. Ultimately, the patient must be able on his or her own to secure services or, if not physically capable, to instruct another person in what must be done. At what point the patient is ready to begin to assume this responsibility is a professional decision. The sheer number of tasks to be accomplished often necessitates a sharing of responsibility by the patient and the social worker. The patient, however, ultimately needs to know exactly how to obtain needed services and what to do if services are not provided. This skill may be only partially or minimally acquired during the inpatient phase of rehabilitation, but eventually the responsibility must be totally assumed by either the patient or a family member. Ideally, the patient will assume the responsibility for knowing the resources available and how to obtain them, even if he or she remains physically incapable of securing them him or herself.

Within a physical rehabilitation setting, the choice of outside resources will be dictated by the needs of patient/family, the discharge plan and in the era of managed care, to some extent, by the managed care provider. Some resources are fairly standardly employed, such as home health services and durable medical equipment. Social security, in the application for SSI or SSDI benefits, is a frequent referral source. Schools and job sites may be important resources in enabling the individual to resume a predisability lifestyle. Attendant care and accessible housing may be critical to a patient's safe discharge. Transportation resources are essential to ensure the individual mobility within the community. Architects and contractors may become involved with the rehabilitation team in designing accessibility modifications within the individual's home environment. Recreational resources, such as accessible swimming pools and wheelchair sports teams, may be significant in resuming an active lifestyle. In general, the entire range of community resources within the individual's own community need to be made accessible in order to afford the greatest opportunity for the resumption of an independent lifestyle.

Reassessment

Reassessment occurs continually within the relationship and is defined by either the social worker or the patient at different times. In general, in a rehabilitation setting, times for reassessment are not preset but occur at natural intervals as a dynamic part of the relationship itself. The most crucial reassessment occurs at the point of discharge from the center. The time spent in anticipation of eventual discharge is a period of high anxiety for the patient and family, and a reassessment of the relationship, goals, and plans for a continuing relationship, if any, occurs repeatedly as discharge becomes imminent.

Transfer or Termination

While planned transfers do occur within a physical rehabilitation setting, the most common causes of termination are external to the relationship and sometimes unplanned by either the social worker or the patient. For example, the most abrupt, disruptive termination during the rehabilitation phase occurs if the patient develops an acute medical problem and is transferred back to a general hospital. The patient may be readmitted later, depending on his or her medical status, but for the acute period, the relationship has been terminated and it is difficult to anticipate when it will be reestablished. Rarely does the social worker contact the patient in a general hospital except perhaps occasionally by telephone. A referral may be made to the social worker in the acute care hospital, but the opportunity for a planned, organized transfer does not exist.

Discharge from the rehabilitation center to return home is a less abrupt, more planned termination; however, it too is usually determined by factors external to the social worker/patient relationship. Plans are often made for continuing the relationship after discharge, but the structure and the frequency of contact will probably be quite different. This type of termination serves as a dynamic to move the relationship to another level.

Outcome measures in rehabilitation are not fully developed and in general relate only to lengths of stay, cost, and physical parameters of function. While of some value, these measures do not address the myriad social and psychological issues related to actual resumption of lifestyle. Knowing that an individual is independent in dressing at discharge and maintains this functional level three months post-discharge, does not address the more crucial issue of the individual's involvement in meaningful activities once he or she is dressed. Magee is a member of Uniform Data System (UDS) for Medical Rehabilitation, a system for measuring outcome in rehabilitation. UDS is a voluntary membership organization, with a current enrollment of approximately 430 rehabilitation units and hospitals. Some 18 different items are scored on a functional independence measure scale (FIM scale) to determine an individual's level of independence at admission to rehabilitation, discharge from rehabilitation, and at 80 to 180 days following discharge. Quarterly reports are produced, which compare Magee's FIM scores with other regional and national data. Data are also generated on cost, so comparisons can be made between FIM change and cost of care. The data are used by the clinical teams to evaluate efficiencies and outcomes within our system and to then alter treatment protocols. While the system does provide some essential evaluative data, the measures are limited by the exclusion of lifestyle or satisfaction parameters.

Case Conclusion

Jeff remained as an inpatient at Magee for approximately two months. Initially, he had some difficulty entering into a relationship with any "shrink type" because he did not see any need for such a relationship. However, the use of the informal, frequent contacts described earlier did eventually allow him to acknowledge some of his own need to talk about his feelings and to look at what had happened to him, what was happening in rehabilitation, and what would happen in the future. We were probably three weeks into the relationship before he was willing to come to my office.

Jeff eventually reached the point where he set the times and the structure of the interviews. As he began to feel the need, he came quite regularly to appointments. His major concerns revolved around relationships with his family and friends and the formulation of his own plans for discharge. Eventually he began to assume a greater sense of responsibility for his own care and his plans for the future. His plan was to go directly from the rehabilitation facility to his own apartment. This plan, while not entirely unrealistic, was certainly not ideal and required the creative coordination of numerous resources to be safe. In addition, his family, the managed care case manager, and many of the staff were opposed to the plan. In order to advocate for Jeff in pursuing his goal, I needed to work with Jeff to process and problem-solve many issues, and I needed to decide if I could realistically support his plan for independence. We decided to try to accomplish his goal and made an outline of all the resources that needed to be in place within the time frame of his anticipated discharge. We divided the tasks between us and during this time touched base almost daily to report progress. This process of working together also provided me with valuable data regarding his resourcefulness, creativity, problem-solving ability, and understanding of and ability to cope with the limitations of his disability. His tasks primarily included finding an apartment that would accept Section 8 certification, identifying friends/family to be trained as attendants, and negotiating financial assistance from his family until SSI benefits were received and Section 8 certification approved. My tasks were to advocate with the case manager, his family, and the team regarding his right to pursue this plan and the feasibility of the plan if all resources were in place. I also pursued numerous referrals for home health care, transportation, SSI, Section 8 housing, and attendant care programs. Teaching was scheduled with his identified family and friends, and eventually I visited his prospective apartment to evaluate accessibility.

Throughout this time, frequent negotiation occurred with the managed care provider regarding certification for his continuing length of stay. While he was continuing to show physical gains in his rehabilitation, the case manager continually evaluated progress and goals as related to the cost of care. These continuous negotiations provided an additional source of stress for Jeff and for me, as we were both aware that funding for a continued rehabilitation stay could be terminated before all our plans were in place. Should this have occurred, Jeff might have been discharged on an interim basis to his parents' home or elsewhere. In addition, the managed care provider had to approve necessary equipment prior to discharge. Fortunately, we were aware at admission that Jeff's coverage for medical equipment was limited and that he had no prescription or software benefits and had immediately completed the Medical Assistance and SSI applications. These additional resources could also provide some cushion if his HMO terminated benefits before all discharge plans were in place. Finally, with the necessary resources in place, Jeff's plan for discharge to his own apartment appeared feasible.

By the date of discharge, Jeff was capable of managing all of his self-care with only minimal assistance. For instance, when dressing he required help only with his shoes and socks and in starting his pants over his feet. With assistance, he was able to transfer from the bed to his wheelchair. He also required assistance with bowel and bladder care. In short, Jeff could manage independently with perhaps three hours of care during each day (two hours in getting up in the morning and one hour in the evening in going to bed). Once he was dressed and in his wheelchair, he appeared exactly as any 19-year-old man might and was capable of going by himself wherever he wanted to go, as long as he was not confronted with steps. The attendants did have to be available at the times he required specific care. His alternative, of course, was to attempt to find someone else to give him a hand, and in fact he often had to telephone friends, his brother, or others. To cover him and provide safety during nighttime hours, we established an accessible telephone system and network of people whom he could call for assistance.

At the time of his discharge, Jeff felt fairly optimistic about his eventual ability to survive and to gradually rebuild his life. The amount of difficulty he would encounter in the process seemed to me to depend heavily on the physical and emotional support system that he had to create (Goldiamond, 1973). His potential support system existed in four major areas: his family; the rehabilitation center; his friends; and the formal support system, that is, the community resources network we had created. In addition, Magee planned for Jeff to return once a week to participate in a spinal cord injury group, see the physician, and receive the general support of the center. At one time or another, each of these support systems failed and occasionally all systems failed simultaneously.

Jeff essentially rejected two potential support systems; his family and the rehabilitation center. Shortly after discharge, he communicated to his parents in particular, but also to his brother, very specific guidelines for their involvement in his life. He made it clear that they were not welcome at his home on any regular basis, and if they appeared, he made his displeasure very clear. Eventually, his family stopped trying to impose their presence on him to offer assistance. Following discharge, Jeff returned to Magee once a week for only about a month, although he maintained close contact by telephone with some staff, including the social worker, for about three months. His primary contact after that period occurred only when he was in a crisis, but even then he rejected coming to the center to talk. The opportunity to go to his home was extremely limited because of distance and because the hospital's defined mission does not include the provision of long-term, intensive counseling services.

The other two support systems, friends and formal network, were intermittent in their support. His friends were not always able to provide the services required, although several demonstrated considerable sensitivity and maturity during extreme crisis. The formal support system, in general, provided the services as originally requested; however, there were times when services were not available and Jeff needed to assume a strong advocacy role. On other occasions, the services were not flexible enough to alter hours of service provision during periods of crisis. The times of major crisis for Jeff occurred when all support systems failed simultaneously or began to impose greater demands than he was able to meet. Since the four systems were separate and uncoordinated, the possibility of all pulling back simultaneously or of making parallel demands on him was increased.

The period since his discharge has been extremely onerous for Jeff and for those of us even peripherally involved. It has been difficult at times to continue to support his need to manage on his own and to direct his own life. His friends were not always responsible as attendants, but although he did not always receive needed care, he has, in fact, remained relatively free of severe medical complications. He was given an eviction notice because of several late night, noisy parties, but he has gone to court on several occasions to appeal the eviction and so far remains in his apartment. On one occasion, he attempted suicide, precipitated, at least in part, by the rejection of a girlfriend (Seligman, 1975). However, he now has a van and is beginning to make plans to attend a community college. Obviously, he has matured considerably throughout this experience. He chose a very difficult route for himself and had to fight to be supported in that choice. He demonstrated the basic survival skills, however, so the plan had a chance of working.

Differential Discussion

The experience of Jeff is illustrative of several key points in the health care and social services system. Particularly for individuals with chronic illness or severe disability, the health care system must be integrated with a system for social and psychological intervention. Within the new health care climate, with more emphasis placed on cost containment, many health care providers are eliminating or limiting the social/psychological component as too expensive or as only providing value-added services. The roots of medical social work are in the linkage of the relationship between health, environment, and social supports. Failure to recognize the relationship between these elements will result in a decrease in the health status of individuals in the community, particularly among the most vulnerable populations, that is, groups such as the elderly, chronically ill, disabled, or at-risk infants. While Jeff did not experience significant medical crisis, he certainly was at high risk, particularly during times when the social systems failed.

In addition, health care today remains a largely fragmented system of disjointed resources. While the goal is to create coordinated systems to meet the health care needs of individuals over time, this goal has yet to be realized. While outpatient, home care, and community care are emphasized as the wave of the future, basic outpatient care remains poorly reimbursed, and coordinated; comprehensive outpatient care, particularly for high-risk populations, is nonexistent. Jeff had no safely net coordinated for him. He needed to assume responsibility for putting the pieces together, and if a piece failed or all failed simultaneously, there were no other resources.

Perhaps case management for at-risk populations will be the safety net of the future. However, the role of the case manager is not well-defined and generally nonreimbursable on the provider side. Even the emerging role definitions of case management contain contradictions. In most definitions, the case manager serves a gatekeeper function to ensure efficient utilization of resources for cost containment. On the other hand, most definitions also encompass advocacy as a role of the case manager. Inherent within these two roles is the possibility of conflict and ethical dilemmas when confronted with individual patient need. The case manager has the potential and the responsibility to coordinate a system of care, but for a long-term, at-risk population, how long does this responsibility last? On the payer side, the responsibility may last as long as the individual is entitled to benefits. However, expiration of benefits may bear no relationship to individual need for such coordination. On the provider side, the responsibility for case management could be based on individual need, but as an unreimbursed service, this is unlikely to occur. As case management continues to grow as a practice model, concerns for social and environmental aspects will, hopefully, be integrated into the definitions of health care.

If confronted in the future with the dilemma of supporting and advocating for a 19-year-old, newly disabled individual living independently in the community, I would probably make the same choice. However, I would be more cognizant of the inherent system failures and do more problem solving regarding potential safety nets. I would probably also define with the individual a more definitive active role for myself as one of the potential safety nets.

The field of physical rehabilitation, as all of health care, needs to work together with the community to create a system of care that addresses the needs of individuals in the community. Hospitals-without-walls can be created and can be cost effective as well as responsive to human needs. Perhaps an eventual partnership of health care and the insurance industry can create such a system, even in the absence of clear national policy or model.

REFERENCES

Amendments to the Rehabilitation Act of 1973. (1978.). Title VII, Part B, P. L. 95-102.

Athelstan, G. T. (1978). Psychological, sexual, social, and vocational aspects of spinal cord injury: A selected bibliography. *Rehabilitation Psychology, XXV*(1), 16-28.

Cook, D. (1979). Psychological adjustment to spinal cord injury: Incidence of denial, depression, and anxiety. *Rehabilitation Psychology, 26*, 97-104.

Crewe, N. M., Athelstan, G. T., and Krumberger, J. (1979). Spinal cord injury: A comparison of pre-injury and post-injury marriages. *Archives of Physical Medicine and Rehabilitation, LX*, 252-256.

David, A., Gur, S., and Rozin, R. (1977-1978). Survival in marriage in the paraplegic couple: Psychological study. *Paraplegia, XV*, 198-201.

Goldiamond, I. (1973). A diary of self-modification. *Psychology Today, I*, 95-102.

Hohmann, G. (1975). Psychological aspects of treatment and rehabilitation of the spinal cord injured person. *Clinical Orthopedics, CXII*, 81-86.

Judd, F. K., Burrows, G. D., and Brown, D. J. (1986). Depression following acute spinal cord injury. *Paraplegia, 24*, 358-363.

Keigher, S. (1995). Managed care's silent seduction of America and the new politics of choice. *Health and Social Work, 20*(2), 146-151.

Kerr, W. and Thompson, M. (1972). Acceptance of disability of sudden onset in paraplegia. *International Journal of Paraplegia, 10*, 94-102.

Lane, H. J. (1975). Working with problems of assault to self-image and life style. *Social Work in Health Care, 1*(2), 191-198.

Orbaan, I. J. C. (1986). Psychological adjustment problems in people with traumatic spinal cord lesions. *Acta Neurochirurgica, 79*, 58-61.

Rabin, B. J. (1980). *The sensuous wheeler: Sexual adjustment for the spinal cord injured.* San Francisco, CA: Multi Media Resource Center.

Richards, J. S. (1986). Psychologic adjustment to spinal cord injury during first postdischarge year. *Archives of Physical Medicine and Rehabilitation, 67,* 362-365.

Seligman, M. (1975). *Helplessness: On depression, development, and death.* San Francisco, CA: Freeman.

Siller, J. (1969). Psychological situation of disabled with spinal cord injuries. *Rehabilitation Literature, 30,* 290-296.

Standards Manual for Organizations Serving People with Disabilities. (1987). Commission on Accreditation of Rehabilitation Facilities, *37,* 47-50.

Trieschmann, R. B. (1978). *The psychological, social, and vocational adjustment to spinal cord injury: A strategy for future research.* Washington, DC: Rehabilitation Services Administration Publication.

Wheeler, D. (1977). Emotional reactions of patients, family and staff in acute care of spinal cord injury. *Social Work in Health Care, 2*(4), 369-378.

Woodrich, F. and Patterson, J. B. (1983, July/August/September). Variables related to acceptance of disability in persons with spinal cord injuries. *Journal of Rehabilitation.*

Zola, I. D. (1981). Communication barriers between able-bodied and the handicapped. *Archives of Physical Medicine and Rehabilitation, 62,* 355-359.

Chapter 17

Mutual Help Group
for Emphysema Patients:
Veterans Administration Medical Center

Zelda Foster
Toba Schwaber Kerson

CONTEXT

Description of the Setting

The program for emphysema patients began at the Brooklyn Veterans Administration (VA) Medical Center in 1966. The medical center, a three-site facility, offers veterans a variety of services, including medicine, surgery, neurology, rehabilitation, and psychiatry for the treatment of acute illness. In addition, the center operates a 420-bed extended care facility at a second location and a large outpatient ambulatory care center at a third location. Medical treatment is offered by full-time physicians, interns, and residents. The interns and residents select the hospital for training in a particular specialty and remain for limited periods of time. There are also extensive programs in social work, nursing, dietetics, psychology, and speech pathology.

The Veterans Administration medical centers and ambulatory care clinics serve veterans with honorable discharges. Eligibility requirements are based on a priority system: service-connected veterans, veterans exposed to Agent Orange, prisoners of war, and World War I veterans are highest; lower priority is given to nonservice-connected veterans with other VA pensions or who meet the established income criteria. More than 40 percent of the priority target group of service-related and low-income veterans use the VA for care. If the veteran's income is over an established amount, a copayment is required to receive services. Space availability determines whether lower-priority veterans are accepted for treatment. Currently, the Veterans Administration is billing private health insurers for nonservice connected patients who are accepted for treatment and have coverage.

The veterans population is aging, and increasing numbers are facing chronic and debilitating illness. Some veterans choose care at a VA hospital because they are not covered by private medical insurance and therefore cannot afford care in other facilities. Outpatient services tend to be narrowly defined, limiting the availability of comprehensive long-term care. Other significant programs offered by the Veterans Administration are domiciliaries, nursing homes, contract nursing homes, VA-operated hospital-based home care programs, and adult day health-care centers. Respite, hospice care, and geriatric evaluation units are offered in some VA facilities.

Initially, in the emphysema program, patients previously assigned to various medical units were instead placed on one unit overseen by a physician specializing in respiratory care and a social worker assigned to address psychosocial concerns (Loveland-Cook, Chediha, Schmidt, and Halloway, 1992). That organizational change provided a cohesive, unifying framework so that these patients were regarded as a group with common needs. Patients were generally hospitalized for treatment of acute episodes of respiratory distress. A team composed of nurses, a social worker, respiratory care therapists, and dietitians was asked to develop an initial plan of care. During a patient's admission or readmission, the social worker engaged the patient in a mutual-help group that defined and addressed psychosocial concerns. The same patients were seen in the emphysema outpatient clinic for follow-up care. This format changed in 1980 when inpatients were dispersed on various units, with the outpatient clinic becoming the major structure for unifying this population. This affected programming and meant that specialized psychosocial services were more often available in ambulatory care.

Policy

Veterans Administration

"If any man shall be sent forth as a soldier and shall return maimed, he shall be maintained competently by the colony during his life," proclaimed the Plymouth Colony pilgrims in 1636 (Becerra and Damron-Rodriguez, 1995). Thus, some form of assistance to veterans has always been present in the United States. Medical facilities for veterans were first established in 1811. Such care was legislated when Congress passed an act for the relief of sick and disabled seamen in 1878, establishing the first merchant marine hospitals that formed the basis for the Public Health Service (Mather and Abel, 1986).

At the present time, veterans are entitled to a vast array of services including health and compensation, education, loan, insurance, pension, and burial benefits, including some for specified survivors and dependents (United States Department of Veterans Affairs, 1996). Because of its missions, vastness, experience, and history, the VA will play many important roles in the reorganization of health care delivery in the United States (Burgess and Stefos, 1991; Demakis et al., 1990; Fisher and Welsh, 1995; Hollingsworth and Bondy, 1990; Holsinger, 1991; Pittman, 1995; Zemberlan, 1990). It is said that it has many assets and liabilities. Among its assets are the development of rehabilitation and long-term care which are two services that are extremely relevant to the general population; its extraordinary contribution to medical education; its research findings and capabilities, which have pioneered efforts in dialysis, liver transplantation, cardiac pacemakers, and radioisotopes; and its special preparation for dealing with national emergencies and helping to manage consequent casualties. Among its liabilities are said to be the lack of clarity about the VA's clinical mission; its very difficult patient population, which includes some of the nation's sickest patients; and a highly centralized, structured and inflexible administration (Fisher and Welsh, 1995). The VA will be different in coming years, but its importance to veterans, their families, and to the U.S. health delivery system will not be diminished.

Policies in Relation to the Mutual Help Group

Policies that support a comprehensive, coordinated approach to patient care grow out of competing priorities, strains between forces, and ambivalent commitments and convictions. Many of the policies and struggles affecting this particular population can be traced to unresolved issues and practices affecting the nature of medical care in the United States. Other policies have more local origins. Interactions between local and larger systems and spheres of influence have affected the growth, course, and survival of the program. A number of policy issues are relevant in tracing the direction that the mutual help group for emphysema patients took, the way it changed, and the ways it survived. For example, the management of long-term chronic illness is, generally, of less interest to physicians except at the times when the illness has a dramatic manifestation. Ongoing manifestations may become less dramatic, less interesting, and, in fact, may stigmatize and demean the patient in the eyes of others. Patients with emphysema require help with long-term management. There are no marvelous cures or advanced technology. Although there are professionals interested in this population, in our cure-oriented system, the resources available and the organization of health care services tend to devalue their contribution.

Most hospitals have an enormous stake in physician training. The nature of this training emphasizes the treatment of singular disease entities with explicit knowledge regarding pathology, specific organicity, and treatment methods. When the needs of patients conflict with currently defined medical training needs, training often takes precedence. Medical training in the treatment of chronic disease is seen as having little desirability. Still, training in disease management supplants training in helping patients to manage complicated physical and psychosocial aspects of illness. This may change as control of the system shifts to managed care entities who are not willing to pay for training. At this time, hospitals tend to restrict programs geared to long-term and continuous care. Health professionals whose role is to meet the needs of these patients are viewed as ancillary. That these health professions have not had enough of a voice in policy development and may not have fought forcefully enough for their imperatives is worth considering as one possible obstacle to policy change. As a result of the federal government's recent emphasis on training for general as opposed to specialty practice, we should see less fragmented training and more generalists capable of treating multiple kinds of illnesses. However, even now, training tends to remain disease-oriented rather than people-oriented.

Self-help and mutual-help groups grow out of consumerism, patient education, and the capacity of patients to help one another. The role of the professional in these groups can be central or peripheral, depending on the purpose, formation, and auspices of the group (Gitterman and Schulman, 1994; Shulman, 1992; Stempler and Glass, 1996). The availability of professionals with an investment in such a group depends on the support, resources, and conceptual orientation of the institution and the disciplines the professionals represent. Each discipline's priorities and concerns with status also affect who gets service, in what form, and for how long. How well the interdisciplinary teams carve out common goals, share in decision making, and invest in each other's contributions depends on complex issues of power, professional competitiveness, territorialism, and institutional sanction (Smith, 1995).

For the VA's emphysema patients, who at the inception of the program were for the most part poor, chronically ill, mainly in their fifties, and employed marginally if at all, the establishment of a special unit represented a marked shift in care. One primary physician and a stable staff knew them intimately. Their breathing and functioning difficulties were acknowledged empathically and viewed as treatable. This hope, consistency of care, and recognition enlisted patients as active participants in their own care. Staff and patients saw the patients as people who had common needs, could help one another, and could collectively participate in and influence their treatment. Patients who were passive, felt victimized, and found dependency comforting were both nurtured and challenged to participate in their own care.

This orientation brought institutional practices into question. Physicians had mixed feelings about how much to encourage patients to raise questions about their illness and treatment. Some nurses were not geared toward patients assuming more self-care. Helping patients to express feelings of anger was threatening to some staff. The patients' eventual interest in promoting day treatment, having a 24-hour respiratory center, seeking ways to bypass admission procedures when in need of hospitalization, and insisting on aftercare from physicians who know them, ran counter to current institutional practices. However, the patients had several successes; they procured clinic care and a small respiratory care center and often were admitted directly to the hospital through the respiratory care physician's intervention. Through their inpatient and outpatient groups, they helped one another to have more say in their own care, assume more responsibility for what happened to them, and become more knowledgeable about their disease.

Although local policy constraints were overcome, more far-reaching health policies continue to constrain practice. Cost-containment policies are shrinking resources available to patients with these kinds of needs. The patients need a 24-hour respiratory care center and day hospital treatment where a consistent staff is attuned to them. Home care services are needed to provide for patients too ill to be transported back and forth to the hospital and who do not have the full and daily help required to keep them stable and comfortable. Emphysema patients now have access to a hospital-based home care program and an adult day health care program. When good preventive and palliative services are not offered, hospitalization becomes a recourse.

As the emphysema program continued, the population served included many of the same patients. The inpatient group became less purposeful, but the outpatient group has continued for many years. More recently, a weekly service for severely disabled emphysema outpatients was instituted, in which patients see the respiratory team physician, nurse, respiratory therapist, and social worker. Each patient comes to the weekly clinic and also joins the group session led by the social worker. The physician and nurse also participate in the group sessions when indicated. This kind of clinic, group, and staffing represents the interests and commitment of specific health care professionals rather than institutional policy and backing. Therefore, it risks discontinuance if the interested professionals leave, the hospital pulls out its already limited resources, or priorities are changed by competing forces. A program that is not in the mainstream risks losing its voice when resources shrink. Questions are raised regarding whether a program is critical, the potential for cure, and its value for physician training. The issue becomes whether we can afford to care for and maintain chronic patients requiring long-term care with minimal potential for recovery or productivity. Similar issues emerge from the hospice movement in regard to the humanistic concerns of offering treatment that is noncure-oriented and that has lesser value in more aggressively oriented medical circles. The difference, of course, is that mandated hospices are to provide service for only the last six months of a patient's life, while living with a chronic illness can last a lifetime.

Reimbursement models further affect care. Payment based on diagnostic-related groupings has resulted in shorter and less frequent hospitalizations. Social workers in hospitals are most often in the role of short-term planners rather than providers of ongoing services. Establishing the appropriate level of care and moving patients along the continuum has value and certainly meets an agreed-upon institutional purpose, but case management and comprehensive treatment services are better ways to provide services to those who are chronically ill and are necessarily large consumers of services (Holle, Rick, Sleifert, and Stephens, 1995). Preventing further erosions of health by maintaining and improving levels of functioning is not yet viewed as offering long-term economic and well-being benefits. Cost containment can be a desirable aim; but one must question shortsighted models of care and payment, which diminish the access to and availability of long-term care and treatment.

Technology

Emphysema is a form of damage to the lungs, in which some of the walls of the lung's air sacs have broken down, trapping stale air in them. Exhaling air puts a squeezing pressure on the air passages. If these are weakened, they may close up and trap more air. The damaged parts of the lungs cannot take the oxygen, which the body needs, out of the fresh air, and they cannot get rid of carbon dioxide by passing it from the blood into the air. Emphysema is generally irreversible, with increasing disability in pulmonary capacity. Relief obtained from medication, breathing apparatus, and respiratory care does not change the course of the disease, which varies in intensity from patient to patient (Kerson, 1985). The roles of pollution, climate, and stress in reducing the effect and the progress of the disease are considerations taken into account when treating it. Smoking is a definite prohibition, and obesity is a handicap because of the increased strain on the lungs and heart.

When medically indicated, patients are admitted to the hospital and followed in the clinic. All receive medication and respiratory therapy and some attend a general monthly outpatient group (Clough et al., 1987; Toshima, Kaplan, and Ries, 1992; Kaplan et al., 1990; Weinbaum, Giles, and Krell, 1991). In addition, nine or ten patients with severe emphysema attend a weekly clinic and outpatient group. Both groups are led by the program social worker with considerable participation from the nurse and physician so that the patient has a framework of care in which to integrate medical treatment and his ability to cope with the illness. This vehicle also allows patients to communicate their needs directly to staff. This connection is not built into the structure of the general emphysema clinic or the monthly outpatient group, where services are offered in more separate and categorical ways. Over the years, the group has served education and social support needs, and its participants view it as a source of support, attention, and connection.

The weekly group has an ongoing agenda that focuses on how patients are coping with severe breathing limitations. It offers its members opportunities to exchange information, share experiences, and discuss upsetting incidents that may have precipitated respiratory crises. There is a social element as patients communicate with others with similar symptoms and concerns. Many of these patients lead isolated lives and feel prevented from participating in many social activities. The group allows for participation and conviviality (Lott, Blazey, and West, 1992). In both groups, the agenda is usually developed by the group. The social worker provides an impetus for the raising of more crucial issues and encourages the kind of group process that will result in a real exchange and sharing of feelings and experiences and a stake in giving help to and receiving it from others. The social worker acts as mediator, enabler, catalyst, and reflector. The aim is to help the group to work on real issues and to further their knowledge of the disease and their capacity to feel greater control and independence. It has been valuable to incorporate the views of other disciplines into this process so that there is a sense of unity, of shared purpose and goals.

Organization

The Brooklyn Veterans Administration Medical Center is one of 172 in the country. In addition, the VA health system has 365 outpatient, community, and outreach clinics; 128 nursing home care units and 37 domiciliaries; and the total system offers a wide spectrum of surgical, medical, and rehabilitative care. Approximately 1,000,000 patients are treated in VA hospitals each year, 79,000 are treated in nursing homes, and 25,000 in domiciliaries. For fiscal year 1995, the cost of the medical programs was $16.5 billion. The VA is affiliated with 105 medical schools and about 900 other schools, participates in the training of about 100,000 professionals each year, and has participated in the professional education of more than one-half of the practicing physicians in the United States (Alexander, 1992; Mirvis et al., 1994; United States Department of Veterans Affairs, 1995; United States Department of Veterans Affairs, 1994).

The VA employs 4,000 social workers, which makes it the largest employer of social workers in the United States. Social workers do discharge planning, case management and care coordination, psychosocial treatment, vocational and financial planning, community services coordination and development, patient education, and post-discharge planning. Social work services are provided to all inpatient and outpatient programs as well as to special programs for the homeless, aged, persons with AIDS, and Persian Gulf War veterans and their families. Social workers work as members of interdisciplinary teams and participate in research in multidisciplinary projects and specific social work research programs (Loveland-Cook et al., 1992). A relatively new emphasis on managed care or coordinated care for older veterans and their caregivers should also be of special help to the patient population, which comprises the "client" in this chapter.

Training approximately 750 to 800 students each year, the VA has the most comprehensive and largest clinical training program for social work students in the United States. As it has done from its beginnings, the VA continues its critical roles in training in health care, establishing standards for social work clinical practice, and determining the functions and roles of social workers working in interdisciplinary teams in the delivery of health care. At present, through a program supported by the Council on Social Work Education and the National Association of Social Workers, it has initiated a 42-site program to help social workers to document and evaluate interventions (United States Department of Veterans Affairs, 1993).

The emphysema clinics are part of the Department of Medicine. Other disciplines assign staff who offer patients a variety of services. The Social Work Department assigns one of its 60 social workers to the program.

Including its homeless outreach program, the department has 82 social workers. Social work has a special stake in this particular program and has offered staff at a somewhat higher ratio than it does on some other services. For the most part, emphysema patients are admitted to general medical wards. The physicians who specialize in the treatment of emphysema may act as consultants or request that the patient be followed on a small inpatient unit or a specialty chest clinic. Social Work Service has had to adapt its program for offering specialized psychosocial services to this population now dispersed on more general medical wards. Defining unique needs, identifying patients, and offering them a collective experience is harder to do.

The emphysema program currently has developed its own inner structure with several unique features. The physician most closely tied to the emphysema patients has carved out a sustained personal and caring role. Because it is personal and individualistic, it also is unstructured at times and reflective of the particular stresses on the one major person. Not tied at this time to the residency training program, the program allows patients ongoing care from the same primary physician. Yet, the potential for the patient to become overly taxed in offering this care clearly exists. The other disciplines assigned to the program share responsibility as colleagues in ways that are also based on preference and style. A more centralized and defined leadership pattern with clear goals and direction might allow for greater accountability and standardization.

DECISIONS ABOUT PRACTICE

Definition of the Client

The outpatient group has been seen from the beginning as the major unit of service. Although various patients and families were seen individually and/or as couples, the group is a focal point because of the social worker's conviction that the patients need and can help one another (Brown, 1991; Henry, 1992; Schopler and Galinsky, 1995). Many are dealing with similar adaptive tasks with a range of coping abilities. With skilled help, it was expected that patients could experience other ways of responding and then broaden the alternatives available to them. Several common patterns are evident. Many patients tend to globalize their problems and patterns of reaction. Subdividing and examining intervening and incremental responses are key areas of work for the group. Extreme anger, fear of anger, and feeling victimized are prevalent themes. These patterns are amenable to change in a group-oriented service. The group represents enough difference in personal style and emotional makeup to allow for the range of feelings and coping patterns needed for a solid and interesting group process. All patients are invited to the group, and they have varying degrees of commitment to the group and differing lengths of involvement. Several assume patient-volunteer status; they contribute to greeting and orienting new patients and participate in the teaching of diaphragmatic breathing.

Goals, Objectives, and Outcome Measures

Goals change and at times conflict during the course of the group's existence. Originally geared to offering patients help in dealing with the management of the illness, medical treatment, family and interpersonal relationships, the hospital system, and vocational concerns, the focus shifted at one point to social change issues (Shapiro, 1991). This posed a threat to the group, polarizing some who wanted to relate only to personal coping issues, and others who did not want to hear or share problems but to struggle for change in the delivery of hospital services. Even throughout this period, a common denominator was the role in helping patients look at typical response patterns and their tendency to feel helpless, overwhelming anger, and fear of reprisal. Patients learned to look at next steps, consider consequences, anticipate renewed efforts, and plan to further their own aims. It was essential to mediate between both factions in the group and to recognize the need for personal change and social action as an integrated process for people who have chronic illness and long-term dependencies on medical institutions.

An important goal is to encourage group members to develop more adequate communication and problem solving with other important people in their environments. Group members clearly develop better communication and problem-solving skills, and aspects of relationship building are enhanced. Health education has become increasingly valued by group members who actively seek more substantial information.

Use of Contract

Patients are identified as having the ongoing task of managing a chronic and stressful illness that affects every aspect of their lives. How they manage will determine to some extent the degree of their disability and the number of problematic respiratory episodes. The agreement is that in a group context they can share concerns, work on them in a mutual and reciprocal way, and identify together how each of them might cope with aspects of their illness with greater control and effectiveness. This broad promise of self-change and systems-change is broken down into specific issues that patients are grappling with in their day-to-day lives.

An important aspect of the agreement is the affirmation of the social worker as helper, mediator, and enabler. The ongoing contract is re-defined as the group process evolves so that it remains sharpened, mutu-ally agreed upon, and continually significant.

Meeting Place

The meeting place has shifted from year to year. The monthly group is now in a large assembly room, which feels too empty and anonymous. Its separateness from the place where medical treatment occurs creates a sense of isolation and disconnection. At the same time, it might be sup-porting increased independence. As staff assess recent problems in assur-ing the vitality of the group, one question is the effect of the meeting place on the group, and whether the separation in spirit and location from the clinic is dulling both purpose and ongoing work. On the other hand, the more intimate setting of the weekly group of more disabled and needy patients has contributed to greater group cohesion.

Use of Time

Most group meetings last approximately one and one-half hours. The patients move very slowly, making for longer beginnings and endings for each session. Although open to changing membership, the group has maintained some members for many years. This has led to questions of how valid and helpful a group with open-ended membership and open-ended duration is for this population (Schopler and Galinsky, 1990; Schopler and Galinsky, 1984). One problem associated with a long-term group is the tendency to slide into ritual and away from content. As this group is now being called upon to examine its very existence, differing stakes in continuity become apparent and must be discussed and resolved.

Interventions and the Stance of the Social Worker

The group approach is based on a mediating role for the social worker (Gitterman and Shulman, 1994). A strong systems orientation has led the social worker to view the group as a system designed to encourage mutual help, which interacts within itself and with other systems. This interactional approach assumes that the patients working together have real work to do in modifying their feelings, thinking, and actions. The social worker's primary concerns are a focus on the here-and-now and how the group process unfolds to permit and support a deepening of the work. The social worker is attuned to issues of commonality and specificity; to feelings and their ambivalence; to content and affect; and to challenging the group members to tune in, to speak, to hear, and to respond. The agenda and the work belong to the group, but the social worker is there as a catalyst, an integrator, and a reflector of the group process ready to encourage unspoken thoughts, to both narrow and deepen the content, to search for affect, and to offer respect and protection. In this sense, the social worker has a very active role.

Use of Outside Resources

Emphysema patients require a vast array of services from financial help to job counseling to changes in living arrangements. Although the Veterans Administration offers benefits counselors, social workers have the best knowledge of and access to state and city programs. The social worker helps patients consider all available options and enhances their ability to seek necessary assistance. How much the social worker directly intervenes depends on his or her judgment regarding the patient's and family's abilities to intervene on their own behalf, and how difficult it is to obtain a response from a particular agency or program. Patients require different degrees of help with concrete planning. Skill is crucial in helping the patient assert himself without either making him feel impotent or abandoning him to forces beyond his ability to manage.

Reassessment, and Transfer or Termination

Reassessment of the group is in process. As medical wards are more geared to general medical diagnoses, the specific identification of this population is more difficult. There is a need in the monthly group to reconnect the patient to his medical treatment to achieve a more dynamic interplay. We have not yet sufficiently focused on the newly diagnosed emphysema patient at the very beginning of what will be an ongoing, disabling process. As the program continued over the years, it emphasized perhaps too much the long-term patient or the very ill patient rather than the newly diagnosed one. The struggle over specific, time-limited, goal-oriented services continues as we feel pulled between the long-term, ongoing needs of patients and the demand on us to hone in on the critical issues with which we can be most effective. Various ongoing management issues will affect our practice as we are required more and more to address outcomes and goal achievement. The role of quality assurance programs and cost-containment pressures will increase, and we are increasingly compelled by our own profession and regulatory agencies to account for and document our work and audit outcomes (Tindill, al Assaf, and Gentling, 1993). As we look at beginnings, middles, and endings in our services to patients, we find that these definitions require a constant assuring of meaningful purpose and process. As reassessment takes place, termination will be a necessary outgrowth, if not for the group itself, perhaps for some members. Termination of the group will be based on how well it is serving a real and needed purpose, whether its purpose can change to meet changing needs, and whether its purpose meshes with agency goals and sanctions. For some patients, the process of the group may not meet their ongoing needs and, together, those patients and staff will have to consider what service might be offered, which would make sense for them. It will be a challenge to identify what is happening, what the remaining needs are, and how we can respond to them.

Differential Discussion

In keeping with the view that social work practice and medical treatment in a hospital should be integrated, one might have reassessed the purpose and life of the ongoing monthly group when it became fragmented from the emphysema clinic. If the social work role is defined as mediating between systems, one might ask whether the internal system of the group began to spin off from the larger system of medical care for which the patient was presumably coming to the hospital. Maintaining connective links is very hard work, and there is some wish, at times, to provide one's own separate service. This understandable wish needs to be addressed when it runs the risk of becoming dysfunctional.

Time-limited and goal-oriented services in the face of chronic and debilitating illness call for difficult decision making. The social worker continually defines and addresses the immediate and more urgent problems within this population. Along the way, the needs of this population can be asserted in ways that will interest the institution and help define meaningful work for the patients. More structured, short-term goals that offer the newly diagnosed patient an opportunity to learn how to manage his illness and deal with adjustment concerns might be considered. Patient education for the more chronic patients might deal with needs for refresher courses and would be even more useful if coupled with a helping experience tied to concerns about reduced functioning. For the end-stage patient, close medical follow-up, the meeting of increased dependency needs, and a socialization experience would be especially helpful.

Patients also need opportunities to teach others, volunteer their services, and be more than consumers and passive recipients of service. The social worker cannot be all things for all patients, nor accept the provision of a service because it is in place; rather, with great creativity, he or she has to examine patients' needs, agency purpose and scope, and perhaps most important of all, be able to expand the kinds of clinical and program skills that can enhance the work.

PRACTICE IN CONTEXT

The decisions that hospital social work departments make about how to carve out and integrate social work practice are becoming increasingly more deliberate and connected to larger hospital goals. The demand in social work to play a vital role in the life of the institution places the responsibility on the profession to offer a focused, goal-oriented service capable of measurement and explicit articulation. The visibility of programs and the support they have from the administration and the medical services are crucial to our vitality within the institution. The creativity and challenge come with translating patient needs in a context to which the institution can lend its sanction, feel a stake, and be encouraged to offer backing and commitment.

REFERENCES

Alexander, C. A. (1992). Physicians in the Department of Veterans Affairs: Another perspective. *Archives of Internal Medicine, 152*(3), 502-504.

Becerra, R. M. and Damron-Rodriguez, J. (1995). Veterans and veterans services. In R. I. Edwards (Ed.), *Encyclopedia of social work*, Nineteenth Edition. Washington, DC: NASW Press, pp. 2431-2439.

Brown, L. N. (1991). Groups for growth and change. New York: Longman.

Burgess, J. F. and Stefos, T. (1991). Federal provision of health care: Creating access for the underinsured. *Journal of Health Care for the Poor and Underserved, 1*(4), 364-387.

Clough, P., Harnisch, L. A., Cebulski, P., and Ross, D. (1987). Method for individualizing patient care for chronic obstructive pulmonary disease patients. *Health and Social Work, 12*(2), 127-133.

Demakis, J. G., Turpin, R. S., Conrad, K. J., Stiers, W. M., Weaver, F. M., Sinacore, J. M., Cowper, D. C., Darcy, L. A., Huck, M. N., and Friedman, B. S. (1990). The whole is greater than the sum of its parts: The anatomy of the Department of

Veterans Affairs Medical District 17 health services research and development field program. *Health Services Research, 25*(Pt. 2), 269-285.

Fisher, E. S. and Welsh, H. G. (1995). The future of the Department of Veterans Affairs health care system. *Journal of the American Medical Association, 273*(8), 651-655.

Gitterman, A. and Schulman, L. (Eds.). (1994). *Mutual aid groups: Vulnerable populations and the life cycle.* New York: Columbia University Press.

Henry, S. (1992). *Group skills in social work: A four dimensional approach,* Second Edition. Pacific Grove, CA: Brooks/Cole.

Holle, M. L., Rick, C., Sleifert, M. K., and Stephens, K. (1995). Integrating patient care delivery. *Journal of Nursing Administration, 25*(7-8), 32-37.

Hollingsworth, J. W., and Bondy, P. M. (1990). The role of Veterans Affairs hospitals in the health care system. *New England Journal of Medicine, 322*(26), 1489-1491.

Holsinger, J. W. (1991). The Veterans Health Administration: A health care model for the nation. *Academic Medicine, 66*(11), 674-675.

Kaplan, R., Toshima, M., Atkins, C. J., and Ries, A. L. (1990). Adherence to prescribed regimens for patients with chronic obstructive pulmonary disease. In S. A. Shumaker, E. B. Schron, J. K. Ockene, C. T. Parker, J. L. Probsfield, and J. M. Wolfe (Eds.), *The handbook of health behavior change.* New York: Springer Publishing Co, pp. 126-143.

Kerson, T. S. (1985.) Respiratory diseases. In *Understanding chronic illness.* New York: The Free Press, pp. 187-219.

Lott, T. F., Blazey, M. E., and West, M. G. (1992). Patient participation in health care: An underused resource. *Nursing Clinics of North America, 27*(1), 61-76.

Loveland-Cook, C. A., Chadiha, L., Schmidt, B., and Holloway, J. (1992). High social risk screening mechanisms: patient characteristics as predictors of social work utilization in the VA. *Social Work in Health Care, 16*(4), 101-117.

Loveland-Cook, C. A., Freedman, J. A., Evans, R. L., Rodell, D., and Taylor, R. M. (1992). Research in social work practice: Benefits of and obstacles to implementation in the Department of Veterans Affairs. *Health and Social Work, 17*(3), 214-222.

Mather, J. H. and Abel, R. W. (1986). Medical care of veterans: A brief history. *Journal of the American Geriatrics Society, 34*, 757-760.

Mirvis, D. M., Ingram, L. A., Kilpatrick, A. O., and Magnetti, S. (1994). Medical school affiliations with Department of Veterans Affairs medical centers, attitudes of medical center leadership. *American Journal of the Medical Sciences, 308*(3), 162-166.

Pittman, J. A. (1995). The future of the VA: Centralization, costs, politics and presentism. *Journal of the American Medical Association, 273*(8), 667-668.

Schopler, J. H., and Galinsky, M. J. (1990). Can open-ended groups move beyond beginnings? *Small Group Research, 21*(4), 435-449.

Schopler, J. H. and Galinsky, M. J. (1995). Group practice overview. In R. L. Edwards (Ed.), *Encyclopedia of social work,* Nineteenth Edition. Washington, DC: NASW Press, pp. 1129-1142.

Schopler, J. H. and Galinsky, M. J. (1984). Meeting practice needs: Conceptualizing the open-ended group. *Social Work with Groups, 7*(1), 3-21.

Shapiro, B. Z. (1991). Social action, the group and society. *Social Work with Groups, 14*(3-4), 7-21.

Shulman, L. (1992). *The skills of helping individuals, families and groups,* Third Edition. Itasca, IL: F. E. Peacock.

Smith, C. S. (1995). The impact of an ambulatory firm system on quality and continuity of care. *Medical Care, 33*(3), 221-226.

Stempler, B. L. and Glass, M. (Eds.). (1996). *Social group work today and tomorrow: Moving from theory to advanced training and practice.* Binghamton, NY: The Haworth Press, Inc.

Tindill, B. S., al Assaf, A. F., and Gentling, S. J. (1993). Total quality improvement: A study of Veterans Affairs Medical Center directions and VA coordinators. *American Journal of Medical Quality, 8*(2), 45-52.

Toshima, M., Kaplan, R. M., and Ries, A. L. (1992). Self-efficacy expectations in chronic obstructive pulmonary disease rehabilitation. In R. Scharzer (Ed.), *Self-efficacy: Thought control of action.* Washington, DC: Hemisphere Publishing Corporation, pp. 325-354.

United States Department of Veterans Affairs. (1995). *VA fact sheet: Facts about the Department of Veterans Affairs.* Washington DC: Office of Public Affairs News Service: Author.

United States Department of Veterans Affairs, (1993). *VA fact sheet: VA social work services.* Washington, DC: Office of Public Affairs News Service, Author.

United States Department of Veterans Affairs. (1994). Annual Report of the Secretary of Veterans Affairs. Washington, DC: Author.

United States Department of Veterans Affairs. (1996). The Veterans Benefits Administration: An organizational history: 1776-1994. Washington, DC: Author.

Weinbaum, G., Giles, R. E., and Krell, D. (Eds.). (1991). *Pulmonary emphysema: The rationale for therapeutic intervention.* New York: New York Academy of Sciences.

Zemberlan, A. (1990). Health services research and development: A tool for hospital management. *Health Services Research, 25*(Pt 2), 169-175.

Chapter 18

Advocacy and Social Action Among Navajo Uranium Workers and Their Families

Susan E. Dawson
Perry H. Charley
Phillip Harrison Jr.

CONTEXT

Description of the Setting

During the Cold War, thousands of uranium miners worked on the Colorado Plateau of Arizona, Colorado, New Mexico, and Utah, mining uranium for the atomic era. Working in largely unventilated mines from the 1940s to the 1970s, mány workers developed lung cancer and nonmalignant respiratory diseases (NMRD), including pneumoconiosis, pulmonary fibrosis, and silicosis (Eichstaedt, 1994). Navajo uranium miners worked both on and off the Navajo Nation throughout this period. The reservation includes a population of 200,000 people living on 25,000 square miles in Arizona, New Mexico, and Utah. Because of the high correlation between respiratory problems and exposures to radiation and silica dust, they are an important group for epidemiologists to study because of their low smoking incidence (Samet et al., 1984; Archer, 1983; Gottlieb and Husen, 1982). This group of older traditional Navajo men also had no understanding of radiation until recently, since there was no word in the Navajo language for it.

The U. S. Public Health Service begán studying uranium miners and the effects of radiation during the 1950s. However, a deliberate decision not to inform the workers about any radiation-induced illnesses was made in exchange for the names of the workers and for entry into the privately owned mining and milling operations. Because the Atomic Energy Commission (AEC) was the sole purchaser of uranium from the companies and bought the uranium for the making of atomic bombs and nuclear energy, the owners of the companies were afraid that if the workers were informed that radiation caused health problems, the companies would no longer have a workforce (Ball, 1993). With this in mind, the Navajo workers believed they were working for the national security interests of the United States.

As a researcher from Utah State University, Susan went to the Navajo Nation in the summer of 1988 to interview uranium miners and their families about the psychosocial effects of not being compensated for occupational illnesses. Susan and a colleague, Gary E. Madsen, returned in 1992 to interview uranium millworkers. Milling of uranium is the second stage of the nuclear fuel cycle, following the mining of uranium ore, in which the ore is crushed, leached, and refined into uranium oxides or yellowcake. During these studies, Susan met Perry Charley and Phil Harrison, both Navajos, who were longtime activists associated with uranium issues. Their fathers had worked in the uranium mines, and Phil had worked as a uranium miner for a summer during high school. When their fathers, Harris Charley and Phillip Harrison Sr., died with illnesses associated with uranium mining, Perry and Phil worked actively to redress the uranium miners' plight.

This chapter will focus on Perry and Phil's advocacy and social action on behalf of the uranium miners, millworkers, and their families. Susan's role as a social work academic involved conducting the two uranium workers' studies of interviews with uranium miners, millworkers, and their families; presenting information at public and professional meetings; publishing the studies' results in scholarly journals and book chapters; and testifying at congressional hearings on behalf of the uranium workers.

Policy

Beginning in the 1960s, illnesses among the Navajo uranium miners became evident with workers becoming critically ill and dying. The ten-year or longer latency period was taking its toll on workers and their families. A series of lawsuits on behalf of nuclear-test downwind victims and underground uranium miners were tried and failed due to the discretionary function exception of the Federal Tort Claims Act. Following the lawsuits, four compensation bills were introduced by Senator Ted Kennedy (D-Massachusetts) in 1979, by Senator Orrin Hatch (R-Utah) in 1981 and 1983, and later by Hatch and Congressman Wayne Owens (D-Utah) in 1989. Finally in 1990, the Hatch-Owens bill became law. It was called the Radiation Exposure Compensation Act (RECA) and provided compassionate payment to underground uranium miners, civilian downwinders of the atomic testing program, and eventually nuclear testsite workers.

Prior to RECA, the only state to compensate uranium miner claims was Colorado. Only those workers who could establish a work record in that state were eligible to apply for and receive benefits. Consequently, until 1990, Navajo uranium miners were ineligible, for the most part, for compensation and suffered greatly economically and emotionally (Dawson, 1992).

Compensation under RECA allows for a payment of $100,000, $75,000, and $50,000 for underground uranium miners, nuclear testsite workers, and downwind atomic victims respectively, and is paid from a $100 million trust fund administered by the U. S. Department of Justice (DOJ). If the claimant is deceased, the payment is made to the widow/widower and/or survivor.

For the uranium miners, the worker or survivor could apply if he had worked in a mine located in Arizona, Colorado, New Mexico, Utah, or Wyoming from January 1, 1947 to December 31, 1971. Working level months (WLM) of exposure to radiation were established in which a nonsmoker needed 200 WLM. A smoker who developed a specific listed respiratory disease or cancer before the age of 45 needed 300 WLM, while a smoker who developed a listed disease after the age of 45, needed 500 WLM. The diseases include any type of lung cancer, fibrosis of the lung, pulmonary fibrosis, corpulmonale related to fibrosis of the lung, or moderate or severe silicosis or moderate or severe pneumoconiosis if the miner worked in a uranium mine within an Indian Reservation. Workers and their survivors may file claims up to 20 years after 1990 (Office of Navajo Uranium Workers).

Technology and Organizations

There are several organizations that offer services and support to uranium workers and their families, including the Indian Health Service (IHS) hospitals, the Office of Navajo Uranium Workers, and four uranium worker support groups. The U.S. Public Health Service operates the IHS hospitals on the Navajo Nation. These hospitals provide health care free of charge to the Navajo people and are staffed generally with family practitioners, internists, and pediatricians. Many of the physicians work at the IHS for a few years and then move off the reservation to private practices. One of the common complaints heard by patients is that they do not have a family doctor who stays long enough to know family members and their medical history. Moreover, the IHS system does not employ pulmonary specialists as a rule. These specialists are needed to fully diagnose respiratory problems. In attempting to document their cases over the years, miners have needed to have health examinations that included chest X rays.

In the past, the tribe brought in its own pulmonary specialist, Dr. Leon S. Gottlieb, who was the first physician to associate and document lung cancer and uranium mining among the Navajo (Gottlieb and Husen, 1982). Since Dr. Gottlieb, there have been no pulmonary specialists associated with the IHS system on the Navajo Nation. When uranium miners were identified as possibly having lung cancer or NMRD, they were referred off the reservation to specialists and hospitals in such places as Albuquerque and Denver. These hospital visits were paid for by the IHS system, including travel to and from the facility; however, lodging and food were not paid for the family member accompanying the patient. This expense often created a hardship for families. Widows and family members told Susan that they would often spend the night in a chair with the miner because they could not afford to stay in a motel. They would also bring their own food or go without. Phil explains,

> My Dad wasn't quite sure if he was going to make it through Christmas and through New Year's, and we had the hardest time there going back and forth to the hospital [about a four-hour drive] . . . We took him in and out for radiation treatment in Albuquerque. We'd leave him there for about two weeks at a time, go pick him up, and bring him back. And it was a lot of work doing that. My other brothers and sisters were still in school. They were small. So finally he passed away in January of 1971 from lung cancer, and from there on it was a lot of responsibility left up to me to take care of my mom and the family.

For the most part, physicians did not speak Navajo, and many patients did not understand their diagnoses and treatment plans. Susan and Gary often heard the miners/millers explain that they had "red lungs" or "uranium on the lungs" in place of the NMRD diagnoses. Also, if treating professionals did not understand the Navajo culture, they might not realize that the patient could believe that a natural event, such as lightning, might be considered responsible for the patient's illness rather than an occupational exposure. A result of the latter would be that the patient and family would not pursue compensation or work-related benefits.

According to Perry and Phil, a comprehensive health care system separate from the IHS, in which a uranium clinic is designed for miners and other uranium workers who are ill, is needed. Phil notes that miners with lung cancer are often too sick to travel off the reservation or to wait in IHS waiting rooms for long periods until they are called. When he visited Japan in 1991 as part of a delegation of American Indians concerned with uranium issues, he toured such a government-funded hospital for the Hibakusha, the bombing victims of Hiroshima and Nagasaki. He said that in addition to treating the Hibakusha, the hospital conducts its own studies of radiation exposure effects.

The IHS has contracted recently with the University of New Mexico School of Medicine and the Miners Colfax Medical Clinic in Raton, New Mexico, to operate a screening van. Miners may receive X rays and testing free of charge through this service. Also, the IHS will take X rays of uranium workers and send them to be read by B readers off the reservation.

The Office of Navajo Uranium Workers, which is a central registry for uranium miners and millworkers funded by the tribe, grew out of a grassroots movement that began in the Red Valley and Cove, Arizona, area of the reservation. Perry's involvement began in 1975 when he noticed that his father began having increasing difficulties with his breathing:

> I was aware that [my father] had spent over twenty years in the underground mines on the Navajo Indian Reservation and the Colorado Plateau. I started making the connections that his previous employment in these mines may have caused his respiratory problems. This prompted me to find out what had actually happened to him. I found out quickly that his was not the only case, that there were countless others with similar disabling and progressive health problems.

Perry worked throughout the 1970s and 1980s in various projects to educate the Navajo people about radiation. After 1975, he was employed as a supervisor for the Community Health Representative (CHR) Program, a grassroots health advocacy program with the tribe. He initiated and revised the program's goals and objectives to emphasize increased public awareness through direct coordination with the Shiprock, New Mexico IHS medical staff and through an intensive educational network with the affected communities. Information was disseminated at chapter house meetings, group presentations, schools, annual fair/events using television networks, radios, and one-on-one contacts with family members in homes. Chapter houses are units of tribal government established for different community areas.

In 1978, Perry worked with Dr. Lora M. Shields, a visiting biology professor at the Shiprock Navajo Community College, on a 12-year March of Dimes Birth Defect Study. Perry also worked with Stewart L. Udall on the attorney's lawsuits, including *Begay vs. United States of America,* on behalf of the Navajo uranium miners and continues to work with him today as claims are processed by DOJ for compassionate payment under RECA.

Beginning in 1978, he gathered mining histories from uranium miners and their surviving families and forwarded the information to Udall's Phoenix office. Perry states,

> Initially, meetings were held at chapter houses for clients. These were much easier than traveling from home to home, though this had to be performed on some difficult cases when necessary. We also had to establish a special office under the Shiprock CHR Program for the specific purpose of obtaining information for Udall's lawsuit when more and more Navajos from all parts of the Navajo Nation started getting involved. This was, in essence, the first Navajo Uranium Office.

Phil noted that when he and others would meet with legislators, tribal officials, or go to conferences, people would ask about the statistics of the uranium workers to justify requests for funding and/or compensation. Trips were made to Washington, DC and in April 1990, during the tribal leadership of Leonard Haskie and Ervin Billy, the Office of Navajo Uranium Workers was established in Red Valley, Arizona.

Four support groups, two for the uranium miners and two for the uranium millworkers, have evolved over the past 20 years. Red Valley's Uranium Radiation Victims Committee was organized in the early 1970s to provide support and technical assistance to uranium miners and their families. In 1978, they invited the CBS television network to document the continued plight of uranium miners. During this visit, a staff member of the Navajo Environmental Protection Commission, using a gamma scintillation counter, noticed that a uranium worker's home was "hot" with radioactivity. Eventually 17 homes in the Oakspring, Arizona, area were discovered to have been built with radioactive materials. Perry was part of a committee that was formed in the Shiprock area specifically for the purpose of identifying any additional habitable structures containing low-level radioactivity. They also prioritized these homes for remediation, locating and acquiring federal monies to replace them and coordinating with tribal and federal agencies in their radiological surveys. Such homes were eventually replaced or renovated to acceptable housing standards. Despite these efforts, Navajo tribal officials were unwilling to assist by obligating tribal monies for replacement homes. This has continued to the present day as homes built in the same fashion continue to be identified in areas affected by past mining experiences.

The Red Valley support group elected Phil as their chairperson in 1982. The group met monthly and worked on organizing around the uranium legislation, health issues, the uranium registry, clean-up of homes, and reclamation of uranium mines and mills. Initially, few people attended the meetings; however, over time the meetings grew to include as many as 100 people. Announcements on the radio and in newspapers were made to advertise the meetings. The committee was instrumental in voicing concerns of the uranium miners and their surviving families to the Navajo tribal government. They also contacted congressional delegates at the federal level in attempts to enact legislation to compensate the workers and their families. At first, tribal officials were not interested, but this slowly changed as the national and international news media continued documenting the problems of the uranium workers.

Perry assisted in starting the Red Mesa/Mexican Water Four Corners Uranium Committee in 1985. This support group had similar intentions as the Red Valley Committee. Their goals were to disseminate information nationally about the plight of the Navajo uranium miners. The committee was further assisted by an elected chairman, who happened to have ties to the Associated Press (AP) through his work with a local TV station. He went on later to become the community's council delegate. The committee was in existence until the enactment of RECA.

Prior to RECA's enactment, Phil and Perry would update the people at chapter house meetings. At one Mexican Water chapter meeting, over 300 people attended to hear the status of the bill and its meaning for them individually. These types of meetings were held throughout the Navajo Nation to apprise people of RECA and to network with each other.

Because the uranium millworkers were excluded from RECA due to a lack of conclusive studies, two support groups were formed among the millers. A Navajo miller approached Phil and asked him if he was interested in developing a millers' group. Organized in 1992 in Shiprock, New Mexico, the Four Corners Uranium Millers Association meets monthly and includes about 100 members. Initially, the group set out to collect data on the millers. They cooperated with Susan and Gary in participating in their study with the millworkers (Dawson and Madsen, in press). The other millworkers' group, the Western Navajo Agency Millers, at Tonalea, Arizona, is located on the western portion of the Navajo Nation, while Shiprock is on the eastern side.

DECISIONS ABOUT PRACTICE

Definition of the Client

Within this context, the client is the group of uranium miners, millworkers, and their families. With over 1,000 uranium mines and four uranium mills on the Navajo Nation, it is estimated that there were over 4,000 miners and 500 to 600 millworkers. The mills averaged 100 workers when they were in operation, and the mines varied. As of August 1995, the Office of Navajo Uranium Workers has registered 2,449 uranium workers, with 1,700 miners and 400 millers identified. The two groups are not mutually exclusive, since 200 of the workers were employed as both miners and millers. According to the director of the Office of Navajo Uranium Workers, 1,500 to 1,600 of the registered miners meet the criteria for RECA eligibility (Benally, 1995).

To date, 280 uranium miners or their survivors have been accepted and compensated. Many of these cases were originally denied and, with the assistance of the Office of Navajo Uranium Workers, their cases were reopened and finally accepted. When a case is denied, the claimant has 60 days to appeal. There are 191 pending cases, and there is no charge for uranium miners to present a claim through the Office (Benally, 1995). When claims are denied, it is usually because of inadequate information, such as insufficient WLM or smoking data and/or lack of proof of compensable disease. When compensation started in 1992, DOJ denied claims without documentation of marriage or death certificate. Many elderly Navajo were married through traditional weddings or lived in common-law arrangements. Death and birth certificates often were unavailable, especially when the worker was born and/or died at home. Mr. Benally, the director of the Office of Navajo Uranium Workers, presented this information to then-president Petersen Zah, and it was arranged in early 1993 that a tribal judge in a tribal court could certify these life events.

In addition to the office, Navajo miners may file their cases on their own or through attorneys. For those who do file through an attorney, it is stipulated that the attorney may receive no more than $10,000 from the claimant's award. (The statistics cited include all cases of Navajo claimants whether they filed with the office, an attorney, or on their own.)

Goals, Objectives, and/or Outcome Measures

While the client is identified as a group, it is important to recognize that the goals that are applied to the group are appropriate in context for individuals within the group. The value of self-determination is an important one for the social work profession (Zastrow, 1993), and it is also important within the Navajo value structure. The practice of social work with American Indians suggests a practice of noninterference (Good Tracks, 1973). Phil illustrates this principle with regard to a uranium miner who had not applied for RECA nor registered with the Office of Navajo Uranium Workers:

I know one person who heard about all the setbacks and all the frustrations that all the people are going through [with RECA] to where he doesn't even want to do anything about it. He hasn't even registered or filed–a miner with some twenty years experience. And I hate to go there and say, "Hey, look, here's what's going on and do you want to file?" I'd be kind of imposing on him. And I don't want to do that unless somebody asks for help, and then I can help them.

One way to address this issue would be through the dissemination of information and education about radiation exposure and RECA through chapter house meetings, congressional hearings, the media, and workshops. In this way, workers and their family members become aware of the information, resources, and options available to them. They may then decide to formulate a plan of action, which may include seeking assistance from others.

Education and dissemination of information about the issues are two important goals for activists working with the uranium workers and their families. Other goals include helping people to register with the Office of Navajo Uranium Workers, to apply for RECA, and to seek technical and emotional support through various support groups, chapter houses, tribal government, and other institutions and networks. In some instances, it is important to go door-to-door to accomplish sharing the information. Phil explains that, within the context of interviewing people for another project, it gave him an opportunity to update them on what was happening with RECA. He notes why going to peoples' homes is important:

And I would say to this day there's a lot of people that have not even filed with the uranium office yet. They have not even started filing a claim for compensation. It's because they're way out there on the reservation. Because of their economic situation, and there's no transportation . . . . There's no money to pay for gas to come out.

In the 1980s, both Perry and Phil went with Dr. Shields to the chapter houses every other month to disseminate educational information. These meetings and Dr. Shields' study were announced on the radio since most families listen to the Navajo station around noontime to hear about chapter and community events. Dr. Shields would define radiation and its potential effects on people. Background information about the history of the atomic age was also presented along with slideshows. Phil believes that this was one of the things that induced people eventually to listen and to attend meetings about RECA.

One other larger environmental community goal is the remediation of abandoned uranium mines and mills. Perry was employed under the Uranium Mill Tailings Remedial Action (UMTRA) Project from 1982 through 1988 under the U.S. Department of Energy to reclaim uranium mill sites located on the Navajo Reservation. In addition to assuring compliance to contract specifications in reclaiming these mill sites, Perry helped to form local citizens' groups at each Navajo UMTRA site to insure adequate citizen involvement throughout the remedial action process. Part of his duties involved informing local residents about remediation activities. To explain technical nuclear terms, Perry assisted in developing a video of various UMTRA activities in the Navajo language.

Perry was then offered employment in Shiprock with the Navajo Abandoned Mine Lands Reclamation (AML) Department in 1988. This is a federally funded tribal department under the U.S. Department of Interior's Office of Surface Mining Control Reclamation and Enforcement. It delegated responsibilities to reclaim mine sites abandoned without adequate reclamation prior to 1977. The AML program established tribal protocol and schemes for the prioritization of abandoned mine sites, and established in-house guidelines for cleanup of radioactively contaminated lands and reclamation of radioactive mine sites. Efforts under AML included taking physical inventory of 1,100 abandoned mine sites located within the boundaries of the Navajo Nation, prioritizing mines according to their degree of physical hazard, and initiating construction activities.

Abandoned mines pose a threat to the Navajo people in that these sites are unreclaimed, unfenced, and accessible. It is not uncommon for children to play in these cavelike spaces and for cattle, sheep, and goats to wander into them for warmth. The sites may be 40 to 50 years old and unstable. In many of the sites, mine waste can travel into washes or streambeds, posing hazards to people and livestock downstream. Perry illustrates:

> We found approximately 500 mines that were used by local shepherds for livestock pens . . . a well-insulated sheep pen, but potentially dangerous to the sheep that used the mines for shelter and lambing. One lady told me in the Tse-Tah area in northwest Arizona, "I always wondered why my lambs were born without fleece and why some were born deformed or with limbs missing." She lived about 200 feet away from a mine for many years, using the mine for a livestock pen. The family was in the process of building an addition to their home using the radioactive mine waste.

Another pathway for human exposure is through ingesting exposed animals' organs, such as the kidneys, in which radioactive elements are concentrated. Eating the livestock's organs is a common practice among the Navajo and therefore of considerable concern.

Use of Contract

While there is no written contract, per se, there is a sense of obligation to work with this group of uranium workers and their families and to obtain compensation through the RECA program. The Office of Navajo Uranium Workers assists uranium mining clients who apply for RECA through the office. Once the client is registered, the process of obtaining compensation is maintained until compensation is either granted or denied.

Hindsight indicates that what has occurred is not unlike the social action campaigns of the 1960 civil rights period. Activists have worked largely on their own, without pay, networking and traveling across the Navajo Nation and to Washington, DC, to promote legislation and the uranium workers' cause. Phil relates:

> Eighty percent of [costs to Washington, DC] is out of our own pockets. All during this time, and we lost a lot of money over this thing, and I don't think I can ever get back the money that I spent on these projects . . . I don't know how long I can stay and put up with this thing. My family's really getting after me for this. They keep asking me to look for a real job that pays. But I said one more year.

Meeting Place

In the above discussion, meeting places include workers' homes, support-group meetings, government agency offices, chapter house meetings, and congressional offices. In addition to the monthly support group and commit-tee meetings, chapter meetings were held periodically to update chapter members on RECA information. These were well-attended meetings, num-bering in the hundreds at the larger chapters, in which information would be presented followed by a question-and-answer period. Other important meet-ing places included congressional hearings in which activists and uranium workers provided testimonies regarding their plight. All three authors have testified on behalf of the uranium workers. Recent hearings of the President's Advisory Committee on Human Radiation Experimentation included testi-monies concerning both the uranium miners and millworkers. Phil has also traveled internationally on behalf of the uranium workers to Japan, as pre-viously discussed, and also to Salzburg, Austria, for the World Uranium Hearings. For the hearings, he and other American Indians presented their stories to "listeners" about the effects of uranium mining on Indian lands. The listeners included nuclear experts and other professionals.

Use of Time

As with many social problems, especially in the environmental area, grassroots social action brings the issue to public awareness. Edelstein notes, "The development of community organizations tends to provide people with a new sense of power in the midst of a situation that otherwise produces an overall sense of loss of control" (Edelstein, 1988, p. 144). The uranium workers and their families have been able to release some of their frustrations and fears through working together with activists, health care professionals, attorneys, social workers, and legislators. All of these resource people have provided technical assistance and social support to these individuals. Moreover, people working in social action campaigns often respond to a multiplicity of events, some of which occur at the same time (Rubin and Rubin, 1992). In some campaigns, activists have the luxury of responding in a well-orchestrated fashion, while in others they find themselves reacting by a "seat-of-the-pants" method. In the Navajo uranium workers' case, there was enough time to organize a grassroots effort to push compensation forward. Activists were able to work both with individuals and institutions to accomplish their agenda for the most part.

In addition to working with other individuals and bureaucracies, the Navajo supported each other. Since the Navajo are clan-based, there is an extended family network that provides social support. Family members ensure that widows and elderly parents are not alone during the difficult period of illness and death. Traditional elders may not have the financial and emotional resources to cope with bureaucracies. In this capacity, older children are able to act as intermediaries between their parents or grandparents and the often complex health, legal, and social systems. Conversely, Perry explains how traditional elders who are ill may act with respect to their families:

> To the Navajos, a house that one dies in should never be used again as the deceased's spirit (chiidi) lingers within. Rather than to condemn a family home, I saw several miners move out of their comfortable houses and reside in shacks or arbor shades. Towards the end, and just before he went into an irreversible coma due to his complete respiratory failure from which he never revived, my father did the same thing. "It makes me breathe better as the house is too confining and out here I can breathe the fresh clean air," he used to

say. A way of making us feel better? Or was he letting us, the family, go gradually?

Interventions and Stance of the Social Worker

Advocacy and social action are the treatment modality and stance of the three authors. A systems approach is also employed, given the role of linking individuals with various institutions on and off the reservation. The goal of advocacy and social action is empowerment of the individual, the group, and the community. The tragedy that has occurred on the Navajo Nation, with regard to the uranium workers and their families, has left many individuals feeling victimized and betrayed (Dawson, 1992). Perry explains,

> I observed [people's] anguish over events they were unknow-ingly subjected to by an uncaring industry and a government whose sole purpose was to procure a potentially hazardous and fatal mate-rial at all costs. Relief in the form of payment for the wrongful injuries sustained in the courses of their employment and in the form of inadequate health care delivery system [is slow]. Close to 20 years has passed and I see very little difference or improvement.

Linking people to needed resources is important and yet difficult on the largely rural reservation. Susan interviewed widows who were eligible for Social Security who had never heard of the benefit. These same widows, many of whom did not speak English, often did not have telephones or money for stamps and stationery. In addition, it is unknown how many workers/families across the reservation have not applied for RECA who may be eligible. Consequently, there is great need for assisting people to access the various systems.

In working one-on-one with patients within the IHS, for example, it was beneficial to not only have someone who understood uranium but also someone who was Navajo. Perry was brought in by an IHS physician at the Shiprock Hospital to assist in informing a 50-year-old miner that he had contracted lung cancer, the deadly oat-cell carcinoma. Perry states,

> The physician felt I could relate better with [the miner] rather than a nurse or a regular hospital staff person. I had to show him his X rays of his chest, pointing out that the dark areas in the photo were cancerous. I explained what cancer was. He had very little comprehension of what this meant . . . I visited him at his home in Sweetwater, Arizona, several times until his death in the summer of 1980. He told me he didn't want to die in "that hospital" but he had to go in . . . He was

also distrustful of the Anglos, the hospitals, and the government that allowed such a thing to happen to him.

In trying to comply with RECA, workers and their families often had to make extra all-day trips, with great hardship, to furnish additional employment documents. In cases where no such documents were available, it would help to refresh people's memories by asking where they worked when a particular child was born. Being knowledgeable about events that took place in tandem with their mining history helped also. In certain cases, revisiting the mines in which they had worked and reestablishing their work history were necessary. The stress of dealing with RECA and the overall situation often took its toll on individuals and families. Perry describes the social stress created from the death of a uranium miner on a Navajo family:

> Wives were hit the hardest when a husband contracted the fatal lung disease. The wife had to assume a role she was taught belonged with the male. Many had very little education, no work experience, and consequently end up on welfare. This was a blow to their ego, their upbringing, and it was embarrassing. Navajos are taught never to "beg" for handouts in order to feed and clothe their children. I recall one wife, rather than face this predicament, chose to divorce the miner. A constant battle to feed the family resulted in the oldest children dropping out of school and starting employment or to care for the father. The father was a strong central figure and when he was no longer available, family stress, disciplinary/emotional problems, and alcoholism developed among the children, and other problems resulted.

Use of Outside Resources

The use of resources off the reservation has helped to support the work being conducted on the Navajo Nation. Work with universities, law firms, and legislators has proven beneficial. Phil would bring experts such as a biology graduate student from the University of New Mexico to chapter meetings to educate the people about radiation issues. Without Perry and Phil's assistance, Susan and Gary would have had great difficulty conducting their work. Perry and Phil provided them with key contacts, information, and support throughout their work as they did with Stewart Udall, Lora Shields, and others. In exchange for their outside contact with individuals and government agencies, Perry and Phil received support and help to further their cause.

Case Conclusion

The struggle of the uranium miners, millworkers, and their families will be concluded partially when compensation from RECA is awarded to the last person who is eligible and when cleanup of the mine and mill sites is completed; however, it is difficult to assess how long it will take for the devastating psychological and social effects to abate. Perry notes that even when compensation is awarded, ". . . my Dad remains dead and I remain bitter, so continues the legacy of the Navajo uranium miners."

All of the people associated with uranium mining, milling, and environmental contamination have participated in a technological disaster. A technological disaster is human-made, as opposed to an act of God such as a tornado or an earthquake. The effects of long-term chronic disasters are often devastating and lingering, creating fear and anxiety not unlike post-traumatic stress syndrome (Dawson, 1993; Roberts, 1993; Baum, 1988; Edelstein, 1988; Vyner, 1988; Baum, Fleming, and Davidson, 1983; Baum, Fleming, and Singer, 1983). While compensation and remediation are addressed, many questions are left unanswered for the uranium victims, such as (1) Will I or a family member become ill? (2) Will my unborn children be affected? (3) Is the water safe to drink? (4) Should we move somewhere else? Until stability is brought to the community through long-term efforts, including counseling and traditional healing ceremonies, these questions remain unanswered.

Differential Discussion

It is difficult to determine what could have been done differently in this effort to obtain social justice for the uranium workers and their families. Given the immense resources of the U.S. government, it is a testament to the Navajo people and the activists that justice was served. Overall, it was a successful effort to obtain compassionate payment and an apology from the government for past wrongdoings. Given the above, still more work needs to be accomplished on the Navajo Nation, including the following recommendations for reform:

1. Tribal leaders should prioritize the needs of the uranium victims over the next five years, ensuring that their needs are met.
2. A full-time Navajo uranium issues lobbyist position should be created and funded by the tribe.
3. Pulmonary specialists should be hired at the IHS hospital facilities.
4. Remediation and cleanup of uranium mine and mill sites should remain high priorities across the Navajo Nation, and such priorities

should not be limited to surface reclamation. Groundwater restoration is needed.

5. Compensation under RECA is slow, and adjustments to the criteria should be rewritten to expedite the program, for example, abolishing the working level months.

6. A comprehensive health care facility, separate from the IHS system and designed specifically for uranium workers and their families, should be established.

7. Epidemiological studies of uranium workers, their families, and communities should be conducted.

8. Outreach services should be provided to uranium families for health, legal, and social services.

PRACTICE IN CONTEXT

Public policy has underscored the lives of the uranium workers and their families since the 1940s. Beginning with the secrecy of the atomic era through the passage of the Radiation Exposure Compensation Act in 1990, the Navajo people have had to react to policies that have threatened the very fabric of their lives. In addition, they have had to respond to large-scale bureaucracies and governmental agencies, which often have not had their best interests in mind. Perry reflects:

> The U.S. government enacted a law (RECA) for "compassionate payment." Many of the uranium miners and their families see little compassion when the very federal agency, the Department of Justice, that had adamantly opposed the establishment of such a law is entrusted to fairly administer the program. These administrators do not have the basic knowledge of the Navajo culture and traditions, and these traditions and values continue to dominate the Navajo way of life.

Reacting to public policies proves constructive when advocacy and social action approaches are utilized successfully, as in the case of the Navajo uranium workers and their families. Working through both conventional and nonconventional methods, a sense of personal and collective control and empowerment was gained. While this social action campaign may appear as though enabled by a few activists and leaders, it actually entails the efforts of all the participants, including the uranium workers, their families, and community residents. As is often the case, those most affected by an issue are often most likely to bring it into the public domain. The activists and helping professionals in this instance worked with the participants as resource people. Within this context, practice becomes a powerful tool to effect change and to encourage social justice.

REFERENCES

Archer, V. E. (1983). Diseases of uranium miners. In Rom, W. M. (Ed.), *Environmental and occupational medicine* (pp. 687-691). Boston, MA: Little, Brown, pp. 687-691.

Ball, H. (1993). *Cancer factories: America's tragic quest for uranium self-sufficiency*. Westport, CT: Greenwood Press.

Baum, A. (1988). Disasters, natural, and otherwise. *Psychology Today, 22*(4), 57-60.

Baum, A., Fleming, R., and Davidson, L. M. (1983). Natural disaster and technological catastrophe. *Environment and Behavior, 15*(3), 333-354.

Baum, A., Fleming, R., and Singer, J. E. (1983). Coping with victimization by technological disaster. *Journal of Social Issues, 39*(2), 117-138.

Benally, T. H. (August 1, 1995). Personal communication with S. E. Dawson.

Dawson, S. E. (1992). Navajo uranium workers and the effects of occupational illnesses: A case study. *Human Organization, 51*(4), 389-397.

Dawson, S. E. (1993). Social work practice and technological disasters: The Navajo uranium experience. *Journal of Sociology and Social Welfare, 20*(2), 5-20.

Dawson, S. E. and Madsen, G. E. (in press). American Indian uranium millworkers: The perceived effects of chronic occupational exposure. *Journal of Health and Social Policy*.

Edelstein, M. R. (1988). *Contaminated communities: The social and psychological impacts of residential toxic exposure*. Boulder, CO: Westview Press.

Eichstaedt, P. H. (1994). *If you poison us: Uranium and Native Americans*. Santa Fe, NM: Red Crane Books.

Good Tracks, J. G. (1973). Native American noninterference. *Social Work, 18*(6), 30-34.

Gottlieb, L. S. and Husen, L. A. (1982). Lung cancer among Navajo uranium miners. *Chest, 8*, 449-452.

Office of Navajo Uranium Workers. (Undated material). Summary of Radiation Exposure Compensation Act. Information Sheet.

Roberts, J. T. (1993). Psychosocial effects of workplace hazardous exposures: Theoretical synthesis and preliminary findings. *Social Problems, 40*(1), 74-89.

Rubin, H. and Rubin, I. (1992). *Community organizing and development*, Second Edition. New York: Maxwell McMillan International.

Samet, J. M., Young, R. A., Morgan, M. V., Humble, C. G., Epler, G. R., and McLoud, T. C. (1984). Prevalence survey of respiratory abnormalities in New Mexico uranium miners. *Health Physics, 46*(2), 361-370.

Vyner, H. M. (1988). *Invisible trauma: The psychosocial effects of the invisible environmental contaminants*. Lexington, MA: Lexington Books.

Zastrow, C. (1993). *Introduction to social work and social welfare*, Fifth Edition. Pacific Grove, CA: Brooks/Cole.

Chapter 19

A Community-Based Response
to the HIV/AIDS Pandemic

George S. Getzel

CONTEXT

Description of the Setting

The Gay Men's Health Crisis (GMHC) is a nonprofit, voluntary organization established in the summer of 1982 by a group of New York City gay professionals who were experiencing a series of deaths of friends and lovers from an increasingly common disease. They saw this disease, without a known etiology, as a threat to themselves and other gay men. The sudden onset and rapid progression of the disease process were of crisis proportions for persons becoming ill with what was to be called Acquired Immune Deficiency Syndrome (AIDS), and those persons caring for them. As persons with AIDS (PWAs) and their loved ones approached the health care system, they typically found confusion, fear, and even the withdrawal of care by professionals and others in hospitals and clinics (Gay Men's Health Crisis, 1995a; Greenly, 1984; Lopez and Getzel, 1984).

The initial efforts of GMHC's founders and early volunteers were to raise money for medical research and to provide support and mutual aid (Kramer, 1989). The early use of social workers and other professionals, as volunteers and later as paid staff, was important because of the far-reaching consequences of the disease process on the social and emotional lives of those diagnosed with AIDS and their caregivers (GMHC, 1995a; Lopez and Getzel, 1987).

GMHC is the oldest and largest nonprofit, voluntary AIDS organization in the world. Its service design has been replicated by other organizations in New York City and in other countries (Altman, 1994, 1986). Advocacy activities on a local and national level have significantly influenced public policy toward people affected by AIDS and HIV prevention strategies.

Policy

As the twentieth century closes, AIDS remains the most significant public health problem in the United States and the world (Mann, Tarantola, and Netter, 1992). AIDS has become a central theme of popular culture and art (Watney, 1989). The stigma and taboos associated with AIDS continue to be obstacles to communities' acceptance of PWAs and the broad dissemination of HIV prevention strategies. Human sexuality and death are subjects where directness and candor may be replaced by fear, shame, and guilt.

The belief that AIDS is an exclusive problem of gay men and drug abusers remains a serious delusion shared by many heterosexual men and women who engage in unsafe sexual practices with partners assumed to be heterosexual and therefore falsely believed to be free of HIV infection (Cox, 1990). Lack of a thorough, ongoing, federal HIV prevention effort at this point in the pandemic's history is scandalous. State and local HIV prevention efforts tend to be influenced by religious and moralistic considerations interfering with effective and nonjudgmental HIV prevention messages to individuals who are sexually active outside marriage or share a gay or lesbian lifestyle (Altman, 1994; Shilts, 1988).

Social work education has been exceedingly slow in incorporating systematic AIDS content in graduate and undergraduate programs, even when located in an urban area with a high incidence of HIV/AIDS. It is apparent that ongoing advocacy is required by interested faculty to update colleagues on changing aspects of the pandemic and its far-reaching consequences to the people that social workers serve. Recruitment of social workers to work with PWAs grows annually. Social workers in the field need constant updating of their knowledge and require emotional support in the workplace to manage the profound stress associated with the delivery of AIDS care (Getzel, 1992; Getzel, 1991a; Shernoff, 1990).

Health care delivery to PWAs illuminates the significant limitations of federal, state, and local funding and service delivery in communities, due to fragmentation of funding streams, the lack of comprehensive benefits, and discontinuities in service availability and coordination. Medicaid benefits provide the largest source of federal spending for the health care of PWAs in poverty or who become medically indigent due to the high cost of private health insurance. Federal contributions to Medicaid are matched by state and local contributions with total benefits packages differing from state to state. New York State, for example, gives enhanced funding to hospitals designated as AIDS centers for the additional costs associated with the care of PWAs. Some states pay for a PWA's private insurance through Medicaid funding (McCormack, 1990).

Social Security Disability Insurance (SSDI) eligibility occurs two years after notification of disability. AIDS is recognized as a disability under the Americans with Disabilities Act. Upon eligibility for SSDI, a PWA can receive Medicare benefits, which unlike Medicaid do not require asset or income tests; that is, if a PWA survives two years after diagnosis. Efforts to make PWAs immediately eligible for Medicare benefits, which is permitted in the cases of persons with renal disease, have been unsuccessful (Bartlett, 1990).

The introduction of managed care by private insurers presents special problems for PWAs and their families. States are beginning to receive waivers from the federal government to put Medicaid recipients under managed care plans. Unless otherwise forbidden by state law, private insurers can refuse to cover a person who has a preexisting condition such as a positive HIV test result or an AIDS diagnosis. The high cost of AIDS treatment and the unpredictability of lifetime medical expenses makes private insurers unwilling to cover such individuals (Fox and Thomas, 1990). Managed care providers are likely to press for mandatory HIV testing of persons seeking coverage in order to determine actuarial risk for populations who are HIV positive or are at risk for infection. Also, innovative and experimental treatments may be excluded from consideration by managed care organizations. Managed care significantly limits use of specialists and choice of physicians, which are impediments to PWAs wanting "cutting edge" treatment options. Managed care for Medicaid recipients may present similar problems of limited treatment choices. Managed care for PWAs is very likely to create high politicalization and conflict in the years ahead.

The AIDS movement in the United States, through its ongoing political activism and advocacy, has been quite successful in protecting the confidentiality of persons seeking HIV antibody testing and making testing voluntary and not compulsory in different states. Voluntary testing and strict confidentiality requirements are meant to encourage trust in people who are wary about human rights violations. The development of anonymous testing sites is one example of an effort to protect the confidentiality of persons receiving voluntary HIV testing (Blendon and Donelon, 1990; Bayer, 1989).

Hospitals influenced by state mandates and managed care directives are increasingly using home health care to deliver services that had been delivered on an inpatient basis, including chemotherapy, artificial nutrition, routine monitoring during acute episodes of illness, and hospice care (Levine, 1990). While in-home care can be highly desirable to PWAs and their families, it also can put severe strains on PWAs' kin and friends, whose presence becomes increasingly important. Social workers in home health services can play a vital role in working both with the PWA and his or her caregivers. Volunteers from community-based organizations such as GMHC can also play a very useful role in assisting PWAs receiving home health services.

The mental health needs of PWAs and their kin have received lagging recognition by health providers. HIV-related dementia is very prevalent, as are other organic disorders associated with opportunistic infections and cancers. Stress disorders and depression are quite common. Younger chronically mentally ill persons with problems of substance abuse are more likely to become HIV infected. Strategies for HIV prevention must be tailored for this population. Unfortunately, the organizational and geographic splitting of medical services from mental health for people with AIDS remains a very significant problem (King, 1993). A policy of "co-location" of AIDS health and mental health service is an absolute necessity to guarantee access to frail and vulnerable mentally ill PWAs.

Technology

AIDS is a condition occasioned by the breakdown of bodily immunity in otherwise healthy persons. There is reduction in the human organism to resist infections from a variety of microorganisms from within and without, resulting in opportunistic infections and cancers. The capacity of the organism to ward off succeeding infections is gradually weakened with HIV's increased replication and the eventual collapse of the immune system (Bateson and Goldsby, 1988).

More than half the persons diagnosed with AIDS since 1981 have died from complications of HIV and AIDS-related opportunistic infections in the United States and throughout the world (Mann, Tarantola, and Netter, 1992). Despite the expenditures of billions of dollars in biomedical research, an effective vaccine has not been produced to prevent HIV infection. Persons with HIV infection have received some limited benefit from antiviral medications that slow down the replication of HIV in the human organism; however, antiviral medications have not stopped successive opportunistic infections (Bartlett and Finkbeiner, 1996).

In the second decade of the pandemic in the United States, the bulk of health care for PWAs focuses on the treatment of opportunistic infections, provision of palliative care and hospice services, and other types of long-term care provision. Significant advances have been made in the treatment of opportunistic infections and cancers such as pneumocystis carrini pneumonia (PCP), cytomegalvirus (CMV), disseminated tuberculosis, Kaposi's sarcoma (KS), and toxoplasmosis. More effective treatments of PCP have decreased the high early mortality, in weeks or months after diagnosis, so common in the early 1980's. While not dying quickly from PCP, PWAs must now make "quality of life decisions" about whether to treat disfiguring KS lesions, CMV-related colitis and blindness, and other chronic and serially fatal opportunistic infections (Bartlett and Finkbeiner, 1996). A variety of mental health conditions associated with the stresses of the disease process, interpersonal problems, and organic disorders are increasingly recognized as a significant aspect of a PWA's well-being (King, 1994; O'Dowd, Natalie, McKegney, and Orr, 1991).

During the course of the disease process, a PWA may develop one or more opportunistic infections that will not be responsive to medical technology. Treatment typically involves the use of powerful chemicals and radiation, which can cause disfigurement, pain, and psychological distress. Artificial nutrition is frequently used to counter the effects of bodily wasting, and infusion machinery and services are also used to administer strong medications. A PWA may become increasingly dependent on medical technology in the hospital or in his or her home. The need for outside assistance with household chores and self-care activities may be needed.

Although AIDS has been recognized for a decade and a half, social workers and other health care professionals continue to see large numbers of men and women in their early adult years and children dying from AIDS-related diseases. The pandemic is no longer the problem of large cities, but every region of the United States has seen a significant increase in the rate of cases. For example, some rural areas have developed social support service for dispersed and isolated PWAs (Rounds, Galinsky, and Stevens, 1991).

Long-term monitoring and care of PWAs call for a collaboration between health care professionals, community-based organizations and informal caregivers such as kin, friends, neighbors, and volunteers. Social workers in their roles as brokers, mediators, and facilitators play an important part in assisting both formal and informal caregivers do their necessary jobs. AIDS as a biopsychosocial condition lends itself to the skills of social workers in community and institutional health care settings (Getzel, 1991a).

The heavy emotional, economic, and physical burdens of AIDS-related symptoms and their treatment typically raise questions of the cessation of treatment (passive euthanasia), as well as assisted suicide (active euthanasia). While assisted suicide is illegal in most jurisdictions, PWAs frequently express the wish to end their lives and may ask for help from loved ones, social workers, and others. The lack of clear societal guidelines make this an emerging area of practice debate and concern (Glick, 1992).

Organization

GMHC has grown from its inception to the present, from one and one-half full-time staff members and few hundred volunteers to a complex service and educational organization with more than 350 full-time staff and 8,000 current volunteers (GMHC, 1995a; GMHC, 1995b). The biopsychosocial perspective of social work has strongly influenced the development of crisis services, use of volunteers, and a multiplicity of support and educational efforts over the first fifteen years of the agency's life. GMHC's strong commitment to advocacy for all people with AIDS is reflected in policy initiatives on the local, state, and national levels.

While initially the use of volunteers was the predominant source of the agency's human resources, the use of paid staff who serve as specialists with programmatic, supervisory, and clinical functions has grown more important. Enhanced federal and state funding earmarked for AIDS service delivery and AIDS education accelerated the agency's organizational and professional expansion. Considerable tensions and conflicts are associated with GMHC's shift from private to more public funding and outreach efforts to intravenous drug users and their partners, persons of color, women and children, immigrants, and other subsets of the general population (Altman, 1994).

As of May 1, 1995, GMHC was serving 5,528 clients with AIDS; since its inception, GMHC has served 16,296 PWAs. Eighty-four percent of current clients are men and 16 percent are women; the number of women served has grown significantly, reflecting the increasing percentage of women diagnosed in the last 10 years in New York City. Black and Latino clients constitute approximately half the clients served, and white, non-Latino clients are 43.2 percent of the client population. Gay, lesbian, and bisexual identifications were revealed by 67.3 percent of clients, heterosexual identification by 27.3 percent, and 5.5 percent did not reveal any sexual orientation (GMHC, 1995d).

GMHC's multiservice approach to working with PWAs and their loved ones has expanded and deepened by reaching out to new populations. In the period 1993 to 1994, 44.5 percent of GMHC's budget went into client programs, 20.6 percent for fund raising, 15.4 percent for AIDS education, 13.2 percent for policy advocacy, and 6.3 percent for management and general expenses (GMHC, 1995a).

The client intake unit is most often the point of first contact with the agency. Using trained volunteers and professionals, the unit collects information about clients' needs for instrumental and social supports, financial status, employment, substance abuse difficulties, housing, sexual history, and recreational interests. PWAs learn about available services and begin to make a connection with a representative of the agency. Data gathered are placed in a computerized file with strict confidentiality guidelines for its use. Intakes occur in the agency, at home, and sometimes on an emergency basis in the hospital (GMHC, 1995c).

The Clinical Services Department provides crisis services that match volunteers with PWAs who need emotional support and assistance managing the tasks of daily living. Services may be long- or short-term in duration and entail assistance with shopping, going to medical appointments, light housework, and other tasks after a hospitalization or on a more sustained basis when a PWA has serious declines in functional capacity. Typically in long-term cases, volunteers work together as teams of "crisis intervention workers" who handle emotional support issues and "buddies" who provide chore assistance. Families with children with AIDS receive individualized crisis intervention and buddy assistance to meet their particular needs. Social workers provide oversight and professional consultation to the volunteers (Lopez and Getzel, 1987).

Social workers and other mental health providers in volunteer capacity lead over 40 support groups for PWAs and their care partners (Grossman and Silverstein, 1993). Groups typically meet on a weekly basis to examine the practical and emotional consequences of AIDS on their lives. Members in groups address their shared concerns about self-revealing their diagnosis, available treatments, changing interpersonal relationships, identity problems, managing the serial crises associated with the disease sequence, and "quality of life" options that surround severe disability, the termination of treatment, and active euthanasia. These themes occur in caregivers' group composed of loved ones of PWAs as well as in groups of PWAs (Gambe and Getzel, 1989; Getzel and Mahony, 1990; Getzel, 1991b). Drop-in groups are also available for PWAs, caregivers, and the recently bereaved who are not prepared to commit to closed membership groups (GMHC, 1995c).

Through public funding, a case management unit has been established to deliver highly individualized services to PWAs with complex service needs. Social workers and other professionals staff the unit. They assist in the planning, referral coordination, and follow-up services requested and needed, such as public assistance, housing, permanency planning for orphaned children, drug treatment services, medical assistance, psychiatric referrals, and the coordination of services within families when more than one person is ill with AIDS (GMHC, 1995a). Other client services include therapeutic recreation, nutritional counseling, a meals program, a children's recreational program to reduce stress in families, legal assistance, health advocacy, financial advocacy, and public entitlement education. GMHC, through legal representation, has challenged human rights violation of PWAs and has lobbied for confidentiality protection and access to entitlement.

AIDS prevention efforts have been an integral component of the services since the agency's inception. In the absence of a vaccine, public health education about the transmission of the Human Immunodeficiency Virus (HIV) and preventive strategies remain the only means to slow the pandemic. Social workers have contributed to the development of safer sex workshops that emphasize the eroticization of condoms and other safer sex behaviors through cognitive-behavioral group interventions (Palacios and Shernoff, 1987). Safer sex workshops for gay and bisexual men, women, people of color, lesbians, and people of different ethnic backgrounds have been developed and are offered throughout New York City. Technical assistance to community and business organizations is also provided. An array of publications are offered in English and other languages on HIV transmission, safer sex techniques, and medical updates on HIV and AIDS treatment. A program on relapse prevention for persons with drug abuse behaviors is also available (GMHC, 1995a).

DECISIONS ABOUT PRACTICE

Client Description

Ben Anderson, 36, worked as a white-collar employee and restaurant worker. Four years ago, Ben discovered that he was HIV positive. Overwhelmed with anxiety about an early death, he entered a drug rehabilitation program for a long-standing problem of heroin abuse and alcoholism. He successfully attended Narcotics Anonymous (NA) and remained clean, except for one "slip" of a few days four years ago. Ben acknowledged that this slip taught him that the process of getting heroin and injecting it was irresistible, but he felt empty immediately afterward.

His upper-middle-class family who lived in Baltimore first learned about his being gay and HIV-positive while he was in rehabilitation. His father and mother became very upset but tended to avoid discussions of Ben's sexual orientation or HIV status. Ben and his brother and sister were college educated. His siblings have children and very successful careers. His parents' silence about his homosexuality and health status was the subject of Ben's ruminative thoughts and stress. Visits to his parents were infrequent and unpleasant. His siblings avoided contact with him, and he was not sure if it was due to pressure from his parents. Members of NA and some women friends that Ben knew prior to recovery became important sources of support for him. Ben's loneliness was chronic, although he had two relationships with lovers of a few years each. He found that he soon got tired of boyfriends, particularly once they showed a great deal of interest in him. Ben ruefully noted that he liked "the hunt more than the prey."

Two years after finding out he was HIV positive, Ben discovered a few KS lesions on his chest. After his AIDS diagnosis was confirmed, Ben decided to go to GMHC. He received encouragement from other HIV-positive members in NA. Increasingly tired and sleeping a good deal of the time during the day, Ben had a hard time finding employment after losing his last job. Ben's money was nearly gone, and he made a decision to no longer ask his parents for help because they had become more distant and remote after his last request. He told the GMHC intake worker, "They can fuck themselves!"

During the intake session, Ben spoke about his financial problems and his wish to know more about KS. Although he spoke fully about his family's lack of ongoing material and emotional support, Ben said he did not want to waste time dealing with them. He told the intake worker that he was very depressed and lonely. The worker indicated that she could refer him to a psychiatrist for medication and a social worker for psychotherapy. Ben was not sure if he should take medication because it could trigger his drug abuse behaviors; he was interested in seeing a social worker for counseling about his tendency to isolate himself. Ben was starting to believe that he was incapable of being sexually intimate.

Ben later attended a monthly medical forum on new treatments for KS and a program on holistic medicine available to PWAs. He decided to apply for Public Assistance and Supplementary Security Income (SSI) to pay his rent and prepared for the eventuality that he would be unable to work due to the continued ill health. His wish was to find employment, if at all possible. Some pressure on him was reduced by knowing that his basic needs would probably be met. Ben was notified that he was eligible for Food Stamps and Medicaid reimbursement of his private insurance plan, which he was unable to pay for on his own.

Referral to an HIV/AIDS counseling program proved very helpful. Ben addressed his ambivalence about going on welfare and being "a failure" in the eyes of his family and others. He said that his talents were squandered on drug abuse and that now he was "soiled goods." Who would want to have a lover with AIDS? Over time, Ben began to recount a history of substance abuse, which began when he was twelve. His parents' remoteness was an old story; they did little to stop him from drinking or get him help when he was younger. He felt that they were more concerned about looking good to their friends and relatives. His parents used money to entice him to do well in school and behave himself. Angrily, Ben would use the money for drugs.

The foci of counseling were the reinforcment of Ben's ongoing recovery and the exploration of how other gay men could find Ben worthy of their attention. His attendance and deepening involvement in NA gave his social worker ample material to explore recovery and his relationship with other men. He often discussed these same concerns with his NA sponsor. Ben's depressed mood significantly improved, and he began dating Ethan who was also in recovery. Ben's anticipation of Ethan's rejection, after revealing he had AIDS, did not occur. Although HIV negative, Ethan said he wanted to date Ben. Quoting a recovery aphorism, Ethan said that they should look at their relationship "one day at a time." Despite some minor ups and downs, Ben and Ethan grew more intimate, in part, because they struggled to communicate with each other, and Ben made effective use of counseling sessions with his social worker.

Thirteen months later, Ben noticed swelling in back of his head and around his eyes. His doctor told him that the KS was growing in cranial cavities and that fluids were collecting, which caused facial swelling and disfigurement. Ben reluctantly agreed to undergo radiation treatment for the lesions in his head and began taking antiviral medication, which he had refused to take after being diagnosed. This first major health crisis after diagnosis stimulated Ben to talk about death and dying with his social worker and Ethan. Ben went to the GMHC's Legal Department and completed his will, a power of attorney, and an advanced directive, which explicated his instructions for medical treatment should he be unable to make these medical decisions himself. Ben named Ethan the executor of his estate, and gave him power of attorney and the right to make medical decisions in his stead.

Ben showed a burst of energy dealing with this health crisis, but he soon became acutely depressed by the amount of time consumed in recovering from radiation and the growing sense that he might die. His preoccupation was expressed in his regret about the burden that he was placing on Ethan, and the thought that death would end their relationship. Ben used counseling to discuss these concerns and was persuaded by his social worker to consider the use of antidepressant medication. GMHC referred Ben for a psychiatric consultation. Ben received much support from Ethan, who became increasingly stressed by the continued progression of lesions in and outside of Ben's body. Ethan joined a GMHC caregivers support group, where he shared his guilt about sometimes having the wish that Ben die quickly and not suffer so much pain.

Ben was hospitalized three months later for recurrent fevers, and after exhaustive testing, he was diagnosed with disseminated tuberculosis. After his release from the hospital, the fevers continued daily and he lost a great deal of weight. Ben had difficulty shopping and going to his doctors. Ben and Ethan decided to ask for a GMHC volunteer buddy and a crisis manager. Fortunately, Ben liked the volunteers, and this provided much needed relief for Ethan.

Ben's social worker and crisis manager encouraged him to call his parents and siblings. He was very resistant to reaching out to them. Family members indicated concern but apparently made a collective decision that they would not visit him. Ben said to the social worker, "Now I can die knowing at least I made the effort. Don't they think that I am going to be buried with them! I want my friends to spread my ashes in Union Square Park near the statue of Mahatma Gandhi."

Ben's weight dropped from 145 to 105 pounds. His bodily wasting was accompanied by KS lesions on his lungs. After a period of some disorientation and agitated depression, Ben began talking to Ethan and his social worker about not wanting chemotherapy and reiterated his wishes not to be resuscitated and not to receive respiratory assistance, antibiotics, hydration, artificial nutrition, or any other extraordinary treatment as written in his living will. Ben and Ethan wept during this discussion, and Ethan pledged to follow Ben's instructions.

The last three months of Ben's life featured increased symptoms of dementia and respiratory difficulties. Ben began taking morphine patches, followed by a morphine drip administered by a home hospice team. He had a few lucid moments when he spoke to Ethan. After two very difficult weeks on the morphine drip, Ben died in Ethan's arms. With the help of friends and the GMHC volunteers, Ethan planned Ben's cremation. A memorial service was held. An AIDS memorial quilt completed in Ben's memory was added to thousands of others.

Definition of the Client

The client system was primarily Ben Anderson, with a secondary emphasis on his partner, Ethan, and those friends who remained important social supports as Ben's functional health deteriorated. GMHC social workers and volunteers received direction from Ben and later from Ethan, Ben's designated proxy for health and related decisions. The involvement of informal and formal providers was dictated by Ben's wish for specific direct or indirect support for emotional, social, and instrumental assistance related to the vicissitudes of the disease process. Ben was seen as an autonomous person wanting and using GMHC services in or outside a hospital setting. Increasingly, GMHC was used as a brokering and mediating function assisting Ben and Ethan to access vital social service, medical, mental health, income maintenance, legal, and other services.

Goals, Objectives, and/or Outcome Measures

The goal of services directed toward Ben Anderson and other PWAs is to enhance their quality of life after diagnosis by providing material and supportive services that allow for maximum individual autonomy, human dignity, and community participation. An array of practical outcomes or objectives flowed from this goal: (1) to stabilize income during periods of disability; (2) to provide medical information and updating; (3) to provide psychiatric consultation for depression; (4) to provide mental health counseling to maintain sobriety, handle family concerns, and overcome social isolation; (5) to provide emotional support and guidance to Ethan, his primary social support; (6) to provide instrumental assistance by volunteers in the home; (7) to assist Ben and Ethan in determining quality-of-life parameters and acting on them during serious illness and the advent of death; and (8) to provide support to Ethan and others during the bereavement process.

Use of Contract

An explicit contract was drawn about service between Ben and all GMHC service providers. A computerized case record allowed for the combining of service notes and clinical oversight by agency staff. Clients have the right to terminate from any and all services provided by GMHC. Clients' rights were detailed in a published client service directory given to Ben during his intake. It was vital that each provider reiterate Ben's right to accept or to reject proffered assistance. Ben had the right to file a complaint with GMHC's quality assurance system if there were evidences of disrespect, lack of responsiveness, breaches of confidentiality, or any other grievance. The development of a clear contract is especially important because it supports clients' rights and entitlements at GMHC, which may be wanting elsewhere because of discrimination toward PWAs, gay men, drug abusers, women, persons of color, and others.

Meeting Place and Use of Time

The strength of GMHC's community-based service approach is its flexibility and informality at times. Social workers and volunteers may meet in agency offices, hospitals, in the client's home, and elsewhere in the community. Service begins with a client's diagnosis and can continue until the client terminates services or dies. Support for caregivers can continue through the bereavement period. Services delivered by volunteers can occur during evenings and weekends based on clients' needs. Clients receiving case management services, because of severe illness and disability, have crisis services available at all times.

Interventions

The general service approach is both multimethod and multidisciplinary. Legal services, medical and public health education, financial advocacy, AIDS counseling, mental health and group support services, intensive case management, crisis management, and chores services were offered to Ben. Social work was the lead discipline for client services working closely with lawyers, health educators, mental health providers, and others. Typically, the use of one service, such as financial advocacy, cogwheels into other client services over the course of months and years. In very complicated cases involving complex interrelated problems, specific case management strategies are used. Services delivered by other specialized agencies for drug treatment, disability services, and long-term care may be brokered by GMHC social workers.

Stance of the Social Worker

In the early phase of intervention with Ben, the worker's stance was supportive and nonconfrontational, allowing for the client's maximum decision making. The focus was "living with AIDS," with a minimum of restriction and, when medically possible, support of Ben's need to not be defined by an AIDS diagnosis and not have all of his life concerns medicalized.

Social workers explored the functional requirements of Ben maintaining independence and biopsychosocial well-being during and after each health crisis. Social workers carefully monitored their own internal responses to the cumulative crises and sense of human tragedy that they experienced through close identification with Ben. A social worker may panic about life-threatening health crises and have an urge to protect a client from further harm by doing too much for the client. The fantasy may develop that if the social worker does as much as possible then the PWA will not succumb to AIDS. Social workers face considerable stress in working with PWAs; they require considerable organizational and peer support, respite, and rewards to sustain their efforts.

Social workers may be gratified through working with PWAs, but they may also receive a good deal of anger from PWAs who are fearful and uncertain about their plight. As Ben became more functionally dependent on others to maintain himself in the community, the social worker and GMHC volunteers made themselves available to bear witness to his grief and sadness about losses of physical well-being and independence. The social worker validated Ben's areas of control, both practical and symbolic, by supporting his plan to limit medical intervention and engaging him in a life review discussion about how he wished to be remembered by others. The worker maintained a balanced perspective during these discussions that did not avoid the discussion of personal mortality, but also focused on day-to-day living.

Use of Outside Resources

Fortunately, GMHC is no longer the "only game in town," as was more the case in an earlier description (Getzel, 1989). Other AIDS organizations exist on the neighborhood and regional levels. Traditional agencies serving the general community have taken on an AIDS focus as part of their programs, which has been abetted by public funding. An array of resources in the community assisted Ben Anderson.

Reassessment and Termination

Ben's case required constant assessment of the record by all GMHC staff and volunteers responsible for his evolving care plan. Toward the end of Ben's life, Ethan was in frequent contact with staff at GMHC. With enhanced contact in the last months of Ben's life, there was almost a daily reassessment of Ben's biopyschosocial condition. Termination from GMHC is associated with the death of the client or his or her transfer to a long-term facility, where further contact is unfeasible. The service objectives listed earlier were met cumulatively over the course of case contact.

PRACTICE IN CONTEXT

The practice approach described in the case illustration represents an effort to address the special needs of PWAs over time. As of this writing, PWAs require complex medical intervention because of the uncertain course of disease patterns culminating in an almost-certain death. Medical care wedded with GMHC's biopsychosocial services serve to relieve the considerable burdens of caregiving in the community. The use of in-home health care services are consonant with the approach developed by GMHC out of dire necessity in the early years of the pandemic. The stigma of HIV/AIDS still weighs heavily on the all those infected and affected, who are also typically coping with an array of prejudices.

The emotional burdens of professionals working with a stigmatized, generally younger population are enormous. Social workers' personal belief systems are strongly challenged. Despite our best efforts, people served meet a tragic end. Sadly, each cohort of PWAs is followed by another. GMHC's approach joins an army of volunteers with professionals. Despite the considerable organizational difficulties this entails, the model of community-based AIDS service organizations provides a growing and viable strategy of outreach and care.

REFERENCES

Altman, D. (1986). *AIDS in the mind of America*. New York: Anchor Book Press.

Altman, D. (1994). *Power and community: Organizational and cultural responses to AIDS*. London, England: Taylor & Francis.

Bartlett, L. (1990). Financing health care for persons with AIDS: balancing public and private responsibilites. In L. O. Gostin (Ed.), *AIDS and the health care system*. New Haven, CT: Yale University Press, pp. 211-220.

Bartlett, J. G. and Finkbeiner, A. K. (1996). *The guide to living with HIV infection*. Baltimore, MD: Johns Hopkins University Press.

Bateson, M. C., and Goldsby, R. (1988). *Thinking AIDS: The social response to the biological threat*. Reading, MA: Addison-Wesley.

Bayer, R. (1989). *Private act, social consequences: AIDS and politics of public health*. New York: The Free Press.

Blendon, R. J. and Donelon, K. (1990). AIDS and discrimination: Public and professional perspectives. In L. O. Gostin (Ed.), *AIDS and the health care system*. New Haven, CT: Yale University Press, pp. 177-184.

Cox, E. (1990). *Thanksgiving: An AIDS journal*. New York: Harper's Press.

Fox, D. M. and Thomas, E. M. (1990). The cost of AIDS: exaggerations, entitlement and economics. In L. O. Gostin (Ed.), *AIDS and the health care system*. New Haven, CT: Yale University Press, pp. 197-210.

Gambe, R. and Getzel, G. S. (1989). Group work with gay men with AIDS. *Social Casework, 70*(3), 172-179.

Gay Men's Health Crisis (1995a). *A pocket history of AIDS and GMHC*. New York: GMHC.

Gay Men's Health Crisis (1995b). *Challenging despair, changing the future 1993/1994 annual report*. New York: GMHC.

Gay Men's Health Crisis (1995c). *Client Programs*. New York: GMHC.

Gay Men's Health Crisis (1995d). *GMHC facts–vital statistics–May 1, 1995*. New York: GMHC.

Getzel, G. S. (1989). Responding effectively to a gay man in crisis. In T. S. Kerson and Associates (Eds.), *Social work in health settings.* Binghamton, NY: The Haworth Press.

Getzel, G. S. (1991a). AIDS. In A. Gitterman (Ed.), *Handbook of social work with vulnerable populations.* New York: Columbia Univerity Press, pp. 35-65.

Getzel, G. S. (1991b). Survival modes of people with AIDS in groups. *Social Work, 36*(1), 7-11.

Getzel, G. S. (1992). AIDS and social work: a decade later. *Social Work in Health Care, 17*(2), 1-9.

Getzel, G. S. and Mahony, K. (1990). Confronting human finitude: group work with people with AIDS. *Journal of Gay and Lesbian Psychotherapy, 1*(1), 105-120.

Glick, H. R. (1992). *The right to die: Policy innovations and its consequences.* New York: Columbia University Press.

Greenly, M. (1984). *Chronicle: The human side of AIDS.* New York: Irvington Publishers.

Grossman, A. H. and Silverstein, C., (1993). Facilitating support groups for professionals working with people with AIDS. *Social Work, 38*(2), 144-151.

King, M. B. (1994). *AIDS, HIV and mental health.* Cambridge, UK: Cambridge University Press.

Kramer, L. (1989). *Reports from the Holocaust.* New York: St. Martin's Press.

Levine, C. (1990). In and out of the hospital. In L. O. Gostin (Ed.), *AIDS and the health care system.* New Haven, CT: Yale, pp. 45-61.

Lopez, D. J. and Getzel, G. S. (1984). Helping gay patients in crisis. *Social Casework, 65,* 387-394.

Lopez, D. J. and Getzel, G. (1987). Strategies for volunteers caring for persons with AIDS. *Social Casework, 68,* 47-53.

Mann, J., Tarantola D. J. M., and Netter, T. W. (1992), *A global report: AIDS in the world.* Cambridge, MA: Harvard.

McCormack, T. P. (1990). *The AIDS benefit handbook*; New Haven, CN: Yale.

O'Dowd, M.A., Natalie, C., Orr, D., and McKegney, F. (1991). Characteristics of patients attending an HIV-related psychiatric outpatient clinic. *Hospital and Community Psychiatry, 42*(6), 615-619.

Palacios-Jimenez, L. and Shernoff, M. (1987). *Eroticizing safer sex.* New York: Gay Men's Health Crisis.

Rounds, K. A., Galinsky, M. J., and Stevens L. S. (1991). Linking people with AIDS in rural communities: the telephone group. *Social Work. 36*(1), 13-18.

Shernoff, M. (1990). Why every social worker should be challenged by AIDS. *Social Work, 35*(1), 5-8.

Shilts, R. (1988). *The band played on: politics, people and AIDS.* New York: St. Martin's Press.

Watney, S. (1989). Taking liberties and introduction. In E. Carter and S. Watney (Eds.) *Taking liberties: AIDS and cultural politics.* London, England: Serpent's Tail, 11-57.

PART IV:
MENTAL HEALTH CARE

Chapter 20

Brief Treatment:
Community Mental Health

Maria DeOca Corwin
Elizabeth Read

CONTEXT

Description of the Setting

The Family and Children's Service Agency is one of the outpatient components of a comprehensive community mental health center that serves a midsize city and surrounding suburban towns. It is a preferred provider for an employee assistance program (EAP) that assesses troubled employees and refers them to treatment for a contracted number of visits. In this case, a particular employee was referred for substance abuse and had three prepaid visits for evaluation under her benefit package. If further treatment were indicated and the client agreed, payment would become the client's responsibility.

"The central task of an EAP is early detection, assessment, and amelioration of worker problems that affect productivity" (Winegar, 1992, p. 64). The client in this case was referred to the agency after she was sent home because she had a hangover. She was required to see a counselor at the EAP to provide assessment, referral, and brief treatment services. The EAP counselor determined that she should be seen for a substance abuse evaluation and selected the family and children's service agency as the appropriate evaluation and treatment resource for this client. The agency provides a variety of outpatient services, including individual, family, and group counseling, psychiatric evaluations, psychological testing, and individual, family, and group substance abuse counseling.

An external-program EAP, such as the one in this case illustration, also manages health care benefits for employers. The EAP monitors the quality, progress, and outcome of the employee's treatment and provides an evaluation summary form that serves as a quality assurance mechanism. The evaluation form ensures that there is a substance abuse evaluation standard—that is, that an adequate amount of clinical information is collected to determine the presence or absence of substance abuse and the degree of impairment, so as to ensure an appropriate level of care. Such substance abuse evaluation forms typically request basic demographic information; a brief description and history of the presenting problem, employment history, health history, and drug/alcohol history; mental status examination, clinical summary, and clinical severity index; and treatment plan (Goodman, Brown, and Deitz, 1992; Winegar, 1992). Although there are a number of rapid assessment instruments for substance abuse, in this instance the evaluation form, coupled with the clinician's experience in substance abuse evaluation, proved sufficient in arriving at a diagnosis and intervention plan.

Managed care has had a major impact on substance abuse treatment programs, where the lack of widely accepted standards of treatment and relatively poor outcomes (rates of relapse range from 25 percent to 90 percent after the first year of completing a program) have led to a demand from employers and insurers for more efficient and effective methods of treatment. The 28-day inpatient treatment program, which had been the standard, has been replaced by partial hospitalization and intensive outpatient treatment. The treatment focus is now on relapse prevention through the treatment of problems in living and through improving social functioning. Managed mental health care organizations have also focused on developing guidelines for determining the appropriate level of care (particularly criteria for determining the necessity of inpatient care) and for selecting outpatient treatment modalities and treatment strategies (Beck, Wright, Newman, and Liese, 1993; Winegar, 1992). The EAP substance abuse evaluation form represents one method for bringing uniformity to the decision-making process. The clinician and external reviewer are more likely to be in agreement on the course of treatment if both are utilizing the same set of evaluation criteria.

Selection of the appropriate level of care is dependent on the degree of biological, psychological, and social impairment. The most severe level of impairment is where the physical dependence would lead to dangerous physical withdrawal symptoms upon stopping usage and where all areas of functioning, including the ability to attend to daily tasks of living, have been negatively impacted. A more moderate level of abuse impairment involves tolerance and psychological dependence with daily negative consequences for the individual's functioning in interpersonal and occupational roles. At a less severe level of impairment, the urge to abuse is present weekly and interferes with optimal attention, concentration, and performance of tasks (Goodman, Brown, and Deitz, 1992).

Assessment of a higher level of impairment would indicate that more restrictive or protective levels of care and a variety of after-care services are appropriate interventions, while the less severe levels of impairment indicate that community-based interventions, shorter-term treatment, and greater levels of client responsibility for goal setting and changes in behavior are appropriate (Heinssen, Levendusky, and Hunter, 1995). The client in this case study met the criteria for a moderate level of impairment, and therefore a community-based, brief therapy approach was indicated.

The family and children's service agency was selected as a preferred provider for the EAP, because it had staff trained in substance abuse evaluation and treatment. It also offers a variety of substance abuse treatment modalities to meet the different needs of clients, as well as mental health services for clients with dual diagnoses or where substance abuse issues are complicated by personality factors or psychological conflicts. As a member of the consortium of agencies that comprise the community mental health center in this area, the client would have easy access to other services, such as vocational counseling, crisis intervention services (inpatient and outpatient), and case management services.

The agency is a part of a decentralized community mental health system. That is, it is a relatively small neighborhood-based office rather than in a downtown center. Clients may be less reluctant to accept a referral to a family and children's service agency located in a converted private home than in a building with the stigmatizing title of a mental health center. Also, decentralized offices tend to have a shorter waiting period for receiving services, which can reduce some of the resentment and anxiety that is associated with being an involuntary client. The agency also has a sliding fee scale, which helps make the cost of treatment more manageable for clients without additional prepaid benefits for mental health/substance abuse services.

Policy

Since the mid-1980s, several factors have contributed to an increased interest in briefer methods of treatment. Foremost among these has been the rapidly rising cost of mental health services. Although only 5 percent of the insured use their mental health/substance abuse benefits, mental health service costs in the recent past have accounted for 25 percent of total health care costs (Goodman, Brown, and Deitz, 1992; Wells, 1994). In an attempt to contain escalating costs, many insurers and employers have turned to managed mental health care approaches. Managed care refers to

> a variety of strategies, systems, and mechanisms that have as their objectives the monitoring and control of the utilization of mental health and substance abuse services while maintaining satisfactory levels of quality of care. Essentially, managed care clients' needs are matched to appropriate treatment resources, and then the delivery and outcome of these resources are monitored. (Winegar, 1992, p. 8)

With the push to contain costs came major shifts in the treatment paradigms for mental health and substance abuse delivery systems. Characteristics of the old systems such as free-choice care, elective admissions, long-term hospitalizations, and open-ended outpatient therapy have shifted to preferred providers, external review, brief hospitalizations, community resources, relapse prevention, and highly focused interventions (Heinssen, Levendusky, and Hunter, 1995). Accountability is a key component of this treatment paradigm shift. That is, with dwindling resources and a shrinking safety net, if costs are to be controlled and mental health benefits preserved, providers must demonstrate the efficiency and effectiveness of their interventions. Accountability means that practitioners "set realistic treatment goals, . . . document progress, recommend new therapy approaches to replace ones that are not successful, and terminate therapy when goals have been achieved." The notion of accountability in the managed care model has also been expanded to include accountability to the managed mental health care firm or employee assistance programs, in addition to the client (Winegar, 1992, p. 158).

Technology

There are other reasons for the emergence of short-term approaches as the treatments of choice during the past decade. First, there has been growing empirical evidence for the effectiveness of short-term, focused, structured interventions. Several studies comparing long-term and time-limited treatment with adult, children, and families have found that the outcomes are equivalent (Budman and Gurman, 1988; Koss and Butcher, 1986; Smyrnios and Kirby, 1993). Research studies have also found that brief therapies appear to fit clients' preferences, in that dropout rates are significantly less in planned short-term treatment. In a study of 149 new patients at a community mental health clinic, the main finding was that the dropout rate for time-limited therapy was half of the rate for open-ended therapies (Sledge, Moras, Hartley, and Levine, 1990). This matches the finding in a nationwide study that the average number of sessions attended is six to eight, even if long-term therapy had been planned (Wells, 1994).

The Community Mental Health Act of 1963 allowed greater availability of mental health services, but there continues to be concern about reaching underserved populations and about effectively meeting the needs of the more diverse client populations that have in recent years been seeking help at community mental health centers. Studies have consistently found that clients of color and working-class and poor clients have underutilized mental health services and have had high rates of attrition when they do seek help (Sue, Zane, and Young, 1994). Research studies on the expectations of such clients about the helping process demonstrate that there has been a clash in perspective between many clinicians and clients about the helping process. These clients come to treatment generally expecting help with specific problems, particularly interpersonal ones, or with states of distress within a relatively short period, while clinicians often have vague or overly ambitious goals and an expectation of an open-ended treatment process. Brief therapy approaches, then, are more congruent with the help-seeking models of culturally diverse, working-class, and poor clients and are being considered as one way of reducing high dropout rates (Wells, 1994).

Budman and Gurman (1988) suggest that the high rate of attrition in planned long-term treatment may not just represent client dissatisfaction, but may be due to the fact that many clients received the help they needed and wanted within a few sessions and were ready to stop, although the clinician may not have deemed the treatment complete. Some studies have found that clinicians tend to evaluate the outcome of their interventions more negatively than their clients, because they focused on their original assessments of significant pathology and thus viewed the client's gain in functioning as insufficient by that standard. Clients tended to have more limited goals, such as improved interpersonal and job functioning, and they felt therapy had been helpful in reaching these goals. Even when the treatment was long-term, the greatest gains in therapy took place in the earliest sessions, with progressively diminishing returns as treatment progressed, contradicting the popular notion that more therapy is always better than less (Wells, 1994).

Strategies for Substance Abuse and Chronic Mental Illness

The shift in treatment strategies for substance abuse treatment programs and services to the chronically mentally ill, stemming from the need for more effective and less costly clinical service systems, has been to more pragmatic and parsimonious interventions. The emphasis in these programs is now as much on improving social functioning and management of problems in living (relapse prevention) as on the illness itself (Heinssen, Levendusky, and Hunter, 1995; Sullivan, Hartmann, Dillon, and Wolk, 1994) Many of the therapeutic techniques of brief therapy, particularly cognitive-behavioral techniques, have been incorporated into substance abuse and psychiatric rehabilitation strategies, because these techniques promote problem-solving and self-efficacy development goals. The shift has been away from viewing the client as a passive participant to one of empowering clients with the skills and resources to manage their illnesses over the course of a lifetime (Hunter, 1995).

The Social Work Philosophy and Value System

Finally, in examining any rationale for brief therapy, it is important to look at the degree to which such a practice approach fits the social work philosophy of practice and its value system. There is a general concern that brief therapy, particularly under managed care, means denial of care and therefore is an unethical way to practice. However, as the previously cited empirical evidence indicates, brief therapy may more closely approximate what clients want from treatment. "Specifically, it is consistent with the notions of the least invasive procedures first, informed patient consent (since treatment is collaborative) and respect for patient autonomy" (Cooper, 1995, p. 28). The brief therapy principles of collaboration, competency, and attending to client meaning systems are also consistent with the values of "affirming . . . uniqueness and individuality" and "affirming problem-solving capacities and self-determination" of clients, which are cardinal social work practice principles. In addition, these principles are akin to the social work techniques of "starting where the client is" and empowerment, as well as the strengths perspective that is marking the paradigm shift from a pathology basis to a competency basis in social work practice (Saleeby, 1992, p. 6).

Social Workers' Competency in Brief Therapy

A central issue as to the adequacy of brief therapy approaches for social work practice relates to the therapist's degree of competence in brief therapy. The lack of graduate programs and comprehensive training programs means that many clinicians are not adequately trained in brief therapy methods. Too often the assumption is made by clinicians that brief therapy requires less skill or that brief therapy means simply a lesser amount of long-term therapy. In actuality, brief therapy requires greater skill, given the rapidity with which the therapist must begin assessment, treatment planning, and intervention and because of the high level of therapist activity, attentiveness, selectivity in focus, intuitiveness, and risk-taking (Cooper, 1995). The following discussion is an introduction to the central tenets and practice techniques of brief therapy, which provide the framework for understanding the kinds of practice decisions that the clinician made in the EAP case described in the main part of the text.

Brief Treatment: Key Features

In the past, brief therapy was defined by a limit on the number of sessions. However, there was little agreement as to what the greatest number of sessions needed to be to qualify as brief treatment (from 15 to 25 sessions being designated as the outer limit). However, recent definitions have focused more on the effective use of time and the systematic use of certain concepts and principles in a strategic manner than on the actual number of sessions. Thus, Wells' (1994) definition of brief therapy emphasizes the limits placed on both goals and length of contact, while Cooper's (1995) description focuses on the "clinical features and value orientation" shared by the many forms of brief therapy. Winegar (1992), describing brief therapy from the managed mental health care perspective, emphasized the guiding principle of the least invasive treatment necessary to bring about the desired change and an intermittent or family practitioner model of treatment.

There are many models of brief therapy, including psychodynamic, crisis intervention, cognitive-behavioral, interpersonal, strategic-structural, and constructivist. While there are significant differences among these models with regard to theoretical formulations of the origins of psychological problems, there are many areas of convergence in certain basic values and assumptions about the treatment process and in treatment techniques. Some of the key practice features and beliefs that are shared by most brief treatment models follow:

1. The rapid establishment of a positive therapeutic alliance involves the creation of a safe environment and encouragement of optimism and motivation. Involuntary and mandated clients are encouraged to become involved clients.
2. Timely response to service requests, rapid assessment, and early intervention means that therapy begins as quickly as possible, with the initial phone call if possible. The assessment and intervention stages are integrated and novelty (a new perspective or a change in

behavior) is introduced early on, usually in the first session, to quickly begin the change process (Budman, Hoyt, and Friedman, 1992).

3. An emphasis on current stresses and symptoms with a "here and now" problem-solving orientation in therapy means that more emphasis is placed on what is currently motivating the client to enter treatment and on what is to be done rather than on the past determinants of problems.

4. Flexible use of time means that therapy is "time-sensitive" or "time-effective;" the length of sessions, the interval between sessions, and the length of contact is a function of the client's needs and what yields the best results in the shortest period of time (Cooper, 1995; Hoyt, 1994)

5. Worker-client collaboration emphasizes early identification of realistic, achievable, measurable goals and objectives. There is an attempt to maintain a clear, specific focus from session to session and frequent reassessment of progress toward goals.

6. There is a high level of worker-client interaction and a clear definition of the responsibilities of each. Client strengths and resources are identified and utilized to address current difficulties. The therapist structures sessions, provides education about resources and skills, and helps in transferring gains in therapy to the client's real life, for example, through the use of homework assignments.

7. An eclecticism of technique and flexibility is used in individual, family, and group modalities. Participation in community resources, for example, self-help groups, is encouraged (Hoyt, 1994).

8. Brief therapies share some values and assumptions. It is generally assumed that change is inevitable and occurs mainly outside of therapy, that clients have capacities and healthy strivings that can be drawn upon for resolving current difficulties, and that pragmatism and the least invasive procedure should determine the level of intervention (Cooper, 1995; Budman, Hoyt, and Friedman, 1992).

Interventions

In general, the therapy process in brief treatment is more structured, focused, and systematic than in longer-term work. In each brief therapy session and in each stage of the treatment process, there are tasks to be accomplished. The first session is a very important one in brief therapy, and it has a number of specific tasks. As Budman, Hoyt, and Friedman note, "the first encounter sets the tone, structure, direction, and foundation of the therapy" (1992, p. 4). First interview tasks include (1) developing a positive working alliance; (2) assessment of client's needs and motivational level to engage in the change process; (3) orientation to the therapy process;

(4) determination of a focus; (5) mutual formulation of goals and criteria for positive outcome; (6) early gain in therapy, usually through introduction to the client of a novel way of thinking, feeling, or doing; and (7) eliciting feedback about the therapy session and homework, if assigned (Cooper, 1995; Hoyt, 1994).

Subsequent therapy sessions have a similar structured quality. The tasks for the middle phase of treatment serve the purpose of maintaining the treatment focus and facilitating the change process. The primary tasks for this phase of the treatment process are (1) intersession bridging, which is a review of the previous session focus, homework, and the client's experience of the problem and attempts at problem resolution during the period between sessions; (2) refinement of focus, if necessary, to ensure efficient use of time; (3) review of progress toward those goals and of time remaining and examination of any obstacles to change, including ineffective intervention strategies; (4) introduction of additional interventions, negotiation of new homework assignments, and transfer to the client's real life of the knowledge and skills gained in therapy; (5) end of session summarizing and bridging to next session; and (6) eliciting of feedback from client on his or her experience of session and homework (Cooper, 1995; Hoyt, 1994).

The final phase of treatment is centered on preparation for termination. The tasks for termination are the following: (1) review of the therapy process, including examination of the therapeutic relationship, gains made, and issues not discussed or not resolved; (2) working through of emotional responses to termination; (3) consolidation and transfer of gains to other areas of the client's life and planning of maintenance strategies; (4) review of and solidification of connections to client's social support system; (5) referral to community resources, if needed; (6) evaluation of practice and documentation of progress and outcomes; and (7) a planned follow-up session or telephone contact (Hepworth and Larsen, 1990; Hoyt, 1994).

Brief Treatment of Substance Abuse

Solution-focused and cognitive-behavioral models are currently the treatment approaches of choice for working with substance abuse within a time-limited framework, although other relapse prevention approaches are emerging, which target clients' social functioning and environmental difficulties and help them to make use of community resources and job opportunities. These approaches employ techniques that address the substance abuser's chronic maladaptive responses to stresses and employ environmental interventions to address environmental (including interpersonal) sources of stress or environmental stimuli to relapse (Hawkins and Fraser, 1987; Miller and Rollnick, 1991; Sullivan et al., 1994).

Cognitive-behavioral interventions focus on behavioral self-control training, cognitive restructuring of addictive beliefs, social skills training, stress management, self-efficacy enhancement, and community reinforcement (12-step programs) (Beck et al., 1993). Solution-focused methods seek to diminish defensiveness about substance abuse through introduction of a tolerable discrepancy between stated goals and behaviors and to engage the client's resources and strengths in moving toward sobriety by having clients identify needs, wishes, and goals for treatment (Selekman, 1993; Berg, 1994). Both of these approaches "emphasize accurate assessment of motivational levels . . . , cooperatively engaging patients at the level they are willing to change and capitalizing on these successes to move toward recovery" (Cooper, 1995, p. 10).

DECISIONS ABOUT PRACTICE

Description of Client and Presenting Problem

The client is a widowed, middle-aged, white woman, who lives alone. Mrs. Spina has two years of college. She has been steadily employed in an administrative position in a business office. She has no children. Her siblings and parents live in other states, and, while they have positive relationships, distance prevents them from being a more active part of her social support network. Since the death of her husband five years ago, when Mrs. Spina began abusing alcohol, she had become more socially isolated, rarely socializing with old friends or with friends from work.

The referral to the EAP was the first time Mrs. Spina had been identified as not performing well on the job. The contact with the agency was her first mental health contact. Mrs. Spina had attended Alcoholics Anonymous (AA) five years previous to this contact but had been uncomfortable with the message and the group process. She had not made any subsequent attempts to return to AA or to seek other help for her drinking problem, although she had been experiencing growing concern about her drinking.

Definition of the Client and Interventions

Mrs. Spina was an involuntary client, who was clearly embarrassed by having to be seen for an alcohol abuse evaluation. The first decision made by the worker was how to respond to the client's resistance, expressed as irritability and annoyance about the process of setting up an appointment. The clinician understood the client's embarrassment and anxiety about having to come in for an evaluation and responded to the covert meanings about setting up an appointment, rather than to the overt difficult behavior, by being accommodating to the client's appointment time needs. This interaction represented two fundamental brief treatment principles. First are that the treatment process should preferably begin before the first interview session. In this instance, the worker began the first session task of establishing the treatment conditions of safety, respect, and rapport during the telephone contact. Second, by the end of the first session clients have been distinguished from nonclients or, in deShazer's terms, "customers" from "visitors" (Cooper, 1995).

Most involuntary and mandated clients begin treatment as nonclients and must be assisted in becoming clients. Attention to the interpersonal context of resistance–that is, the ability of the worker to hear the client's unspoken fears and to manage negative countertransference reactions to provocative or hostile behaviors–is one method of dealing with resistance to becoming a client. Clarity and honesty about the referral process is another way of dealing with the client's concerns about and reluctance to become involved in treatment (Rooney, 1988). In this case, there were issues around confidentiality, job security, and clinician responsibility to the referral source, the EAP, which needed to be acknowledged and addressed. In the first session, the clinician first addressed the issue of confidentiality and what would have to be reported back to the EAP. This was essentially the diagnosis, recommendations for treatment, and the outcome of the evaluation–brief treatment contact. The issue of job jeopardy was also addressed, as were the client's feelings about the referral. Having the opportunity to express her anger and embarrassment about being caught appeared to have allowed Mrs. Spina to look at the issue for which she was being referred and to reflect upon what she wanted to get from the contact. The time frame of three allotted sessions was also reviewed with the client. Her acceptance of the time frame may have served as a motivating force for her.

A major determination that has to be made in the first session in a brief therapy substance abuse case is the level of the client's motivation to make changes in his or her addictive behavior, in order to tailor the brief intervention to fit what the client is actually able to do rather than what the clinician thinks would be a worthy goal or outcome. Thus, the worker must assess who in the client's system is willing and able to change, what he or she is willing to do to make the necessary changes or adaptations, and whether the appropriate interventions to meet the client's needs can be offered within the time frame available to the client.

Prochaska, DiClemente, and Norcross developed a model of how people change, based on their research of self-initiated and professionally facilitated changes in addictive behaviors. In their model, "modification of addictive behaviors involves progression through five stages–precontemplation, contemplation, preparation, action, and maintenance" (1992, p. 1102). In the precontemplation stage, there is no motivation to change. Rather the client is unaware or "underaware" that substance abuse is a problem for him or her. In the contemplation stage, the person is aware that a problem exists and is considering doing something about the problem, but has not made the commitment to take action. Weighing the pros and cons and possible solutions is an important part of this stage. In the preparation stage, the individual either intends to take action shortly or has made an unsuccessful recent attempt at change. Action is where patients actively modify "their behavior, experiences, or environment in order to overcome their problem . . . and maintenance is the stage in which people work to prevent relapse and consolidate the gains attained during action" (Prochaska, DiClemente, and Norcross, 1992, p. 1104).

Mrs. Spina moved from the precontemplation stage to the contemplation stage by the end of the first session. It appeared that Mrs. Spina had been poised to move in that direction and that the crisis of being in jeopardy of losing her job and in a counseling situation, in which she could be assisted to progress from precontemplation to contemplation, made it possible for her to move to the next stage rapidly. In the evaluation of the client's alcohol usage, the clinician was able to accurately empathize and reflect back to the client the thoughts, feelings, and conflicts she was experiencing about her drinking (a form of motivational interviewing) (Miller and Rollnick, 1991). This raised the client's awareness of the centrality that drinking had assumed in her life and of its negative consequences for her without arousing feelings of guilt, shame, or embarrassment that can lead to defensiveness and denial. Mrs. Spina's initial guarded stance shifted to an openness to self-evaluation and to an examination of her options for dealing with her acknowledged drinking problem.

Treatment Goals and Objectives

Having weighed the pros and cons of addressing her drinking problem and having learned the worker's assessment of her current situation and treatment needs, Mrs. Spina was able to define treatment goals and objectives for the remaining two sessions. She agreed that taking steps to alter her drinking behavior would be the goal for this contact. Attending AA and making use of behavioral management strategies were objectives to achieve the goal of changing addictive behaviors. The worker helped her to identify internal and external triggers, her personal warning signs that she was likely to drink again, and to formulate a plan of how she might manage these situations. That is, the clinician helped the client to restructure her day, which had been structured around drinking, and gave her the behavioral strategies to manage cravings and stresses (Liftik, 1995). Attending AA would also address the risk factor of social isolation for Mrs. Spina's female pattern of problem drinking, that is, drinking alone and covering up the problem drinking (Turner, 1989).

Contract

The contract between the worker and client consisted then of the mutually agreed upon definition of the problem to be worked on, the agreed-upon level of care, and the goals and objectives for the three-session contact and follow-up contact. They agreed that Mrs. Spina did not need detoxification or rehabilitation and that her treatment needs could be met on an outpatient basis. She agreed to try AA again and to attend a meeting before the second scheduled interview. The worker provided her with a list of AA meeting places and times. At the end of the first session, Mrs. Spina had moved from the contemplation stage to the preparation stage of change. She had also gained some of the tools needed for taking the next step toward change in addictive behaviors (Prochaska, DiClemente, and Norcross, 1992).

Use of Time

The time limit of three sessions shaped the nature of the therapeutic relationship and the goals and intervention strategies selected. The worker had to quickly overcome the client's anger and reluctance and rapidly establish a positive working alliance if anything were to be accomplished within this time frame. The goals had to be realistic and achievable within the time frame, and the intervention strategies had to be precisely matched to the goal and objectives (Wells, 1994). Although the worker recognized that Mrs. Spina probably had unresolved bereavement issues that would continue to constitute a risk factor for abuse of alcohol, the client wanted and could only pursue the goal of sobriety at this point in her recovery. Therefore, bereavement work would have to be postponed or become part of her AA work. The client was seeking guidance on how to manage the day-to-day urge to drink, not insight about why she drinks,

FIGURE 20.1. Ecomap for Mrs. Spina

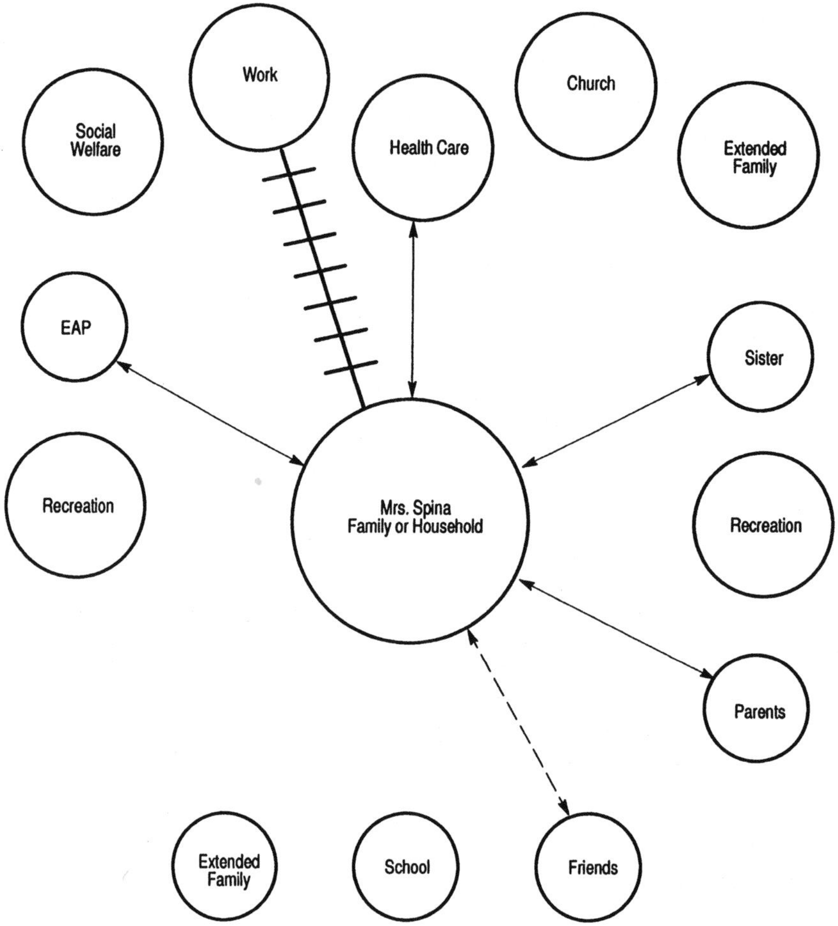

and therefore that had to be the focus of interventions for this treatment contact.

By the second session, Mrs. Spina had moved from the preparation stage to the action stage of change. She had attended several meetings since the first session and had established a daily schedule of attendance. She had bought the "Big Book" and she was ready this time to hear the message and to respond to the support of the group in her struggle for sobriety. She reported not having drunk alcohol during the previous week. Therefore, the worker's interventions in this session centered on relapse prevention through the monitoring of such risk factors as boredom, sadness, isolation, and unrealistic expectations about the recovery process.

By the third and last session, Mrs. Spina was firmly established in her connection to AA. She was attending meetings on a daily basis and had identified a potential sponsor. She reported that she had not done any drinking in the three weeks since the first session and expressed some confidence that she would be able to continue to be sober. The foci, then, in the final session were on the review and consolidation of gains made and on termination issues. Mrs. Spina wanted to continue her focus on maintaining sobriety and on decreasing her social isolation. She was disinclined to seek additional therapy for unresolved issues and feelings. A follow-up telephone contact was planned and agreed to by worker and client.

Stance of the Social Worker

"Addressing alcoholism requires that [the worker] play multiple roles, such as coach, teacher (transmitting information about addiction and recovery), counselor, and therapist" (Zweben, 1995, p. 198). In the stage of early recovery, the worker generally adopts an active role, and in substance abuse brief therapy an activist role is essential. The worker in this case study was, by training and inclination, more likely to favor introspection and exploration of underlying, causal issues. To meet the treatment needs and expectations of this client, the worker adopted an activist, educative, guiding stance. The worker provided information about the agency, confidentiality issues, the agency's obligation to the EAP, AA meetings, and behavior management techniques. She also educated the client about the process of addiction and recovery and about risk factors for relapse. The worker saw the referral to AA as a way of addressing both the client's alcoholism and her need for a social support network.

Termination

While the client desired no further clinical services, Mrs. Spina was given information about the use of therapy with addictive behaviors, treatment resources, and the role of the agency in assisting her in getting services in the future should she desire to do so. In reviewing the course of the treatment, worker and client were in agreement about the progress that had been made. In terms of measurable, behavioral criteria, Mrs. Spina had achieved the goals of reducing her drinking and becoming involved with AA. In terms of less observable gains, the client demonstrated improvements in self-esteem, in her sense of efficacy, and in a sense of optimism that changes could be made with a problem that she had felt hopeless about before treatment. While there were differences in perspective of worker and client regarding the need for further therapy, both worker and client were in agreement that maintaining sobriety was the first order of business; therefore, the client's involvement with AA was the most appropriate ongoing level of care for her.

Differential Discussion

This three-session intervention demonstrates the utility of employing brief therapy principles to effect a positive outcome. The key brief therapy features that appear to have been most useful in this case were (1) client determination of goals and client definition of positive outcome; (2) rapid establishment of a positive working alliance; (3) client-worker agreement on specific, achievable goals; (4) an active, structured, and focused intervention approach; and (5) connection to community resources. The brief treatment of substance abuse features that appeared to have contributed to the positive outcome were (1) successful assessment of the client's motivation level for change in addictive behaviors, (2) interventions geared to that level of motivation, and (3) relapse prevention interventions.

It was also helpful that the worker could adapt her therapeutic style to match the client's needs and expectations and that the worker could join the client in feeling there had been a successful outcome to the intervention, in spite of the client's disinclination to get additional therapy for underlying problems. The worker concluded that the client was likely to return for additional help in the future if she needed it, because of her experience of success with brief therapy. This intermittent treatment model matches most clients' use of clinical services and therefore is an important perspective for brief therapists to foster. At follow-up, the client reported that she had maintained her sobriety and remained committed to attending AA.

REFERENCES

Beck, A. T., Wright, F. D., Newman, C. F., and Liese, B. S. (1993). *Cognitive therapy of substance abuse*. New York: Guilford Press.
Berg, I. K. (1994). *Family based services*. New York: W.W. Norton.
Budman, S. H. and Gurman, A. S. (1988). *Theory and practice of brief psychotherapy*. New York: Guilford Press.

Budman, S. H., Hoyt, M. F., and Friedman, S. (Eds.). (1992). *The first session in brief therapy.* New York: Guilford Press.

Cooper, J. F. (1995). *A primer of brief psychotherapy.* New York: W. W. Norton.

Goodman, M., Brown, J., and Dietz, P. (1992). *Managing managed care: A mental health practitioner's survival guide.* Washington, DC: American Psychiatric Press.

Hawkins, J. D. and Fraser, M. W. (1987). The social networks of drug abusers before and after treatment. *The International Journal of the Addictions, 22*(11), 343-355.

Heinssen, R. K., Levendusky, P. G., and Hunter, R. H. (1995). Client as colleague: Therapeutic contracting with the seriously mentally ill. *American Psychologist, 50*(7), 522-532.

Hepworth, D. H. and Larsen, J. (1990). *Direct social work practice: Theory and skills.* Belmont, CA: Wadsworth.

Hoyt, M. F. (1994). Characteristics of psychotherapy under managed behavioral healthcare. *Behavioral Healthcare Tomorrow, 3*(5), 59-62.

Hunter, R. H. (1995). Benefits of competency-based treatment programs. *American Psychologist, 50*(7), 509-513.

Koss, M. P. and Butcher, J. N. (1986). Research on brief psychotherapy. In S. L. Garfield and A. E. Bergin (Eds.), *Handbook of psychotherapy and behavior change,* Third Edition. New York: John Wiley & Sons, pp. 627-670.

Liftik, J. (1995). Assessment. In S. Brown (Ed.), *Treating alcoholism.* San Francisco: Jossey-Bass, 57-94.

Miller, W. R. and Rollnick, S. (1991). *Motivational interviewing: Preparing people to change addictive behavior.* New York: Guilford Press.

Prochaska, J. O., DiClemente, C. C., and Norcross, J. C. (1992). In search of how people change: Applications to addictive behavior. *American Psychologist, 47*(9), 1102-1113.

Rooney, R. H. (1988). Socialization strategies for involuntary clients. *Social Casework, 69*(March), 131-140.

Saleeby, D. (Ed.). (1992). *The strengths perspective in social work practice.* New York: Longman.

Selekman, M. D. (1993). *Pathways to change: Brief therapy solutions with difficult adolescents.* New York: Guilford Press.

Sledge, W. H., Moras, K., Hartley, D., and Levine, M. (1990). Effect of time-limited psychotherapy on patient dropout rates. *American Journal of Psychiatry, 147*(10), 1341-1347.

Smyrnios, K. X. and Kirkby, R. J. (1993). Long-term comparison of brief versus unlimited psychodynamic treatments with children and their parents. *Journal of Consulting and Clinical Psychology, 61*(6), 1020-1027.

Sue, S., Zane, N., and Young, K. (1994). Research on psychotherapy with culturally diverse populations. In A. E. Bergin and S. I. Garfield (Eds.), *Handbook of psychotherapy and behavior change,* Fourth Edition. New York: John Wiley & Sons, pp. 783-817.

Sullivan, W. P., Hartmann, D. J., Dillon, D., and Wolk, J. L. (1994). Implementing case management in alcohol and drug treatment. *Families in Society,* 75(1), 67-73.

Turner, J. (1989). Treatment issues for alcoholic women. *Social Casework,* 70(6), 354-369.

Wells, R. A. (1994). *Planned short-term treatment.* New York: The Free Press.

Winegar, N. (1992). *The clinician's guide to managed mental health care.* Binghamton, NY: The Haworth Press, Inc.

Zweben, J. E. (1995). The therapist's role in early and ongoing recovery. In S. Brown (Ed.), *Treating alcoholism.* San Francisco: Jossey-Bass, pp. 197-230.

Chapter 21

"Would You Abandon Your Child?" An Inpatient Psychiatric Staff Confront Change, a Difficult Case–and Each Other

Sherri Alper
Toba Schwaber Kerson

CONTEXT

Description of the Setting

The Department of Psychiatric Services at Southwestern Vermont Medical Center (SVMC) in Bennington, Vermont, provides psychiatric care to area adolescents and adults. Formerly named The Special Management Unit (SMU), the service admitted both psychiatric patients and elderly patients with senile dementia whose behavior proved too disruptive for care on the medical floors of the hospital. The unit originally functioned solely as a nursing unit, but through the vision of a senior administrator who recognized the need for state-of-the-art psychiatric care, a psychiatrist was hired to assess the needs of the community and develop responsive psychiatric services.

By the time the client described in the chapter was admitted, the 10-bed unit had developed to include a range of services and an expanded interdisciplinary staff. Under the direction of the clinical director (the psychiatrist) and the administrative director (a social worker), the unit initiated an alcohol detoxification program and a partial hospitalization program. All patients were served within the context of the 10-bed unit, which occupied a separate wing on the fourth floor of the hospital. While staff expressed initial concern regarding the impact of a diverse diagnostic mix on treatment, productive clinical use of disparate diagnoses increased the effectiveness of the therapeutic milieu (Walker, 1994). Upon discharge, patients often commented that they gained a greater understanding of themselves through getting to know others who were either more fully recovered or more seriously ill than they were.

The unit is codirected by the clinical and administrative directors. A master's-level psychiatric nurse practitioner oversees nursing care, which is provided by registered nurses assisted by licensed practical nurses. A master's-level expressive arts therapist leads daily art therapy groups and is responsible for the development and coordination of recreational activities for patients. A master's level clinical social worker and the psychiatric nurse practitioner share the primary responsibility for individual, family, and group psychotherapy. A part-time MSW and certified alcohol and drug counselor provide direct service to patients admitted for detoxification and assist all staff in working with addicted clients. On a consultation basis, a psychologist in the community provides psychological testing as a component of patient evaluation. During the academic year, a student from an area graduate program in psychology interns on the unit.

Evolution from a Nursing Unit
to a Multidisciplinary Team

During the period of evolution from a nursing unit to a true multidisciplinary team, weekly staff meetings often focused on the clarification of roles, overlapping responsibilities, and unique expertise of each discipline in an effort to ensure a consistent and unified approach to the care of each patient (Bendicsen and Carlton, 1990; Rideout and Richardson, 1989; Yurkovich, 1990). Daily morning team meetings provided a forum for informal education between the disciplines regarding their respective roles and perspectives on patient care. For example, evening and night nursing staff often contributed valuable information and insight, since patients frequently interacted differently on the "off shift," after the structured activities of the day.

Policy

The laws relating to deinstitutionalization and the turning away from hospitalization have affected all inpatient work. Because they limited so drastically the number of days for which they are willing to pay for inpatient psychiatric care, Medicare, Medicaid, managed care companies, and other forms of insurance have made it less possible to provide sound treatment other than crisis work in inpatient settings (Strumwasser et al., 1991). The shift in federal policy from an emphasis on mental health needs in the 1960s and 1970s to drug and alcohol abuse in the 1980s and 1990s also influenced the psychiatric inpatient service.

Like community hospital psychiatric units in many states, the SMU unit complied with many state laws having to do with maintaining proper procedures and the protection of patients; for example, there are laws governing the use of chemical and physical restraints, informed consent, and involuntary hospitalization and treatment ((Bentley, 1993; Reamer, 1987; Rosenson, 1993). Such laws vary from state to state and complicate the provision of care in institutions such as SVMC, which serves patients from the neighboring states of New York and Massachusetts. The state of Vermont appoints a patient advocate to support patients hospitalized on psychiatric units (Annas, 1989; Protection and Advocacy for Mentally Ill Individuals Act, 1986). The SMU staff developed a collaborative and mutually respectful relationship with the state patient advocate who visited inpatient units throughout the state on a monthly basis and met with patients to discuss their care.

In addition to adhering to laws governing the treatment of the mentally ill, psychiatric units must also ensure that they are in compliance with Joint Commission on Accreditation of Health Care Organizations (JCAHO) guidelines for accreditation. Guidelines for psychiatric units include careful attention to issues such as the provision of a safe physical environment as well as specific protocols for interdisciplinary collaboration, treatment planning, and quality assurance. JCAHO accreditation has profound implications for third-party reimbursement, public opinion of quality of care, and program development.

The ethics and values of the various professions represented acted as important supports to the policies developed for the unit. Both nursing and social work staffs often referred to their own professional guidelines in decision making about patient care (Joseph and Conrad, 1989). The social worker referred specifically to the National Association of Social Workers (NASW) Code of Ethics (NASW, 1994).

In recent decades, the consumer advocacy movement has had an enormous impact on patient care (National Alliance for the Mentally Ill, 1995). Consumer advocacy organizations who work on behalf of the mentally ill and their families provide copies of "A Patient's Bill of Rights" and additional information, and advocate to ensure that state laws are obeyed and quality of care disputes are addressed.

Implications of Managed Care

The role that most managed care companies have defined for themselves is twofold: (1) to increase access to quality care for subscribers and

(2) to maintain cost-effective utilization for the payer (Monahan, 1994). Sources of conflict between caregivers and managed care services have primarily been related to the issue of clinically appropriate duration of services. The evolution of managed care has affected the delivery of psychiatric services in a number of important aspects. First, the average length of stay for an acute inpatient psychiatric admission at SVMC is now nine days, generally enforced by utilization reviewers from third-party payers (sometimes referred to by staff as a fiscogenic recovery). Second, clinical staff have needed to clarify treatment goals on a daily basis, as a result of both managed care review and continuous quality improvement. Third, patients admitted for acute psychiatric care are increasingly more seriously ill, especially with the downsizing or closing of state hospitals. Fourth, the ability to provide reliable outcome data has become increasingly important. Fifth, collaboration with outpatient providers of mental health services to create a seamless delivery system is more frequent. Finally, the survival of inpatient psychiatric units in community hospitals may depend in the future on the ability to provide a range of services in addition to short-term acute hospitalization.

In response to the dictates of a changing behavioral healthcare environment in Vermont, The Department of Psychiatric Services began several years ago to expand its services to include the partial hospitalization (day-treatment) program; the alcohol detoxification consultation/liaison services with area colleges, high schools, and nursing homes; as well as improved outreach education and public relations including workshops, a periodic newspaper column, radio programs on mental health, community screenings, and a concerted effort to develop an increasingly positive collaborative relationship with area physicians, the community mental health center, private practitioners, and area HMOs.

Social work education frequently emphasizes the potential strengths possible in unifying similar systems for advocacy and political action (Haynes and Mickelson, 1991; Richan, 1991). The administrative director, spurred by concern over the long-term well-being of small psychiatric units in community hospitals, founded an organization of psychiatrists and administrators from similar programs throughout the state, which met quarterly to address areas of mutual concern and share resources. Discussion often focused on political changes at the state level affecting the delivery of mental health services, program development, and practice issues. Occasionally, speakers from tertiary care facilities were invited to meet with the group to discuss collaborative opportunities for seamless delivery of care.

It is important to note that despite many of the legitimate concerns about the intrusion of managed care into the professional clinical arena, there have been positive developments as well. Clarity of treatment plans, accountability in relation to outcome, and increased interagency and interdisciplinary collaboration continue to improve the delivery of care (Sabin, 1991).

Technology

The primary technological advance in psychiatric care in recent years has been the development of several classes of drugs that have heralded major changes in the lives of two categories, in particular, of psychiatric disorders. Clozaril and resperidone have been used successfully in treating some patients with severe psychotic disorders who previously might have spent their lives in state institutions (Gerhart, 1990). Electroencephalography (EEG), brain mapping, and the adjunct use of computers have provided a glimpse into the potential for diagnostic accuracy and treatment efficiency (Squire, Stout, and Ruben, 1993). The development of selective serotonin reuptake inhibitors, successful weapons against depression, has promoted the successful treatment of clinical depression, without many of the bothersome side effects that previously characterized older medication

The primary technology, however, remains intervention that is not purely biological or medical. State-of-the-art psychiatric services in the 1990s provide staff with the knowledge base to use a variety of sophisticated interventions. Crisis intervention; individual, family, and group psychotherapy; behavior modification; cognitive therapy; the therapeutic milieu; and patient/family education provide the basis of technology to promote healing (Hogarty et al., 1991). It is often the role of the social worker to educate others in medical settings that "technology" is different in mental health services. The ability to cite research regarding various therapeutic modalities is often the most effective means of helping others understand that mental health is not unscientific and that acute inpatient psychiatric programs provide treatment rather than custodial care (Hobfoll and Shlomo, 1986; Rubin, 1985).

Organization

Southwestern Vermont Medical Center is a 140-bed community hospital in Bennington, Vermont, a town of about 13,000 people. Located in the southwestern corner of Vermont, SVMC services the local community and neighboring towns in Massachusetts and New York. The hospital has a well-developed community outreach program, which provides education and wellness services to the surrounding communities, generally free of charge. The Department of Psychiatric Services has played an important role in the delivery of workshops through the Wellness Connection. Typical mental health offerings have included workshops on menopause, stress reduction, anger management, parenting, and separation and divorce. Free community screenings for addictions and depression have been successfully hosted for several years.

The Department of Psychiatric Services reports directly to the senior vice president, who is a strong advocate for the interests of the service within the institution and in the community. The collaborative relationship with the senior vice president promotes creativity and program development, and serves as an important resource for the bolstering of staff morale during difficult fiscal times. The department has expanded its services within the organizational context over the past several years. In an effort to promote its role within the host institution, psychiatric services social workers and nursing staff have served as consultants to other departments. This role evolved in collaboration with the director of education of the hospital, who began to utilize psychiatric services staff in the delivery of educational programming for the institution. Recent examples include a workshop on "Coping with Difficult People," which is presented to hospital support staff during Secretaries' Week; "Assertiveness Training" for new nursing preceptors; bereavement process sessions for oncology nurses; and team building/communication workshops for other departments using the Myers-Briggs Type Indicator (Allen, 1994; Carlson, 1989; Nelson and Stake, 1994).

When the unit changed its name from "The Special Management Unit" to "The Department of Psychiatric Services," the staff struggled with how it could concurrently meet the needs of patients admitted with true psychiatric diagnoses and assist medical caregivers in behavioral intervention and medication with difficult, generally demented patients not appropriate for admission to the unit, while still increasing the average daily census so that the service would remain financially viable. A decision was made to admit only patients with psychiatric diagnoses who would benefit from acute hospitalization services. Admitting diagnoses most often included depression and suicidality, schizophrenia, bipolar disorder, dissociative identity disorder, and alcohol detoxification. Dual-diagnosed patients are well-served by the unit's expertise in both mental illness and addictions. In order to fulfill an important need in the organization, the staff has developed a collaborative program of consultation/liaison services to other departments and area nursing homes to provide consultation to patients who were not able to participate in the therapeutic milieu of a psychiatric unit.

Finally, it is important to consider the hospital culture in which the department exists. Within the catchment area of the hospital, many people refer to the Department of Psychiatric Services as "The Fourth Floor." Patients report that they feel stigmatized by dint of their admission to the psychiatric unit; they fear that their reputation as being "crazy" will have a profound impact on their lives. This issue is addressed often during the course of an inpatient admission.

PRACTICE DECISIONS

Defining the Social Worker's Role on the Psychiatric Unit

Social work practice in inpatient psychiatric programs varies according to the context of professional practice and the role definition of the clinical social worker. At SVMC, both the psychiatric unit management and the senior vice president encourage the creative development of the social work function within the unit itself, the broader organization of the hospital, and the community.

The social worker's role in psychiatry, therefore, is collaboratively defined and includes many of the functions described by Walker-O'Keefe (1993): the development and implementation of a therapeutic relationship; diagnosis, generally using the medical model and *DSM IV* as a guide, (American Psychiatric Association, 1994); individual, family, and group psychotherapy; disposition planning; crisis intervention; and resource development. In addition, within the institution the social worker is a patient advocate; consultant to other hospital services, psychiatric unit representative on various hospital committees such as Quality Assurance, Ethics, and Oncology Care, and Education and Outreach; and participates in the hospital's continuous quality improvement programs. Finally, as the primary therapist, the social worker also facilitates managed care clinical reviews.

As the psychiatric unit has evolved from a nursing service, it has become important for the social workers and nurses to define exclusive and overlapping areas of expertise (Friedman, 1993; Kanter, 1991). In the model that has evolved, nurses assume primary responsibility for case management services and nursing management, including assessment, patient education, and nursing care plans. The clinical social worker coordinates psychotherapeutic intervention including individual, family, and group psychotherapy and is also responsible for the coordination of care with patients' outpatient psychotherapists (Farley, 1991).

Description of the Client

Sarah Reinhart was a 16-year-old high school sophomore who was admitted following an overdose of over-the-counter medications in an attempt at suicide (Doyle, 1990; Linehan, 1981). Sarah had taken several handfuls of an analgesic and fallen asleep in her room. The empty bottle was beside her for her mother to find easily. She was brought to the emergency room by her mother and was transferred to the psychiatric unit as soon as she was pronounced medically clear. The provisional admitting diagnoses included the following: major depression, post-traumatic stress disorder, and panic (Wolfe, Sas, and Wekerle, 1994; Wozencraft, Wagner and Pellegrin, 1991). Upon admission, Sarah was tearful, withdrawn, and mistrustful of staff. In the initial assessment interview, the patient and her mother were interviewed conjointly since Mrs. Reinhart refused to leave her daughter alone. Mrs. Reinhart also made it immediately clear that she would not tolerate having her daughter "doped up" on medication.

Sarah had an apparently normal developmental course through infancy, latency, and early adolescence. She lived with her mother, father, and 11-year-old brother. She also frequently stayed overnight with her maternal grandmother who lived nearby, a place where she always felt safe. She was an average student, with no difficulties in school, had not previously had any serious medical illnesses, and had never received counseling prior to her admission to the hospital. She denied substance abuse. Sarah's current suicidality brought to light sexual abuse by a paternal uncle who lived nearby, which had been ongoing for several years. Sarah reported that she had been raped in her bedroom on occasions when her family was not at home, and that her uncle threatened her life if she reported the abuse. She had become increasingly fearful of being alone, especially after dark, and she awoke with frequent nightmares (Lyon, 1993).

Definition of the Client

Sarah's admission immediately raised the issue of defining the client. Mrs. Reinhart adamantly refused to leave her daughter's side, and was frequently tearful herself at the disclosure of Sarah's abuse. Sarah had informed the emergency room physician in her mother's presence of the sexual abuse as the precipitant for her suicidality. Mrs. Reinhart appeared alternately somewhat dazed and angry and, upon arrival on the psychiatric unit, informed a nurse that she had always suspected that the uncle in question was "weird." She berated herself for not paying attention to her gut and protecting her daughter. She was extremely protective of her daughter, and stroked her hair frequently. She refused to leave the unit when evening visiting hours were over. On the first evening of admission, she requested, and was granted with Sarah's consent, permission to spend the night in the unit's living area. Mrs. Reinhart's behavior escalated daily. Despite agreements made with staff that she would abide by the visiting hours and return home at night, she was unable to fulfill her agreement when it was time to leave. She became her daughter's shadow, frustrating the efforts of the psychiatrist, the social worker, and the nursing staff to carry out the unit's guidelines for visitation. Sarah's roommate and other patients began to complain about the intrusion of Mrs. Reinhart into the therapeutic milieu, and they angrily confronted staff about their perception of unequal treatment. Mrs. Reinhart became increasingly threatening, stating that if she were forced to leave she would discharge her daughter against medical advice, and that she would hold the unit staff "legally and morally responsible" for whatever happened. Sarah remained somewhat regressed and passively accepting of her mother's attention. In the morning team meeting, the staff wondered whether the mother/daughter interaction on the unit reflected their normal style of interaction or whether what they were witnessing was truly crisis behavior. They agreed to adopt a "wait and see" perspective, acknowledging that during a short, crisis-oriented admission it was not appropriate to attempt to diagnose and modify potential enmeshment.

Sarah had no visitors other than her mother. Her father declined an invitation by the social worker to come to the hospital for a planning meeting because he was employed at both a day and evening job to support the family. Mr. Reinhart reported that he hoped he would not see his brother before the legal issues were addressed because he feared he would try to kill him. He also noted that his wife generally handled family problems because of his heavy work schedule. The social worker and psychiatric nurse decided that while it was important to encourage Mr. Reinhart to be involved, it was equally crucial to respect historic family relationships, gender differences, and roles. The social worker and psychiatrist decided that it was not appropriate to invite Sarah's younger brother to participate in family treatment.

Therefore, the client became both Sarah and Mrs. Reinhart. This decision caused dissension among the staff, some of whom believed that if Mrs. Reinhart could not respect staff's request for adherence to unit policies, Sarah should not be treated. Other staff believed that Mrs. Reinhart herself needed treatment and that there was an ethical obligation to her as well. This issue was discussed daily at morning treatment planning meetings. The clinical social worker and clinical nurse specialist worked collaboratively in the treatment and coordination of care of Sarah and Mrs. Reinhart.

Goals, Objectives, and/or Outcomes

Because of the short-term nature of the admission, which was dictated primarily by Sarah's insurer, the team decided on a crisis-intervention approach (Golan, 1978; Mor-Barak, 1988; Parad and Parad, 1990; Slaikeu, 1990). The complex and troubling aspects of the family system would need to be addressed in outpatient psychotherapy and not during the height of the current crisis. The goals, therefore, were the following: (1) to provide crisis intervention and restabilization for Sarah and her mother; (2) to report the abuse to the appropriate authorities as dictated by state law (Sempke, Stowell, and Durgin, 1993); (3) to facilitate the initial legal interventions; and (4) to educate Sarah and her mother regarding the legal process, psychological responses to abuse, and community resources to which they could turn. Sarah and her mother both agreed with the treatment goals, and neither wished to add anything specific to the list.

Use of Contract

Contracting is a common form of intervention on inpatient psychiatric units. For example, patients who are permitted to have passes to freely leave the unit when they do not have specific treatment obligations and move about the grounds of the hospital must agree to specific guidelines to insure their safe return. During Sarah's admission, attempts by the staff to develop a workable contract with Mrs. Reinhart were repeatedly frustrated; she would agree to whatever was requested during the day, but when evening came she refused to abide by any of the agreements that had been negotiated. The evening and night staff became increasingly frustrated by her attitude and their inability to enforce visitation rules.

Meeting Place

The SMU is small, consisting of only five double rooms for patients, rooms for seclusion, group therapy, art therapy, several offices, a nurses' station, and a common living room. Because of the limitations of the physical milieu, all patients were acutely aware of Mrs. Reinhart's presence. One patient reported that Mrs. Reinhart's constant presence made her feel "invaded."

Theory Informing the Work

The hospitalization of adolescents requires that the social worker attend concurrently to psychiatric issues, normative adolescent development, and the multiple systems in which teenagers live. Developmental theory supports the notion that the task of the adolescent is self-definition and individuation from family of origin, a process bound to be impeded by hospitalization and some regression. In this case, attempts at discussion with Mrs. Reinhart resulted repeatedly in her challenge to staff: "Would you abandon your child if she had been raped and traumatized?" The staff speculated that Mrs. Reinhart's extremely protective and intrusive stance were related to her feelings about having inadequately protected her daughter from the abuse, but the social worker's efforts to raise the issue with Mrs. Reinhart as a clinical issue were met with glares and a stony silence.

Stance of the Social Worker and Clinical Nurse Specialist Collaboration

The social worker and clinical nurse specialist (CNS) collaborated to (1) coordinate work with various agencies and professionals; (2) monitor issues of patient confidentiality as the various systems became involved in her care, including frequent telephone calls from the reviewer for the family's healthcare insurance; (3) provide assessment, treatment planning, and therapeutic intervention for both Sarah and her mother; (4) serve as Mrs. Reinhart's advocate with staff; (5) develop a plan to address the concerns of other patients reactive to Mrs. Reinhart's behavior; and (6) develop and implement a comprehensive discharge plan to provide ongoing treatment and support for Sarah and her family. Sarah was supported by her mother, the nursing staff, the social worker, and the clinical nurse specialist through the investigative process, which included her first pelvic examination, during her eight-day hospitalization.

Rather than act as therapist for both Sarah and Mrs. Reinhart, the social worker quickly decided to request that the CNS act as Mrs. Reinhart's therapist. This strategy enabled the social worker to evaluate Sarah without her mother's intrusion. While Mrs. Reinhart was generally mistrustful and unwilling to leave her daughter's side, occupying Mrs. Reinhart under the guise of addressing the legal and reporting issues freed Sarah for individual intervention. In addition to her individual work with Sarah and collaborative work with the CNS in relation to Mrs. Reinhart, the social worker also assumed a leadership role in team discussions regarding how to handle the intrusiveness of Mrs. Reinhart. As supervisor, the CNS supported the nursing staff as they addressed repeated contract failures and their feelings of frustration and powerlessness.

Use of Outside Resources

Because of Sarah's age and status as a minor, and because of state-mandated reporting guidelines, the many community agencies pictured in the ecomap following this section were a part of the service delivery system. Neither Mrs. Reinhart nor Sarah chose to disclose to Sarah's school what had happened. The social worker worked with them regarding informing the guidance office that Sarah had been hospitalized, for a reason they did not wish to discuss, and would return to school when she was able. Because Sarah had been sexually assaulted, the social worker was mandated to report the abuse to Social and Rehabilitative Services (SRS), who in turn required an investigation by the police. A state trooper, experienced in such cases, was assigned to interview Sarah and discuss with Sarah and her mother the legal options open to them. Southwestern Vermont is lucky to have a Social and Rehabilitation Services that is accessible, skilled, and collaborative. Once the abuse was reported to the SRS worker, she assumed all further reporting responsibility and coordination of the investigation. She chose a police investigator who had worked with many such cases, and she was present at all interviews. She collaborated with the psychiatric services team through the social worker and clinical nurse specialist. Sarah and her mother were both educated about a local abuse advocacy group, Project Against Violent Encounters (PAVE). They were given PAVE literature and offered the option of a PAVE volunteer to support them through the investigatory and legal process. Mrs. Reinhart declined the use of PAVE for the duration of Sarah's hospitalization.

It is important to note that Sarah's maternal grandmother is included in the ecomap. While she was not actively involved during Sarah's hospitalization, her home was identified repeatedly by Sarah as her safe place. Upon discharge, Sarah elected not to return to her home, the setting of the abuse, but to return instead to her grandmother's. Needless to say, her mother went with her.

Use of Time

Among the changes in the provision of inpatient psychiatric services in an era of managed care has been the trend toward shorter lengths of stay. It was clear upon admission that Sarah's admission would be assessed by the managed care utilization reviewer every other day. It was also readily apparent that Sarah and her mother would not be able to tolerate an extended admission. Finally, the administrative director understood that this case had the potential to cause dissension among both unit staff and

FIGURE 21.1. Ecomap for Sarah Reinhart

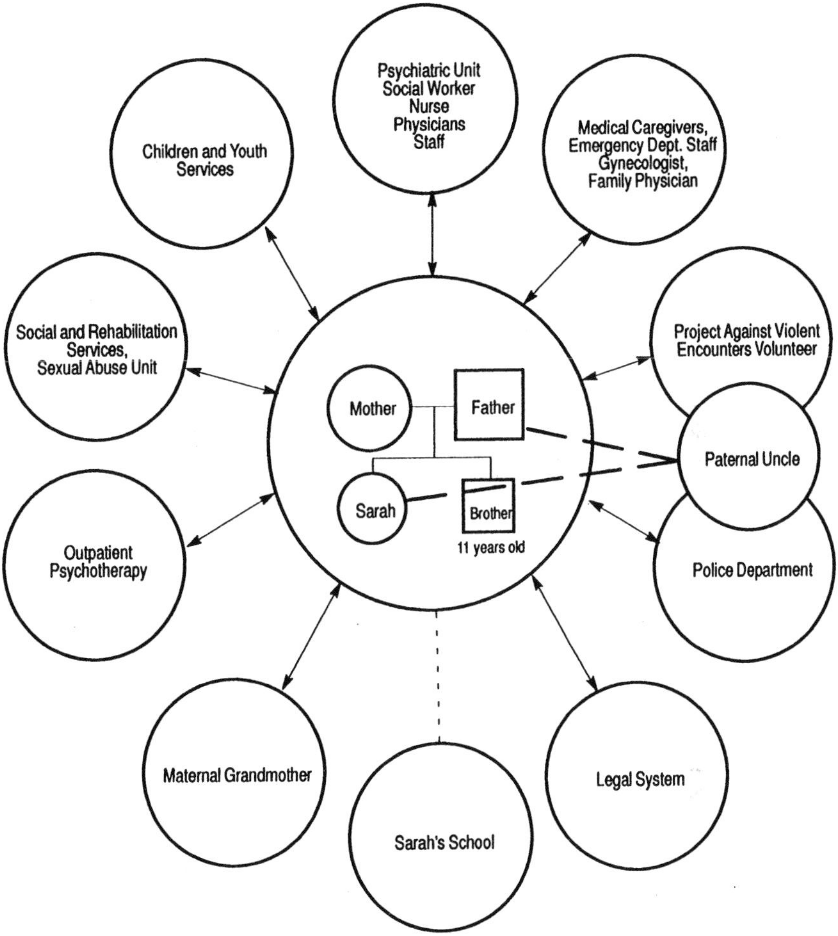

Sarah's fellow patients. The use of time in this case became an integral part of the treatment plan for Mrs. Reinhart. After several days, the staff were able to encourage Mrs. Reinhart to leave Sarah for brief periods to go home to get personal articles. The intervention involved explaining to Mrs. Reinhart what activities Sarah would be involved in during her absence and appointing the exact time of her return. This became part of the daily negotiations between Mrs. Reinhart and the treatment team.

Case Conclusion

Sarah's case illuminates the complexities of inpatient psychiatric care and the opportunities for collaborative practice. The challenge to provide the highest quality, most empathic care for the patient (here defined as Sarah and her mother) was contingent on the following: the presence of managed care in the clinical arena; the necessity for a seamless behavioral health delivery system; the ability of a team with disparate points of view to successfully conceptualize and deliver treatment; and the inclusion of community agencies and the legal system in treatment planning.

Upon follow-up six months later, Sarah reported that she was participating in individual therapy and that her family was being treated in weekly family therapy as well. She had returned to school, although she still had occasional nightmares and would not stay alone at home even for brief periods. Sarah's uncle who had perpetrated the abuse moved to another state. Sarah and her family declined to press criminal charges.

Differential Discussion

This case raised many issues that required thoughtful and collaborative discussion among staff. Among the questions raised were the following: (1) Who is the patient? (2) What good are unit policies if they are not enforced? (3) How could the treatment team deal with the powerful countertransference issues triggered by Mrs. Reinhart's behavior? (4) Was the staff seeing regressive, crisis-induced behavior on the part of Sarah and her mother, or was their current enmeshment characteristic of their relationship? (5) How could the staff process their disparate perspectives about how this case was to be approached and still provide a unified treatment plan? (6) What was the appropriate relationship between empathy and limit-setting?

This case provided one of the first real challenges to the collaborative atmosphere so carefully nurtured between the disciplines on the unit. Since it was difficult to attend to such issues fully during Sarah's hospitalization, care was taken subsequent to discharge to provide a forum for staff to vent their frustration about the case and their anger at Mrs. Reinhart's power to polarize the staff. Even now when there is a disagreement among staff on the unit, someone is likely to laugh and say, "Remember Sarah?"

* Special acknowledgment is due to Ana Rosales, MSN, CNS, and Alice Wislocki, LICSW, the clinicians who so ably rose to the challenge of this complex case.

REFERENCES

Allen, J. (1994). Using the Myers-Briggs Type Indicators–part of the solution. *British Journal of Nursing, 3*(9), 473-477.

American Psychiatric Association. (1994). *Diagnostic and Statistical Manual of Mental Disorders,* Fourth Edition Revised. Washington, DC: American Psychiatric Association.

Annas, G. (1989). *The rights of patients.* Carbondale, IL: University of Illinois Press.

Bendicsen, H. and Carlton S. (1990). Clinical team building: A neglected ingredient in the therapeutic milieu. Residential Treatment for it. *Children and Youth, 8*(1), 5-21.

Bentley, K. J. (1993). The right of psychiatric patients to refuse medication. *Social Work, 38*(1), 101-106.

Carlson, J. G. (1989). Affirmative: In support of researching the Myers-Briggs Type Indicator. *Journal of Counseling and Development, 67*(8), 484-486.

Doyle, B. B. (1990). Crisis management of the suicidal patient. In S. J. Blumenthal and D. J. Kupfer (Eds.), *Suicide over the life cycle.* Washington, DC: American Psychiatric Press, pp. 381-423.

Farley, J. (1991). Transitions in psychiatric inpatient social work. *Social Work, 39*(2), 207-212.

Friedman, S. (Ed.). (1993). *The new language of change: Constructive collaboration in psychotherapy.* New York: Guilford Press.

Gerhart, U. C. (1990). *Caring for the chronic mentally ill.* Itasca, IL: F. E. Peacock.

Golan, N. (1978). *Treatment in crisis situations.* New York: The Free Press.

Haynes, K. S. and Mickelson, J. S. (1991). *Affecting change: Social workers in the political arena,* Second Edition. New York: Longman.

Hobfoll, S. E. and Shlomo, W. (1986). Stressful events, mastery and depression: An evaluation of crisis theory. *Journal of Community Psychology, 14,* 183-195.

Hogarty, G. E., Anderson, C. M., Reiss, D. J., Kornblith, S. J., Greenwald, D. P. , Ulrich, R. F., and Carter, M. (1991). Family psychoeducation, social skills training and maintenance chemotherapy in the aftercare treatment of schizophrenia: Two-year effects of a controlled study on relapse and adjustment. *Archives of General Psychiatry, 48,* 340-347.

Joseph, M. V. and Conrad, A. (1989). Social work influence on interdisciplinary ethical decision making in health care settings. *Health and Social Work, 14,* 22-30.

Kanter, J. S. (1991). Integrating case management and psychiatric hospitalization. *Health and Social Work, 16*(1), 34-42.

Linehan, M. M. (1981). A social-behavioral analysis of suicide and parasuicide: Implications for assessment and treatment. In G. H. Glazer and J. F. Clarkin (Eds.), *Depression: Behavioral and directive intervention strategies.* New York: Guilford Press, pp. 147-169.

Lyon, E. (1993). Hospital staff reactions to accounts by survivors of childhod abuse. *American Journal of Orthopsychiatry, 63*(3), 410-16.

Monahan, M. J. (1994). The role of the social worker: The clinician's view. In R. K. Schreter, S. S. Sharfstein, and C. A. Schreter (Eds.), *Allies and adversaries: The impact of managed care on mental health services.* Washington, DC: American Psychiatric Press.

Mor-Barak, M. E. (1988). Support systems intervention in crisis situations: Theory, strategies and a case illustration. *International Social Work, 31*(4), 285-304.

National Alliance for the Mentally Ill. (1995). Annual report. Washington, DC: National Alliance for the Mentally Ill.

National Association of Social Workers. (1994). *Code of ethics.* Washington, DC: NASW Press.

Nelson, B. A. and Stake, J. E. (1994). The Myers-Briggs Type Indicator personality dimensions and perceptions of quality of therapy relationships. *Psychotherapy, 31*(3), 449-455.

Parad, H. J. and Parad, L. G. (1990). *Crisis intervention, Book 2: The practitioner's sourcebook for brief therapy.* Milwaukee, WI: Families International.

Protection and Advocacy for Mentally Ill Individuals Act of 1986, P.L. 99-319, 100 Stat. 478.

Reamer, F. (1987). Informed consent in social work. *Social Work, 32*(5), 425-429.

Reamer, F. (1995). *Social work values and ethics.* New York: Columbia University Press.

Richan, W. C. (1991). *Lobbying for social change.* Binghamton, NY: The Haworth Press, Inc.

Rideout, C. A. and Richardson, S. A. (1989). A team building model: Appreciating differences using the Myers-Briggs Type Inventory with development theory. *Journal of Counseling and Development, 67*(9), 529-533.

Rosenson, M. K. (1993). Social work and the right of psychiatric patients to refuse medication: A family advocate's response. *Social Work, 38*, 107-112.

Rubin, A. (1985). Practice effectiveness: More grounds for optimism. *Social Work, 30*, 469-476.

Sabin, J. E. (1991). Clinical skills for the 1990s: Six lessons from HMO practice. *Hospital and Community Psychiatry, 42*, 605-608.

Semke, J., Stowell, M., and Durgin, J. (1993). Influences on social work time expenditure in a voluntary psychiatric unit. *Health and Social Work, 18*(1), 32-39.

Slaikeu, K. A. (1990). *Crisis intervention: A handbook for practice and research,* Second Edition. Boston: Allyn and Bacon.

Squire, M., Stout, C., and Ruben, D. (1993). *Current advances in psychiatric care.* Westport, CT: Greenwood Press.

Strumwasser, I., Paranjpe, N., Udow, M., and Share, D. (1991). Appropriateness of psychiatric and substance abuse hospitalization: Implications for payment and utilization management. *Medical Care, 29*(8), Supplement.

Walker, M. (1994). Principles of a therapeutic milieu: An overview. *Perspectives in Psychiatric Care, 30*(3), 5-8.

Walker-O'Keefe, J. (1993). The role of clinical social work in inpatient psychiatric care. In M. B. Squire, C. E. Stout, and D. H. Ruben (Eds.), *Current advances in inpatient psychiatric care: A handbook.* Westport, CN: Greenwood Publishing.

Wolfe, D., Sas, L., and Wekerle, C. (1994). Factors associated with the development of posttraumatic stress disorder among child victims of sexual abuse. *Child Abuse and Neglect, 18*, 37-50.

Wozencraft, T., Wagner, W., and Pellegrin, A. (1991). Depression and suicidal ideation in sexually abused children, *Child Abuse and Neglect, 14*, 505-510.

Yurkovich, E. (1990). Patient and nurse roles in the therapeutic community. *Perspectives on Psychiatric Care, 25*(3-4) 18-22.

Chapter 22

Placement of a Developmentally Disabled Man

Susan B. Freeman
Beth Wrightson

CONTEXT

Description of the Setting

The Regional Center of the East Bay (RCEB) is one of 21 regional centers throughout the state of California providing comprehensive assessment and specialized services for developmentally disabled individuals. Regional centers are central points for developmentally disabled people ("consumers") to obtain or be referred for necessary services. To be considered developmentally disabled, a person must be substantially handicapped by mental retardation, autism, epilepsy, cerebral palsy, or a condition closely related to mental retardation or requiring similar treatment (Budley, 1983; Dudley, 1987). Handicaps that are solely physical are excluded. The handicap must have occurred prior to the age of 18 and continue or be expected to continue indefinitely (Grossman, 1984; Lanterman Act, Sec. 4512).

Consumers may be referred at any age by various sources, including schools, hospitals, parents, or community agencies. Their eligibility is determined by an assessment team usually consisting of a social worker and a physician, but which may also include a psychologist, an occupational therapist, a nurse, and a nutritionist. Once a consumer is determined eligible, the case is transferred to a case manager.

A case manager working for RCEB is responsible for advocating, counseling, coordinating, and obtaining necessary services for the developmentally disabled consumer (Harris and Bergman, 1987; Keenan, 1983;

Kurtz, Baggarozzi, and Pollane, 1984). A case manager is additionally responsible for coordinating the development of an individual program plan for each consumer, which may include calling participants to come to the meeting, facilitating the meeting, and assisting the consumer in determining his or her goals. Since the process is supposed to be person-centered, however, the consumer has the choice of who will do these tasks.

According to the Resource Manual of the California Department of Developmental Services, person-centered planning is an approach to determining, planning for, and working toward the preferred future of a person with developmental disabilities and her or his family. The preferred future is what the person and family want to do in the future based on their strengths, capabilities, preferences, lifestyle, and cultural background. Person-centered planning is a framework for planning and making decisions. It is not a collection of methods or procedures. Person-centered planning is based on an awareness of, and sensitivity to, the lifestyle and cultural background of the consumer and family.

The process for an individualized program plan must include the following procedures:

1. Gather information and conduct assessments to determine the life goals, capabilities and strengths, preferences, barriers, and concerns or problems of the person with developmental disabilities. Assessments shall be conducted by qualified individuals and performed in natural environments whenever possible. Information shall be taken from the consumer, his or her parents and other family members, his or her friends, advocates, providers of services and supports, and other agencies. The assessment process shall reflect awareness of, and sensitivity to, the lifestyle and cultural background of the consumer and the family.

2. Develop a statement of goals, based upon the needs, preferences, and life choices of the individual with developmental disabilities, and a statement of specific, time-limited objectives for implementing the person's goals and addressing his or her needs. These objectives shall be stated in terms that allow measurement of progress or monitoring of service delivery. These goals and objectives should maximize opportunities for the consumer to develop relationships; be part of community life in the areas of community participation, housing, work, school, and leisure; gain increased control over his or her life; acquire increasing positive roles in community life; and develop competencies to help accomplish these goals.

3. Establish a schedule of regular, periodic review and reevaluation to ascertain that planned services have been provided, that objectives

have been fulfilled within the time specified, and that consumers and families are satisfied with the individual program plan and its implementation and reassessment. (Lanterman Act, Sec. 4646.5)

The policies would be excellent guides to practice if each case manager did not carry between 80 and 85 cases. Often, case managers feel like case managees, since all of the people involved tell them what to do (Intagliata, 1982). A minimum of four consumer contacts annually is required. There is generally no fee for services; however, families with incomes over $70,000 may pay a small percentage of case management costs.

Policy

State Law

California established the regional center system with the enactment of the Lanterman Developmental Services Act in 1977. The intent of this law was to provide service to developmentally disabled individuals in their local community in the least restrictive manner and the most normal environment possible (Rothman and Rothman, 1984). Prior to this act, services were provided only at the time of institutionalization (Boggs, 1984; DeWeaver, 1983). The law explicitly states who is to be considered developmentally disabled (Winkler and Keenan, 1983). In addition, once an individual is so diagnosed and accepted into the system, with rare exceptions as long as he or she remains in California, that individual is a regional center consumer. A 17-year-old accident victim with severe brain damage, for example, is eligible for regional center services for as long as he or she lives. Had the accident occurred a year later, he or she would be ineligible. Numerous accountability procedures, such as the individual program plan, are mandated by law, thereby placing an emphasis on paperwork and limiting direct consumer contact. Each year, the California Legislature determines the funds to be allocated to each regional center. While the legislature is cutting social services for all other populations in the state, the funding for developmentally disabled consumers has remained stable. Although funding has not been cut, it has also not kept up with current costs of living, so that residential and program operators have not had their rates increased in the last eight years.

The policy of each local regional center determines how these funds will be used. Funding priorities for the Regional Center of the East Bay range from a high priority for residential placement and day programming to a lower priority for respite, speech therapy, and equipment purchases. Also,

RCEB's policy has been to increase caseloads in order to stay within funding limitations. Caseloads are now at 85, and this drastically affects case managers' abilities to provide services.

RCEB's policies affect the social worker's relationship with the consumer. Thus, the center hires people with master's degrees in the human services to be case managers and hires others with bachelor's degrees and experience to assist the case managers. The fact that this agency does not require all case managers to be educated in the same discipline affects consistency of services to the consumers as well as the professional environment for the case manager.

Insurance

Except for the few consumers who have significant assets or family insurance policies with HMOs, managed care has not greatly affected the developmentally disabled population. Most consumers of the center's services receive Medi-Cal or Medicare. We expect that as managed care becomes more prevalent in these public insurance programs, it will increasingly impact consumers. In addition to customary fee-for-service insurance programs, the federal government also provides a Medicaid waiver program for consumers in the community. This provides monies to the RCEB in return for time spent by staff case managing in community care facilities.

Technology

A comprehensive assessment of the individual's developmental status and needs is the basis for designing and maintaining a program of services. In making these assessments, professionals use a variety of IQ and social functioning scales, as well as the *DSM IV*. In delivering these services, special emphasis is given to the social integration of the person and to the least restrictive, effective service alternative. Services are continuously coordinated, reflecting planned and active participation by the individual and/or the family, the provider of service, and the case manager (Slater and Winkler, 1986).

Much of the treatment is purchased or provided by other community agencies that specialize in services to the developmentally disabled population. These services might include infant stimulation programs, behavioral consultation, residential services, speech therapy, and, less often, individual psychotherapy. Genetic counseling services are sometimes provided by outside specialists, and this helps both to advance the knowledge about various genetic disorders and to enable families to understand the risks entailed in having more children (Mealey, 1984).

In some instances, recent technological advances have enabled the developmentally disabled consumer to make significant progress. This is clearly evident for the nonverbal cerebral palsy consumer whose world is changed by an electronic communication device. Other examples include computers that were originally adapted for people with physical disabilities and can be activated by a voice, a single switch, or a turn of the head. Another youngster with severe cerebral palsy but superior intelligence is nonverbal and spastic. She is being evaluated for a computerized device that will produce words on tape. A case manager might arrange for consultation with a speech therapist and evaluation by a rehabilitation engineer to determine the most useful device. A regional center can usually help to purchase this very costly equipment.

Many RCEB consumers carry a dual diagnosis of developmental disability and mental illness. They are often followed by psychiatrists and treated with behavioral interventions and a variety of drugs (Carr, 1994). Consumers with epilepsy also receive a combination of drugs for seizure control from their general physician or their neurologist (Kerson, 1985).

Organization

Formal Dimensions

The regional centers were organized by the California legislature as part of a network of private, nonprofit agencies under contract to the California Department of Developmental Services. The RCEB is governed by a board of trustees representing various categories of developmental disabilities and reflecting the geographic and ethnic characteristics of the regional center's population. At least one-third of the board must be composed of people with developmental disabilities or members of their families. The board appoints a director who sets policies with the help of his or her administrative staff. The current director is in the process of reengineering the structure of the agency from a "flat" management team approach to a more hierarchical model. This will concentrate most of the power in a few top administrators.

RCEB is highly bureaucratized. Requests for services often must go through several channels before they are approved, and all services are extensively documented. Recently, there has been recognition that case managers, with their heavy caseloads, need more support in the form of supervision and training, and there has been a move in this direction.

Informal Dimensions

In a bureaucracy such as RCEB's, structure is increasingly formal. For example, previously, extraordinary purchases had to be approved by supervisors and directors, and case managers would have to appeal to their superiors, with whom they might or might not have a good relationship, on a case-by-case basis. Recently, this process has become more formalized, with a set of written consumer service standards and a peer review committee that hears requests for exceptions to the standards. As in any organization, knowing the right people and having physical proximity to them can smooth the way in many situations.

Interorganizational Dimensions

An established network of organizations advocates for consumers with developmental disabilities. In addition to 21 regional centers, there are residential institutions, called state developmental centers, across the state. Each country has a developmental disabilities council, which raises awareness about and advocates for consumers. The federal government has provided for two advocacy and monitoring bodies. A series of area boards–federally funded agencies mandated to perform a broad variety of advocacy functions–monitor regional center policies, while Protection and Advocacy, a legal agency, protects the rights of both mentally ill and developmentally disabled consumers. These organizations give resources to both the case managers and consumers–resources to turn to when they disagree with regional center decisions or policies.

Other social service agencies important to the work with consumers include adult protective services, licensing agencies, Social Security Administration, Medi-Cal offices, the Department of Developmental Services, and the Department of Vocational Services. Case managers work with these agencies to assure continuous service delivery to consumers on their caseload.

DECISIONS ABOUT PRACTICE

Description of the Client

Joseph Wolfe is a 29-year-old, mild to moderately retarded white man, with a diagnosis of Williams syndrome. In addition to retardation, Joseph has many features consistent with Williams syndrome. He is short; microcephalic; has coarse features; and has an open mouth with a prominent, thick lower lip and a dental malalignment. Joseph is neat, clean, and well-dressed, and although he is unusual looking, he is not really unattractive. His personality is also typical of those with Williams syndrome in that after initial nervousness subsides, he exhibits what is sometimes described as a "cocktail party personality." Joseph is a warm, outgoing, "huggy-touchy" person. Despite his graying hair and crow's feet, he gives the impression of a young, vulnerable boy. People tend to feel protective and maternal toward him and find him very likeable. A challenge to serving Joseph is that he frequently vomits copiously in response to stress.

Joseph was referred to the regional center by his mother at the suggestion of a physician from a genetics clinic. Mrs. Wolfe explained that for the past six years, Joseph had been living at a convalescent hospital with geriatric patients (Kruzich, 1986). He had no day programming. She was requesting the regional center's services to help find a more appropriate living situation and a day program. In the convalescent hospital, the majority of patients are nonambulatory. A limited activity program is geared to the elderly, including, for example, throwing a softball from one wheelchair to the next. This type of facility is structured for the chronically ill patient; it makes someone like Joseph appear chronically ill. He received a lot of attention, being the only young patient, and was the "pet" of the nurses and many other patients.

Mrs. Wolfe is 51 years old with bleached-blond, highly teased hair. She dresses in tight-fitting, seductive clothing, and is a hostess in a cocktail lounge. She treats Joseph like a child, always referring to him as a "boy" and reinforcing his medical needs and his dependence on her (Falck, 1984; Schilling, Gilchrist, and Schinke, 1984; Winkler, Wasow, and Hatfield, 1983). She triggers much of his vomiting. Her last words to him as she left the first placement in a family-care home were, "Now darling, don't disappoint Mommy and vomit." She is not a particularly likeable person because she is domineering and pushy.

Mrs. Wolfe provided sketchy information about Joseph's early years. He was the product of a full-term pregnancy. Labor was induced after Mrs. Wolfe slipped and fell down a flight of stairs. Joseph was born with the cord wrapped around his neck and required resuscitation. As a baby, he had severe feeding problems, including frequent vomiting, and he failed to gain weight. Developmental milestones included holding his head up early, walking without support at 13 months, and speaking single words at 30 months.

Medically, Joseph had frequent serious respiratory illnesses requiring hospitalization as a child. At 16, he had a severe drug reaction with hypertension and a stroke that resulted in paralysis of the left side. He shows some neurological difficulties, particularly in fine motor coordination, visual perceptual abilities, and mild left-handed ataxia that may be related to Williams syndrome, birth trauma, or the residuals of the stroke. His only current health problem is diverticulitis. It is recommended, however, that Joseph have his blood pressure checked frequently, since individuals with Williams syndrome often have renal failure stenosis, which is a closing of the arteries that lead to the kidneys.

Joseph's parents were divorced when he was young, and he has no contact with his father. He sees his mother frequently and maintains contact with his sister. As a child, Joseph was placed in various residential schools for mentally retarded youngsters. He carried the diagnosis of isolated mental retardation until the age of 21, when he was referred by a friend to a genetics clinic and diagnosed as having Williams syndrome.

Joseph has good self-care skills, is able to read and write simple words, print his name, and order from a menu. He speaks clearly and has good receptive language skills. He is weakest in community-living skills such as using public transportation, crossing the street, cooking, and managing money.

Once Joseph was accepted as an RCEB consumer, the assessment worker arranged placement at a small family care home near Joseph's sister (Agusta and Bradley, 1985); the home is a private, licensed residence shared with three other men, which is run by a couple. There were shared bedrooms, home-cooked meals eaten in the kitchen, and a weekly "family" outing to a restaurant and to a shopping center. There were no planned activities in the home, although the residents were taken to the local handicapped recreation program one night a week. A joint visit by the assessment worker and the case manager was made at the time of the placement. This was the most normal, homelike type of environment available. A disadvantage was that this particular couple tended to overprotect and control their residents.

Immediately after placement, Joseph began vomiting and crying. His vomiting was not polite or controlled. He sat at the dinner table and threw up all over the food (not only his) and then continued to throw up anywhere and everywhere so that everyone knew he was vomiting and in distress. The caretaker felt she could not keep him. He was sent to his sister's for a brief time and then returned to the convalescent hospital because his mother, stressing his medical needs, refused to accept any other option for his care.

A team conference was set up soon after and was attended by the case manager, the assessment worker, a regional center psychologist, and the regional center physician. It became clear during this meeting that Mrs. Wolfe had been brought up in foster homes and viewed Joseph's placement in a small care facility as a reenactment of her childhood and a threat to her own mothering abilities. The team decided to pursue day programming and consider placement only at a large residential facility.

Plans were made, working with Mrs. Wolfe and Joseph, to have Joseph attend a workshop and travel by a bus, with both activities funded by the regional center. The workshop coordinator visited Joseph at the convalescent home prior to placement. In addition, Mrs. Wolfe and Joseph went to visit a large residential facility for mentally retarded consumers in the area and were placed on a two-year waiting list.

The facility is a self-contained residence and program for 76 developmentally disabled adults, who live in cottages in a countrylike setting at a distance from the town. The residents all work in the workshops on the campus, which has a collegelike quality. There are different personnel for different shifts, allowing staff the strength to deal with more difficult consumers. Disadvantages of the facility are the isolation and the institutional atmosphere. For example, meals are taken in an impersonal central dining room with little homelike character. There is also significant staff turnover.

The workshop in which Joseph was placed is one of a number of workshops sponsored by a county association for the retarded. Generally, it is a place for people unable to function in competitive employment. The workshop program has educational and training components with classes in, for example, sex education, food skills, and self-help skills, as well as assembly-line type jobs for which the employee is paid on the basis of what he or she produces (a percentage of the minimum wage based on what a nondisabled worker could produce). There is also a social component with events such as dances, camping trips, and lunches at restaurants.

Once Joseph had begun at the workshop, the case manager contracted behavioral services for him (Yule and Carr, 1980). The program that was set up stressed Joseph's "manliness" and "healthiness" and was monitored by Joseph and the workshop staff. It included a daily notebook that was scored morning and afternoon on "manliness" and "healthiness" at the day program. The scoring was done by Joseph and checked by his teacher with a goal of gradually decreasing any statements suggesting weakness, ill health, nervousness, or lack of ability. It was gradually extended to the convalescent hospital and withdrawn from the day program. An additional program was set up by the behavior specialist to improve Joseph's physical strength and included jogging with the behavior specialist and participation in the special olympics.

After several months at the workshop, placement needs were again explored. It was decided, with Joseph's and his mother's concurrence, to place him at a middle-sized board and care facility where other consumers from his workshop lived. The new residential facility houses 20 people and consists of a series of cottages behind a larger home, in a residential area in the same city as the convalescent hospital. There is different supervision for different shifts, although the owner/manager is there during the day and sleeps close by. Each cottage has several shared bedrooms and an occasional single room, as well as a TV room. All residents eat together in a central dining room. During the day, the residents go to their programs, which include various workshops as well as a special adult education school. Some go by public transportation, some are transported in minibuses. There is active programming many evenings and weekends. It includes movies, scouts, dances, and adult education by teachers from the local school district who provide classes in singing and crafts. It is somewhere between the small family home and the large residential facility. It certainly does not have the warmth or homelike atmosphere of a smaller facility; yet, it provides an active, stimulating environment.

After a series of preplacement visits, placement was successfully completed. Joseph was able to make the transition from the convalescent hospital to the residence not so much because he knew other people from the workshop but because he had developed social skills and a better self-image from his workshop and behavior program (Hall, 1983).

Definition of the Client

According to strict policy terms, a regional center consumer is defined only as the developmentally disabled individual. In practice, however, a family member or a board and care facility operator is often also a consumer. Families can play a critical role in helping their developmentally disabled member live more independently (McCallion and Toseland, 1993). In Joseph's case, it would have been impossible to do successful planning without considering his mother as a consumer (Mueller and Leviton, 1986). This became clear after her needs were not taken into account in the first placement. If a relationship had not been established with Mrs. Wolfe, she could have sabotaged any future programming.

Goals, Objectives, and Outcome Measures

Goals or objectives of the RCEB consumer are formally written into the individual program plan, which is developed with the consumer and significant community and family members; reviewed quarterly or semi-annually; and rewritten triannually, or more frequently, if the planning team calls for a new plan. Since the case manager is not only the direct provider of service but often the coordinator as well, Joseph's goals depend on the relationship between himself and the case manager, the behavior specialist, the workshop staff, and the convalescent hospital staff. Joseph's initial goals were less refined and broader-based, becoming more focused once he entered the workshop program.

Use of Contract

The contracts or plans for achieving the goals are also explicitly stated in the individual program plan. This plan is exact, with clear reference as to who is responsible for implementing the goals and in what way. In Joseph's case, the behavior specialist developed an additional contract with Joseph to increase his feelings of healthiness and reinforce his being a responsible adult.

Meeting Place

Meetings often take place in the consumer's home, school, or day program and, less rarely, in the agency. As noted above, the Lanterman Act calls for meetings to be held in "natural settings" (Lanterman Act, Sec. 4646.5). For Joseph, all visits took place at the convalescent hospital or the workshop. Because our meetings required a feeling of warmth, support, and attention, and one of the goals was to increase Joseph's sense of healthiness, we met on the patio outside the sterile atmosphere of the convalescent hospital.

Use of Time

Duration and frequency of visits vary, depending on the consumer's need and the case manager's time restrictions. Joseph was anxious and often talkative, requiring long visits, particularly in the initial phase of the relationship. As he became more comfortable and familiar with the case manager, visits were shorter. This intervention with Joseph lasted seven months.

Regional center policy dictates that once an individual is accepted as a developmentally disabled consumer, in most instances he remains a consumer as long as he is living in California. If the regional center is not funding any services and if there is no need for case manager intervention, the case can become inactive. At one point, when Mrs. Wolfe was rejecting all alternatives and seemed intent on sabotaging plans, the option to make Joseph inactive was considered, though it was never used.

Interventions

For Joseph, the most effective treatment was a behavioral approach to deal directly with his vomiting and to enable him to integrate successfully into a day program. A strenuous exercise program (Carr, 1994) and relaxation techniques were also utilized (Hams and Bergman, 1987; Peveler and Johnston, 1986; Blumenthal, 1985; Herson and Bellack, 1985; Thyer, 1983). It was recommended to Mrs. Wolfe that she and Joseph receive some family therapy to help them deal with their symbiotic relationship, but thus far this has not occurred (Boyer, 1986).

Stance of the Social Worker

It was important to take an active role with Joseph. Since he lived in a convalescent hospital, he had assumed the role of a weak, sick person. His resistance to giving up that role required active intervention to effect any change. Mrs. Wolfe had ambivalent feelings about making any change in Joseph's lifestyle and needed direct confrontation, as well as recognition of her feelings. She needed to feel that control was in her hands, and not the social worker's (McCallion and Toseland, 1993). Joseph profited more from a warm, supportive approach, since any confrontation made him anxious and immobile. While an active stance remains necessary with Joseph, currently, the social worker's stance with Mrs. Wolfe can be more passive, taking her into consideration when important changes are to take place in Joseph's life. Neither Joseph nor Mrs. Wolfe would benefit from sharing the case manager's life experience, since each would view such sharing as an imposition on their needs.

Use of Outside Resources

Joseph required the use of many resources from the onset of his relationship with the assessment worker. These included arranging for the placement, having the RCEB fund it, and actually transporting Joseph to the home. Once the case manager became involved, concrete services were again needed (McCallion and Toseland, 1993; Miller, 1983). These included setting up the workshop program, arranging for transportation to the workshop, and arranging for behavior consultation. Because of

Joseph's retardation and his childlike self-image, these services had to be carefully arranged by the social worker, explained clearly both to Joseph and his mother, and required much support and coordination. For example, prior to Joseph's entering the workshop, the workshop coordinator visited him at the convalescent hospital to reassure him and explain the program. Figure 22.1 is an ecomap of Joseph's support system.

FIGURE 22.1. Ecomap for Joseph Wolfe

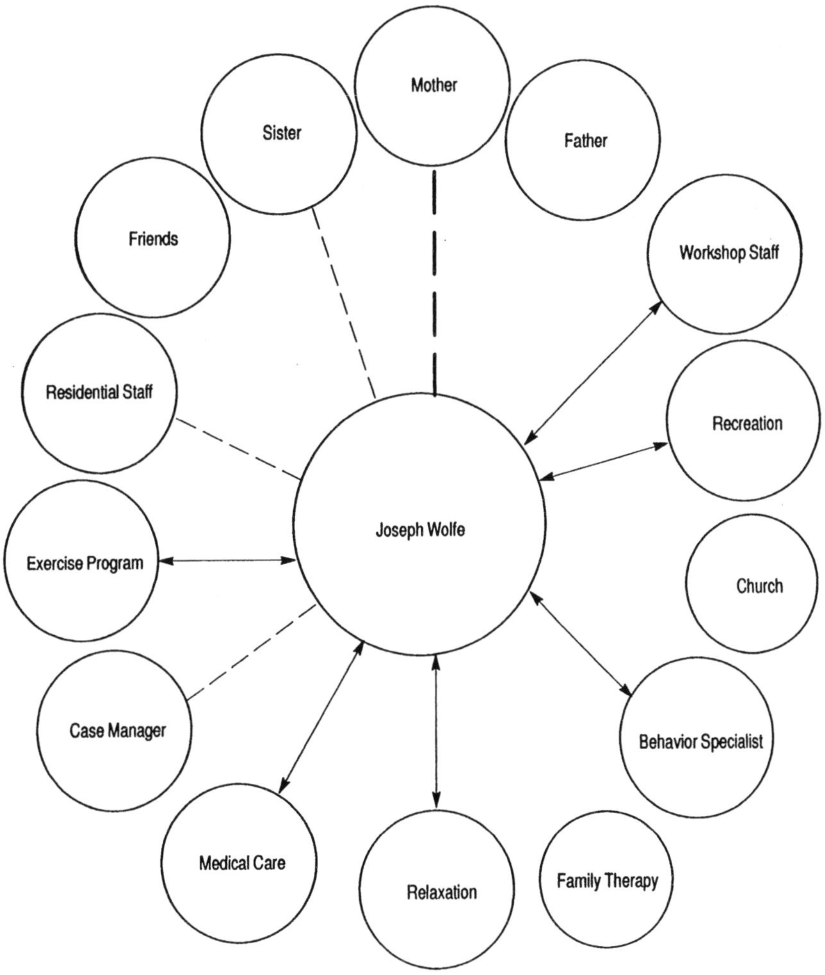

Reassessment

Reassessment of needs and goals takes place quarterly or semiannually, according to the individual program plan. In Joseph's case, a reassessment and then a change of goals took place after the failure of the original placement. At that point, it was decided by the regional center team and the case manager to slow down and place the highest priorities on programming and therapeutic intervention in order to prepare Joseph for placement.

Transfer or Termination

Joseph was transferred to another case manager for geographic reasons. He and his mother require frequent intervention. When there are large caseloads, localizing consumers can help provide more effective service. The decision to transfer Joseph was made once it was felt he had sufficient support in his life to be able to accept the change. Once he was in the workshop, adjusting well, and involved in a behavior program, the transfer took place. The actual transfer occurred in the workshop with a joint visit by both the old and new case managers.

Case Conclusion

Joseph has so far adjusted well to the new residential facility. Mrs. Wolfe does not view the new caretaker as a threat to her mothering ability. The behavioral program terminated successfully.

Differential Discussion

Different practice decisions might have resulted in a different outcome. Mrs. Wolfe's involvement was critical to the success of any placement for Joseph. Additionally, had the goals and contract been drawn with placement as the first priority, Joseph would probably not have had the social skills to interact successfully with peers and would have returned to the convalescent hospital. The workshop setting allowed him to develop and incorporate these skills at his own pace. In addition, larger homes, such as the one Joseph seems to be more comfortable in, are becoming very scarce as philosophies about living situations change. The trend today is toward smaller homes that approximate a more normal, shared living situation, such as one in which college students or other roommates might reside. The next step for Joseph might be to one of these smaller licensed residences or even to a supported living situation where he has his own apartment and receives personal assistance.

If the therapeutic approach had been to involve Mrs. Wolfe and Joseph in psychotherapy with the exclusion of a behavioral approach, progress would have been slower or limited. The key factor is not Joseph's level of retardation, but his emotional dependence on his mother and his consequent lack of sense of self as a competent adult. If he were not retarded, Joseph might have benefitted from other treatment techniques requiring more insight.

Another approach to this case would be to urge the family as a unit, and Mrs. Wolfe as an individual, to receive psychotherapy (Munro, 1985; Falck, 1984). Certainly, Mrs. Wolfe remains a needy woman with many unresolved conflicts. She has gained absolutely no understanding of her relationship with Joseph and could still sabotage treatment. When she dies, Joseph's sister will probably assume Mrs. Wolfe's role. His mother is preparing his sister for this eventuality and creating enough guilt so she will feel responsible for Joseph. Joseph's sister allies with his mother and could not have helped Mrs. Wolfe gain perspective. Our range of options is not as great as it seems, given both Joseph's and his mother's needs, program openings, transportation, and other limitations.

Given more time and resources, the case manager could have used a more active intervention with Mrs. Wolfe, perhaps modeling for her and guiding her to be more competent at advocating for Joseph (McCallion and Toseland, 1993). Again, caseload and time limitations can limit the extent to which a case manager can work with family members.

PRACTICE IN CONTEXT

RCEB is influenced by technology, policy, and organization. The basic policy goal is to create the most normal, least restrictive environment, which means many fewer state hospitalizations. Continually changing policy also seems to have a major effect, particularly in terms of priorities for service, caseloads, and accountability procedures. When a caseload jumps from 45 to above 80 and continues to creep upward, it is impossible to provide consumers the same quality of service. Technology has also had its effect. A changing service model, more refined behavior intervention techniques, electronic communication devices, psychotropic drugs, and a more advanced body of genetic knowledge have profoundly influenced the progress of many of our consumers. Both formal and informal factors of organization influence practice.

These, then, are some of the factors that have influenced the case manager's relationship with Joseph. Joseph probably would not have been a consumer of RCEB had he not been referred to a genetics clinic that recognized his Williams syndrome and referred him to us. The policies of striving for normalcy and of choosing the least restrictive alternatives most certainly led to an emphasis on a workshop and a move from the convalescent home. Both day programming and residential placement are high priorities within the regional center system, so Joseph was assured of funding for these programs. On the other hand, the size of caseloads and paperwork requirements are both policy decisions that definitely limited the time Joseph spent with the case manager and also made a transfer based on geographic centralization imperative. If the case manager had maintained a strict definition of Joseph as the only consumer, not including his mother, no progress could have taken place. The relationship benefitted from having a flexible meeting place and variable durations and frequencies of meetings. Meetings could take place outside the sterile atmosphere of the convalescent hospital and thereby not reinforce Joseph's illness, and could occur as often and for as long as needed. Both an active stance in dealing with Joseph and a continuous provision of concrete services were necessary because of Joseph's retardation and his image of himself as a child. Although there are many ways in which any case manager will always have to act assertively on Joseph's behalf, it is hoped that as he gains more emotional distance from his mother, he can better advocate and provide for himself. It is that emotional dependence that severely limits his abilities to act more independently and assertively on his own behalf.

REFERENCES

Agosta, J. M. and V. J. Bradley (1985). *Family care for persons with developmental disabilities: A growing commitment.* Boston, MA: Human Services Research Institute.

Blumenthal, J. A. (1985). Relaxation theory, biofeedback, and behavioral medicine. *Psychotherapy, 22*(3), 516-530.

Boggs, E. (1984). Feds and families: Some observations on the impact of federal economic policies on families with children who have disabilities. In M. A. Slater and P. Mitchell (Eds.), *Family support services: A parent professional partnership.* Stillwater, OK: National Clearinghouse of Rehabilitation Training Materials, pp. 63-84.

Boyer, P. A. (1986). The role of the family therapist in supportive services to families with handicapped children. *Clinical Social Work Journal, 14*(3), 250-261.

Budley, J. (1983). *Living and stigma: The lives of people who we label mentally retarded.* Springfield, IL: Charles C. Thomas.

Carr, E. G. (1994). Emerging themes in the functional analysis of problem behavior. *Journal of Applied Behavior Analysis, 2,* 383-399.

DeWeaver, K. L. (1982). Producing social workers for practice with the developmentally disabled. *Arete, 7,* 59.

DeWeaver, K. L. (1983). Deinstitutionalization of the developmentally disabled. *Social Work, 26*(11), 435-439.

Dudley, J. R. (1987). Speaking for themselves: People who are labelled as mentally retarded. *Social Work, 32*(1), 80-82.

Falck, H. (1984). Mental retardation: A family crisis. In T. O. Carlton (Ed.), *Clinical social work in health settings.* New York: Springer, pp. 198-207.

Grossman, H. (1984). *Manual on terminology and classification on mental retardation.* Washington, DC: American Association on Mental Deficiency.

Hall, J. A. (1983, May 27). *Evaluation of group treatment for improving the social skills of mentally retarded adults.* Paper presented at the Annual Convention of the Association for Behavioral Analysis. Milwaukee, WI.

Hams, M. and Bergman, H. C. (1987). Case management with the chronically mentally ill: A clinical perspective. *American Journal of Orthopsychiatry, 57*(2), 296-302.

Herson, M. and Bellack, A. S. (1985). *Dictionary of behavioral assessment techniques and methods.* New York: Pergamon Press.

Intagliata, J. (1982). Improving the quality of community care for the chronically mentally disabled: The role of case management. *Administration in Mental Health, 8*(4), 655-674.

Keenan, M. P. (1983). Standards for social workers in developmental disabilities. In L. Winkler and M. P. Keenan (Eds.), *Developmental disabilities: No longer a private tragedy.* Silver Spring, MD: NASW Press.

Kerson, T. S. (1989). *Understanding chronic illness.* New York: The Free Press.

Kruzich, J. M. (1986). The chronically mentally ill in nursing homes: Issues in policy and practice. *Health and Social Work, 11*(1), 5-14.

Kurtz, L. F., Bagarzzi, D. A., and Pollane, L. P. (1984). Case management in mental health. *Health and Social Work, 9*(3), 201-211.

Kusserow, R. P. (1984). *A program inspection on transition of developmentally disabled young adults from school to adult services.* Washington, DC: U. S. Department of Health and Human Services.

Lanterman Act (1977 including 1993 Amendments). Welfare and Institutions Code (Sections 4500-4850) State of California Code.

McCallion, P. and Toseland, R. W. (1993). Empowering families of adolescents and adults with developmental disabilities. *Families in Society, 74*(12), 579-587.

McDonald-Wikler, L. (1987). Disabilities: Developmental. In A. Minahan (Ed.), *Encyclopedia of social work* (Eighteenth Edition). Silver Spring, MD: NASW Press.

Mealey, L. (1984). Decision making and adjustment in genetic counseling. *Health and Social Work, 9*, 124-133.

Miller, G. (1983). Case management: The essential services. In C. J. Sanburn (Ed.), *Case management in mental health service*. Binghamton, NY: The Haworth Press, Inc.

Mueller, M. and Leviton, A. (1986). In-home vs. clinic-based services for the developmentally disabled child: Who is the primary consumer-parent or child? *Social Work in Health Care, 11*(3), 75-88.

Munro, J. D. (1985). Counseling severely dysfunctional families of mentally and physically disabled persons. *Clinical Journal of Social Work, 13*(1), 13-31.

Peveler, R. C. and Johnston, D. W. (1986). Subjective and cognitive effects of relaxation. *Behavior Research and Therapy, 24*(4), 413-414.

Rothman, D. J. and Rothman, S. M. (1984). *The Willowbrook wars: A decade of struggle for social justice*. New York: Harper & Row.

Schilling, R. F., Gilchrist, L. D., and Schinke, S. P. (1984). Coping and social support in families with a developmentally disabled child. *Family Relations, 33*, 47-55.

Slater, M. A. and Winkler, L. (1986). Normalized family resources with a developmentally disabled child. *Social Work, 31*(5), 385-390.

Thyer, B. A. (1983). Behavior modification in social work practice. In G. Herson, R. M. Eisler, and P. M. Miller (Eds.), *Progress in behavior modification*. New York: Academic Press, pp. 173-216.

Winkler, L. and Keenan, M. P. (Eds.). (1983). *Developmental disabilities: No longer a private tragedy*. Silver Spring, MD: NASW Press.

Winkler, L., Wasow, M., and Hatfield, A. (1983). Seeking strengths in families of developmentally disabled children. *Social Work, 28*, 313-315.

Yule, W. and Carr, J. (Eds.). (1980). *Behavior modification for the mentally handicapped*. London, England: Croom-Helm.

Chapter 23

A Transitional Residence
for the Mentally Ill:
To Achieve Independent Living

Carey Donovan
Edward Blanchard
Toba Schwaber Kerson

CONTEXT

Description of the Setting

Shalom House, Inc.

Shalom House is part of an umbrella organization, Shalom House, Inc., which oversees a variety of housing options and support services for adults with severe and prolonged mental illness. Included in this continuum are three rooming houses (two are McKinney-grant-funded facilities); three intensive group homes; two HUD 202 congregate apartment projects; three HUD Shelter Plus Care programs, which provide housing subsidies throughout Maine for homeless individuals with mental illness, substance abuse, or AIDS; and a state-funded Bridging Rental Assistance Program providing subsidies statewide for mental health consumers (Rafferty, 1995; Johnson, 1994; Levine and Rog, 1990; Gore, 1990). A team of community support caseworkers provides comprehensive case management services for all clients. To supplement these services, in-home, one-on-one support is available to individuals who require such intense intervention to enable them to successfully remain in independent housing. In-home support can mean emotional help at difficult times or assistance in managing the activities of apartment life, such as cooking or cleaning. Similar in-home assistance has been available for other disabled populations, such as the physically handicapped, and is now seen as a critical element in helping some people with mental illness to live successfully in the community (Ridgeway and Zipple, 1990). Shalom House continues to expand services in keeping with its mission.

Shalom House

Shalom House is a psychiatric transitional residence in Portland, Maine. Founded in 1972 by local churches and synagogues concerned about deinstitutionalization, it was the first independent facility for psychiatric patients in our state (Budson, 1978; Golomb and Kocsis, 1990; Stoner, 1988). The house itself is large, old, comfortable, and located in the heart of Portland, within walking distance of the hospital, mental health and social service agencies, the downtown area, a campus of the University of Maine, the city library, a major art museum, and many potential places of employment. It has room for 12 residents and operates at 95 percent capacity. Residents are adults with serious mental health problems who need a transitional program that will prepare them for more independent living, which is the purpose of Shalom House (Chacko, 1985; Deegan, 1992). All residents accepted to the program are presumed to be capable of leaving Shalom House and living more independently in the community within 12 to 18 months. Shalom House is the one remaining transitional program in the agency. All others offer permanent housing.

Policy

It is thought that those who are mentally ill comprise 25 to 50 percent of the homeless population (Johnson, 1994; Levine and Rog, 1990; Gore, 1990; Lindbloom, 1991; Posey, 1990). The policies discussed in this section relate to both homelessness and mental illness.

Deinstitutionalization

Shalom House was created because a group of private citizens was concerned that the process of deinstitutionalization was causing former mental hospital patients to live in communities that were unprepared to deal with them (Menninger and Hannah, 1987; Talbott, 1979, 1986; Wilson, 1975). Deinstitutionalization is the process of (1) preventing both unnecessary admission to and retention in institutions; (2) finding and developing appropriate alternatives in the community for housing, treatment, training, education, and rehabilitation of [persons] who do not need to be in institutions; and (3) improving conditions, care, and treatment for those who need to have institutional care (U.S. General Accounting Office, 1977). This approach is based on the principle that persons are entitled to live in the least restrictive environment necessary and lead lives as normally as they can (Flexer and Solomon, 1993; Levy and Rubenstein, 1996; Liberman, 1987).

Policies related to deinstitutionalization came about during the decades of the 1960s and the 1970s for many reasons including (1) the civil rights movement's emphasis on the protection of due process and least restrictive care, (2) the increasing costs of institutionalization, (3) the development of more effective and efficient psychotropic drugs and other social and psychological interventions, and (4) the availability of increased levels of public assistance for those who were unable to work as the result of illness (Segal, 1995). At the same time, in Maine and other states, patients of state hospitals sued states for inadequate and neglectful treatment in the state hospitals. The settlements of these lawsuits led to a number of consent decrees mandating states to further downsize the state hospitals and in some instances to close them entirely. Court decisions began to affect the conditions of mental hospitalizaition by defining (1) parameters of overcrowding and patient-to-staff ratios, and (2) involuntarily detained patients' rights to specific treatments, as well as the types of treatment they may refuse and the methods through which a child could be declared disabled and thus eligible for Supplemental Security Income (Johnson, Kreuger, and Stretch, 1989; *Bartley v. Kremens,* 1975; *Donaldson v. O'Connor,* 1974; *Wyatt v. Stickney,* 1972). Thus, major changes in the law restricted the states' power to and means for holding and treating mentally ill persons. Unless they were proven to be dangerous to themselves or others, mentally ill people could not be confined against their will and could be confined only for short periods of time. Their treatment had to be meaningful, and in addition, it was illegal to require patients to work in any area of their institution without pay. Currently in Maine, two-thirds of the patients who are admitted to the state hospital are sent home within two weeks. There are more services available in the community, but there is no centralized coordinating body (Johnson and Castengera, 1994; Johnson and Banerjee, 1992).

Supplemental Security Income Program

In 1974, the federal goverment assumed responsibility for former state programs for Old Age Assistance, Aid to the Blind, and Aid to the Permanently and Totally Disabled and created, instead, the Supplemental Security Income program for those who have medical verification of "the inability to engage in any 'substantial gainful activity' by reason of any medically determinable physical or mental impairment[s] which can be expected to result in death or which has lasted or is expected to last for a continuous period of not less than 12 months" (Supplemental Security Income Modernization Project, 1992, p. 84). The benefit levels of SSI increase automatically with inflation. The federal government provides the basic SSI benefit and some states provide supplemental monies. Recipients also automatically receive Medicaid and food stamps or a cash supplement equal to the value of food stamps for which they would have been eligible. Thus, with the federal government paying a large percentage of the costs of Supplemental Security Income, Social Security Disability payments, Medicaid and Medicare, states had a great incentive to discharge patients from mental hospitals to nursing homes, boarding homes, and the community. In 1990, the conditions for providing Supplemental Security Income to children were also determined (Meyer, 1995; *Sullivan v. Zebley,* 1990; Lawyers Cooperative, 1991).

The Social Security Income program is an improvement from the past, but it still has many problems because supplemental benefits vary with each state, the eligibility standards are outdated, benefits are inadequate, there are disincentives to marry and to live with others, and many who appear to be eligible do not receive benefits (Meyer, 1995). In addition, the federal government established a funding mechanism for start-up costs for regional community mental health centers, which would provide care for patients closer to home and in a less restrictive setting than the state hospital.

McKinney and Shelter Plus Care Grants

Federal programs such as McKinney and Shelter Plus Care grants were enacted from 1987 to 1995 to provide much needed housing subsidies for homeless mentally ill people. The Stewart B. McKinney Homeless Assistance Act of 1987 (PL. 100-77) establishes competitive programs for transitional housing, housing for disabled homeless people, the rehabilitation of single-room occupancy buildings, and the prevention of homelessness. However, these programs are poorly funded, administratively fragmented, and are located in ten different federal departments. The Interagency Council on the Homeless, which was to act as a clearinghouse for all programs, cannot possibly manage the problems (Interagency Council on the Homeless, 1991; Stoner, 1989). There is great concern that decreases in federal funding and the increased authority of the states will further erode the program.

Parents of the mentally ill are shocked to learn that they cannot get treatment for their desperately ill offspring (Wasow, 1978). Police are reluctant to transport the mentally unstable; and hospitals are full or are reluctant to process an involuntary commitment. When families finally succeed in having an ill relative committed, they find he or she is discharged a few days later. At the heart of this situation is a conflict between an individual's right to refuse treatment and the ability of a psychotic person to make sound judgments on his or her own behalf. (Belcher, 1988; For a discussion of this issue, see Wasow, pp. 523-538).

The concept of "community care," which seemed so bright in the 1960s, has now faded. There are many more mental health services available in communities, but mentally ill people who live in the community must be sufficiently functional and motivated to comply with the care that is available. Often, the nature of their illnesses prevents them from following medical regimens or coming to a mental health center for regular appointments. Assertive Community Treatment (ACT) teams, a new model for aggressive outreach to people who are difficult to engage, are effective but costly (Bond et al., 1990; McGraw et al., 1995; Olfson, 1990; Santos et al., 1993). Many more need this service than there are teams to provide it. Also, while mental illness can be a very long-term problem, no one agency is assigned continuous responsibility for the mentally ill. In practice, "community care" looks a lot like "let people fend for themselves."

Family Activism

One result of these changes has been the growing activism of the families of the mentally ill. Family groups have been established all over the country, and a national network–The National Alliance for the Mentally Ill–has grown dramatically in regard to membership and political voice. These groups provide education and support to families, lobby for services and changes in legislation, and at times organize and run their own service-providing agencies. At the same time, patients have become active and formed their own groups. They have lobbied for changes in the way services are provided and for more dignity in their treatment. As activists, they want more control over treatment and are adamantly opposed to any encroachments on their right to refuse care. Consumer groups with the aid of public advocates now have considerable power in influencing how service providers respond to their needs. With both groups, professionals can be in the uncomfortable position of not knowing whether they are considered friend or enemy. It is within this complex environment that Shalom House operates as a Transitional Residence for the mentally ill.

Technology

The technological developments that are relevant to the mentally ill are those related to diagnosis, treatment, and psychosocial rehabilitation. Most dramatic is the development of new psychotropic medications that have made many symptoms of mental illness more manageable, so much so that most people with major mental illnesses can live in the community. It is important to remember, however, that comprehensive care of the mentally ill transcends technology and includes a variety of concrete, supportive, and educative services in addition to medical treatment. Although great strides have been made in the treatment of the mentally ill, great problems remain. To some extent, the problem lies not with the technology, but with the way it is used. Mental illness can be a long-term problem and patients often suffer as the result of a lack of treatment continuity.

Most people who are referred to Shalom House have already been in several hospitals or treatment facilities. They are likely to have a different diagnosis from each, because mental illness is truly difficult to diagnose and hospitals tend to have policies that require a diagnosis to be recorded on admission but not necessarily reevaluated at a later date. As a result, diagnosis tends to take place when the doctor knows the least about the patient. Inaccurate diagnosis and lack of continuity contribute to problems in prescribing medication. There are many possible medications and dosage levels. Each facility may go through a trial-and-error process with the patient rather than build on the knowledge gained in the previous facility (Sheehan, 1983). A greater emphasis on documentation would be one way to alleviate this problem (McDougall, Adair-Bischoff, and Grant, 1995).

The right medication can make an almost unbelievable difference in a patient's functioning. Of concern is the patient's ability or willingness to take the medicine as prescribed. This is one of the many reasons why the patient and family have to be included and educated in the process of treatment. At the present time, there are many approaches and therapies available to clients. Most have something to offer, but it is very easy for a patient and family to become confused about and estranged from a mental health "system" that has a new theory or therapy at every turn. Patients can be helped enormously when they receive an accurate diagnosis, helpful medication, supportive therapy, continuity of care, education, and concrete services. Psychosocial Rehabilitation is a very helpful philosophical base for many programs working with this population (McFarlane, Shirley, and Deakins, 1992; Peterson, Patrick, and Rissmeyer, 1990). This strengths model involves the consumer in determining and working toward goals and deemphasizes the limitations and symptoms of mental illness.

Organization

Shalom House, Inc. has an executive director and clinical (MSW), finance, and housing directors. About 40 staff serve approximately 140 clients in the various settings. Shalom House employs a coordinator (MSW), two full-time, BA-level caseworkers and two live-in residential managers. A social work student generally completes a field placement here each year. Shalom House provides a comfortable, secure, and informal environment for consumers and staff. Although the environment is highly structured with many rules and consequences, and the staff carries a great deal of authority including the right to expel a client, the atmosphere remains relaxed and egalitarian. Each staff member has a specific job description, but roles are flexible and everyone is involved in a little bit of everything. Many informal conversations between staff and residents occur in the kitchen, dining room, and hallways. The offices for Shalom House are located on the second floor of the house, interspersed with bedrooms, bathrooms, and the laundry area. Most of the business (other than confidential matters) is conducted within earshot of the residents.

Shalom House is known as a supportive place to work. Live-in positions turn over every 18 months or so, but other staff positions are held for periods of five to ten years. Some permanent staff have risen through the ranks of students, back-up house managers, and house managers before assuming case manager positions. Shalom House has a cooperative arrangement with Portland's major hospital, which has a residency program in psychiatry and a full range of psychiatric services including an inpatient unit, emergency room with psychiatrists on call 24 hours a day, a day treatment program, and an outpatient clinic providing medication and treatment. A medication clinic funded by the state and a private psychiatric hospital offering inpatient and outpatient services are also available. Staff at Shalom House are educated to know when a client needs to be evaluated for medication or treatment or taken to the hospital when an emergency arises.

There are cooperative arrangements with other agencies in Portland, including the Bureau of Rehabilitation, which is the major community support provider; a social club for the mentally ill; the Portland Coalition for the Psychiatrically Labeled, which is a consumer advocacy group; and a crisis intervention unit. Since Shalom House accepts clients from all over Maine and sometimes from out of state, we communicate with treatment centers all over New England.

Case Description

Bill Jones is a 31-year-old veteran, who has a primary diagnosis of chronic undifferentiated schizophrenia and a secondary diagnosis of alcohol abuse (Torney, 1988; Winerip, 1994). He has had six psychiatric hospitalizations. All occurred within the past three years, and none lasted more than two weeks. Bill's personal difficulties date back further. In fact, he reports a suicide attempt at the age of 11 and feeling "different" in high school. He was in the armed services for five years before being given a dishonorable discharge for being absent without leave for three months. Apparently, Bill drank heavily while in the service and during this time was briefly married and divorced. For the seven years since leaving the service, Bill has been a transient. During that time, he had one job that lasted two years, but none of his other jobs have lasted more than a few months. He has gone through periods of heavy drinking and minor involvement with the law, and was charged once with disorderly conduct and once with forging identification (Calsyn and Morse, 1991). He has not been involved with Alcoholics Anonymous and does not consider himself an alcoholic.

Bill's first psychiatric admission occurred three years ago. He was traveling on a bus from Massachusetts to Maine and created a disturbance when he got into a fight with a man he thought was making advances. The bus driver put him off the bus, called the sheriff, and Bill, paranoid and delusional, was admitted to a hospital in New Hampshire with a diagnosis of acute schizophrenic episode. Bill remembers being paranoid and delusional a couple of years before that, but he received no treatment and the feelings went away. During the last three years, Bill has drifted around Maine, living with relatives, holding jobs for a week or a month at a time, and being admitted to local psychiatric units. He has overdosed twice when despondent about not working and not being able to support himself. He was referred to Shalom House from a community mental health center. At that time, he had no means of support other than the largesse of relatives, was having increasing difficulty holding a job, and had been hospitalized four times in the previous year.

Definition of the Client

At Shalom House, our client is the individual resident, not the family or community. Unlike many social agencies, we choose our clients. Once accepted, the prospective resident may have to wait for a room to become available. Over the years, Shalom House has developed a specific profile of an acceptable client: someone who is judged to be currently incapable of independent living but who is felt to have both the ability and motivation to achieve independent living within 18 months; someone who can assume responsibility for his or her own medication; and someone who can adjust to group living, including having a roommate, and is in reasonably good health. Screened out are those under 18 or those with active drug or alcohol problems, violent behavior, or suicidal impulses that are not under control.

Bill is an example of the flexibility of Shalom House's admissions guidelines. The program coordinator, a social worker, decides whether to admit an applicant in consultation with the rest of the staff. Although Bill had a history of alcohol abuse and suicide attempts, the referring agency felt he was not presently suicidal; and he had been abstinent from alcohol for three months. We decided to offer Bill a place at Shalom House if he agreed not to drink in the house. Making this agreement gives us the latitude to offer a place to someone whose admission is considered risky, knowing that if he or she breaks the agreement, we can ask the individual to leave the program. Mental illness is often intertwined with drug or alcohol problems and episodes of harm or threat to self or others. If we screened out everyone with these experiences, we would have no admissions; so we use our best judgment.

A complicating factor in these assessments is the anecdotal nature of psychiatric records. We have often received records stating that a person was "violent" or "very violent." In order to understand what that means, we have had to call the person who wrote the record and say, "What exactly did this person do that was violent?" Bill's records were a case in point. His application to Shalom House was at first denied without an interview because his hospital records indicated a severe drinking problem and an arrest for attempted murder. Upon receiving this letter, Bill called me and denied that he had ever been arrested. In the ensuing interview, he was open and cooperative and denied the charges without being defensive or showing any hostility. We requested records from hospitals that had treated him previously to look for evidence of such charges. A hospital in New Hampshire responded and described the incident in which Bill was psychotic, created a disturbance on a bus, and was brought to the hospital by the sheriff. There was no arrest, and no injuries were reported. Apparently, this was the incident that, when told by Bill to a doctor two years later, sounded like an arrest for attempted murder.

Contract

A new Shalom House resident enters into an elaborate set of agreements. Shalom House is probably the most demanding environment the resident could choose—more demanding than being in an institution or living alone. Every day, residents weigh the benefits against the effort. No drugs, alcohol, violence, stealing, sexual relations, or suicide gestures are allowed at Shalom House. Violation of any of these cardinal rules leads to immediate dismissal; a resident who has violated one of those rules is given one week's notice to leave. However, unless a contract specifically stipulates that a resident may not drink, individuals are free to drink outside of the house, as long as the drinking is not disruptive to the house and does not interfere with the resident's progress.

There is no curfew at Shalom House. Residents can come and go anytime. Each resident has his or her own key to the front door. Residents are free to go away on weekends. They are, however, expected to be at Shalom House during the week and required to be at house meetings Monday evenings and to be at dinner Monday through Thursday, unless excused. Everyone must cook for the house and clean up one night a week together with another resident. Everyone has one assigned house duty a week, for example, cleaning the second floor bathroom. These duties are checked twice a week. Failure to complete a house duty results in being assigned extra duty the following week. Staff gives assistance as needed to help residents complete tasks.

Each resident must maintain a day program, which can be working, going to school or day treatment, doing volunteer work or sheltered work, or looking for work. In any case, residents are required to do something constructive during the day. We discourage people from using sickness as an excuse to stay home. If a resident's day program is looking for work, the resident is expected to make a minimum of two job contacts a day and to hand in a job contact sheet describing these activities at the end of the week. Residents are also expected to take their medication as prescribed. In certain instances, staff may help residents with medication by using means such as reminders or pill caddies. The ultimate goal is for residents to take their medication more reliably by themselves.

The first six weeks are a trial period. At the end of that time, the staff makes a decision regarding whether the person should be fully accepted into the program. If the person is found unready to meet the demands of the program, he or she is asked to move out. The contract between the resident and the agency is complex and remains very much a live issue during the course of the resident's stay. All of these policies are discussed at the time the individual comes for an initial tour, again at the interview, and again at the time of admission. New residents are given a handbook.

The agreement between the resident and the case workers is that they will meet regularly during the resident's stay to set goals, review progress, and deal with whatever personal matters are at issue. In addition, the social worker will direct the resident toward needed community resources and, if necessary, advocate for the client. Residents are told when they come in that anything they say will be shared freely with other Shalom House staff. The staff provides skill teaching in areas needed for clients to become more independent. Skills to cope with recurrent symptoms are particularly important.

Goals

The general goal for each Shalom House resident is to achieve independent living within 18 months. Goals that fall under this general guide are specific to each client. Each has a community living plan. "Independent living" is a general phrase that means living in the community as opposed to living in an institution or in the parents' home. It begs the question of work and does not mean that one is no longer mentally ill or no longer needs medication and treatment. In fact, it may be defined broadly enough to include infrequent, brief, and self-initiated psychiatric hospitalizations.

In Bill's case, his initial goals in coming to Shalom House were to find work and to rely on the support of the house to overcome the nervousness that had already caused him to lose or leave several jobs. His longer-range goals that related to living independently were to develop a support system and save money for an apartment (Maines and Markowitz, 1979; Markowitz and Nitzberg, 1982). The following is the service plan that was developed after Bill moved into Shalom House.

Service Plan

Goal: To achieve independent living

Objectives:

1. Obtain employment.
   a. Make at least two job contacts every day.
   b. Register with two vocational development programs.
   c. Apply to the office of vocational rehabilitation.
   d. Attend occupational meetings on Monday afternoons.
2. Maintain employment.
   a. Attend work regularly despite feelings of nervousness.
   b. Discuss work problems with Shalom House staff.
3. Develop a support system.
   a. Continue to spend two hours every day in common areas of the house.

   b. Make an effort to stay up until at least 8:00 p.m. four nights a week.

   c. Once income is obtained, do at least one recreational activity every week.

   d. Work with the social worker on developing interests and hobbies.

 4. Save money.

   a. Develop a budget with the social worker.

   b. Open a savings account and save for an apartment.

 5. Watch for early symptoms of illness.

   a. Discuss with staff any concerns in this area.

   b. Develop additional ways to handle stress.

Meeting Place

Usually the social worker meets with residents in his or her office. Interviews with prospective residents and more informal contacts with residents are held downstairs in the manager's apartment, which is more comfortable and more accessible to the common rooms. Informal conversations with residents are also held in the common areas. This leaves the office as the most formal of available settings. The formality of the office is preserved to emphasize that it is a place to converse seriously. When residents want to see the social worker, they generally ask whether the social worker is free or make an appointment rather than use the office as a drop-in center. The house managers are encouraged to do the opposite, to almost always have open conversation with residents discussing common issues and concerns in the common areas.

Use of Time

The maximum stay at Shalom House is 18 months. The highly structured expectations of the house and the constant turnover tend to assure that as residents' lives become stabilized, they will want to move out of Shalom House and be on their own. We discourage residents from making hasty, unplanned exits from the house. We hope they will stay at Shalom House until they have a steady means of financial support, some sort of routine for daily living, some friends in the community, significant progress toward the goals with which they entered Shalom House, and that their illness is stable. We want them to maintain a new job for three months before leaving. Finally, we want them to notify the rest of the group that they are leaving rather than to move out suddenly.

The social worker meets with each resident once or twice a week during his or her stay and for a few weeks afterward. Former residents may be followed by the Shalom House, Inc.'s Community Support Team after discharge if they wish. In-house meetings vary from a few minutes to an hour. The limiting factor is the resident's own tolerance for extended conversation. Only a handful of residents at Shalom House can tolerate an hour's conversation. My first sessions with Bill lasted only five or ten minutes. While being completely direct and to the point, he would answer questions with as few words as possible and introduce no new topics of conversation. Then he would fidget and ask, "Anything else?" Recently, he has become more relaxed and spontaneous, and it has been possible to converse with him for a half hour.

Reassessment

A major reassessment occurred with Bill one month after he arrived at Shalom House. After looking for a month, he finally found a job washing dishes in a restaurant. He only held the job for a day. When I sat down with Bill he had just missed several days of work, calling in sick. He opened the discussion by saying he thought he should go back to the hospital. It was difficult to elicit from Bill how he was feeling and why, because at this point he was still very nonverbal. Gradually, however, the picture emerged that he had been feeling suicidal for two weeks without telling anyone and that if he were to do anything to harm himself, it would probably be by overdosing. He said that his grandmother, with whom he had previously been living, had sold her home and he would not be able to go back there, that there were long waiting lists for the vocational programs, and that he simply could not tolerate the dishwashing job. If he could not do that, he did not know what else there was for him.

Rehospitalization was seriously considered, but I proposed an alternate plan for Bill to stay at Shalom House and be in a full-time day treatment program. Bill was willing to consider it and to make a contract that he would not make any suicide attempts. He agreed to come to the staff if he became too depressed to control his suicidal impulses so that we could get him to a hospital. Bill's doctor supported this plan and facilitated a speedy referral. Within a day, Bill was in a full-time day treatment program. While still depressed, he appeared to have found some relief almost immediately from having brought his feelings out into the open and through experiencing this change of plan.

The focus of the plan changed from vocation to treatment. It was suggested to Bill that he apply for Social Security Disability (SSDI) and Supplemental Security Income (SSI), and procedures for doing so were explained. This option seemed reasonable since he had not been able to maintain a job in five years. This remained the general plan for a couple of months. However, the process of getting on SSI and SSDI is a long one, and as Bill began to feel better, there began a gradual refocusing back in the vocational direction. He was encouraged to try vocational activities again and to try to determine what his tolerance for working might be. A medication change was also made, with good results; Bill began to feel less uncomfortable and to be more relaxed and spontaneous. The day treatment program was able to place patients in volunteer jobs, and a job in the hospital kitchen was arranged. Bolstered by his positive experience doing volunteer work, Bill applied for a paying job in the hospital kitchen, and after several interviews he was hired as a full-time dishwasher. He began this job while keeping his case active with SSI and SSDI in the event it turned out that he could not successfully hold this job.

Another reassessment occurred on the issue of alcohol use. Bill confessed occasional limited use of alcohol to me but denied it was a problem, saying that before he would have kept drinking all night but now he was able to stop at two beers and come home. The staff decided to change his contract to allow very limited drinking. The issue of interests and hobbies was also reassessed. Bill insisted that he had no interests and hobbies and no intention of developing any. He maintained that this simply was the way he was and that he could live with it. I agreed to drop any mention of hobbies from his service plan. Service plans must reflect client choice even if staff believe different goals would be good to work on.

Treatment Modality

In trying to define the type of treatment Bill received at Shalom House, it is easy to overlook the obvious. Concrete services are possibly the largest part of what makes Shalom House therapeutic. Many adults recovering from mental illness simply need a place to start. A temporary, no-rent, safe place to live within walking distance of potential jobs may be all that is needed.

In addition, the milieu of Shalom House has been carefully crafted for therapeutic benefit. Everyone has structured chores and duties. The natural desire to be like everyone else in the group tends to reinforce higher levels of functioning. Since everyone has psychiatric problems, it also circumvents the argument, "I'm a sick person; you can't really expect me to do all this." Teaching of daily living skills is also an important part of the Shalom House program. Shalom House residents should leave the program with some proficiency at cooking, cleaning, shopping, budgeting, banking, making friends, coping with their mental illness and structuring their free time. If they do not have a car, they should be familiar with the bus system. They should also be familiar with the social service system and know what services are available and how to obtain them. Shalom House also serves an educational function: residents should leave with some understanding of their illness and how to manage it, both in terms of medication and of awareness of vulnerable areas.

The work that goes on between social worker and client consists largely of emotional support, but also includes goal setting, referrals, education, limit setting, and contracting. Many mentally ill adults desperately need someone to recognize their strengths as well as their disabilities and to treat them with respect. In addition, it is up to the social worker to provide focus to the efforts of client and agency by developing, with the client, a comprehensive service plan. Case worker and client review progress and write a new plan every three months.

Drawing up a community living plan requires the case worker to accurately assess thé needs, abilities, and motivations of the client. It does not do much good to write "find a job" on the service plan of a client who has no intention of doing so. The case worker must be skilled at matching the complex resources of the community to the complex needs of the client. This is not simply an intellectual exercise; it involves facilitation and preparing the client for the service and the service for the client. It is often the job of the social worker to better educate the client about his or her mental illness. It is also up to the social worker to enforce the expectations of the program since clients must fulfill certain responsibilities in order to remain at Shalom House. Contracting can be a useful tool. Thus, the treatment offered by the social worker at Shalom House includes assessment, emotional support, skill teaching, appropriate referrals, written comprehensive service plans with periodic review and revision, education, enforcement of program expectations, and contracting. It must be admitted, however, that clients tend to be more impressed with the concrete services provided, such as food, shelter, small loans of money, and someone to talk to, than they are with the aspects of the program that are prized by the staff.

Stance of the Case Worker

I have to be active with Bill and draw him out. I must also listen very closely for clues, since he gives out so little that indicates how he is feeling, or what he is thinking. Drawing him out and sustaining a conversation is a goal in itself. I also have to work hard with Bill to get him to link feelings to events. He tends to experience feelings as facts that have no connection to any reality. For example, when he was suicidal and considering hospitalization, he had no idea why. He said, "I'm just depressed, that's all." It was only through a lot of probing that I was able to put together the puzzle and say, "Gee, Bill, no wonder you're depressed. Your grandmother sold your home, you couldn't get into the vocational programs, it took you a month to find a job, and now you're not able to do it." Also helping Bill to see that there are other ways to cope with his feelings than to be hospitalized is an important step.

Outside Resources

Overall, one makes more headway with Bill manipulating the objective realities of his life than talking to him about his feelings. Bill's timely referral to day treatment can be considered a concrete service. Clearly SSI and SSDI are concrete services. Bill did the footwork on his own, but we provided him with the information he needed to pursue it. Unfortunately, the system is set up in a way that just about guarantees that if you walk in there naive, you will end up with nothing. Bill has sometimes been without spending money, and Shalom House has provided him with funds to fill his prescriptions.

Residence at Shalom House is itself a concrete service. We provide shelter in an urban setting and charge 51 percent of a person's income for room and board. This allows a high priority status when applying for subsidized housing. A person with no income is charged nothing. We also provide a subsidy to people who are just beginning to work, since we are cheaper than alternative living arrangements. This allows a resident to leave Shalom House with a security deposit, the first month's rent, and some savings. Figure 23.1 is an ecomap of Bill's support system.

Transfer or Termination

We knew the decision to allow Bill to do some drinking and remain in the program was risky. I began to get feedback from house managers that Bill was drinking too much. This was discussed with Bill, but he minimized it as a problem. The behavior continued and one night Bill was discovered drinking in his room. He was discharged from the program with one week's notice. While this was difficult for Bill, it was necessary to enforce the rule of no drugs in the house, to keep it a safe environment for other residents.

Bill did leave Shalom House with a full-time job. He had no particular difficulty finding a new place to live. He occasionally returned to Shalom House as an ex-resident visitor. He was referred to the Community Support Team and accepted their services. He held his job in the hospital kitchen for approximately two years, then was fired. During this time he

FIGURE 23.1 Ecomap for Bill Jones

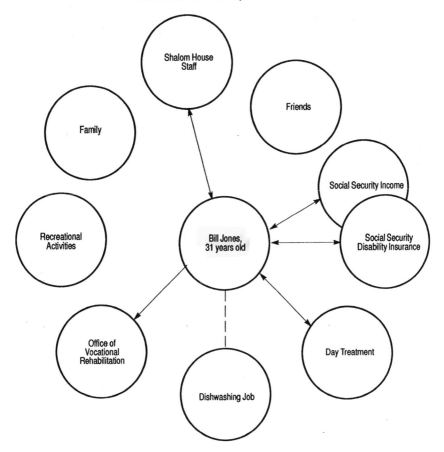

reportedly became increasingly involved in drug and alcohol abuse. Clearly, the dual disorder of alcoholism was underestimated by his care providers and himself.

Differential Discussion

Five major decisions affected Bill's stay at Shalom House. The first was the decision to admit him to the program. This was a judgment call, but our finding was that he met the program guidelines and could be admitted to the program under a contract for no alcohol abuse. The second decision involved what course of action to take when he quit his first job and became suicidal. In retrospect, the plan of full-time day treatment, a medication review, a contract not to act on suicidal feelings, applications to SSI and SSDI, and continuing at Shalom House worked very well. It is important to realize that this decision, like every other, was a gamble. Despite his contract, he could have impulsively taken an overdose, precipitating another hospitalization and dismissal from Shalom House. I believe the plan we implemented addressed his concerns directly, taking away his need to make a dramatic statement by overdosing. The next two decisions were somewhat contradictory: urging applications to SSI and SSDI and encouraging continued vocational involvement. The first move creates for Bill a possible way out of the destructive cycle he has been in for the past few years: attempting work, failing, become psychotic, suicidal, or alcoholic; being admitted to a hospital, and recovering; and starting the cycle all over again. The second suggestion allows for some more testing in this area, for keeping options open, and for clarifying what his problem with work really is.

The fifth and most risky decision was to allow some alcohol use while in the program. If we had enforced our original no-alcohol contract with him, he would have been asked to leave even earlier. This would have upheld the sanctity of contracts at Shalom House and saved us the future trauma of having to ask him to leave for drinking on the premises. It might have undercut his denial and minimalization of alcohol as a problem in his life. However, it also would have denied him the opportunity to try drinking in a responsible way. Since he was certain to try drinking when on his own, and since he was not at all interested in alcoholism treatment, it seemed reasonable to have him do his experimenting with us. The fact that he came on his own and told me that he had done some drinking made it harder for me to respond to his honesty by asking him to leave. In social work, there is not always a right answer.

PRACTICE IN CONTEXT

The case of Bill Jones at Shalom House was clearly affected by technology, policy, and organization. Without effective medication, Bill would not have been a candidate for a house like ours. Furthermore, a change of medication during his stay allowed him to feel much more relaxed and probably contributed to his being able to work again.

Bill's experience with us was shaped by the organization of Shalom House. Once here, Bill faced a series of nonnegotiable expectations that included maintaining a day program, participating in house responsibilities, and continuing to take medication. Shalom House creates a very therapeutic environment for persons recovering from mental illness with its focus on responsibility with support.

Some questions should be raised regarding the overall care Bill has received as a mentally ill person. Although we were able to coordinate a variety of services for him while he was at Shalom House, these were only minimally integrated with anything that has happened before or since. One problem with Shalom House is that it is a short-term solution to a long-term problem. Clients are here on the average for nine months, but they are mentally ill for much longer. Within our whole national system of health care and mental health care, there is a bias toward short-term care. The mentally ill and their families are subjected to many short-term interventions such as brief therapy or brief hospitalization, each of which "reinvents the wheel." In some cases, a client is served by the same agency for many years, but the workers turn over every year or two, creating a series of fresh starts. Perhaps if we had had more of a history with Bill we would have known that it was a mistake to condone any drinking. Was he "set up for failure" due to our ignorance? Conversely, in the 12 years that have passed since Bill left Shalom House, no one has ever written to us for information, despite the fact that we now know quite a bit about him.

When Shalom House was founded, it was hoped that our efforts at education and rehabilitation would be effective in interrupting the pattern of recurring hospitalizations for our clients. Unfortunately, the more serious forms of mental illness tend to be more cyclical than we wanted to believe. Over the years, Shalom House has adapted to this reality by taking clients back two or three times and by developing other, permanent, residential and support programs. Our expectations now are that client skills will be strengthened but they will continue to deal with their illness for many years.

As illustrated by the case of Bill Jones, mental illness is very often compounded by drug or alcohol problems. This is extremely common and very difficult to treat. Mental health programs often miss the boat on this issue. On the other hand, traditional drug and alcohol programs are very structured and have almost no ability to accommodate adults who are mentally ill. In recent years in Maine, there has been an effort to provide more training on drug and alcohol abuse for mental health personnel, to have alcohol counselors employed in mental health settings, and to develop new programs for the mentally ill substance-abusing client. An innovative Robert Wood Johnson-funded Dual Diagnosis Collaborative has been formed in Portland to encourage integration of care for both problems

(Goldman, Morrissey, and Ridgeley, 1994; Goldman, 1995; Shore and Cohen, 1990).

As noted, the function of Shalom House is to prepare clients for "independent living." This concept has also been called into question as Shalom House has evolved. In the past 20 years, Portland has changed from being an economically semidepressed area to being a very popular and expensive place to live. It has become increasingly difficult for our clients to find any housing they can afford, and the housing they do find is often substandard. At the same time, mental health services are becoming less available. Hospitals fill their beds and stop accepting voluntary patients. Community support workers have full caseloads and cannot accept new clients. When clients are left to struggle under unfavorable circumstances, the question arises, "What's so great about independent living?" It is often difficult to convince the parents of a mentally ill young adult that this is a desirable goal. They prefer to see their family member taken care of somewhere.

Future Trends

Several significant trends will continue to influence and change the systems of care for individuals living with mental illness:

1. The consumer movement and its increased input into the form that treatment takes will grow. Having adequate supports and housing subsidies to live where one chooses will push the system into providing supports for people in their own homes. There may be less reliance on transitional group facilities.
2. The pace of research into new psychotropic medications is quickening. Entirely new drugs with different actions on the brain have helped people for whom no medication has been effective. As the biochemical basis of mental illness is more firmly established, stigma will decrease.
3. Research in the area of family psychoeducation has underlined the effectiveness of educating families, clients, and mental health staff about modifying the environment in ways that lower stress, particularly with individuals suffering from schizophrenia. This approach coupled with adequate medication has shown itself to lower relapse significantly.
4. Family groups will continue to advocate for more active treatment interventions. Outpatient commitment laws are being enacted in many states despite concerns about violation of individual rights.

5. Changes in how health and mental health services are delivered is
   beginning to impact those with serious mental illness. The advent of
   managed care even in the public sector (Medicaid) will effect services in unknown ways. The decision by the federal government to
   reduce deficits by capping Medicare and Medicaid benefits and
   reinstating block grants to the states will have dramatic consequences for this population. It is important that we not lose sight of
   the fact that long-term flexible supports are critical in ensuring an
   acceptable quality of life for people who just 30 years ago were
   institutionalized. Not to provide such support will lead to the tragedy of more homeless, mentally ill who are disenfranchised from
   American life.

REFERENCES

Bachrach, L. L. (1991). Psychosocial rehabilitation in the care of long term
patients. Revised version of a paper presented at the Institute on the role of
community psychiatry in psychiatric rehabilitation. Boston, MA. June 1,
1991. American Psychiatric Association.

Bartley v. Kremens, 402 F. Supp. 1039 (E.D. Pa. 1975).

Belcher, J. R. (1988). Rights vs. needs of homeless mentally ill. *Social Work,*
33(4), 398-402.

Bernheim, K. and Lewine, R. (1979). *Schizophrenia: Symptoms, causes and*
treatments. New York: Norton.

Bernheim, K., Lewine, R., and Beale, C. (1982). *The caring family.* New York:
Random House.

Bond, G. R., Wetheridege, T. F., Dincin, J., Wasmer, D., Webb, J., and De-Graff-
Kaser, R. (1990). Assertive community treatment for frequent users of psy-
chiatric hospitals in a large city: A controlled study. *American Journal of*
Community Psychiatry, 18(6), 865-891.

Budson, R. (1978). *The psychiatric halfway house: A handbook of theory and*
practice. Pittsburgh, PA: University of Pittsburgh Press.

Calsyn, R. J. and Morse, G. A. (1991). Correlates of problem drinking among
homeless men. *Hospital and Community Psychiatry, 42*(7), 721-725.

Chacko, R. (1985). *The chronic mental patient in a community context.* Washington, DC: American Psychiatric Press.

Deegan, P. E. (1988). Recovering: The lived experience of rehabilitation. *Psycho-*
social Rehabilitation, 11(4), 11-19.

Deegan, P. E. (1992). The independent living movement and people with psychiatric disabilities: Taking back control of our lives. *Psychosocial Rehabilita-*
tion Journal, 15(3), 3-19.

Donaldson v. O'Connor, 493 F. 2nd 507 (5th Cir. 1974).

Flexer, R. W. and Solomon, P. L. (1993). Psychiatric rehabilitation in practice.
Boston, MA: Medical Publishers.

Goldman, H. H. (1995). Evaluating the Johnson Foundation program on chronic mental illness. *Psychiatric Services, 46*(5), 501-503.

Goldman, H. H., Morrisey, J. P., and Ridgeley, M. S. (1994). Evaluating the Robert Wood Johnson Foundation program on chronic mental illness. *Milbank Quarterly, 72*(1), 37-47.

Golomb, S., and Kocsis, A. (1990). *The halfway house on the road to independence.* New York: Bruner-Mazel.

Gore, A. (1990). Public policy and the homeless. *American Psychologist, 45*(8), 960-962.

Interagency Council on the Homeless. (1991). *Federal programs to help homeless people.* Washington, DC: Author.

Johnson, A. K. (1994). Homelessness policy in the United States. *Social Policy and Administration, 28*(2), 151-163.

Johnson, A. K. and Banerjee, M. (1992). Purchase of service contracts for the homeless: The development of a city-wide network. *Journal of Applied Social Sciences, 16*(2), 129-141.

Johnson, A. K. and Castengera, A. R. (1994). Integrated program development: A model for meeting the complex needs of homeless persons. *Community Practice, 1*(3), 29-47.

Johnson, A. K., Kreuger, L. W., and Stretch, J. J. (1989). A court-ordered consent decree for the homeless: Process, conflicts and control. *Journal of Sociology and Social Welfare, 16*(3), 29-42.

Lawyers Cooperative. (1991). Sullivan v. Zebley. *U. S. Supreme Court Reports, 107*, 967-983.

Levy, R. M. and Rubenstein, L. S. (1996). *The rights of people with mental disabilities: The basic ACLU guide to the rights of people with mental illness and mental retardation,* Carbondale, IL: Southern Illinois University Press.

Levine, I. S. and Rog, D. J. (1990). Mental health services for homeless mentally ill persons: Federal initiatives and current service trends. *American Psychologist, 45*(8), 963-968.

Liberman, R. (Ed.). (1987). *Psychiatric rehabilitation of the chronic mental patient.* Washington, DC: American Psychiatric Press.

Lindblom, E. (1991). Toward a comprehensive homelessness-prevention strategy. *Housing Policy Debate, 2*(3), 957-1025.

Maines, D. and Markowitz, M. A. (1979). Elements of the perpetuation of dependency in a psychiatric halfway house. *Journal of Sociology and Social Welfare, 6*, 52-69.

Markowitz, M. A. and Nitzberg, M. L. (1982). Communication in the psychiatric halfway house and the double bind. *Clinical Social Work Journal, 10*(3), 176-189.

McDougall, G. M., Adair-Bischoff, C. E., and Grant, E. (1995). Development of an integrated clinical database system for a regional mental health service. *Psychiatric Services, 46*(8), 826-828.

McFarlane, W. R., Stastny, P., and Deakins, S. (1992) *Family-aided assertive community treatment: A comprehensive rehabilitation and intensive case management approach for persons with schizophrenia disorders*. San Francisco: Jossey-Bass.

McGraw, J. H., Bond, G. R., Dietzen, L., McKasson, M., and Miller, L. D. (1995). A multisite study of client outcomes in assertive community treatment. *Psychiatric Services, 46*(7), 696-701.

Menninger, W. and Hannah, G. (1987). *The chronic mental patient/II*. Washington, DC: American Psychiatric Press.

Meyer, D. R. (1995). Supplemental security income. In R. L. Edwards (Ed.)., *Encyclopedia of social work*, Nineteenth Edition. Washington, DC: NASW Press.

Olfson, M. (1990). Assertive community treatment: An evaluation of the experimental evidence. *Hospital and Community Psychiatry, 11*(6), 634-641.

Peterson, C. L., Patrick, S. L., Rissmeyer, D. J. (1990). Social work's contribution to psychosocial rehabilitation. *Social Work, 35*(5), 468-472.

Posey, T. (1990). A home, not housing. *Psychological Rehabilitation, 13*, 3-4.

Rafferty, Y. (1995). The legal rights and educational problems of homeless children and youth. *Educational Evaluation and Policy Analysis, 17*(1), 39-61.

Ridgway, P. and Zipple, A. M. (1990). The paradigm shift in residential services from the linear continuum to supported housing approaches. *Psychosocial Rehabilitation Journal, 13*(4), 11-31.

Santos, A. B., Hawkins, G. D., Julius, B., Dica, P. A., Hills, T. H., and Burns, B. J. (1993). A pilot study of assertive community treatment for patients with chronic psychotic disorders. *American Journal of Psychiatry, 150*(3), 501-504.

Segal, S. P. (1995). Deinstitutionalization. In R. L. Edwards (Ed.). *Encyclopedia of social work*, Nineteenth Edition. Washington, DC: NASW Press.

Sheehan, S. (1983). *Is there no place on earth for me?* New York: Random House.

Shore, M. F. and Cohen, M. D. (1990). The Robert Wood Johnson Program on Chronic Mental Illness: An overview. *Hospital and Community Psychiatry, 41*(11), 1212-1216.

Stewart B. McKinney Homeless Assistance Act of 1987, P.L. 100-77, 101 Stat. 482.

Stoner, M. R. (1988). The voluntary sector leads the way in delivering health care to the homeless ill. *Journal of Voluntary Action Research, 17*(1), 24-35.

Stoner, M. R. (1989). *Inventing a non-homeless future: A public policy agenda for preventing homelessness*. New York: Peter Lang.

Sullivan v. Zebley. (1990). 493 US 521, 106 L. Ed 2d 967, 110 S Ct 885.

Supplemental Security Income Modernization Project (1992). *Final report of the experts*, Baltimore, MD: SSI Modernization Project.

Talbott, J. (Ed.). (1986). *Our patients' future in a changing world*. Washington, DC: American Psychiatric Press.

Talbott, J. (Ed.). (1979). *The chronic mental patient: problems, solutions, and recommendations for a public policy*. Washington, DC: American Psychiatric Press.

Torney, E. F. (1988). *Surviving schizophrenia: A family manual.* New York: Harper and Row.

U.S. General Accounting Office. (1977). Returning the mentally ill to the community: The government needs to do more. Washington, DC: U.S. Government Printing Office.

Wasow, M. (1978). For my beloved son David Jonathan: A professional plea. *Health and Social Work, 3,* 127-145.

Winerip, M. (1994). *9 Highland Road.* New York: Pantheon Books.

Wilson, D. C. (1975). *Stranger and Traveler: The story of Dorothea Dix, an American reformer.* Boston, MA: Little, Brown and Company.

Wyatt v. Stickney, 493 F. Supp. 521,522 (1972).

Chapter 24

Intensive Case Management for People with Serious and Persistent Mental Illness

Carolyn S. Weiss
Toba Schwaber Kerson

CONTEXT

Description of the Setting

The setting is a comprehensive community mental health/mental retardation center in Philadelphia, which is made up of approximately 390 full- and part-time employees representing a wide array of disciplines and expertise. The agency provides mental health, mental retardation, and drug and alcohol programs. Funding is provided primarily through the state and county Offices of Mental Health, Mental Retardation, and Drug and Alcohol. Certain programs also receive federal funding. Fees for service are determined on a sliding scale, and some clients do pay toward their treatment costs.

The Intensive Case Management (ICM) program is in the mental health department of the agency. The ICM program consists of two supervisors, nine intensive case managers, one intensive case management support staff person, and one administrative assistant. One of the supervisors is the ICM program director who supervises one ICM team that consists of two case managers who work primarily with children (LeCroy, 1992), two case managers who work primarily with adults, and one case manager who works primarily with Russian-speaking adults. She also supervises the other department supervisor, a program manager, who in turn, supervises the ICM support staff and a team of four case managers who work primarily with adults. That manager does not carry a caseload, but works with clients and staff from both teams.

Intensive case managers (ICMs) maintain relatively small caseloads, which usually do not exceed 30 clients. Thus ICMs have the time to develop close working relationships with their clients and work with them toward achieving identified goals and outcomes. Intensive case managers are expected to have contact with their clients at least every two weeks, however most clients are seen much more frequently.

Policy

Various policies mandate the services that ICMs provide. Many years ago, people with a major mental illness were left in large institutions with limited active treatment and little or no hope of ever returning to the community. With the introduction of psychotropic medication, the civil rights movement, which asserted the right of the severely mentally ill to live and be protected in the community, as well as the realization that such long-term hospitalization was extremely expensive, deinstitutionalization began in the 1960s and has continued into the 1990s. Legislation in the 1960s gave birth to the development of community mental health centers, which in addition to other services, provided the follow-up treatment for people with a major mental illness (Bloom, 1984). The patients who were discharged into the community required follow-up care to minimize future hospitalizations (Homstra et al., 1993).

Through the years, the focus of treatment programs has changed to address issues unique to certain populations. At one time, outpatient therapy for the "worried well" was more the focus of treatment dollars. The focus now is on people with serious and persistent mental illness who tend to have frequent psychiatric inpatient hospitalizations or frequent contact with psychiatric emergency services (Cohen, 1990). As a result, the Intensive Case Management program is mandated and monitored by the state (Rothman, 1994). Although ICM is a very expensive program, it is still less expensive than inpatient hospitalizations (Dorwart and Hoover, 1994). The ICM is expected to work closely with clients, their families, supports, and other service providers to decrease the number and length of hospitalizations and to help clients develop the skills necessary to function as independently as possible in the community (Bigelow and Young, 1991). ICMs can accomplish these goals by referring clients to programs that are alternatives to hospitalization (Budson, 1994).

Currently in Pennsylvania, the law provides for two types of admission to a psychiatric hospital. People can be admitted either voluntarily or involuntarily. A voluntary admission is referred to as a "201" under the

Mental Health Procedures Act. This type of admission can take place when a client and psychiatrist together agree that psychiatric hospitalization is indicated. The client can sign into the hospital and is required to give 72 hours notice prior to signing out of the hospital.

Involuntary admission under the Mental Health Procedures Act is referred to as a "302." In order for a 302 to be approved by the county delegate, the petitioner must be able to testify that he or she witnessed the person exhibit signs of mental illness and that he or she has witnessed behavior that demonstrates that the person is a danger to him or herself or others. If those criteria are met and if a psychiatrist then concurs that inpatient hospitalization is necessary, then the person can be admitted for up to five days. At that point, he or she will have a hearing to determine whether continued involuntary inpatient hospitalization is appropriate.

Criteria have been established to determine who should receive ICM services. Title 55 of the Pennsylvania Code (Office of Mental Health, 1991) addresses consumer eligibility for ICM as follows.

(a) Persons eligible for intensive case management are:

    1.   Adults, 18 years of age or older, who have a serious and persistent mental illness

    A person shall be considered to have a serious and persistent mental illness when two of the following criteria are met:

    (i)   Diagnosis—Schizophrenia or chronic major mood disorder (diagnosis codes 295 and 296 in the DSM III-R)

    (ii)   Treatment history—One of the following:

        (A) Admission to state mental hospitals totaling 60 days within the past two years

        (B) Two admissions to community inpatient psychiatric units totaling 20 or more days within the past two years

        (C) Five or more face-to-face encounters with emergency services personnel within the past two years.

        (D) Three or more years of continuous attendance in a community mental health service, at least one unit of service per quarter

        (E) History of a sporadic course of treatment as evidenced by at least three missed appointments within the past six months, inability to or unwillingness to

maintain medication regimen, or involuntary commitment to outpatient treatment

(iii) Functioning level—One of the following:

*(A) Global assessment of functioning scale (*DSM-III-R, *pages 12 and 20) ratings of 40 and below*

(B) A rating of 60 and below if the person is 35 years of age or younger or has a history of aggressive or violent behaviors

2. *Adults who were receiving intensive case management services as children and were reviewed by the provider and approved by the county administrator as needing intensive case management services beyond the date of transition from child to adult*

3. *Children who are mentally ill or emotionally disturbed and who meet one of the criteria described as follows:*

(i) Children, six years of age or younger, who are enrolled in or require early intervention services under section 671 of the Education of the Handicapped Act

(ii) Children who, with their families, are receiving services from three or more publicly funded programs such as, Medical Assistance, Aid to Families with Dependent Children, and Special Education

(iii) Children who are returning from state mental hospitals, community inpatient units, or other out-of-home placements, including foster homes and juvenile court placements

(iv) Children who are recommended as needing mental health services by a local interagency team that shall include county agency representatives

4. *Families of eligible children who are receiving intensive case management services*

(b) Exceptions—An adult or child who is receiving, or who needs to receive, mental health services, but who does not meet the requirements of this section is eligible for intensive case management upon review and recommendation by the county administrator and written approval by the department's area Office of Mental Health.

Managed care has had a significant impact on the entire mental health system (Boyle and Callahan, 1995). Its impact on the ICM program has been increasing over time. The Medicaid (MA) program is converting to an HMO system. Currently in Pennsylvania, MA recipients can voluntarily choose to switch to an HMO through MA, and eventually the switch will be mandated. At this time, MA recipients can continue with MA coverage as they have known it, sign up for an MA HMO, or sign up for an MA HMO and change their MA HMO every month. The difficulty that this presents to ICM is that some MA HMOs do not pay for ICM services. If they do pay, prior authorization must be obtained from the HMO. One of the problems is that the client may not always inform the ICM of the insurance change, thereby risking reimbursement for ICM. When an HMO does authorize ICM, it does so by limiting the number of 15-minute units of service per month. The HMO then closely monitors the client's progress and the units of service used by the ICMs. If ICMs use more units of service than approved in a given month, the HMO decides whether it will authorize payment for those units.

Technology

Varied technologies apply to ICM. The Management Information System (MIS) Department oversees much of the computer-related technology. A computer system is used to compile the data obtained daily from clinicians regarding clients and the services that they receive. Reports are generated regularly to describe the frequency of contacts with clients or others with regard to clients, location, activity, outcome, time spent, etc.

Medication is a critical aspect of positive treatment outcomes. New medications are being used with well-documented benefits. Some require closer medical follow-up, such as regular blood tests, and the ICMs assist their clients in that process. All ICMs carry a beeper with them so that they can be reached when out in the community. In addition, ICMs use crisis beepers to provide 24-hour emergency coverage to clients. Intensive case managers complete strength-based service plans with clients at least once every six months. They also complete treatment plans every three months, as well as annual psychosocial evaluations. Psychiatrists meet with clients to complete psychiatric evaluations and assure that medication is appropriate. Medical tests and imaging might be needed to rule out organic disorders. For some clients the use of electroconvulsive therapy (ECT) is beneficial. ICMs use agency vans to transport clients when necessary. The vans are equipped with mobile phones so that the case managers can communicate with clients and staff as needed.

Organization

The process of teaming in the provision of ICM services is relatively new in Philadelphia. Previously, case managers would be assigned a caseload and would be responsible for those specific clients. When an ICM was out sick or on vacation, other ICMs would fill in as needed. If an ICM left his or her job, the caseload would be temporarily assigned to other case managers. Clients, their family members, and other supports would work closely with just one ICM. If that ICM left his or her job, it was difficult for other staff to know how to proceed with that client and for client and family to feel comfortable working with new staff.

Teaming in ICM has been a tremendous asset in coping with these issues (Abramson, 1989). Clients are now assigned a primary ICM who is responsible to assure that paperwork is completed on time and that the client's needs are met; however, the primary is not the only ICM who works with the client. Each ICM has his or her own unique style, experiences, areas of interest, and expertise. Exposing clients to a diverse group of professionals seems to be enriching for them and allows the ICMs to enrich their experience. In this way, when ICMs leave, client's relationships with other ICMs may lessen the loss and ease the transition. It is also much easier for ICM staff, who are already accustomed to working with a particular client and his or her supports. Teaming in ICM also has helped to decrease staff burnout. When case managers become increasingly frustrated by manipulative and high-risk behaviors or threats, they do not have to deal with these situations alone.

Weekly, in addition to individual supervision, each ICM team meets with a consulting psychiatrist, and both teams meet together to discuss ongoing issues, monitor progress, and share resources. ICMs also meet with each other informally on a daily basis to review current status and crisis situations. The team shares the responsibility for developing and revising ongoing plans.

The ICMs are mandated by the state to attend a certain number of training days each year. Each ICM is required to attend a one-time ICM basic training, which teaches the referral process for many programs and familiarizes him or her with resources available to clients. As long as that training mandate is met, ICMs can choose from a variety of other training topics based on their own interests. Some ICM trainings address issues such as motivating unmotivated people, working with people who have a mental illness and drug and alcohol problem, establishing boundaries, developing effective and unique service/treatment plans, managing aggressive behaviors, exploring cultural differences, assessing risk of suicide, as well as other issues ranging from sexual abuse to psychopharmacology.

The ICM program functions 24 hours per day, seven days per week, 365 days per year. Intensive case managers are on call and can be reached by beeper at any time during the workday. In addition, each team has one emergency beeper that is rotated among all team members, allowing each staff person to be on call approximately one week per month. Also, because ICM serves an area with many Russian immigrants, there is one emergency beeper for Russian-speaking clients. The supervisors also participate in on-call coverage.

Intensive case managers work very closely with staff from other programs in the mental health system and with members of the community (Moore, 1992). Developing strong working relationships with other providers is critical to the ICM role (Florentine and Grusky, 1990). Clients are informed by their ICM that they can be referred to services throughout the mental health system, not only at the particular agency that the ICM represents. When clients are referred, the ICM follows up regularly to monitor and reassess their progress. For example, when a client goes to a vocational or day program, the ICM will meet regularly with the client and the appropriate staff to coordinate treatment. The same holds true whether the client is in the community or in a short- or long-term psychiatric hospital (Kanter, 1991). ICMs provide such continuity to assure that all members of the client's treatment team are aware of progress or any concerns, if the client appears to be decompensating.

PRACTICE DECISIONS

Description of the Client

The client is Butch Gills, a 42-year-old, divorced, white male who currently lives in a community residential rehabilitation (CRR) program at the maximum-care level. He is relatively short, with a medium build and blonde hair. His ex-wife refuses to have any contact with him. After his divorce, he lived with his parents before moving into the CRR. They had difficulty managing his behaviors, mood swings, complaints, threats, and obsessive thoughts at home (Torrey, 1995). He visits his family and calls them more often than they would like. He shares a CRR townhouse apartment with two roommates with whom he does not get along very well. He views himself as higher functioning and less ill than they are, and so he is often rude and disrespectful to them. Staff at the CRR encourage Butch to work toward the goal of learning to cook, but he seems to feel that is "beneath" him.

He supports himself on his SSI benefits (approximately $496.00 per month) and some financial assistance from his family. He is also a Medical Assistance (MA) recipient. At this point in time, he has not signed up for an MA HMO, but if he does, that could have a significant impact on the mental health services that he receives. When angry with ICMs or with other mental health professionals, he threatens to "get an HMO" so that he can "get rid of" us, because at times he claims that we have done nothing for him. (Boyle and Callahan, 1995)

Butch is the second oldest of four siblings—three boys and one girl. His relationships with each of his siblings is filled with conflict. They (and his parents) don't seem to have a good understanding of mental illness and how it affects Butch specifically (Mueser and Gingerich, 1994). ICMs have tried to educate family members, but they have only been minimally receptive. Butch's father has been more sympathetic to the stresses facing his son. Butch's mother is admittedly a recovering alcoholic and is over-whelmed by the challenges she faces in her own recovery. He seems to strive for approval from both of his parents and becomes angry and frustrated when he does not get it. He is extremely demanding and needy of their time and attention. They try to divide their time among their children, but Butch becomes extremely jealous when he is not the focus of their attention. That seems to only add to their continued frustration and results in their distancing themselves from him.

Butch has made some friends, but has found it almost impossible to maintain them. He demands all of their time and attention and spends much of the time with his friends talking about his obsessive thoughts. He does not seem as interested in others as he is in himself. He wants to participate in activities that interest him and does not seem to care if others enjoy the activity or not.

Intensive case managers are trained to find strengths within each of our clients. Butch has many strengths. He is friendly, outgoing, has a good sense of humor, and is quite personable. He keeps himself and his apartment clean. He is resourceful and utilizes the supports that he has. Butch has good communication skills and is often able to make his needs known.

Definition of the Client

This client was assigned to ICM because he met several of the criteria. He has been diagnosed with schizoaffective disorder (American Psychiatric Association, 1994), has been in a state mental hospital for more than 60 days, has had multiple inpatient community psychiatric hospitalizations, multiple face-to-face contacts with psychiatric emergency personnel, several years of continuous attendance in a community mental health service, and a global assessment of functioning below 40. (Bush, Langford, and Rosen, 1990)

At times, when he shows less insight, Butch does not see himself as a client. He blames the fact that he is labeled as a "client" for his problems. He sometimes states that if he never came for treatment, never took psychotropic medication, and never went into the hospital, he never would have had the types of problems he has, which result in his being the identified client (Bernheim and Lewine, 1979). He often prefers to blame others rather than take responsibility for helping himself improve.

During the course of treatment, his family has also been encouraged to obtain various mental health services. There are several problem areas for this family, and ICMs have offered to refer them to individual and/or family therapy. Additionally, they have been referred to the agency's education and support program for family members. The family has refused these services because they see Butch as the only one requiring services. (Mueser and Gingerich, 1994; Torrey, 1995)

Goals, Objectives, and/or Outcome Measures

When discussing goals, the first thing one should pay attention to is whose goals are being established. It is clear that the goals that the ICM has for Butch are often very different from the goals he has for himself. In addition, it is also clear that his parents have goals that they would like him to achieve. The program that he attends and the staff who work with him in those programs may also have their own goals for Butch to achieve. However, more than likely, the only goals that he will achieve are the ones that are his, not the ICM's, his parents', or anyone else's. Furthermore, the fact that others have their own agenda of goals for Butch does influence the work they do with him and the content of the contacts.

Some conflicts with his parents are a result of his not achieving or working toward their goals. Many of the ICM's frustrations with Butch also stem from the fact that he does not seem to be striving for that which we want (and assume he wants) to achieve. For example, a goal of ICM is to decrease the number of inpatient psychiatric hospitalization days. Butch has had a high frequency of hospitalizations over the past few years, in particular. An ICM goal is to help set up supports that will aid in avoiding unnecessary hospitalizations (Hornstra, Bruce-Wolfe, Sagduyu, and Riffle, 1993). Based on his behaviors, avoiding hospitalizations does not seem to be his goal. There are many occasions when he comes in requesting hospitalization, yet is evaluated by a psychiatrist and the recommendation is for him to remain in the community with additional support, an increase in medication, or with close supervision for a short time. Often, if he is not admitted upon his request, he will leave and go directly to a psychiatric emergency service at a hospital and request hospitalization from them without telling them that he had just been denied admission. At that time, he will often tell them that he is suicidal, even though he may not be. He can give them a description of a suicide plan and they usually will admit him. Upon closer scrutiny of the situation, one can often learn that Butch had no plans for the weekend, so he went into the hospital. When that is the true reason for admission, he often signs himself out of the hospital in just a few days. His manipulation of the mental health system is extremely frustrating to those who work with him.

One consistent goal for Butch is to increase contact with his family. This is in complete contrast to his parents' goal that he have less contact with them. Again, this is a major source of conflict between them. Butch also seems interested in getting a job as a retail sales clerk, but at this time, due to his shifts in mood and his thought disorder, this is an unrealistic goal (Hatfield and Lefley, 1993). ICMs encourage Butch to see this as a long-term goal and urge him to set smaller goals that will ultimately help him achieve the goal of a job as a sales person. He has difficulty focusing on the more achievable short-term goals. He gets impatient and wants to "just go out and get a job." ICMs do not want to see him fail, but we are clear with him that the choice is his, not ours.

Use of Contract

There are both written and unwritten contracts with Butch. He knows that he does not have to talk to an ICM if he doesn't want to on a particular day. If he does want to talk to or meet with an ICM, he can do that without a scheduled appointment. Since he is usually so needy of time from ICMs, he has met with most members of both ICM teams and seems comfortable talking to all of them. Butch has given the ICMs written permission to talk to his family and other treatment providers. He is aware that periodically the ICM does contact others to monitor his progress.

The more formal written contract between Butch and the ICM team is his strength-based service plan, which is updated at least every six months. The service plan can address the following areas: mental health, drug and alcohol, physical health, living situation, daily living, household, financial management, education, vocation/employment, legal, social support, leisure, and mobility. In order to complete the service plan, the ICM discusses each of the areas with Butch. They talk about the current status and Butch's strengths in each area, then Butch decides whether he wants to develop a goal and what the goal is. He and the ICM then outline the specific measurable action steps needed to achieve the goal, who is responsible for each step, and what the time frame for completion will be.

Meeting Place

ICMs meet with Butch in the partial hospital day program, which Butch attends four to five days per week; the ICM office; his apartment; his parents' home; the community; at medical appointments; in psychiatric emergency rooms; and in the various psychiatric hospitals to which he has been admitted. Experience has shown that it is best to see each client in as many different settings as possible. It allows the case manager to see a different perspective each time. It is also helpful to see clients interact with other people. Some people behave differently in one setting versus another. Paying close attention to those sometimes subtle changes can provide valuable information. Meeting in various settings has also helped to build the working relationship with Butch because he sees the ICMs in all of those situations as well. Many clients have expressed a great deal of appreciation to ICMs for "being there" with them in so many settings. It allows the ICM to see the client at his or her best and worst.

Use of Time

Time can be difficult to manage for ICMs working with Butch. He is, by his own admission, very attention-seeking with family, peers, and service providers. Whether he is inpatient or outpatient at a particular time makes no difference in his need for time and attention. Sometimes just spending a few minutes is enough, but usually he feels the need for more time. As a result, ICM and other members of the treatment team have felt "burned out" from working so closely with him. The team model for providing ICM services has been useful. Butch meets with his primary ICM as well as other members of the ICM team on a rotating basis. Therefore, no one ICM is expected to meet all of his demands for attention. We set clear boundaries with him and assist him in developing coping skills. He is redirected to utilize other supports, when appropriate, in an effort to empower him toward independence. We have tried to help him better articulate what he actually wants or needs, so that he can advocate on his own behalf. Since he often seeks attention when he is bored, ICMs assist him in structuring his leisure time. This usually includes developing a detailed schedule with him.

Interventions

Clients' problems and their individual coping skills and supports vary widely, as do the types of interventions used by case managers. ICMs are trained in intervention techniques. Intensive case managers are flexible, supportive, and have engagement, assessment, and advocacy skills. The ICM approach is strength-based and views clients in all aspects of their lives (Sullivan, 1992). We assess and reassess our clients regularly to determine strengths and needs in all areas addressed in the ICM service plan. In addition, we need to look for and assess any other areas as they arise.

One of the main points of intervention for ICMs with Butch is in the psychiatric emergency room when he presents himself for hospital admission. We work closely with emergency service staff in assessing Butch and making recommendations for treatment. The assessment and plan at this point is often critical to the outcome. The ICM team members are proactive and help him develop alternatives to hospitalization. We encourage him to agree to the least restrictive appropriate treatment.

Stance of the Social Worker

The stance taken by ICMs with Butch has changed over time. Butch's problems have also changed, to a certain degree, and different patterns of behavior have been established. We want to assist him in learning to tolerate boredom and to find constructive ways to spend his time. This results in decreased hospitalizations.

Intensive case managers have tried to be a "constant" in Butch's life. Many people who come to a mental health center for treatment are referred from one program to the next. They have different clinicians working with them in each program. For some individuals, this is very difficult. Some clients have said that it is difficult to start to build a relationship with one clinician, then to be referred to another and start over again. Butch is one of those people who have that difficulty. Having an ICM team who works with a client regardless of which program or mental health center he or she attends, where he or she lives, whether or not he or she is cooperative, or has other supports, is a powerful dimension to treatment (Raiff and Shore, 1993). Each ICM client knows that wherever he or she goes, whatever he or she does, the ICM team will be there to offer support. ICMs help clients identify and gain access to their support systems (Biegel, Tracy, and Corvo, 1994). It is much healthier for clients to call a responsible friend or a family member to socialize or talk to about certain things, rather than to call the ICM.

Consistency and familiarity are important to clients and to family members who also receive support, time, information, education, and attention from the team (Rubin, 1992). Many family members report that they are comforted by knowing that the ICM is a constant for their loved one. This is particularly important to parents who are concerned about what will happen to their mentally ill son or daughter once the parents are no longer able to care for them.

Each ICM has a different personality, style, and approach in working with clients, and each has strengths in particular areas. Some are firmer with clients and better able to set clear boundaries and limits, while others are more supportive and empathic. Some are more formal with clients and others, less formal. Fine clinicians blend styles and develop the clinical skills necessary to alter the approach as the client's needs change (Anthony, Cohen, and Farkas, 1988). Teaming in ICM allows for clients to receive the best from each case manager.

Many clients seem to feel that people view them in terms of their mental illness; consequently, that one aspect of their lives often becomes their identity. Intensive case managers do not see them that way. We see them as people with strengths and weaknesses, hopes and dreams, and with qualities of all human beings. Not all of their issues are a result of their mental illness. Many times they are confronting the same developmental hurdles with which we all must manage. Unfortunately, many of their hopes and dreams have been robbed from them by mental illness. They often have difficulty with developing relationships, tolerating stress, and learning effective coping skills (Hatfield and Lefley, 1993). Many people lose sight of their strengths and only focus on their illness. As professionals, we help our clients and their loved ones see the strengths within and work to bring them out.

Use of Outside Resources

Over time, Butch has been referred to inpatient psychiatric hospitals, respite programs, partial hospital and social rehabilitation day programs (Garvin, 1992), vocational programs, drop-in centers for consumers of mental health services, programs and services for adult children of alcoholics, medical appointments, boarding homes, community residential rehabilitation programs, Social Security, and Medicaid. Butch prefers to receive services close to home and therefore tends to refuse referrals that are not in the immediate geographic area.

Within the past year, Butch agreed to be referred to a companion program. This program matches a client with a volunteer who is able to spend one-to-one time in social contact with the client (Biegel, Tracy, and Corvo, 1994). Overall, the match between Butch and his companion seems to have been a success. However, at times Butch will talk about his companion in unkind ways. His feelings about and reactions to others shift with his moods. This is very frustrating for Butch's companion and the ICM team.

The city of Philadelphia has adopted a community support program approach to working with people with serious and persistent mental illness (Macias et al., 1994). This model places the client at the center and the ICM directly around him or her. The ICM is viewed as the link between the client and a variety of services and supports including client identification and outreach, mental health treatment, crisis response services, health and dental care, housing, income support and entitlements, peer support, family and community support, rehabilitation services, and protection and advocacy. The ICM assesses the client, determines appropriate outside resources, makes the referrals, and monitors the client's progress on an ongoing basis. Figure 24.1 is an ecomap for Butch Gills, which outlines available resources.

Reassessment

Reassessment is an integral aspect of ICM. Since in many situations our clients are generally involved in a wide variety of programs on a daily or weekly basis, we meet with them in those environments, and monitor and assess their progress (Bedell, 1994). Butch is scheduled to attend a partial hospital day program four to five days each week. ICMs meet with him and staff regularly to reassess his progress in the program. When there is a problem, program staff inform the ICM so they can also assess the client and make recommendations. As valuable members of the treatment team, staff in these programs work closely with our clients, respond to situations as they arise, and help the ICMs determine when the client is ready to move to the next level of treatment. Reassessment helps the client and staff be aware of stressful situations that could result in the client decompensating. The psychiatrist can be consulted to adjust medications as needed. This proactive approach can reduce pressures and support the client through a potentially difficult time. Therefore, reassessment is an essential tool for decreasing psychiatric hospitalizations.

Transfer or Termination

According to the Pennsylvania Code (Office of Mental Health, 1991), Section 5221.12 continues:

(c) Termination–Intensive case management may be terminated for one of the following reasons:

    1. Determination by the consumer or the parent of a child receiving the service that intensive case management is no longer needed or wanted

   2. *Determination by the intensive case manager in consultation with his supervisor or the director of intensive case management, and with written concurrence by the county administrator that intensive case management is no longer necessary or appropriate for the adult or child receiving the services*

As part of the mandate for the ICM program, cases may not be closed unless the above mentioned criteria are met. ICMs have been working with Butch for many years. Many of us have established a strong working relationship with him and his family. More than likely, Butch's case will not be closed to ICM in the near future. When his current ICM leaves her position, Butch will be reassigned. Knowing other ICM team members will ease his initial anxiety about working with a new ICM who will use the existing service plan for further continuity.

Case Conclusion

Coping with a mental illness is an overwhelming prospect, and Butch and his family rely on the entire ICM team for support and encouragement (Hatfield and Lefley, 1993). The relationship has grown over the years and although Butch complains about the ICMs at times, he continues to turn to us when things are not going well. He also shares successes with the ICM team. Overall, Butch and his family agree that having an ICM is a true asset in his life (Rubin, 1992). We will continue to help him gain insight, overcome obstacles, and achieve success.

Differential Discussion

In retrospect, it seems that several conflicts in Butch's life are as a result of power struggles with his family, friends, and mental health professionals. His family and friends have pushed him to be the type of son/brother/friend that they want, rather than truly listening to what he wants and needs. They have been reluctant to find a reasonable compromise or to just "give-in" on some issues that are not worth arguing about. Butch, his family, and friends have placed a lot of importance on "winning each argument." Perhaps the treatment team could have found other ways to help Butch and his family get to the point where they could share feelings, openly discuss issues, and develop better strategies for problem solving and communication.

Mental health professionals have struggled to help Butch gain insight into his illness, take responsibility for his actions, and decrease psychiat-

FIGURE 24.1. Ecomap for Butch Gills

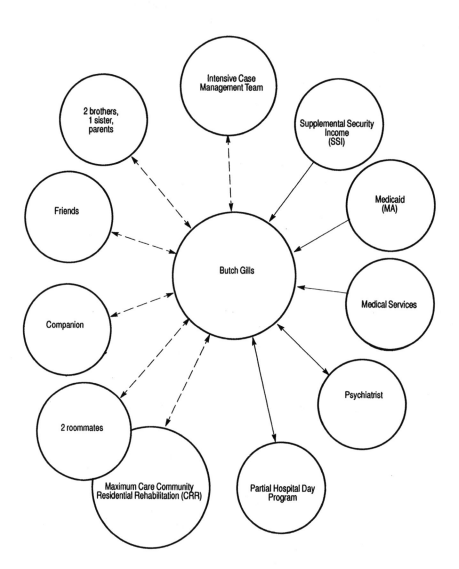

ric hospitalizations. As a result, we put pressure on him to achieve our goals of decreasing hospitalizations and finding appropriate ways to get attention from others. It is important to be aware of whose goals are being addressed—the client's or the treatment team's. More than likely, he will only achieve the goals that are his, not goals that others have for him.

REFERENCES

Abramson, J. S. (1989). Making teams work. *Social Work with Groups, 12*(4), 45-63.

American Psychiatric Association. (1994). *Diagnostic and statistical manual of mental disorders,* Fourth Edition. Washington, DC: American Psychiatric Association.

Anthony, W. A., Cohen, M., and Farkas, M. (1988). The chronically mentally ill: Case management—more than a response to dysfunctional system. *Community Mental Health Journal, 24,* 219-228.

Bedell, J. R. (Ed.). (1994). *Psychological assessment and treatment of persons with severe mental disorders.* Washington, DC: Taylor and Francis.

Bernheim, K. F. and Lewine, R. R. (1979). *Schizophrenia: Symptoms, causes, treatments.* New York: W. W. Norton and Company.

Biegel, D. E., Tracy, E. M., and Corvo, K. N. (1994). Strengthening social networks: Intervention strategies for mental health case managers. *Health and Social Work, 19*(3), 206-216.

Bigelow, D. A. and Young, D. J. (1991). Effectiveness of a case management program. *Community Mental Health Journal, 27,* 115-123.

Bloom, B. L. (1984). *Community mental health: A general introduction,* Second Edition. Monterey, CA: Brooks/Cole.

Boyle, P. J. and Callahan, D. (1995). Managed care in mental health: The ethical issues. *Health Affairs, 14*(3), 7-22.

Budson, R. D. (1994). Community residential and partial hospital care: Low-cost alternative systems in the spectrum of care. *Psychiatric Quarterly, 65*(3), 209-220.

Bush, C., Langford, M., and Rosen, P., and Gott, W. (1990). Operation outreach: Intensive case management for severely psychiatrically disabled adults. *Hospital and Community Psychiatry, 41,* 647-651.

Cohen, N. L. (Ed.). (1990). *Psychiatry takes to the streets: Outreach and crisis intervention for the mentally ill.* New York: The Guilford Press.

Dorwart, R. A. and Hoover, C. W. (1994). A national study of transitional hospital services in mental health. *American Journal of Public Health, 84*(8), 1229-1234.

Florentine, R. and Grusky, O. (1990). When case managers manage seriously mentally ill: A role-contingency approach. *Social Service Review, 64,* 79-93.

Garvin, C. (1992). A task centered group approach to work with the chronically mentally ill. *Social Work with Groups, 15*(2/3), 67-80.

Hatfield, A. B. and Lefley, H. P. (1993). *Surviving mental illness: Stress, coping and adaptation.* New York: The Guilford Press.

Hornstra, R. K., Bruce-Wolfe, V., Sagduyu, K., and Riffle, D. W. (1993). The effect of intensive case management on hospitalization of patients with schizophrenia. *Hospital and Community Psychiatry, 44*(9), 844-847.

Kanter, J. S. (1991). Integrating case management and psychiatric hospitalization. *Health and Social Work, 16*(1), 34-42.

LeCroy, C. W. (1992). Enhancing the delivery of effective mental health services to children. *Journal of the National Association of Social Workers, 37*(3), 225-231.

Macias, C., Kinney, R., Farley, O. W., Jackson, R., and Vos, B. (1994). The role of case management within a community support system: Partnership with psychosocial rehabilitation. *Community Mental Health Journal, 30*(4), 323-339.

Moore, S. (1992). Case management and the integration of services: How services delivery systems shape case management. *Social Work, 37*, 418-423.

Mueser, K. T. and Gingerich, S. (1994). *Coping with schizophrenia: A guide for families*. Oakland, CA: New Harbinger Publications.

Office of Mental Health–Commonwealth of Pennsylvania. (1991, May). Pennsylvania Code. Title 55-Public Welfare. Department of Public Welfare, Chapter 5221–Mental Health Intensive Case Management.

Raiff, N. R. and Shore, B. K. (1993). *Advanced case management: New strategies for the nineties*. Newbury Park, CA: Sage.

Rothman, J. (1994). *Practice with highly vulnerable clients: Case management and community-based service*. Englewood Cliffs, NJ: Prentice Hall.

Rubin, A. (1992). Is case management effective for people with serious mental illness? A research review. *Health and Social Work, 17*(2), 138-150.

Sullivan, W. P. (1992). Reclaiming the community: The strengths perspective and deinstitutionalization. *Journal of the National Association of Social Workers, 37*(3), 204-209.

Torrey, E. F. (1995). *Surviving schizophrenia: A manual for families, consumers, and providers*, third edition. New York: Harper & Row.

Chapter 25

He's Schizophrenic
and the System Is Not Helping:
Reflections of a Troubled Parent
and Professional

Mona Wasow

INTRODUCTION

This chapter is written by a person who wears three hats: first and foremost, the hat of an endlessly grieving parent of a son who has schizophrenia; second, that of an educator in the area of serious mental illness; and, third, as a clinician. The three hats are sometimes in serious conflict with each other.

Fifteen years ago, when this chapter was first written, I had many more answers than I have now! Schizophrenia is a dreadful disease with no known cure, and it leaves many victims in its path of destruction. Just as cancer is a generic term for many different illnesses with multiple etiologies and multiple outcomes, so schizophrenia is a generic term for many different serious mental illnesses (SMI) that probably have different etiologies, and most surely have different outcomes. The schizophrenias strike 1 to 1.5 percent of the population the world over, and there is ample evidence that these illnesses are brain diseases, albeit ones that are exquisitely sensitive to environmental stresses.

With most serious diseases, parents usually get prompt and sympathetic help when they ask for it. Sometimes there is little that can be done, but the medical model is used to intervene as soon as possible to prevent further deterioration. Only in SMI is this reversed in a strange and terrible way. Mental illness seems to have fallen into the hands of the legal profession, under the name of civil rights. In our zeal to protect human freedoms, we have created a legal climate in which mentally ill patients are free to "die with their rights on." Mental health laws prevent involuntary medications and involuntary hospitalizations. They were designed out of a scientific and humane concern "to protect the rights of mental patients and to insure that unwanted, difficult people are not dumped into mental hospitals to be forgotten" (Wasow, 1978, p. 128). This, in principal, is a good idea and no doubt has spared unnecessary loss of freedoms for many people; but the law has gone to an extreme that now prevents help to those in desperate need (Ennis, 1973).

MANAGED CARE

"How does managed care affect people with SMI?" I asked the director of an institution for people with schizophrenia. "Oh, yes, 'mangled care.' . . ." she responded. The basic premises behind managed care are sound. Health care should be well coordinated and provided efficiently. Economic crises call for greater effort at providing low-cost care. It also makes sense to evaluate the work being done to look for progress and results. In reality, however, there are monumental problems with managed care in the SMI area. Some case managers do not know what they are doing. Money that should be going into treatment and care often goes into management costs. Management is very time-consuming. Not only does money get diverted away from treatment, but so too does time. As one case manager succinctly put it, "There is so much bureaucracy to deal with. Today, I spent three hours on the telephone with insurance companies and ten minutes with the client."

Specific to SMIs is the issue of time. Perhaps it is realistic to estimate six days of hospital time for the treatment of certain kidney problems, but such time estimate for SMIs are totally unrealistic. Because of the nature of the illness, SMIs are not treated on a par with other serious illness. No one says you have a $10,000 limit on cancer treatment, for example, but that is exactly what is done in the area of SMI. Many policies have a $10,000 limit; others limit outpatient visits to 20 per year, and so on. In order to keep some people with SMI in the community, weekly visits are a must, and the year has 52 weeks. So instead of adequate care, we get the revolving-door phenomenon. Managed care insists on periodic reviews to look for progress and results. Again, in principle this makes sense. In reality, it puts people with a SMI in a "Catch 22" position. If there is improvement, people are discharged, which often means that deterioration follows. If there is no improvement, they are discharged, which means further deterioration. The nature of many SMIs does not fit the desired course of illness as perceived by managed care.

PERSONAL INVOLVEMENT

My son David was born in 1957, a beautiful, big, healthy, brown-eyed boy. It was surely one of the most joyous days of my life. My first personal encounter with the mental health system came in 1972, the year David was 15. Something was wrong: despite his desire to do well, our lovely, bright son was failing in school. He was behaving very erratically, and his moods swung from extreme happiness to acute depression. I took him to see Dr. A, a well-known psychiatrist in town. Dr. A spent one hour with the boy and referred him to a child psychiatrist. The specialist spent two hours, charged us $100, and declared David to be "a fine, intact youngster." "What a relief," I thought, "the specialist must be right!"

By the next year, however, things were much worse. David was now a truant, and his mood swings were even greater. He was also actively hallucinating and thought that "people" were planning to destroy him. He told us with great agitation that he was going to take a gun and go north where he would find food to save all the starving people of the world.

David began to wander away from the house for days at a time–usually barefoot and without money or food. He offered no explanation of where he had been except to say that he was headed for Alaska. He looked exhausted. We were all badly frightened and felt we had lost control over the situation. I took David back to Dr. A, who told me, "Your son has an inability to screen out sensory perceptions." A year later, however, he admitted to us that he had realized that David was schizophrenic at that time. Was he afraid of labeling our son? He never shared that diagnosis with us, he only spoke of "sensory perceptions." Ignorance helped neither our son nor us. A paragraph from my personal journal reads,

> My God, what is happening to our little David? Those were hallu-
> cinations last night! Is this what R.D. Laing calls "a different way of
> looking at life?" Or is David mentally ill? Is it bad genes, or bad
> parenting? I know these are futile, irrelevant questions. But we must
> get help! I'm so scared. (Wasow, 1978, pp. 135-136)

My case, unfortunately, is all too typical. In 1973, when David was 16 and "schizophrenia" was finally diagnosed, we were told that medications were an absolute necessity to prevent further deterioration. At that time, David was still able to function reasonably well. He said, rather typically for a person with schizophrenia, "I will not take meds. I am not sick."

Following is an excerpt from a letter I wrote to "that month's" psychiatrist, during a period when we were able to get David admitted to the hospital "through the back door."

Dear Dr. B.,

A note of explanation as to why I've temporarily stopped coming to family therapy session on Tuesdays. I've lost hope–it seems so futile. I'd like to suggest we try something new.

You say that David has a lifelong pattern of holding other people responsible for his life. Therefore, you will attempt to get him to take responsibility by not taking it for him. As a theory, that makes sense. But suppose he really is *not* capable of this? Then it's like insisting that a cripple walk. I've thought about this a great deal, trying to understand the pattern of David and our family over the past 16 years, and I think you have cause and effect mixed up. Perhaps other people have always directed David's life because he's been unable to cope himself. There is another case of schizophrenia in the family, and there may be a genetic component here. It seems to me, and to others I've talked to who have known David since birth, that he never "would have made it," even to age 12, without the extra protection he was given.

The reason I dwell on this is because of the rapid deterioration that has set in since we withdrew our support and direction. To me, David's deterioration indicates that we're on the wrong track. In January 1973, my husband and I gave up control, and David was essentially on his own. We were friendly, but there was very little contact with David. We did stay out of his life at this time, just as you are doing at the hospital. It was between January and June that he went from "intact" to really sick.

When we put him in the hospital, he still was largely intact. It seems to us the last three months have seen steady deterioration. I was shocked when he came home last weekend–he eats like an animal, he takes no care of himself physically (unbathed, hair matted and filthy), he doesn't talk at all, and he seems profoundly depressed. Also, he has active hallucinations.

I know that there are no correct answers for this kind of mental problem. I am panicked. I love my kid, and I want us to try another direction before it's too late. There's nothing to lose. I truly believe (and, I guess, this is a professional difference of opinion between us) that it would be helpful to David to be told: "I am the doctor. You are the patient. Let me help." The kid is panicked and feels hopeless and helpless. I think that at this point he needs someone to take control temporarily, because he doesn't seem to have the hope, faith, or ability to do it on his own. Please let me hear from you soon. I am writing instead of talking because I'm so terribly upset. (Wasow, 1978, pp. 139-141)

For the following four years, we lived an indescribable nightmare as we watched our beloved son turn into a suffering, terrified person. Every doctor said he must have medicine. Everywhere we turned the law said, "No, we must protect his civil rights." Can you imagine the law determining whether or not you could give antibiotics or a blood transfusion to a child in need of surgery (Knee, 1977)? After four years, our son was a psychotic vegetable, unable to feed or clothe himself, wandering about on highways in front of traffic. There really are no words to describe the pain, suffering, panic, and destruction of those days, for all of us. Madness reigned supreme, both in our son and in the mental health care system. The dominant concern of the mental health system was to follow the law, not to help David. Finally, David stepped in front of a car on the highway and was officially judged "incompetent" under the Wisconsin mental health law that provides for involuntary commitment for treatment—four years too late. He was committed to a hospital and responded beautifully to medications. Within a few days, he was without psychotic symptoms, feeling deep relief, and able to take care of his basic needs. He was certainly not normal, but he was greatly improved and remained so for the next six months (Wasow, 1986).

Under the new mental health laws, a case must be reviewed in the courts every six months. Even after having gone through it twice in the last four years, I cannot quite believe what followed: David was declared "competent." He went off his medications and slowly but surely became desperately ill again. In the next three years, the cycle was repeated; only it was even worse. Pleading with doctors and lawyers about what had happened in the past and what was obviously happening again was in vain.

Let me skip the horror of those seven years and get to the details of May 1980. David was wandering about in a psychotic state, eating out of garbage cans, hallucinating, living in a terror I do not suppose I understand. One night, perhaps, as a desperate plea for help, he attempted to jump out of a tenth story window. Good news! Now he could be declared "dangerous to self or others," and the crisis intervention team was called. They were called at 8 p.m. and arrived at midnight. But now there was a new problem: by midnight, David was catatonic. As such, he was not considered "dangerous," and the crisis team left. The following day was a repeat, and this time the crisis team said, "hospitalize him." He was then handcuffed and put in a police car, where he spent the next six hours being rejected by every major hospital in Madison, Wisconsin. Finally, he was accepted into a hospital 20 miles outside of the city. The following week, two court hearings were held to determine whether or not he was mentally ill and in need of care. The local mental health board had lawyers there to look after his civil rights. There was no physician there to look after his health. Therein lies the crux of this issue: the battle is civil rights versus health care. In every other illness, medical intervention is used at the earliest possible moment. Only in mental illness does the law dictate that such intervention can only be used voluntarily or at the end stage of the illness. Now it is 1995, 23 years since our first encounter with the mental health and legal systems. At the moment, David is considered a success statistic in a model community treatment program. He is a "success" because he has not been rehospitalized in the past three years, and because he is quiet and unobtrusive and does not bother anyone.

Once it was suggested that he live on his own, but within a few months, he was very skinny, had boils on his body, and was essentially mute. There was no toilet paper in his bathroom, no food, no sheets on the mattress, and the chaos in his room was congruent with the chaos in his poor, sick mind. He had lived in 15 different places in 12 years: three times with relatives, four times in a room by himself, twice at the YMCA, in two different group homes, once in jail for six weeks while waiting for a court hearing to determine placement (that was his only crime: truancy—no place to live), once in a room with a roommate, once in an unlocked institution for 130 mentally ill people, and then off to an NIMH project. There were also six hospitalizations, but I do not count those. His case is quite typical for a SMI person. Moves are stressful even for people in good health. Imagine what all that moving does to a frightened, fragile, mentally ill person.

None of our model community treatment programs would consider my son or others like him a "success." They understand that rehospitalization should not be the only outcome criterion—that quality of life, patient satisfaction, and social functioning all need to be considered. But the reality of the situation is that despite massive deterioration, the mental health system as a whole does not provide him asylum. So unless he commits an outwardly violent act, my son gets listed as a "success" in the deinstitutionalization movement. That is not how he looks to me. I think he looks like a giant, broken, plastic throwaway toy. And he breaks my heart (Wasow, 1978, pp. 162-167). The deinstitutionalization movement has been a success in that most people with SMIs are no longer locked up in hospitals, and that is a very good thing. What has failed is adequate community care. There is nothing more I can say or do for my poor, desperately ill son or the thousands upon thousands of others who suffer like him.

DIFFERENT PERSPECTIVES

"People with mental illnesses, family members, educators, researchers, clinicians, religious leaders, and policymakers have multiple perspectives on SMI and what needs to be done in every conceivable situation" (Wasow, 1995, p. 171). There are major and understandably different perspectives on the issues of deinstitutionalization vs. asylum, medications and/or involuntary commitment, autonomy vs. dependence, confidentiality vs. information sharing, and so on. There are many different values, beliefs, and multiple agendas. Some people focus on treatment, some on social change, others on education, advocacy, research, or on housing. "Some of us are fired by pain, others by rage, political convictions, intellectual curiosity, religious belief, status, or a combination of these things. Some are no longer fired up but rather burned out" (Wasow, 1995, p. 195).

SMIs are devastating illnesses that evoke strong feelings of upset in all concerned. We are still in the dark ages in our understanding of what causes these illnesses, and how to adequately treat them. This is the ideal fermenting ground for disagreement and upset. The less we know, the greater the tendency to argue and not listen well to others. It is hard to live with ambiguity. But if all these different groups could do a better job of listening to each other to try and understand each other's different perspectives, to try and stand in the shoes of the others, there might be possibilities for creative compromise and maybe even a few solutions.

WHY SUCH ANGER?

Why do parents of people with SMI experience so much anger? The first thought that comes to mind is that the tendency to be angry and frustrated is just there for parents of *all* defective children–the "Why me, oh God?" syndrome. While part of this may be true, it is not enough to explain the extent of rage toward professionals found among parents of people with schizophrenia. In fact, in a study done on parental versus professional views of the adjustment of parents of mentally retarded (MR) children, just the opposite was found to be true (Wikler, Wasow, and Hatfield, 1981). That is, the professionals, in this case social workers, were feeling frustrated that they could not be more helpful to the parents. The parents, however, perceived the professionals as being quite helpful. The parents were not only not angry, they were grateful for the help.

What, then, are the differences? I would suggest several. In the first place, mental retardation is rightfully seen as a largely fixed condition. You can maximize what potential there is, but you cannot change the condition. With schizophrenia, some professionals are still thinking in terms of rehabilitation and "cure." But there is, at this point, no cure for schizophrenia (Mendel, 1976), and to lead parents to believe in one is an unending cruelty. Parents are constantly being led into false hopes: "If only I did this . . . or that. If only . . ."

There is another marked difference. Parents of MR children are not blamed for the retardation. It is accepted and known that it could happen to anyone. But parents of schizophrenic people are blamed by society, sometimes overtly, more often subtly. However it is done, that guilt-producing blame is clearly the greatest heartache of them all, next to actually losing the child to mental illness. Another major complaint from parents is the lack of knowledge about the disease on the part of many professionals. Information about schizophrenia is one of the things parents need most. Thankfully, there are organizations that provide it and more.

ORGANIZATIONS THAT HAVE PROVED HELPFUL

The National Alliance for the Mentally Ill

On September 7 through 9, 1979, 275 representatives of parent support and advocacy groups for the SMI from 28 states and Canada met in Madison, Wisconsin. In a remarkable display of unity and concern, they established the first National Alliance for the Mentally Ill. This alliance and the hundreds of local chapters from which it grew developed in large part out of dissatisfaction both with professionals and with the mental health delivery system. Its objectives are two-fold: (1) to fight for better care for the mentally ill through better legislation, better housing, adequate money, increased research, etc., and (2) to provide emotional support for families of the mentally ill. It is essential that professionals know about these alliances, work with them, and make appropriate referrals (Westman, 1979).

Nonprofessionals May Be Better Than Professionals

There are many examples of helpful and impressive work coming out of nonprofessional groups: Alcoholics Anonymous, Al-Anon, groups of parents of the developmentally disabled, AIDS support groups, and so many more. What makes them helpful? There is one obvious explanation. Most of these groups are made up of people who share in the experience—they have "been there." Thus, there is no credibility gap. But there may be other reasons, which relate to our training of professionals. Fisher (1975) feels that graduate schools of social work have the potential of training *out* of their students interpersonal skills that have been shown to lead to effective practice. Hence, some nonprofessionals, unaffected by such training, may communicate higher levels of interpersonal skills, especially in their understanding of and empathy with the client. The current attack on professionalism derives in part from the consumer-advocacy movements of the 1960s and 1970s. None of the professions has escaped attack. But the most hopeless of all professionals in the present climate have been those belonging to the so-called "helping professions"—the social workers, psychologists, guidance counselors, and others who run the so-called service agencies that deal with people in distress of one kind or another. The scientific basis of these professions, assuming there is one, is rather shaky, resting as it does on the social sciences, which offer only sandy footing, and developmental psychology and psychiatry, which are not much firmer. (Glazer, 1978, pp. 39-40)

Eighty-nine parents of schizophrenic people, all members of a self-help group in the Washington, DC area, were asked to describe how they got help (Hatfield, 1978). To meet the problems of coping with schizophrenia in the family, these parents sought out an array of professional and nonprofessional supports. They reported friends, relatives, self-help group members, and books as being most helpful, and various forms of therapy as least helpful. In fact, nearly half of this sample found no value at all in therapy. These findings are better understood when needs of families are expressed. Of highest priority are understanding of the illness, practical guidance, inpatient management, and community resources such as housing. These are not typical functions of therapy. Self-help groups may serve these needs better (Hatfield, 1978a). One reason that mental health professionals have been so limited in their capacities to meet the needs of these families is because these needs are not known. As Hatfield says, "Little is known about the crises of mental illness, how families cope with this devastation, to whom they turn for help, and how adequate is the help received. Little effort has been made to go to these families and find out" (Hatfield, 1978a).

One of the particularly salient findings of Hatfield's study is that parents found books so helpful. Clearly this was their best source of information about the disease. Why was this information not coming from the professionals? Are they perhaps ignorant? Is it still easier and perhaps more popular to learn about the psychodynamic theories of schizophrenia? If this is the case, then parents would indeed do better to turn to the books, for it is there that the more recent biochemical and genetic explanations of schizophrenia are to be found. It should be mentioned here that most self-help groups are primarily committed to the biochemical explanation of schizophrenia, and they keep their members informed of new research developments.

Parents of schizophrenic children say they learned about self-help organizations primarily through friends, by word of mouth, and from the telephone book. Only rarely were mental health professionals a referring source. Again, one has to ask why, since professionals often refer alcoholics to AA, parents of the mentally retarded to self-help groups, and so on. This has been a negative tirade against professionals. When parent and professional are suspicious of each other, the patient is the loser. Unfortunately, professionals have not been trained to develop a working alliance with patient's relatives (Hatfield, 1978b). The ideal would be professionals and parents working together as allies and as mutually respected collaborators—the professionals as experts in the disease, as advocates linking patients to needed resources, and as developers of new resources; and the parents as experts on their child and as critical resources for the child's well-being. Quite apart from the ideal, one must also acknowledge the fact that many schizophrenic people do not have any family or friends who can look after them. There may be no one around who loves them. The state and its professionals are then better than no one at all.

SOME SUGGESTIONS FOR NEW DIRECTIONS

Parents of Adult Schizophrenic People of San Mateo County have said that most of their children have experienced all sorts of treatment, from total isolation and being stripped of their clothes, to massive dosages of tranquilizers rendering them vegetables. Thus, they decided to fight for better care and better treatment. Families of people with SMI contend with formidable and heartrending burdens. They have fewer social supports and services than exist for almost any other illness. In addition, there is still a great deal of ignorance about the illness, and much prejudice is directed against both the mentally ill and their parents. What follows are several suggestions that could alleviate the burdens both experience.

Self-Help Groups

Self-help groups appear to offer more in the way of social supports and crisis intervention than anything else in our society, at the moment. Self-help groups give more credence to the biochemical explanation of schizophrenia; this fact alone makes them invaluable to parents, as it takes some of the onus off their backs. In addition, by participating in self-help groups, families can support each other emotionally, exchange practical management hints, and serve as advocates for needed resources.

Professional Training

We need to update the training of professionals, especially in educating them about what is known and not known about schizophrenia. If this were accomplished, more realistic and helpful treatment goals could be set up. In our training and teaching of professionals, perhaps we can find ways of better sensitizing them to the pain and stress that parents of SMI people experience, so that they can develop the same understanding and compassion usually shown to families coping with other major disabilities. Toward this end, I would suggest making use of some family members to do part of the training. Wikler (1979) found this method useful when she used parents of the mentally retarded to help sensitize and teach social work students about what the parents were experiencing. We could do the same in the area of SMI.

Hospitalization

Some people really do need hospitalization. Under our present "progressive" mental health laws, it has become virtually impossible to involuntarily hospitalize many in desperate need of such protection. There are those who really cannot care for themselves, no matter how good the community resources, and who may have no family to pick up the pieces. We need long-term, humane facilities for them. It is presently unrealistic to think in terms of "cure," and it is outrageous to have them dumped out in the streets with inadequate resources. Admittedly, in the past, too many people were indiscriminately locked up. But now we have swung to the other extreme, and many people with SMIs are living in appalling isolation and neglect. In addition to those who need long-term care, there are many who need short-term crisis hospitalization. This, too, has become a complex legal issue, often to the detriment of the mentally ill, their families, and the community. The present mode of leaving the decision about commitment up to the mentally ill themselves often makes no sense. My suggestion, then, is for revision of the new mental health laws, making it possible to hospitalize those in desperate need. Proving that a person is "harmful to self or others" is too arbitrarily defined. In its present form, deinstitutionalization has become an indiscriminate method by which the government washes its hands of the responsibility for its most dependent citizens. We need to develop a better way.

Community Resources

Community resources should be better developed. Community medicine in its present form throughout the United States is not working well. Lack of money, resources, community preparation, and trained people seem to be the main reason. The basic concept of community medicine–that patients will deteriorate less outside of institutions–is a good one. We still have a problem, however, with an erroneous assumption based on the notion of "cure." Recent research concerning social-psychological rehabilitation of people with SMI indicates that we should change our thrust from "preparing" to "sustaining" in the community. A good model for this has been developed in Madison, Wisconsin. Called Program of Assertive Community Treatment (PACT), its basic thrusts are the following:

1. Develop assertiveness with SMI people and involve them in programming. They regress when they are on their own.
2. Design individualized programming.
3. Provide enough supports to keep SMI people going, but not so much as to smother them.
4. Develop and sustain relationships with SMI people as responsible citizens.
5. Utilize the assertive approach to working with community resources.
6. Provide and/or attend community education concerning SMI.
7. Advocate the retention of responsibility for patient care and follow up when referrals are made.

As was stated almost 30 years ago, "We know that with some intervention people can be kept off the bottle–off the needle–off the hallucination–off the whatever–even though they cannot be made over . . . [and] cannot be cured. They can be sustained" (Loeb, 1967, p. 10).

Social Supports

The following kinds of social supports need to be developed:

1. *Crisis services.* Just as we recognize that crises develop among heart patients, diabetics, and cancer patients, for example, we should recognize that crises often occur for SMI people and their families. With recognition would come the building of services to help cope with crises.
2. *Respite care for families.* This service is available for parents of the mentally retarded. We should be doing no less for parents of SMI people.
3. *Professional advocates for services for SMI people.* The law has become so complex and help so difficult to get that many parents need assistance in getting protection and care for their children.
4. Further development of parent advocacy and support groups is needed, as well as more referrals made to them by professionals.

Interorganizational Relationships

Mention has been made of the need for better cooperation between professionals and families. Throughout the 1980s and 1990s, we have seen a healthy rise of the consumer movement (consumers refers to people with SMIs). The rise of this movement means a big shift in professional relationships with both SMI people and their families. The strict medical model is being seen as limited in value as consumers gain more control to speak out for themselves. Health care providers need to make a shift related to the emerging societal emphasis on consumer power and autonomy. This results in changes in roles and boundaries. The patient is viewed as a competent individual and as his or her own agent of change, and practitioners are asked to see the patient less as a patient or client and more as a colleague (Haiman, 1995, p. 443). Medical models of treatment deal with medications, and these are key elements for effective symptom control, but rehabilitation, education, and social models are taking on much more importance as more collaborative ways of dealing with SMI people are being used. Just as people with cancer are much more than just their illness, so people with SMI are much more than their illnesses. Increasingly, we are seeing the importance of integrating caring, holistic, scientific, and artistic ways of trying to help people with all kinds of illnesses.

Outcome Measures and Interventions

As was mentioned under the topic of managed care, the nature of SMIs do not fit into our usual concepts of progress or cure. SMIs have unpredictable ups and downs. We cannot yet think in terms of cure, and probably should be thinking in terms of *habilitation*, as opposed to rehabilitation. How can we best help people to live life as fully and satisfactorily as possible, given their particular SMI? Interventions need to occur on all levels. Mass education of the public is needed to cut down on the agonies caused by prejudice and stigma against SMI people. A continuum of care is needed, all the way from hospital care to independent living, to reflect the heterogeneity of these illnesses, as well as the unpredictability of their course. Better communication and coordination of efforts are needed between all kinds of different groups: SMI people, families, clinicians, researchers, policy makers, educators, police, and the population as a whole. As for outcome measures, it would be good to see more emphasis on quality-of-life issues. We can and should measure such things as reduced symptoms, staying off drugs and alcohol, keeping out of trouble with the law, and reduced homelessness. But let us not forget to ask consumers what is important to them, and what would help to reduce the pain in their lives—to say nothing of what might add some peace and satisfaction to those lives.

SUMMARY

With the possible exception of persons with AIDS, there probably is no group of people so badly hurt by the prejudices and stigma of society as those who must live with SMIs. No group of parents have been so badly hurt and misunderstood by professionals either, although thanks to the National Alliance for the Mentally Ill (NAMI) and a new generation of professionals, that picture is beginning to change for the better. Schizophrenia and other SMIs are terrible, debilitating, and chronic illnesses. Little is known about their causes, preventions, or treatments. All this leaves professionals feeling terribly frustrated, discouraged, and insecure. It leaves parents feeling overwhelmed, angry, and heartbroken. Needless to say, such a combination of feelings tends to bring out the worst in everybody. Even so, is it possible that parents and professionals can pull together better than they have been? This might best be accomplished by an updating of our knowledge, or lack of it, about these diseases; training professionals to be more sensitive toward the agonies of parents and other family members; and better utilizing both family and consumer advocacy groups. It would help to get the care of SMI people at least partially out of the courts. Developing better community resources with more social supports for SMI people would go a long way in alleviating some of their terrible social isolation.

In short, we need a holistic, comprehensive approach to the care of people with SMIs–one that encompasses both the medical/scientific, and the creative/artistic forms of helping. We know so little about these horrible illnesses, but we do know that almost all human beings respond well to kindness, respect, and genuine care. People with SMIs deserve no less.

REFERENCES

Ennis, B. (1978). *The rights of mental patients: The basic ACLU guide to a mental patient's rights*. New York: Avon.

Fisher, J. (1975). Training for effective therapeutic practice. *Psychotherapy: Theory, Research and Practice, 12*, 118-23.

Glazer, N. (1978, November). The attack on the professions. *Commentary, 65*(5), 34-41.

Haiman, S. (1995). Dilemmas in professional collaboration with consumers. *Psychiatric Services, 46*(5), 443-445.

Hatfield, A. (1978a). *Help-seeking behavior in families of schizophrenics*. Paper presented at the 55th annual meeting of the American Orthopsychiatric Association, San Francisco, CA.

Hatfield, A. (1978b). *Providing social supports for the families of the mentally ill*. Paper presented for the President's Commission of Mental Health, Washington, DC.

Knee, R. I. (1977). Health care: patients' rights. In J. B. Turner (Ed.), *Encyclopedia of social work*. Washington, DC: National Association of Social Workers, pp. 541-544.

Loeb, M. B. (1967). *Social worker's responsibility in community mental health centers*. Paper presented at the Community Mental Health Conference, Saratoga Springs, NY.

Mendel, W. M. (Ed.). (1976). *Schizophrenia: The experience and its treatment*. San Francisco: Jossey-Bass.

Test, M. A. and Stein, L. I. (1978). Community treatment of the chronic patient: Research overview. *Schizophrenia Bulletin, 3* (4), 350-364.

Wasow, M. *Professionals have hurt us: Parents of schizophrenics speak out*. Unpublished manuscript. University of Wisconsin School of Social Work, Madison.

Wasow, M. (1978). For my beloved son David Jonathan: A Professional Plea. *Health and Social Work, 3*(1), 126-146.

Wasow, M. (1986). The need for asylum for the chronically mentally ill. *Schizophrenia Bulletin, 12*(2), 162-167.

Wasow, M. (1995). *The skipping stone: Ripple effects of mental illness on the family.*, Palo Alto, CA: Science and Behavior Books.

Westman, J. C. (1979). *Child advocacy: New professional roles for helping families.* New York: Free Press.

Whitmer, G. E. (1980). From hospitals to jail: The fate of California's deinstitutionalized mentally ill. *American Journal of Orthopsychiatry, 50*(1), 65-75.

Wikler, L. (1979). Consumer involvement in the training of social work students. *Social Casework, 40*(3), 145-149.

Wikler, L., Wasow, M., and Hatfield, A. (1981). Chronic sorrow revisited: Parent vs. professional depiction of the adjustment of parents of mentally retarded children. *American Journal of Orthopsychiatry, 51*(1), 63-70.

Williams, D. H., Bellis, E. C., and Wellington, S. W. (1980). Deinstitutionalization and social policy: Historical perspectives and present dilemmas. *American Journal of Orthopsychiatry, 50*(1), 54-64.

Chapter 26

Children's Intensive Case Management in an Urban Community Mental Health Center

Diane Frankel
Lyne Iris Harmon
Toba Schwaber Kerson

CONTEXT

Description of the Setting

The agency that provided services is a large, comprehensive community mental health/mental retardation center covering a catchment area that spans a wide range of communities in Philadelphia County, from the poor to the affluent. The agency provides mental health outpatient and partial hospitalization services, case management services for the mental retardation (MR) population, drug and alcohol outpatient treatment, case management services to children and adults, and residential facilities for the mental health (MH) and mental retardation (MR) populations. The Child and Family Division, under which these services were provided, is located in the agency's main building, which is in a neighborhood in the middle of the catchment area and is readily accessible to public transportation. The stable, integrated neighborhood acts as a bridge between the poorest and wealthiest individuals who live in the catchment area.

Policy

Community Mental Health Act Amended

In October 1963, Congress enacted the Community Mental Health Act (Public Law 88-164), which authorized federal funds for community mental health centers to be located in communities or "catchment areas," with each center being responsible for a range of mental health services designed to help the mentally ill to remain in their communities. In 1975, an amendment to the Community Mental Health Act added children's services to those already extant (Larsen, 1986). Initially, community mental health centers were established with the premise that the federal government would provide seed money for the first eight years of operation, after which centers were expected to be financially self-sufficient (Goplerud, Walfish, and Aspey, 1983). To survive, the centers had to develop programs that generated increasing amounts of nonfederal funding.

Child and Adolescent Service System Program

In 1984, in response to the number of children nationwide who were unserved or receiving inappropriate restrictive care due to the lack of community-based services, the National Institute of Mental Health (NIMH) initiated a federally funded program to improve the service system for children and adolescents with severe emotional disturbances. The patchwork categorical system that existed for provision of children's services was failing, and a coordinated system of care had to be developed (CASSP Annual Report, 1995; Lourie and Katz-Leavy, 1991). Services failed especially when the needs of child and family cut across agencies and systems, and the NIMH launched the Child and Adolescent Service System Program (CASSP) to assist states and communities in developing such community-based systems of care (England and Cole, 1992; Day and Roberts, 1991; Lourie and Katz-Leavy, 1991). Until the early 1990s, few local systems provided a continuum of care that combined an array of community-based services with other essential elements, including interagency collaboration and case management. At that time, the state of Pennsylvania also moved away from institutional placement, especially after studies showed a disproportionate representation of children and adolescents in psychiatric hospitals and residential treatment settings (Annie E. Casey Foundation, 1992).

CASSP principles led to significant changes in the philosophy of service provision to children with mental health problems and their families. Changes occurred in service system development, components of the system of care, and, importantly, in the role of families in the system and in the care of their children (Lourie and Katz-Leavy, 1991). CASSP encouraged the development of systems of care based on (1) mobilization of community members, (2) respect for the autonomy and interdependence of the systems, (3) appreciation of divergent perspectives, and (4) commitment to shared goals (Homonoff and Maltz, 1991).

Intensive Case Management

Clearly, clients who required services from a variety of different systems and providers needed help with coordination of these services. Consistent with CASSP principles, Intensive Case Management (ICM) services were begun in Philadelphia in 1989. Services were developed to coordinate all systems such as mental health, child welfare, juvenile justice, and drug and alcohol. The ICM social worker's coordinating role is critical to service delivery as he or she acts as a single point of contact for the client and family, assessing client's needs and dealing with resource allocation and distribution (Werrbach, 1996; 1994). In addition to coordination of services, the ICM program, working with CASSP principles as their foundation, emphasized client and family strengths, self-determination, parent-professional collaboration, and facilitating the highest level of functioning possible within the community (Weick and Saleeby, 1995). All match the social worker's approach, which is based in person-in-environment theory (Germain, 1991; Austin, 1990). These ICM services in Philadelphia County were initially provided on a regional basis with the Northwest Center being one of four community mental health centers in the city with a children's ICM unit. The ICMs at the Northwest Center provided services for three catchment areas in the northwest section of the city, in addition to the catchment area served by the Northwest Center.

Among the many defined roles of the children's ICM are assessment provider, resource coordinator, resource developer, educator, advocate, crisis intervention provider, and counselor/therapist (Wolk, Sullivan, and Hartman, 1994; Indyk et al., 1993; Raiff with Shore, 1993; Moore, 1992; Rothman, 1991; Young, 1990; Moore, 1990; Johnson and Rubin, 1983). The ICMs could identify needs and, with the family's input, design plans to enable the children to remain in the community and improve their level of functioning; however, many necessary resources were limited or lacking.

Early Periodic Screening, Diagnosis, and Treatment

In 1992, the problem of limited resources changed in Pennsylvania with the implementation of the federally mandated Early Periodic Screening, Diagnosis, and Treatment Program (EPSDT), which allowed the development of systems of care based on individual need rather than program availability (Copeland, 1995). Up to that point, services for children were restricted to outpatient, inpatient, and partial hospitalization programs, which were all on the Medical Assistance (MA) fee schedule. The available MA-funded programs and services dictated which interventions an individual child could receive. With the advent of expanded services, the individual child's needs now dictated the interventions that would be implemented. Under the EPSDT funding stream, care can be provided for individuals up to 21 years of age who are eligible for Medical Assistance, and each state defines how EPSDT funding is accessed. The Philadelphia Office of Mental Health used this opportunity to improve services using a wraparound service model for children and their families (Karp, 1996; Fitler, 1994; Dore, 1993). Individually tailored wraparound services include, but are not limited to, behavior specialists, therapeutic staff support, and mobile therapists. Interagency meetings in which all the service providers and the family planned jointly in deciding which services would best fit a particular child's needs are critical in this approach. For the first time, mental health services could be provided to children in their natural environment, including home, school, and community, whether or not such services were covered under the preexisting state medical assistance funding. The Northwest Center was one of the lead agencies in the implemention of EPSDT-funded services.

EPSDT state regulations require that a psychiatrist or licensed psychologist prescribe the recommended services to meet the criteria for medical necessity. Next, a behavioral specialist designs a behavioral plan to be utilized by the parent, teachers, or mental health staff support person; a therapeutic staff support person implements the behavioral plan on a one-to-one basis with the child in the environment in which he or she is having difficulties; and mobile therapy allows payment for psychotherapeutic intervention wherever it might be helpful.

For each referral, a request packet is submitted to the state, which includes the mental health treatment evaluation, a plan of care summary, and until January of 1995, a request for prior authorization. As of January 1995, the state placed those services provided by the behavior specialist, mobile therapist, and therapeutic staff support on the medical assistance (MA) fee schedule. These services could then be accessed without prior authorization from the state for a period of four months, except when the cost of these services amounted to more than $10,000 per month or for continuation of therapeutic staff support services past the initial four-month period.

At the time services were delivered to this client and his family, plans were being made on the state level to shift all MA-funded mental health and physical health services from a fee-for-service model to a mandated managed-care system. EPSDT-funded services may then be part of the managed care contracts, and the funding for the ICM services may also be shifted to a managed-care model. Although the case being presented here was not part of a managed-care contract, the shift could have occurred at any time. This potential policy change created a feeling of uncertainty about the funding streams supporting these new programs.

Technology

The technologies utilized by the service provider in this case were varied. A sophisticated management information system and charting system to track the service provided had been established to gather data that could be used in evaluating the value of the interventions being utilized. Consideration was given to the possibility of medicating the client, but his foster parents and the foster care agency were hesitant. The social work supervisor and the ICM social worker worked from a person-in-environment perspective. The in-home behavioral specialist worked from a behavioral modification/social learning theory base. The in-home therapist used a systems approach in working directly with the family as well as the system providers.

Organization

The Northwest Center is a subsidiary of the Northwestern Corporation, a provider of mental health, mental retardation, residential, home health, early intervention, and drug and alcohol services. The corporation also provides EPSDT-funded services throughout Philadelphia, the five surrounding counties and throughout the Commonwealth of Pennsylvania. A community action advisory board organized in 1974 continues to advise the center. In order to respond to the advent of voluntary managed care and the proposed implementation of mandated managed care, the Northwestern Corporation developed Pennsylvania Behavioral Health in July 1994, whose mandate was to eventually centralize access to a continuum of services throughout the Philadelphia area and the surrounding five counties. Pennsylvania Behavioral Health negotiates managed-care contracts and handles intake, utilization management, scheduling, and credentialing for all of the subsidiaries. Referrals for outpatient services are done via Pennsylvania Behavioral Health, which handles all managed-care referrals for the Northwest Center as well as for other subsidiaries in the Northwestern Corporation.

DECISIONS ABOUT PRACTICE

Description of the Client

Charles Smith Williams is a handsome, physically age-appropriate ten-year-old African-American male who is always neatly dressed and groomed. Charles is the middle child in a family of three, including a brother, Peter, 12 years old, and a sister, Jennifer, 9 years old. These siblings reside with their adoptive parents, Mr. and Mrs. Williams. The children have lived with Mr. and Mrs. Williams since Jennifer was several months old. They were placed in this long-term foster care home with the Williams couple who hoped to and eventually did adopt them. The children's birth parents lost custody because of a history of abuse and neglect as a consequence of substance abuse. Mr. and Mrs. Williams are a working-class couple in their forties who own their own home in an urban area in Philadelphia. They had no children of their own and had not been foster parents prior to the arrival of the three children. The social worker never had a clear idea of what led them to become foster parents or why they so strongly desired to adopt these children. Mrs. Williams, especially, is a very private person. By the time they first presented at the agency, it was clear that the three children and Mrs. Williams were very closely bonded. Mrs. Williams was the primary caretaker as Mr. Williams worked very long hours. On weekends, Mr. Williams played a peripheral role in some family activities such as attending church, taking walks in the park, and playing ball. Generally, though, Mrs. Williams functioned like a single parent, focusing much of her energy to meet the needs of the children.

Prior to referral for ICM- and EPSDT-funded services, Charles and his family were known to the Northwest Center for four years. Initially, Charles was referred to the agency's Developmental Disabilities Unit because at the age of three-and-one-half, he demonstrated delays in development that were thought to be, in part, emotionally based. He participated in the agency's preschool program for children with emotional disturbances until he entered public school. In addition, on her own initiative, Mrs. Williams referred Charles' older brother, Peter, to Northwest Center's outpatient services when his behavior at home became very difficult to manage. At different intervals, Charles, his older brother, and other family members received individual and/or family therapy interventions at the agency-based site for the years preceding the referral for ICM services.

Four months prior to the referral for in-home wraparound services, Charles was hospitalized in a children's psychiatric inpatient facility. At the time, he was diagnosed as oppositional, defiant disorder, rule out attention deficit/hyperactivity disorder. He had been very physically aggressive with his siblings and was oppositional and nonresponsive to his foster parents when they set limits or expressed affection. Charles often beat up his younger sister, had frequent confrontations and conflicts with his older brother, and would not respond to his parents' attempts to limit his behavior and structure his life. The foster care agency was deeply concerned about the challenging emotional problems Charles presented in the family, and the foster care worker thought that hospitalization would allow for a comprehensive psychiatric assessment of Charles and a regrouping and stabilization of the family.

As Charles' hospital discharge was considered, both the hospital and foster care agency social workers requested ICM services for the family because they recognized that case management across many systems was critical for establishing and maintaining stability. Even with the continued presence of the foster care social worker, both social workers thought that mental health case management was necessary to assure access to and utilization of all necessary services. Shortly after the referral for intensive case management was made, the child advocate assigned to the children requested that NWC provide wraparound services to help Charles to control his aggressive behavior toward his siblings and to develop more positive interaction among the family members. The child advocate was involved because of the adoptive/foster care status of these children. The psychiatric hospital social worker agreed with this recommendation. At the time of referral, Charles had no significant problems in school, although his academic achievement was marginal; thus, the interventions were all home-based (Hodges and Blythe, 1992).

Shortly after in-home, EPSDT-funded services were requested for Charles, EPSDT wraparound services were also requested for Jennifer, who had a two-month stay at the same psychiatric inpatient facility as a result of overly-withdrawn behavior. Jennifer was acutely shy, refused to talk or communicate, and looked forlorn. Her inability to communicate her needs or feelings was seen as a signal that an intensive mental health intervention was necessary. It was thought that Jennifer may have been traumatized by her physically aggressive older brother but was unable to verbalize her feelings about this experience. Jennifer had not had previous individual mental health treatment.

The outpatient therapist who had worked with the family, the psychiatric hospital social worker, and the foster care social worker all concurred that they had difficulty engaging Mr. Williams in the family treatment, and the couple did not work together to create a sense of consistency and stability for the children. Mrs. Williams would set up expectations, and Mr. Williams in his attempt to endear himself to the children would undermine the structure being established. There was concern that if these children were not more emotionally stable, the foster care arrangement might have to be disrupted and the siblings separated. Thus, a referral was made with a request to provide in-home behavioral and family therapy interventions in order to avoid disruption in the foster care arrangement.

Mr. and Mrs. Williams agreed that they had difficulty working as a team. It was felt that the dynamics between the family members needed to be addressed in the environment where the difficulties were experienced. Consequently, Mr. and Mrs. Williams' adoption request was put on hold. It became clear that the systemic issues that involved all family members had not been adequately addressed in either the outpatient setting or in the inpatient setting, and an alternative approach needed to be attempted.

As the Situation Evolved

In the abstract, both of the Williamses had rather rigid expectations of how children should behave, but in practice they were loving, flexible, and sometimes overly solicitous. Approximately two years after the initiation of the ICM services, Mr. Williams had a massive heart attack. This created a tremendous upheaval in the family. Initially, Mr. Williams was not sure whether he would resume his normal life or be incapacitated. He recovered sufficiently to return home, but he could no longer work. Being home full-time upset the consistency in and balance of daily activities established by Mrs. Williams. Initially, the children were excited by his presence, especially since he was less of a disciplinarian than his wife; but, over time, the family situation became increasingly strained. Mrs. Williams decided to go to work, first part-time, then full-time, in order to add to the family income and possibly, although this was not articulated, to withdraw from the intensity of meeting the daily needs in this family. At this point, Mr. Williams became the primary caretaker.

Another significant change that the family experienced was the assignment of a new foster care worker. Mrs. Williams had had a very strong, supportive relationship with a male foster care worker who left the agency for another job. She was never able to establish a comfortable relationship with the new worker, a young and less-experienced woman whom Mrs. Williams thought to be unsupportive, intrusive, and critical. As a result, Mrs. Williams withdrew and spent a lot of time in family therapy expressing her discomfort with the foster care agency. The ICM social worker's perspective was that the foster care agency had to closely monitor the progress of the children in order to act responsibly, but the foster care agency did not recognize how this monitoring was perceived nor how the increasingly conflictual relationship between foster parents and foster care agency affected the children (Singer, Powers, and Olson, 1996).

Due to the children's dependent status and the foster care agency's concern about the stability of these children, the Child Advocates Office raised its level of involvement. A social worker and a pro bono attorney were assigned and took the position that these children were bonded to their foster parents, were in a loving family, and could benefit from additional services to help the parents and others in the environment help the children. Instead of seeing the children as the problem, the child advocates saw altering dimensions in the environment as the solution.

Definition of the Client

Both the ICM and EPSDT funding streams require that individual children be identified as the focus of the mental health treatment interventions and defined as the client. Thus, wraparound services are child-centered and family-focused. Treatment plans and goals and all supporting documentation must focus on an individual child and his or her behavioral problems, which will be addressed through recommended interventions (Rogg, 1992). In this case, the ICM clients were Charles, Jennifer, and their family.

Goals, Objectives, and Outcome Measures

The initial objective was to stabilize Charles so that he would be able to remain in his foster placement and, ultimately, he and his siblings could be adopted by the couple. To reach the objective, mental health interventions were initially provided in the home and subsequently in the school, making the environment more consistent so that Charles could learn to deal with his anger, aggressive acting-out behavior, and aggressive and oppositional relationships with his siblings and foster parents. Mr. and Mrs. Williams were intensely involved in the in-home interventions and worked to develop additional parenting skills. The ICM social worker's goals, which were ongoing, were to (1) assess needs, (2) identify service providers, (3) help the client and family to access services, (4) monitor the use of the services, (5) link all of the service providers, (6) coordinate the provisions of services, and (7) assess progress and reassess needs. Outcomes were measured by Charles' ability to function at home and later at school, demonstrated through acceptable behaviors as observed and reported by the family and the foster care social worker who were part of the interagency team (Ellmer, Lein, and Hormuth, 1995). When Charles' level of aggression was reduced, when he was more responsive and cooperative at home, and when the foster care worker and County Office Children and Youth social workers who had contracted with the foster care agency to provide care felt that the situation was stabilized, the request for formal adoption could proceed.

Use of Contract

There were multiple contracts; the overriding one was the service plan developed by the ICM social worker in conjunction with Charles' foster parents and the foster care social worker. This plan outlined the significant areas in Charles' life, the goals in each area, the available strengths and resources, and who was responsible for accomplishing each goal in a particular time frame. The responsibilities of the ICM social worker and foster parents were outlined. This contract was reviewed at least once every six months or as needed. Due to the constantly changing needs, the service plan was updated every several months. Each time the service plan was signed by the ICM social worker, client, and family, and reviewed and signed by the social worker's supervisor.

In addition to the service plan, there were multiple additional contracts and treatment plans. Formal contracts were established between the Northwest Center and the various service providers for the wraparound services in the home and school. Specific treatment plans were defined; objectives, goals, means for achieving the goals, and time frames for each of the different mental health/behavioral interventions being utilized were described. For example, the in-home family therapist developed a specific treatment plan focused on improving the quality of the relationships between Charles and his siblings and Charles and his foster parents, especially his foster father. Later, when in-school interventions were initiated, a behavioral specialist helped design a behavioral management plan. This plan was agreed to by the child, foster parents, school personnel, foster care social worker, and therapeutic staff support implementing the plan in an interagency meeting, a key component of wrap-around services. It was the responsibility of the ICM social worker to make sure that the overall service plan incorporated the individual treatment plans and that all services were coordinated.

Meeting Place

Wraparound services were provided at home, in the school, and in the community. The ICM social worker met with the child and family in their home, at the agency, and in any community-based setting, such as the school where services were provided. The ICM social worker also used agency conference rooms to facilitate larger interagency meetings, which usually included the foster parents and the professionals from the many child-serving systems involved in providing services to this client and family. At the agency, four ICMs shared space. Smaller offices were available for private meetings, but the majority of the ICM social worker's work was in the field.

Use of Time

Time was flexible in working with clients and service providers. State regulations dictated minimum amounts of time required to meet the criteria for this level of service; for example, a client on an ICM caseload must be seen twice a month in face-to-face contact. There were no time restrictions. Since the social worker working with Charles and his family was identified as an ICM and wraparound services were for clients in crisis, twice-a-month contact was considered a baseline minimum. In reality, more frequent and extensive contact was needed.

Initially upon referral for wraparound services, the ICM social worker spent many hours on the telephone with the foster care agency, the Child Advocates Office, and other mental health professionals in order to coordinate services and support the foster parents in dealing with multiple interventions. She met at least once a week with the foster parents to explore their willingness to participate in all of the intensive services. All professionals and the foster parents agreed with the wraparound intervention plan, and this was formalized at an interagency meeting facilitated by the social worker. Next, the ICM social worker spent considerable time contacting potential wraparound service providers. She then helped create an environment in which the family could be sufficiently accepting and engaged to support in-home wraparound services. After these services were established, the ICM social worker reduced her time on the case, continuing to assess needs and monitor progress. In case of a crisis, the ICM social worker continued to be available by beeper. The social worker updated all involved agencies weekly.

When Charles settled down at home, he began exhibiting oppositional behavior in school, and the ICM social worker again increased her involvement, spending up to two days per week making an assessment, establishing the necessary services, and working with Charles, his family and the school personnel to facilitate smooth transitions with the new service providers. In addition, many hours were spent every four months when a prior authorization packet had to be completed and submitted to the state for continued funding.

Stance of the Social Worker

In this situation, the role of the ICM social worker involved planning, implementing, and monitoring EPSDT-funded wraparound services, as well as coordinating the other services this child was receiving. The stance of the social worker in this case depended on the time, the place, and the people with whom she was interacting. Overall, the social worker was supportive, encouraging, and facilitating. She listened to Mr. and Mrs. Williams' concerns, questions, confusion, and anger, and worked at providing a stable, consistent place where they could better deal with the overwhelming nature of all the services being provided. Although the foster parents agreed to and initially welcomed the wraparound services, they sometimes felt that the need for multiple services was a statement that the foster care agency lacked confidence in their ability to parent these children.

The social worker's stance required specific skills and maturity in working with a complicated system. Her ability to maintain clear boundaries and keep from becoming enmeshed helped to ameliorate any potential negative effects of splitting, triangulation, and/or projection and displacement (Kramer, 1985; Framo, 1981). In doing so, she was able to help the foster parents to avoid displacing their frustration onto the children. Her involvement was also critical to the professionals/service providers. The conflicts, challenges, and disagreements, which existed among the agencies, seemed to negatively affect the children's problems.

Although the social worker did quite well in managing boundaries, maintaining her multiple roles remained a struggle. The role of the ICM is to support the child and the family; thus, it was critical that she support the Williamses and especially validate Mrs. Williams' caring, responsible, and loving parenting. The social worker labored around issues of confidentiality and how to maintain viable working relationships with all of the professionals involved when she could not always support and affirm their point of view. In addition to maintaining boundaries, she had to remain tactful to a point that sometimes clearly tested all of her inner resources. The social worker's stance with the Williamses was also educative and confrontive. She modeled ways for them to set reasonable expectations and boundaries in a caring and empathetic way.

The social worker established and maintained multiple relationships with all the professionals and service providers involved with the family. She also had to maintain a strong sense of her own clinical and professional skills, an awareness of her strengths, and knowledge and understanding of this client, his family, and the system dynamics. Frequently, the social worker had to manage displaced and projected anger and frustration because there were so many different professionals and agencies involved with different alliances, responsibilities, and viewpoints about what was best for this child. The social worker again took the stance of listener, providing support, suggestions, directions, setting appropriate boundaries, and gently confronting when it seemed appropriate.

Interventions

Due to the varied and complicated issues involved in this case and the multiple service providers engaged in helping Charles and his family, the intervention strategies used by the social worker addressed issues on the micro, meso, exo, and macro levels of practice. The initial interventions focused on needs assessment and the provision of information about in-home wraparound services. After more than one year of outpatient therapy, Charles was hospitalized in an inpatient psychiatric facility. The hospitalization was prompted by a sudden and severe deterioration in his functioning in the home environment, which led to extreme concern about the safety of all the children. At the time of discharge from the psychiatric inpatient facility, it was apparent that Charles' needs were greater than outpatient therapy could provide and that his family would have to be helped to provide the consistency that would allow him to control his anger and be a more cooperative family member. After the assessment phase, when an in-home behavior specialist (who was also a family therapist) was assigned to the case, clear goals for working with the family were outlined.

It became clear that the home environment lacked the level of consistent structure and clearly stated expectations and consequences that were needed to help Charles control his impulses. Since Mr. and Mrs. Williams also recognized that they had difficulty working together and that Charles' behavior was negatively affected by the lack of consistency, the family agreed to intensive family therapy. A system of positive reinforcements was introduced, with Charles first receiving small toys or games each day he could control his behavior and, eventually, with his receiving a larger reward each week he could do the same. The rewards were never food or candy, and they were chosen to be somewhat educational and to reinforce positive parent-child relationships. While the family therapist was working with the systemic issues, the social worker kept daily contact with the foster parents to monitor progress, met with Charles once a week, and received weekly reports from the behavior specialist. This monitoring allowed the foster parents an opportunity to ventilate, as they were at times overwhelmed by the number of different professionals coming in as experts.

After one year of in-home therapeutic interventions, when Charles was eight years old, his behavior at home improved, but he developed severe behavioral problems at school. Again, his behavior was overly aggressive toward other children and he refused to follow adult's instructions and directions. The ICM social worker therefore increased her contact with Charles and his foster parents, and additional wraparound services, including therapeutic staff support, as well as behavioral consultation were initiated at the school setting. Around this time, the in-home family therapy was ended and the focus shifted to in-school interventions. Again, interventions and rewards were kept consistent between home and school.

During the school year, Charles had had five different teachers in a single classroom. Since Charles' deterioration in school was evaluated to be at least partially in response to this succession of temporary teachers, the ICM social worker conferred with the Williamses and helped to initiate a request for a school transfer. Charles' behavior improved significantly in the new school setting with additional support, consistency, and structure being an integral part of his learning experience. However, as he got older, the academic demands increased and his developmental limitations became more apparent. His frustration with learning then compounded his emotional and behavioral problems. Charles continued with the in-school services for two school years with a gradual reduction in frequency and intensity the second year. During the summer months Charles attended a day partial hospitalization program for elementary school children. The social worker functioned as a facilitator, liaison, interpreter, and advocate for the family with all service providers.

The ICM social worker had many responsibilities on the meso and exo levels of practice. She maintained contact with all of the professional agencies and service providers involved in Charles' life and facilitated communication among them by organizing and facilitating both interagency meetings and interdisciplinary team meetings and by acting as a conduit for the passage of the information between professionals. This role had been agreed upon by all of the professionals involved and the family at the first interagency meeting. The ICM social worker was also responsible for completing application packets that were submitted to the Philadelphia County Office of Mental Health/Mental Retardation and to the State Office of the Department of Public Welfare in order to access and continue the funding that supported the wraparound services. At this point in time, the state was just beginning to work out its procedures for handling these applications, and much time and energy were spent in ensuring that the services were not disrupted. The ICM social worker had working relationships with the Children and Youth Agency, the child advocates, the numerous mental health service providers, and personnel from the Philadelphia School District (teachers, principals, school psychologists, and special education staff). The social worker and the social worker's supervisor functioned also on the macro level, attending county and statewide meetings focused on policy and program planning and monitoring the new EPSDT-funded services. Feedback to the EPSDT-funded wraparound services was then incorporated into the evaluation and planning process at a policy level.

After over three years of ICM social work services and three years of EPSDT funded wraparound services, which were initially intense and gradually reduced, Charles and his siblings were adopted by the Williamses. The wraparound services were ended, and the family started to participate in outpatient family therapy. The ICM social worker continues to carry the case, monitoring progress, being available in case of a crisis, and continuing the multiple interventions she has provided throughout her involvement with Charles and his family.

Use of Outside Resources

There were multiple resources available to this child and family, including those already involved and those brought in to implement wraparound services. The agencies already involved, which were able to devote some resources to this child and family, were the foster care agency; the County Children and Youth Agency, which contracted for the foster care services; Child Advocates; and the School District of Philadelphia, which provided special education services. In addition, Charles and his family were active in church-related activities, and Charles was enrolled in various community-based after-school activities. In order to provide wraparound services, the ICM social worker accessed EPSDT funding through the State Office of Medical Assistance and contracted with an agency to provide some of the specialized in-home/in-school services recommended for Charles. After Mr. Williams became ill and unable to work, Mrs. Williams returned to work in the community close to home and Mr. Williams was helped to apply for disability benefits to provide some additional financial support for the family. Figure 26.1 provides an ecomap for Charles Williams.

Reassessment

Reassessment was linked to the stated goals, objectives, and contracts, and progress was reassessed at least twice a month and every time the

FIGURE 26.1. Ecomap for Charles Williams

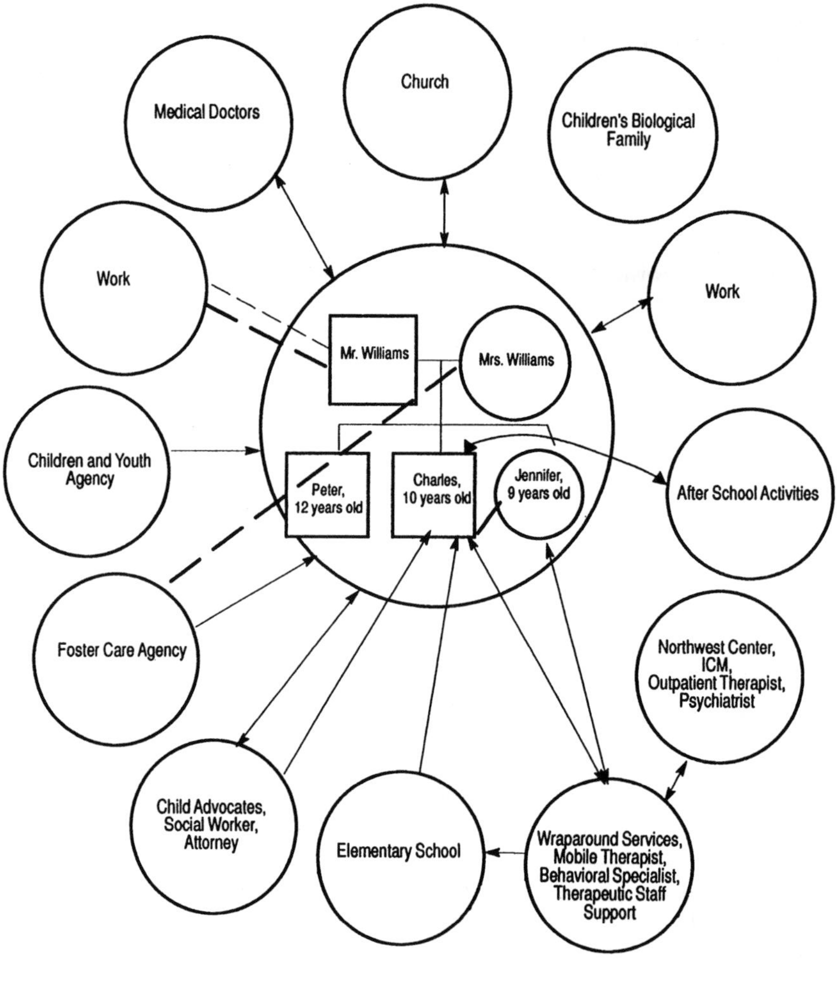

social worker had contact with Charles and his family. When the ICM social worker contacted service providers to document progress, each agency used its contact with the social worker to assess progress as outlined in its individual service plans. The reassessment process was activated whenever a crisis arose, and plans were altered as needed. Significant changes in the overall plan were considered and approved by the entire interagency team at a meeting called by the ICM social worker.

Alterations in the mental health treatment plan were implemented in a timely fashion, and the social worker was responsible for notifying the rest of the interagency team of the changes.

At times, Mrs. Williams expressed her frustration and anger at the multiple intrusions in her life and her being made to feel less than capable. The social worker acknowledged these feelings with empathy and used this as an opportunity to review with Mrs. Williams her commitment to work toward adopting the children. She emerged with a renewed vigor to accept the challenges, both directly with the children and with all of the agencies involved to work toward adoption. She also recognized how important it was for her husband to take a more active role with the children.

Transfer or Termination

Charles has been receiving ICM services for over five years. The services were initially quite intensive, reduced to moderate, became intensive again, and have for the past year been gradually reduced. The intensity of the ICM services parallels the intensity of the wraparound services provided for Charles. Presently, Charles has therapeutic staff support in school on a very limited basis, with a plan to completely eliminate this service in the next four months. The behavior specialist's services will also be discontinued at that time because his services will no longer be necessary. In-home family therapy was ended two years earlier when a shift was made to focus on school problems. All of these decisions were agreed upon by the entire interagency team as everyone felt that Charles' functioning at home was much improved. The family was somewhat relieved at the discontinuation of the in-home wraparound services because they felt the services were intrusive at times. The Williamses officially adopted Charles and his siblings, accomplishing what was a significant part of the initial objectives.

As the wraparound services are being terminated, the family has agreed to return to outpatient treatment to further reinforce and consolidate the gains made as a result of the wraparound interventions. This also provides a forum to address reactions to finalizing the adoption process. The ICM social worker will continue to carry the case, to monitor the child's and family's adjustment to the termination of wraparound services, and to manage their transfer to outpatient services at the Northwest Center. The family requested that the ICM social worker remain available as a support and resource, especially when Charles moves to middle school next year. In addition, the Philadelphia County Offices of Mental Health and Mental Retardation strongly recommends that the ICM stays involved for a minimum of six months after all the goals have been achieved. If Charles' progress continues and the family remains stable for six months, the case can be transferred to a less intense level of case management called Resource Coordination.

DIFFERENTIAL DISCUSSION

The ICM social worker and her supervisor found working with Charles and his family and the multiple systems especially intense and challenging. The challenges were compounded by the fact that the funding stream was new. Although these creative and individualized services could be recommended and funded, the service providers, who were to implement all the services, needed to be identified and trained. Also, at the beginning of the case, the entire process to access, provide, and document these services had not yet been formalized.

The child advocate and the foster care social worker and their agencies were very enthusiastic about the new mental health funding stream and the opportunities it presented to meet the needs of Charles in order to stabilize his foster placement. The Northwest Center administration was highly motivated to begin to use this funding stream to expand the services they could provide to the children who presented at their center. Due to this pressure to provide services for Charles, the social worker supervisor committed to facilitating, developing, and implementing a wraparound plan before appropriate service providers were identified, screened, contracted, and available. The ICM social worker fielded many calls from the child advocate, the foster care social worker, and the family, all of whom were anxious to begin the in-home interventions. The ICM supervisor had to immediately interview and contract with appropriate mental health professionals who had the expertise and experience to meet the specific needs of Charles and his family. Having learned from this experience, in subsequent cases, two significant changes were made. First, the ICM social worker set more realistic time frames for starting wraparound services based upon availability of appropriate staff for each specific case, thereby establishing more realistic expectations. Secondly, the Northwest Center assigned other staff to interview, screen, and contract with wraparound providers so that the ICM would have a list of potential providers at her disposal. It was clear that a plan could be developed quickly but that the implementation of the plan was dependent upon the availability of behavior specialists, mobile therapists, and therapeutic staff support all properly trained to work with this new model.

Although case management services traditionally have functioned to facilitate interagency systems collaboration, historically, the child serving systems in Philadelphia County had not worked intensively together. For the first time, this new funding stream required that different service systems work closely together and integrate parent-professional collaboration. These collaborations highlighted the many divergent perspectives held by the various child-serving systems: the ICM model is one based on a biopsychosocial ecosystem approach; the EPSDT funding stream is based on a medical model; and the child advocate office is based on a model of legal advocacy. As the ICM social worker gained more experience planning and providing these services, she became more aware of how important it is to understand and work with the missions that define the operations of different systems.

The ICM social worker learned by experience that she had to focus more attention in subsequent cases on who was in charge of the case management when case managers from other systems were also involved, who had the control, the power, the authority, and the ultimate responsibility. There were many times when decisions were independently made by various individuals, which negated the ability of the ICM social worker to coordinate services. Subsequent to this case, the ICM social worker clarified the issues of responsibility, control, and authority at the onset before the wraparound services began. This was accomplished at the initial interagency meeting.

As we look back on this case, the question still remains whether the professionals completed a truly comprehensive assessment of the strengths and limitations of the home and the foster parents, and the availability of other resources. It is clear, however, that after decades of stagnation in availability of new and expanded individualized children's services, the eagerness to test the new system overshadowed all else. In this case, the MH funding stream became the primary provider of services for Charles and his family.

Now that the adoption is finalized, the relationship with the ICM social worker and the availability of in-home and community-based mental health services provide an opportunity to stabilize this family, and for Charles and his siblings to be adopted by parents with whom they are strongly bonded. Charles and the siblings are now part of a loving family who will benefit from continued support from the ICM social worker and the mental health system as the children reach the developmental challenges of adolescence.

REFERENCES

Annie E. Casey Foundation. (1992). *Focus, 2,* 2-6.

Austin, C. (1990). Case management myths and realities. *Families in Society, 71*(7), 398-405.

CASSP Annual Report. (1995). Sensitivities, skills and services: Mental health roles in the implementation of part H of PL-99-457. Appendix D,19-20.

Copeland, V. C. (1995). A programmatic approach to improving the health of poor children. *Journal of Health and Social Policy, 6*(4), 53-72.

Day, C. and Roberts, M. C. (1991). Activities of the child and adolescent service system program for improving mental health services for children and families. Special section: Disadvantaged children and their families. *Journal of Clinical Child Psychology, 20*(4), 340-350.

Dore, M. M. (1993). Family-based services in children's mental health care. Special issue: Family treatment. *Child and Adolescent Mental Health Care, 3*(3), 175-189.

Ellmer, R., Lein, L., and Hormuth, P. (1995). Coordinated services for children's mental health: A process evaluation. *Journal of Mental Health Administration, 22*(4), 346-357.

England, M. J. and Cole, R. F. (1992). Building systems of care for youth with serious mental illness. Special section: Treatment and service systems for adolescents. *Hospital and Community Psychiatry, 43*(6), 630-633.

Fitler, T. M. (1994). The contribution of collaborative planning and wrap-around support services to the adjustment level of severely emotionally disturbed children. *Dissertation Abstracts International, 455*(4), 1114-A-1115A. (University Microfilms No. DA9422280.)

Framo, J. (1981). The integration of marital therapy with sessions with family of origin. In A. Gurman and D. Kniskern (Eds.), *Handbook of family therapy.* Brunner/Mazel, New York, pp. 135-139.

Germain, C. (1991). *Human behavior in the social environment: An ecological view.* New York: Columbia University Press.

Goplerud, E., Walfish, N., and Aspey, M. (1983). Surviving cutbacks in community mental health. *Community Mental Health Journal, 19*(1), 62-76.

Hodges, V. and Blythe, B. (1992). Improving service delivery to high risk families: Home based practice, *Families in Society, 73*(5), 259-265.

Homonoff, E. and Maltz, P. (1991). Developing and maintaining a coordinated system of community-based services to children. *Community Mental Health Journal, 27*(5), 347-357.

Indyk, D., Bellville, R., Lachapelle, S., Grodon, G., and Dewart, T. (1993). A community-based approach to HIV case management: Systematizing the unmanageable. *Social Work, 38*(4), 380-387.

Johnson, P. and Rubin, A. (1983). Case management in mental health: A social work domain? *Social Work 28*(1), 49-55.

Karp, N. (1996). Individualizing wrap-around services for children with emotional, behavioral and mental disorders. In G. H. S. Singer, L. E. Powers, and

A. L. Olson (Eds.), *Redefining family support: Innovations in public-private partnerships*. Baltimore: Paul H. Brookes Publishing Co, pp. 291-310.

Kramer, J. (1985). *Family interfaces: Transgenerational patterns*. New York: Brunner/Mazel.

Larsen, J. (1986). Local mental health agencies in transition. *American Behavioral Scientist, 30*, 174-187.

Lourie, I. and Katz-Leavy, J. (1991). New directions for mental health services for families and children. *Families in Society, 72*(5), 277-285.

Moore, S. (1990). A social work practice model of case management: The case management grid. *Social Work, 35*(5), 444-448.

Moore, S. (1992). Case management and the integration of services: How service delivery systems shape case management. *Social Work, 37*(5), 418-423.

Raiff, N. with Shore, B. (1993). *Advanced case management: New strategies for the 90s*. Newbury Park, CA: Sage Publications.

Rogg, D. J. (1992). Child and adolescent mental health services: Evaluation challenges. *New Directions for Program Evaluation, 54*, 5-16.

Rothman, J. (1991). A model of case management: Toward empirically based practice. *Social Work, 36*(6), 520-528.

Singer, G. H. S., Powers, L. E., and Olson, A. L. (Eds.). (1996). Redefining family support: Innovations in public-private partnerships. Baltimore, MD: Paul H. Brookes Publishing Co.

Weick, A. and Saleeby, D. (1995). Supporting family strengths: Orienting policy and practice toward the 21st century. *Families in Society, 76*(3), 141-149.

Werrbach, G. B. (1994). Intensive child case management: Work roles and activities. *Child and Adolescent Social Work Journal, 11*(4), 325-341.

Werrbach, G. (1996). Family strengths-based intensive child case management. *Families in Society, 77*(4), 216-226.

Wolk, J., Sullivan, P., and Hartmann, D. (1994). The managerial nature of case management. *Social Work, 39*(2), 152-159.

Young, T. (1990). Therapeutic case advocacy: A model for interagency collaboration in serving emotionally disturbed children and their families. *American Journal of Orthopsychiatry, 60*(1), 118-124.

Chapter 27

Mental Health Care in a Combat Environment: The Application of Small Unit Stress Debriefings

James A. Martin

CONTEXT

Military duties often involve exposure to extremely stressful events: training accidents, combat, peacekeeping, or humanitarian deployments. Many individuals exposed to traumatic stress will suffer short-term physical, psychological, and/or social stress symptoms. Initial symptoms, in some circumstances, evolve into long-term dysfunction affecting the individual's physical health, emotional well-being, and social relationships. Group functioning can also be affected by traumatic stress, causing diminished unit performance, lower morale, and less cohesion. Small unit stress debriefings provide "first aid" for those exposed to traumatic stress.

INTRODUCTION

During the 1991 Persian Gulf War, approximately 700,000 American service men and women deployed to Southwest Asia (Department of Defense Report, 1995). For most of these soldiers–sailors, marines, and Air Force service members–the Persian Gulf War was the highlight of their military service. Collectively, they share in the pride and glory associated with a historic military victory.

Many of these Gulf War veterans experienced prolonged separation from family and loved ones, as well as military duty in a foreign environment that exposed them to a range of physical, psychological, and social stressors (Wright et al., 1995; Stokes, 1992). For some, these exposures were associated with the development of measurable physical and/or psychological symptoms (Marlowe, 1994). Since the end of the Gulf War, a relatively small number of veterans have developed what is referred to as "a mystery illness"–a collection of physical symptoms that do not seem to be related to one individual (or even cluster) of Gulf War zone exposures (Department of Defense, 1995).

Individuals who represent what has been referred to as "pockets of trauma" (Martin, 1992) are among those who experienced significant stress during the Gulf War. These are the individuals and small groups who directly encountered the most profound horrors of combat, including the death of comrades (Holmes, 1985). This chapter addresses a battlefield response to combat-related mental health needs of military personnel. The application of small unit stress debriefings offers an example of an intervention designed to prevent or diminish the biopsychosocial sequelae of combat-related trauma. This approach, first used in a formal way by S.L.A. Marshall (1947) in World War II has now been adapted and applied in a variety of civilian settings around the world (Shalev and Ursano, 1990).

Description of the Setting

The location was a desert area in southern Iraq. Earlier in the week, it was the scene of three days of violent confrontation between Iraqi and U.S. combat units. A unilateral cease-fire had been in effect for the past two days and a devastated Iraqi military had been offered an opportunity for unconditional surrender.

The combat arms organization ("parent unit") referred to in this chapter contained approximately 9,500 soldiers organized in a number of smaller combat and combat support units. By the nature of its combat role, most of the soldiers were men. There were a few women attached to the combat support units serving just behind the forward combat units. (These women were mostly medical, communication, logistical, and transportation personnel.) The focus of the intervention described here involves a small unit stress debriefing that took place in one of the combat arms units at a time when it was deployed in the Iraqi desert in a defensive position waiting for its next mission. These tired soldiers had set up tentage, and much of their time was being spent trying to catch up on sleep and generally just "wind down" from the excitement and stress associated with the past few days of combat. There were no "creature comforts" in this setting. The weather was overcast but mild. It had been a few weeks since these soldiers had showered or had a hot meal. Some mail had been delivered, but it was already a few weeks old. There was no access to commercial phones. Some current information was available from the U.S. Armed Forces Radio station in Saudi Arabia via portable radios. Like all soldiers in combat, these men and women knew a lot about the current operational activities going on right around them, but they knew very little about events and conditions outside of their small piece of the battlefield.

The U.S. Army (like the other branches of the armed services and many foreign militaries) is very concerned about "combat stress" (Ingraham and Manning, 1986). The prevention and treatment of combat-stress-related battle fatigue casualties are the stated responsibility of all military leaders and a primary focus of military medical doctrine and military mental health services. Historically, combat-stress-related battle fatigue causalties have accounted for a substantial percentage of all combat causalties. Combat stress is an important component of all combat-related illnesses and injuries (Copp and McAndrew, 1990), including combat-related post-traumatic stress disorder (Green, 1994).

One type of mental health response to the stress of combat is the application of a crisis-intervention approach referred to here by the term "small unit stress debriefing" and now in the civilian stress-related literature by the term "critical incident stress debriefing" (Mitchell, 1981). This intervention is rooted in the history of combat psychiatry (Shalev, 1994). In its most generic form, a stress debriefing is "a group-oriented intervention in which the major elements of a trauma are reviewed by the participants shortly after the event" (Shalev, 1994, p. 201). Regardless of its form, debriefings are viewed as methods of preventing stress exposure from producing subsequent physical, psychological, and/or social dysfunction (Brom and Kleber, 1989). The general goals of stress debriefings (in military or civilian settings) are to "decrease overwhelming emotions, decrease cognitive disorganization, enhance self-efficacy, facilitate emotional disclosure and return of pleasure, disengage from the disaster role, learn new coping skills, initiate the grief process, legitimize feelings and emotions, and correct inaccurate information" (Shalev, 1994, p. 216).

Policy

U.S. Army medical doctrine states the following regarding policy:

... following any especially traumatic event (such as combat deaths or accidental deaths in a unit, or harm by friendly fire, or observed harm to innocent noncombatants), debriefing teams ... will deploy to the affected units to conduct critical incident debriefings. These debriefings should be accomplished within days of the terrible event, as lulls in the action permit. (Stokes [1992], unpublished paper, p. 17)

During the early phases of the Gulf War deployment, the concept and method of small unit stress debriefing was taught to mental health personnel (and some chaplains) as part of the ground preparations for combat. Many of the mental health personnel in the Gulf, especially those from U.S. Army Reserve Component personnel, did not have adequate training or preparation for what they might reasonably expect to encounter in combat (Holsenbeck, 1992).

Technology

Even before the Persian Gulf War, from 1990 to 1991, there was a flourishing literature on the prevention of post-traumatic stress disorders (Brom and Kleber, 1989). Critical incident stress debriefing had its own literature, primarily in the emergency medicine-health services area (Mitchell, 1986) and in the disaster response literature (Raphael, 1986). When the Gulf War began, the Army Medical Department was in the final stages of adopting a version of this intervention.

The U.S. Army Medical Center and School in San Antonio, Texas, had developed an extensive set of handouts (small cards) providing step-by-step instructions on managing stress in combat, treating battle fatigue, and providing after-action stress debriefings in small groups. These aids had been widely distributed among Active Component and many Reserve Component Army mental health personnel. The approach suggested for stress debriefings was modeled after Mitchell's (1983) guide for critical incident stress debriefings. There are seven phases: introductory, facts, thought, reaction, symptoms, teaching, and reentry. In the introductory phase, the group is brought together and provided a brief explanation about the nature and purpose of the debriefing, including a discussion of confidentiality and privacy. During the facts phase, the group reconstructs the event in detail and in chronological order. In the thought phase, the leader attempts to personalize the event and shift focus from the factual to a focus on the emotions associated with the facts. The reaction phase is one in which the leader works to help participants identify and ventilate their feelings and emotions. In the symptoms phase, the group discusses physical and psychological stress responses. During the teaching phase, the leader educates participants about normal reactions to abnormal stressors. The reentry phase completes and closes the debriefing by asking for final comments and helps group members define self-help activities, as well as identifying local mental health resources available for follow-up.

The intervention described in this chapter includes the core components of this model. It also contains components of S.L.A. Marshall's "historical group debriefing" (Shalev, 1994). Brigadier General Marshall was an Army historian whose field work spanned World War II, Korea, and the Vietnam War. In the course of developing a method for documenting soldiers' experiences in battle, Marshall recognized that his debriefing techniques resulted in profound psychological changes among those debriefed (Shalev, 1994). The following principles highlight the core components adapted from Marshall and applied in the debriefing described in this chapter (Belenky and Martin, 1996; Marshall, 1947).

1. The debriefing is carried out in the operational environment.
2. The intervention occurs immediately after combat.
3. All members of the small group (unit) take part in the debriefing.
4. Rank/status is "put aside" during the debriefing; all members are considered equal witnesses.
5. The structure of the debriefing follows a chronological reconstruction of the event(s).
6. Details are solicited from each participant and conflicting information is tolerated.
7. There is no fixed time limit on the session.

Organization

Mental health personnel typically conduct combat stress debriefings in a "host" setting. This means that the mental health provider comes into the situation as an outsider and must gain the trust and support of the host leadership in order to obtain access to those requiring debriefing services. Access to these soldiers requires support from both the formal organizational leadership and the informal unit "gatekeepers" (unit chaplains, unit medical officers, and senior sergeants who lead many of the sections within units). It is often of immeasurable help when the mental health professional has experience with and/or knowledge of the methods of the organization and a strong positive identification with the organization's goals. The mental health officer's demonstration of the requisite knowledge of basic soldier skills provides a critical basis for acceptance by both soldiers and their leaders.

My colleague and I were senior military officers and experienced mental health professionals. By virtue of age and military rank, we were legitimate peers of the senior unit-level leaders, and slightly older and more senior than the unit gatekeepers. In addition, we had considerable experience as scientists working with similar combat arms units in a variety of garrison and field training settings. We had no previous combat experience, but we were knowledgeable soldiers, personally and professionally comfortable in this environment.

While training, experience, and willingness to share the hardships of the combat environment were important factors in obtaining access to combat units, establishing opportunities to actually implement debriefings services following combat involved a number of other considerations.

In the typical post-combat situation, small units are spread over very large geographical areas. Initially, it was necessary to obtain a combat vehicle and the required navigational equipment (and the skill to use this equipment) in order to move independently into the areas where soldiers were in need of debriefing services. When tactical equipment is scarce and/or in great demand, as it was in the early phases of the Gulf War, obtaining these logistical resources requires the same kind of organizational skills and creative determination that social workers must employ in civilian settings when they are competing for scarce agency resources.

Second, it was necessary to establish effective precombat relationships with critical unit gatekeepers. Groups exposed to traumatic stress typically wall themselves off and resist the approaches of outsiders. In order to overcome this natural tendency, the author made numerous pre-combat visits to the small component units in this military organization during the weeks and days before the start of the actual combat operations. These "circuit-riding" visits to unit medical personnel, chaplains, and senior noncommissioned officers were opportunities to introduce and/or reinforce unit-level knowledge about prevention and treatment of combat stress. In all of these visits, the author and his colleagues presented themselves as members of the organization, not as "outside experts" coming to take over. It was important to take time to listen when gatekeepers and/or unit leaders wanted to discuss soldiers who were experiencing some type of stress-related problem. The issues were typically a family-related concern or some type of phobic reaction to their (chemical/biological) protective mask. The mental health personnel did not "take over," rather they provided leaders and gatekeepers with the requisite information and/or support that allowed them to continue working with the soldier. Only in a few cases was it necessary to move a soldier to a less stressful environment. Typically, this involved allowing the affected soldier a chance to sleep, rehydrate, and the opportunity to talk to a concerned listener about the issue(s) that precipitated the current symptom(s). In most cases, the soldier returned to his unit within 24 to 36 hours.

By spending time on a regular basis "circuit riding," we were able to overcome the label of stranger. We were able to educate gatekeepers and unit leaders concerning the nature and value of postcombat debriefings and the critical importance of debriefings for those who might experience severe combat trauma. When the time came for interventions, we were there as promised.

DESCRIPTION OF THE TRAUMATIC INCIDENT AND THE CLIENTS

On the evening that the cease-fire went into effect, soldiers from the headquarters unit of the parent organization had arrived in a new area and were beginning to establish camp for the night. They had moved their combat vehicles into a coil, which means a circular defense arrangement with tanks and fighting vehicles facing outward. The sixteen men in the advanced group (ten enlisted soldiers in their early twenties, four senior enlisted soldiers in their late twenties and early thirties, and two young officers in their mid-twenties) were digging foxholes in front of their vehicles.

Doug, a young enlisted soldier, and a member of a fighting vehicle crew, was digging his foxhole when his vehicle commander called him back to the commander's vehicle. Doug turned, shouldered his shovel, and accidentally stepped on a sand-covered, unexploded munition. The munition, commonly referred to as a bomblet, exploded. The rifle grenades that Doug was carrying in a bandoleer across his chest exploded as well, and Doug was probably killed outright. The area in which this occurred was open desert terrain and the soldiers in this group were spread out in an area about half the size of a football field. While not everyone saw the actual explosion, everyone was immediately present at the scene.

Two very young enlisted medics in the group tried to resuscitate Doug. They had finished their basic military medical training in the United States just a few months earlier; thus, they were very inexperienced soldiers and medics. Both soldiers had only been with this unit a few weeks and, in many ways, were still strangers in this unit. The resuscitation was gruesome. As they tried to ventilate Doug, air escaped from his cheek, so someone put a hand there. Then air escaped from his chest, so someone put a hand there. Then air escaped from the abdomen, so someone put a hand there. Finally, air escaped from one eye socket. The medics, surrounded and watched by their fellow unit members, continued their efforts for about 20 minutes, at which point a physician from the medical section arrived, assessed the situation as hopeless, and called off the resuscitation.

The group dispersed in shock and disbelief. Over the next two days, there was very little discussion among those present, and the medics kept to their own tent and work area. Doug's body was evacuated to a regional holding area for transportation back to the United States. The unit leaders planned to set up a memorial service in a few days, once the unit moved to a more permanent location.

PRACTICE DECISIONS

Two days after the event, while circuit-riding in the area, the author and his psychiatrist colleague stopped by to visit this unit in response to information that there had been an accidental death. After discussing the event with one of the senior officers, a junior officer in charge of the section where the dead soldier, Doug, had been assigned approached and asked us to see one of his soldiers, a medic, because this soldier "appeared still upset" by what had happened. We responded that we would see him, and discussed that if he was obviously distressed this probably was indicative of less obvious but still significant distress in others who had been involved in and/or present at the resuscitation, in the soldier's comrades who were not present, and in the soldier's immediate chain of command. We proposed to assemble all involved do a debriefing and reconstruction of the accident, the resuscitation, and relevant events before and after. The section leader agreed to this approach and about one hour later we met with the members of Doug's section, along with a few other individuals who had been present at Doug's traumatic death.

Definition of the Clients

While this situation evolved from a leader's concern about a particular soldier's apparent emotional distress that was associated with a horrible post-combat incident, this was a traumatic event that clearly warranted a supportive group-level intervention. The debriefing included all members of Doug's section–those individuals who were at the scene, as well as a couple of soldiers with an immediate personal and/or professional relationship with Doug. The question of any necessary individual interventions for the identified medic (or others in the unit) would be considered subsequent to the debriefing. This approach follows Army doctrine (and professional practice models) that encourage the avoidance of labeling individuals as patients in the context of normal human response to an abnormal life experience (Copp and McAndrew, 1990; Brom and Kleber, 1989). In addition, this approach clearly takes advantage of the military group as a potential natural helping network and the power of military unit cohesion as a buffer against the stress associated with combat experiences (Belenky, Noy, and Solomon, 1987).

Goals, Objectives, and Outcome Measures

Many individuals exposed to traumatic stress experience short-term physical, psychological, and social stress symptoms. In some circumstances, these initial symptoms can evolve into long-term dysfunction, that affects the individual's physical health, psychological well-being, and social relationships. Group functioning can also be affected by traumatic stress exposure, causing diminished performance, lower group morale, and less group cohesion (Holmes, 1985).

Small unit stress debriefings can be thought of as "emotional first aid," a mental health intervention for otherwise normal individuals exposed to extreme stress. A debriefing involves a group reconstruction of experiences after exposure to a traumatic event. The group retells their experiences around a historical timeline as a means of identifying and clarifying important aspects of the event. The group is also provided an opportunity to deal with the traumatic experience and any associated stress. Small group stress debriefings provide a safe, supportive environment in which individuals have an opportunity to share their traumatic experience with others similarly exposed. Following are the primary goals and objectives of this approach (Martin, 1995).

1. Clarify any misconceptions of the event and its consequences.
2. Recognize and acknowledge feelings and discuss associated emotions.
3. Reduce symptomatology that could result in prolonged stress symptoms, illness, or behavioral dysfunction.
4. Enhance individuals' ability to help themselves.
5. Encourage and inform individuals of where to go if they need additional help.
6. Facilitate any grief process.
7. Improve communication among group members.
8. Enhance group cohesion.
9. Prepare the group for any future exposure.

Various types of debriefings are being applied worldwide to a broad range of traumatic events. While intuitively helpful, it is necessary to emphasize that there is very little empirical research to support the effectiveness of debriefings and there is danger in unreasonable expectations for debriefing's universal effectiveness (Shalev, 1994).

Use of Contract

There were two therapeutic contracts involved in this mental health intervention. The first was a promise to address the unit leader's concern about the medic who seemed to be experiencing considerable distress. The second contract was established with group members once they were assembled as a group. In order to set a debriefing contract with this group, we explained both the nature and purpose of our presence and the group debriefing. This was done using examples of other debriefings that we had recently conducted in response to a variety of combat-related traumatic events. We directly addressed the issue of confidentiality and privacy by making our mental health role clear and emphasizing that identifying information from any of our debriefings would not go to senior members of the units involved. We made it clear that as in any group process, we expected group members to respect the privacy and confidentiality of fellow group members. As Lewis (1994, p. 90) has pointed out, being able to talk to others (spouse, friends, clergy, etc.) about the traumatic experience is one of the curative methods of coping with the stress associated with a traumatic event. With this in mind, group members need only to be asked to "limit their discussions to significant others, do not talk to the media, and (in general) respect the rights and privacy of the others who have participated in the debriefing" (Lewis, 1994, p. 91). We began the debriefings by making it clear that individuals were free to choose not to participate, they could choose to leave at any time, and no one will be forced or coerced to say or reveal any information that they prefer not to discuss.

Meeting Place

Debriefings should be conducted in a safe and secure place, preferably in a familiar location for the group. For example, in a military context, if the traumatic event occurred in a tactical setting, a discrete location within the unit's field site would be an ideal location for the debriefing. If the debriefing takes place in garrison, a unit area would be more appropriate than a hospital or other clinical setting. The idea is to use a location that provides some degree of privacy, where the debriefing process will not be interrupted, and where participants feel "at home."

The debriefing described in this chapter took place in an open area behind one of the supply tents. It was an area that was out of the way from other activities and offered a reasonable degree of privacy. A few folding chairs and some boxes provided places to sit. Seating was by choice except that the two mental health officers sat at opposite sides of the circle. This was done to provide us (the group leaders) with full vision of all participants at all times during the group process. If there had been the likelihood of interruptions and/or the weather required it, the session could have been held in a large tent (the substitute for a conference room). Again, the critical issue is to hold the session in an area that limits distractions and/or interruptions like phones ringing or people coming in and out. If you are in a closed setting, you also want to locate one of the group leaders in front of the primary access in and out of the room. This will inhibit individuals from leaving when things become stressful. It also allows the group leader to control any outsider interruptions. Once begun, the session continues without a break. Individuals are asked to quietly leave and return if they have to use the bathroom, etc. If someone leaves because he or she is upset, one of the group leaders always follows to help ensure that the individual is able to gather enough composure to return to the group. None of these issues developed in this debriefing.

Use of Time

Stress debriefings must be conducted as soon as possible after the traumatic event. It is important that basic human needs (hydration, food, sleep) are considered first. Mitchell (1983), in his discussion of interventions with fire-rescue personnel, recommends the use of a brief "defusing" immediately after the traumatic event in order to help the individual regain some composure and to offer some practical information designed to assist the physical and emotional transition from the site to home. In this model, individuals are typically brought back together as a group the next day for a formal debriefing once their need for rest and replenishment has been met.

The actual time allotted to the stress debriefing is not fixed. Sessions lasting two to three hours are common. The debriefing described in this chapter lasted two and one-half hours. On the other hand, the historical group debriefings performed by S.L.A. Marshal during World War II and Korea (Shalev, 1994) often went on for hours (and sometimes days). It must be remembered that Marshall was primarily a historian and his task was recording highly complex information about combat events that often involved a day or more of intense fighting. Marshall believed that "sessions should be limited only by the time it takes to achieve the desired results" (Shalev, 1994, p. 207). As Shalev points out, "This attitude toward time, that the unfolding of the process determined the (amount of) time for the debriefing, is similar to that of traditional psychodynamic therapy, where the length of the treatment is determined by its course" (Shalev, 1994, p 208).

Interventions

Debriefing group leaders typically use a chronology to help the group identify and establish "a road map" of the critical events associated with the trauma. At each step along the time line, leaders ask group members to review the who, what, when, where, and sometimes the possible whys of the event. It is important to allow the group to establish the facts, examine key stressors, and surface feelings. Leaders do not dispute discrepancies between personal accounts but do try to bring about a mutual clarification of the facts as they are known or perceived by the group members. The leaders ensure that all participants are treated as equal witnesses. Rank or title has no special significance in reviewing or establishing events as they happened. Experience of the event becomes the primary source of one's position in the group process at any given point in the session.

In the debriefing described in this chapter, we used the reconstruction of the event to facilitate a discussion of thoughts, feelings, and actions of the participants. The objective was to encourage individuals to take an active role in coping with their own stress. We encouraged emotional ventilation and facilitated the grief process. We also looked for signs and symptoms of dysfunction that would require further intervention and we provided group members with information on normal reactions to trauma and information on self-help coping measures.

In the course of this debriefing, the events of the resuscitation, as described earlier, were presented in vivid detail. A few of Doug's friends who were not present at the death, initially expressed reservations about the competency of the medics and whether all that could be done to try to save him was done. In response to these expressed misgivings, one of the medics (the one we had been asked to see earlier) stood in the center of the group and described the resuscitation. During his vivid and detailed recounting, it became obvious to Doug's friends who had not been present at the time of the accident that the two medics had done the best they could and that they had done more than Doug's friends could imagine themselves doing. As he spoke, the young medic visibly became less distressed and he appeared to gain confidence and self-assurance. The group clearly identified with this medic's pain. Their praise for his heroism and their expressions of support were responses that demonstrated to the medic that he was a welcomed member of the primary group. He was no longer a distrusted outsider.

Doug's sergeant and platoon leader raised another issue. Just before the ground war, Doug's wife had given birth. The mother and child were fine, but by Army regulation, Doug met the requirements to be granted emergency leave to go home to visit his spouse and child. The chain of command (this sergeant and platoon leader) and Doug discussed this, and mutually agreed that since there was no problem at home, he should stay with the unit, go through the ground war with his comrades, and then go home.

This decision was reexamined by the group in the light of Doug's subsequent death. In retrospect, everyone wished Doug had gone home. However, the group consensus was that the decision was the correct one at the time, and that faced with similar circumstances in the future the decision would likely be the same. In the process of this discussion, it was obvious that these two section leaders were feeling guilty and somewhat responsible for this decision and the subsequent tragedy. After all, they could have insisted that he return home. The presentation of the facts and support from Doug's peers helped these leaders recognize that the decision for Doug to remain with the group was a correct decision and was not related to Doug's subsequent death.

By the end of the debriefing everyone had a clearer view of the accident, its antecedents, and the resuscitation. For the medic who was most affected, the debriefing was a turning point in how he viewed himself and how his comrades viewed him. This medic had dealt directly with his personal distress over this incident and understood the respect with which his comrades viewed him.

Stance of the Social Worker

The social worker's approach as a stress debriefing leader is guided by some basic mental health beliefs that provide a context and framework for the process. Debriefings are intended to quickly restore individual emotional equilibrium and to enhance group cohesion and mutual support. The debriefing should help to reduce short- and long-term emotional and associated physical distress. The debriefing participants are considered normal persons who have experienced an abnormal, severe stressor. While therapeutic in nature, the debriefing is not considered "therapy." Every effort is made to cast the debriefing and those being debriefed as "non-patients." Rather, the debriefing is presented as a type of preventive maintenance for the human mind, like changing the oil and filter in a car after a long, demanding trip. The leaders' approach is similar to that used in most classical group interventions. It involves setting the stage and facilitating the process. As discussed earlier, a focus on a timeline and the use of phases (Mitchell, 1983) provides the necessary structure for this process.

Use of Outside Resources

It is critical to have the sanction of the organization or group that is the host for the debriefing. In the case highlighted in this chapter, sanction came from the senior military chain of command in the parent organization. Without this support, it is usually impossible to effectively offer these services. The organization usually provides the resources (location and employee's time) that allow the debriefing to occur. It is also important to have the sanction of gatekeepers in the organization that can effectively control or block access. In this case, it was also necessary to gain the local unit commander's support. This is analogous to having a school principal's support even when the school superintendent had agreed to the intervention. The primary resource used in the debriefing process is the group itself. This includes the mutual support members offer one another during the debriefing, as well as the practical advice, guidance, and tangible help that group members may be able to provide one another during and subsequent to the group debriefing.

Reassessment

A formal follow-up to a small group stress debriefing is very unusual. Typically, the debriefer attempts to obtain an informal reading on the subsequent well-being of group members. This is usually done via contacts with someone in the organization in a position to know about group member status. For example, in a military unit this might be the unit chaplain or medical officer. Sometimes it might be the unit commander. In this case, feedback came a few weeks later from the unit commander. He was no longer concerned about the medic and he reported that the unit was doing very well overall. We were also provided follow-up information concerning the young medic, from the medical officer responsible for his technical supervision. He reported a noticeable change in this soldier's overall attitude. The medic was described as being more mature and enthusiastically planning to continue a military career, including applying for advanced-level military training upon his return to the United States. This was in contrast to a pre-event description of this medic as immature and unmotivated.

Transfer or Termination

In most debriefings it is not necessary to refer participants for additional mental health intervention. During the debriefing process participants are told about various support services that exist in their communities (or military units), including counseling and other mental health services. Also, during the debriefing process, the group leaders typically talk about the biological, psychological, and social symptoms that often accompany exposure to severe stress. Participants are told about the normal nature and duration of these symptoms, and how to deal with them using various self-help techniques and informal social supports. Participants are also told how to recognize when symptoms have become abnormal, and how and where to seek professional assistance. In this debriefing, we made it clear to participants that our mental health team would remain with their parent organization until the command's redeployment out of the combat zone. We also discussed the process of obtaining mental health care via referral from unit medical officer.

Consultation

Individuals conducting debriefings require their own source of emotional support. The debriefing process is often very stressful for the debriefer. It is critically important that mental health personnel conducting debriefings have the opportunity to talk about their experience. This is accomplished in two ways. First, those doing group debriefings need to work in teams of two or three. After the debriefing, these individuals process the group experience with each other. This is a critical component of the overall process. It allows an emotional release from the intense stress that results from the debriefing experience. The sharing of thoughts and feelings among and between the debriefers also allows them to discharge some of their own reactions to the event, as well as their experiences and feelings toward the participants. In addition to debriefing one another, it is helpful for emotional well-being, as well as for the enhancement of technical skill and teamwork, for the debriefers to review their work with an outside supervisor and/or consultant. This is commonly referred to as "debriefing the debriefer." In this particular case, we had an opportunity to review this debriefing session among ourselves, and subsequently with the rest of our mental health team. As always, during this review process, we identified things that worked out well and we considered things that might be done differently in future debriefings. We also allowed ourselves a moment to feel the intense sadness that unit members had shared with us over the loss of a good soldier and a good friend.

Case Conclusion

By the end of this debriefing, everyone had gained a clearer view of the accident, its antecedents, and the resuscitation. Unit members openly shared their grief with one another. The unit leaders, who had questioned their decision about sending Doug home when his spouse delivered their baby, had heard Doug's peers reinforce the fact that they made the correct decision. There was no need to continue second guessing themselves. It was a positive turning point for the medic who was most affected. By the end of the debriefing, this medic was clearly free of the doubt and emotional distress that he had been experiencing and his comrades obviously viewed him with a new respect. We were later told that from that point, he became a valued and well-thought-of member of the unit, whereas before, he reportedly had been treated as peripheral.

Differential Discussion

In retrospect, we recognize that we were fortunate to have this debriefing opportunity. When our mental health team was attached to this command, a few weeks before the start of the ground war, there were many predictions that a United Nations advance into Iraq would result in hundreds, if not thousands, of American casualties. We had joined the organization whose role was to lead the entire invasion, engage the main body of Iraq elite infantry and armor, and allow an even larger and more powerful American force to sweep around and destroy the powerful Iraqi Army. Among other threats, we were worried about the use of chemical and biological weapons and the likelihood of numerous physical and psychological casualties.

When we invaded Iraq, we found an army whose morale was broken. Iraqi soldiers were more inclined to surrender or flee than fight. American forces were extremely successful and incurred only a few casualties. Fortunately, chemical and biological agents were not used. While the number of American dead and injured was small (148 in a force of 700,000), some of these combat deaths and injuries were the result of the common combat experience of friendly fire (units mistakenly attacking some of their own personnel). Friendly fire deaths became one of the issues that we had to deal with in our command. As a result of the overall small number of American dead and wounded, and the corresponding very small number of battle fatigue causalities, our small mental health team was able to adequately support our command. In addition, because the actual ground fighting ended so quickly, we were able to rapidly get to units that required our services.

If the actual events of the Persian Gulf War had been as predicted, we would have been overwhelmed by battle fatigue casualties and unit debriefings would have been put off until events and direct service demands allowed us the time and the access to units in need of debriefing services. Under these circumstances, involving conditions that could easily occur in any future conflict or even in any major national disaster, it is clear that one of the vital tasks required as part of combat (and emergency service) preparations is the training of selected group members in debriefing methods. Unit chaplains, senior medical technicians, and paraprofessionals with good people skills could be trained to provide critical services under these dramatic circumstances. This approach is also in keeping with the concept that debriefings represent emotional "first aid," somewhat analogous to Red Cross Cardiopulmonary Resuscitation (CPR) training. In hindsight, more of our precombat time and energies could have been focused on developing a basic debriefing capability in every major subordinate unit in our command.

PRACTICE IN CONTEXT

The mental health aspects of military operations and the consequences of combat stress have been recognized for a long time (Copp and McAndrew, 1990; Elder and Clipp, 1988). Many veterans of World War II, Korea, Vietnam, and the Persian Gulf War bring to their civilian lives enduring memories of a beneficial military experience in which they developed important life skills and friendships that have been sustained across a lifetime. For other veterans, memories of combat (and the other stressors associated with military experiences) cast a dark, persistent shadow on their lives and on the lives of those closest to then. The prevention and treatment of combat stress casualties have been the basis for the development of a variety of mental health approaches that have been adopted and adapted to civilian settings. The use of small group stress debriefings is one example of a prevention technique that evolved from the military experiences and has now been recognized as a valuable approach across a variety of life-stress exposures.

REFERENCES

Belenky, G., Noy, S., and Solomon, Z. (1987). Battle stress, morale, cohesion, combat effectiveness, and psychiatric casualties: The Israeli experience. In G. Belenky (Ed.), *Contemporary studies in combat psychiatry.* New York: Greenwood Press, pp. 11-20.

Brom, D. and Kleber, R. J. (1989). Prevention of post-traumatic stress disorders. *Journal of Traumatic Stress, 2*(3), 335-351.

Copp, T. and McAndrew, B. (1990). *Battle exhaustion*. Montreal: McGill-Queen's University Press.

Department of Defense (DOD) Report (1995). Comprehensive clinical evaluation program (CCEP) for Gulf War veterans: report on 10,020 participants. Washington, DC: Office of the Assistant Secretary of Defense for Health Affairs, The Pentagon.

Elder, G. H. and Clipp, E. C. (1988). Combat experience, comradeship, and psychological health. In J. P. Wilson, Z. Harel, and B. Kahana (Eds.), *Human adaptation to extreme stress*. New York: Plenum Press, pp. 131-156.

Green, B. L. (1994). Psychosocial research in traumatic stress: an update. Journal of Traumatic Stress, 7(3), 341-362.

Holmes, R. (1985). *Acts of war*. New York: The Free Press.

Holsenbeck, L. S. (1992). Psych-force 90: The OM team in the Gulf. *The Journal of the U.S. Army Medical Department*, PB8-92-3/4, March/April, pp. 32-38.

Ingraham, L. and Manning, F. (1986). American military psychiatry. In R.A. Gabriel (Ed.), *Military psychiatry*. Westport, CT: Greenwood Publishing Group, pp. 25-65.

Lewis, G. W. (1994). *Critical incident stress*. Bristol, PA: Accelerated Development.

Marlowe, D. H. (1994). The general well-being of Gulf War era service personnel from the states of Pennsylvania and Hawaii: A survey. Frederick, MD: U.S. Army Medical Research, Development, Acquisition and Logistics Command.

Marshall, S. L. A. (1947). *Men under fire: The problem of battle command in future war*. New York: William Morrow.

Martin, J. A. (1992). Mental health issues: Lessons learned from Operation Desert Shield/Storm. Proceedings of the Psychology in the Department of Defense Symposium, pp. 221-225. Colorado Springs, CO: U.S. Air Force Academy.

Martin, J. A. (1995). Responding to trauma and disaster: Applying psychosocial "first aid." Spring Session: Continuing education for professional social workers. Bryn Mawr, PA: Bryn Mawr College, Graduate School of Social Work and Social Research.

Martin, J. A., Sparacino, L. R., and Belenky, G. (1996). (Eds.). *The Gulf War and mental health: A comprehensive guide*. Westport, CT: Praeger.

Mitchell, J. T. (1981). *Emergency response to crisis: A crisis intervention guidebook of emergency service personnel*. Bowie, MD: R. J. Brady Co.

Mitchell, J. T. (1983). When disaster strikes: The critical incident stress debriefing process. *American Journal of Emergency Services, 8*, 36-39.

Mitchell, J. T. (1986). Critical incident stress management. *Response!, 5*, 24-25.

Raphael, B. (1986). *When disaster strikes*. London: Hutchinson.

Shalev, A. Y. (1994). Debriefing following traumatic exposure. In R. J. Ursano, B. G. McCaughey, and C. S. Fullerton (Eds.), *Individual and community responses to trauma and disaster: The structure of human chaos*. New York: Cambridge University Press, pp. 201-219.

Shalev, A. Y. and Ursano, R. (1990). Group debriefing following exposure to traumatic stress. Proceedings of the Wartime Medical Services, Second

International Conference (pp. 192-207). IFS Institute for Hospital Planning, Stockholm; 33 Stermalsgatan; S-11426 Stockholm, Sweden.

Stokes, J. (1992). Coordinating draft, field manual (FM) 8-51: Combat stress control in a theater of operations. Chapter 7. Fort Sam Houston, TX: U.S. Army Medical Department School and Center.

Wright, K. M., Marlowe, D. H., Martin, J. A., Gifford, R. K., Belenky, G. L., and Manning, F. J. (1994). Operation Desert Shield and Desert Storm: A summary report. Washington, DC: Department of Military Psychiatry, Walter Reed Army Institute of Research.

Chapter 28

A Woman Addresses Her Recurrent Depression in Psychotherapy: Private Practice

Carol Silbergeld
Toba Schwaber Kerson

Clinical social workers are the majority of mental health professionals providing services to the general public in agencies, clinics, and private practice (American Board of Examiners in Clinical Social Work, 1995). They are increasingly recognized as autonomous mental health professionals. According to recent National Association of Social Work estimates, 30 percent of clinical social workers are engaged in some form of independent practice at least part of the time (Gibelman and Schervish, 1993). The number has greatly increased over the past two decades; it is thought that about 18,000 social workers identify themselves as private practitioners and more than 10,000 social workers who identify themselves by their agency jobs also see clients privately (Barker, 1992; Barker, 1984; Social Workers Vault . . . , 1985). This growth has been aided by trends encouraging private practice of all kinds, increased professional endorsement, cutbacks in agency budgets, increased third-party financing, and the willingness of many social workers to view themselves as autonomous (Wallace, 1982).

Policy

Licensing

The independent practice of social work is increasingly regulated by state governmental agencies. In 1945, California became the first state to register social workers. In the mid 1960s, Oklahoma, Virginia, and California became the first states to license clinical social workers. Currently, all states regulate the practice of social work through licensure or certification (DeAngelis, 1993; National Association of Social Workers, 1985).

Licensing raises many issues for social workers (Land, 1987; Johnson and Huff, 1987). Professional licensure, certification and registration (referred to here as licensing) serve to protect the consumer, practitioner, and profession. Proponents of licensing argue that it encourages the highest standards of professional performance (Barker, 1987), enhances social work status by subscribing to the more autonomous medical model, and ultimately increases possibilities for third-party reimbursement. In addition, it increases the likelihood of having a middle- and upper-middle class clientele. Historically, focusing on the egalitarian roots of social work and its commitment to the eradication of racism and poverty, opponents within the social work community have thought that social workers should not be competing with other mental health professionals for middle-class clientele. However, since 1964, the National Association of Social Workers has officially recognized private practice as a legitimate area for social workers, but stated the position that practice within agencies should remain the primary avenue for the implementation of the goals of the profession (Kelley and Alexander, 1985).

Licensing, with its often concomitant requirements for continuing education, postgraduate training, and supervision, also compels clinical social workers to acquire advanced skills (Goldmeier, 1986). Along with a small but growing number of graduate schools, a number of institutes and clinics have developed educational programs that enable the master's-level-prepared social worker to earn a clinical doctorate or a postgraduate certificate. The evolution of such programs seems to parallel the spread of licensing across the country.

Health Insurance

Health Insurance greatly affects the provision of health care. Clinical social workers have increasingly been included by law in health plans, disability plans, self-insured employee welfare benefit plans, and hospital service contracts offering mental health care (Barker, 1987; Barker, 1983). In 1977, California passed the Torres Bill, the first state vendorship bill requiring insurance policies that included mental health coverage to recognize licensed clinical social workers as reimbursable providers. Such laws vary from one state to another. Some require a referral from a licensed physician, others may require documentation of supervision or specified periodic consultation with a licensed psychiatrist or psychologist. Coverage for out-of-state vendorship also varies (Cutler, 1995). Most social workers strive for maximal autonomy.

Third-party reimbursement is critical for most people to be able to afford private psychotherapy and for independent social work practitioners to compete with other professionals for clients. Insurance plans expand the client pool to include lower and middle-income groups. Receiving substantial payments for most cases also permits the private practitioner to reduce fees for financially needy patients (Barker, 1982) and those who are not insured. However, the health insurance industry has undergone drastic changes in the last decade and these changes are having a profound impact on the independent practice of psychotherapy. Prior to the 1980s, health benefits were typically indemnity plans. Although traditional indemnity plans still exist, they are rapidly being replaced by managed care. With indemnity plans, insurance companies generally limit their reimbursement for psychotherapeutic services by setting a maximum hourly fee, limiting the client's total dollar expenditure, defining the treatment modes, or restricting qualifying diagnoses (Lechnyr, 1984). However, there is minimal insurance company involvement in the case management, and therapists' communications with insurance companies are generally confined to bookkeeping. Therapists' bills need to include dates of treatment, type of therapy provided, and a diagnosis. Insurance plans vary as to total dollar expenditures allowed, but they are often liberal, paying from 50 to 80 percent of customary charges, and except for ceilings on annual expenditures per patient, are generally not intrusive in the treatment process. Treatment is sometimes terminated because some patients are unable to continue treatment when they are no longer eligible for reimbursement (Jackson, 1987; Sharfstein, Maszynski, and Meyers, 1984). Issues related to diagnosis sometimes create conflicts for the therapist, especially when diagnoses such as psychoses, substance abuse, and sexual perversions are particularly stigmatizing. At the other end of the diagnosis quandary are the clients who may have wanted to discuss a social or situational problem but who had to receive a psychiatric diagnosis in order to receive reimbursement. For example, many insurance companies will not reimburse for treatment of transient situational disturbances, marital, or parent-child problems, since the current *Diagnostic and Statistical Manual* does not consider these to be psychiatric diagnoses (American Psychiatric Association, 1994). People coping with life-circumstance problems such as divorce, death, problems with spouse, child, or job may be experiencing prolonged emotional stress and be in need of psychotherapeutic help. If therapists determine that their patient(s) warrant a psychiatric diagnosis, they must discuss the diagnosis and the release of the diagnosis to the insurance company with the patient. Issues relating to informed consent and release of information are complex (Applebaum, 1993; Reamer, 1987, 1983).

Managed Care

Health insurance is extremely costly. The cost of health care in the United States has risen drastically over the last decade to over 12 percent of the nation's gross national product (Kelton-Locke, 1992). As a result, a variety of mechanisms have been developed by insurance companies and corporations to contain the rising costs (Grahm, 1992-1993). Health maintenance organizations (HMOs), such as Kaiser Permanente, were early responses to the fee-for-service models of health care delivery, which were created in order to contain the rising costs of health care for large groups of employees. Preferred provider organizations (PPOs) offer discounted fee-for service arrangements to those chosen providers who agree to the terms and conditions required by contracting entities. PPOs are not a radical departure from traditional fee-for-service practice; however, they interpose a layer of administrative intervention that usually takes the form of concurrent review with a case manager. Forms need to be completed, conversations need to be had with reviewers, and billing mechanisms vary among PPOs. Proper authorizations must be obtained and are usually provided for a limited number of sessions. Membership in many PPOs with varied rules and procedures can be administratively overwhelming.

The main goal shared by all managed care approaches is the reduction in the cost of health care (Esposito, 1995; Brown, 1994; Austad and Hoyt, 1992; Austad and Berman, 1991). This is accomplished with pretreatment authorization, concurrent utilization review, increased cost sharing by the insured, limited fees for the participating providers, and closer scrutiny of claims with the power to deny payment for care thought to be unnecessary or not cost-effective (Kelton-Locke, 1992). Many companies are forming exclusive relationships with large multidisciplinary group practices and making capitated arrangements whereby the groups share the financial risks and perform the case management themselves. Increasingly, PPO panels are closed to new applicants, and potential clients may well decline services if the therapist is not on their preferred provider panel. In addition, ongoing patients frequently find their insurance policies are altered, and, for financial reasons, they are forced to transfer to a therapist on their insurance policy's list of providers.

The ever increasing third-party involvement in treatment authorizations and reviews is also having a major impact on the length of treatment and consequently on the kind of work that can be done in a brief time period (Dorwart, 1990; Riemersma, 1992; Tischler, 1990). In a recent survey of the experiences of California psychologists with managed care (Clifford and Denkers, 1994), clinicians found that the reviewers often have inadequate or inappropriate credentials and are often hostile and authoritarian to them. Many reviewers responded with rote approaches, such as "depressed clients need to be on medication." Denials based on "lack of medical necessity" are common. It is also very difficult to engage in a therapeutic process with the ever present threat of termination of services. Additionally, many practitioners believe that the majority of managed care companies hold a strong antipsychoanalytic bias and that managed care is incompatible with the practice of psychoanalytic psychotherapy (Alperin, 1994). A 1995 survey conducted by the California Society of Clinical Social Work found that 90 percent of clinical social workers rated managed care experiences as negative (Goldman 1995). Concerns most often cited were about violations of patient confidentiality, the overuse of medications in order to shorten treatment, and the lack of interest in in-depth treatment. Clinicians are increasingly facing ethical dilemmas when treatment is being terminated at a time when they believe their patient to be at emotional risk. This also raises legal liability issues that have yet to be resolved (Kurzman, 1995; Phillips, 1995; Reamer, 1994).

The need for therapists to provide detailed accounts of patients' treatments to managed care personnel greatly impacts on therapist-patient confidentiality (Gothard, 1995). Insurance companies require that patients sign forms consenting to the release of information regarding their treatment. In addition to diagnosis, many insurers request detailed treatment summaries in order to justify continued reimbursement. This information may be on file and/or accessible to the patient's employer and insurance company personnel. Patients' concerns about what is being shared often hinders their trust and comfort in sharing very personal or potentially damaging information for fear of it getting into the wrong hands. The Bennett-Leahy Bill, which is currently under Congressional consideration, proposes to address some of these problems, but may in fact "precipitate a confidentiality disaster" (Scarf, 1996, p. 38). Clinicians are finding that the utilization reviews are too frequent and too lengthy, there is a lack of varied orientations, treatment planning decisions often appear to be made by formula rather than sound judgment or compassion, and treatment is increasingly fragmented. Thus, the increasing intrusion of an ever present third party hinders the relationship between social worker and patient. These trends are very problematic for our profession and are obstacles to the mental health of our patients. We are faced with the challenge of reducing the costs of mental health services and providing adequate treatment. Hopefully, we are in a transition phase, and other more creative solutions lie ahead.

Organization

With the exception of third-party involvement, which is escalating and appears to be increasingly unavoidable, clinical social workers in private practice are not guided or controlled by agency or supervisory mission or structure and consequently are free to make their own decisions about case selection, treatment, and fees. Consequently, patients who don't have mental health benefits or choose not to use them are not under any constraints regarding length of treatment or amount of fee. Basically, one must establish one's own organization with a sound structure, referral base, consultant network, physical environment, accounting system, contractual arrangements, malpractice insurance, and means of accountability.

Because they function autonomously, private practitioners must find alternate routes for maintaining referrals and for professional consultation. Successful private practitioners establish a network of referral sources and market themselves as a small business (Borenzweig, 1981; Levin, 1984). One aspect of marketing means defining oneself clearly to possible sources of referral. Defining oneself as a specialist is often helpful. For example, one may hold oneself out to the public as a specialist in a particular treatment mode such as family or group treatment; a certain problem area such as divorce-adjustment, depression, or substance abuse; or a particular type of client such as children or adolescents. In terms of professional consultation, clinical social workers utilize specialists in areas such as psychiatry, psychology, neurology, speech and hearing pathology, neuropsychology, educational psychology, and medicine when other kinds of diagnostic information is needed.

To organize a private practice, one needs to have an accounting and billing system, a tax plan, and policies about delinquent fees and malpractice (Barker, 1995, Bernstein, 1981). The manner in which the patient handles fee payment is an important communication to the therapist. Close scrutiny of the meaning of unpaid bills, late payments, or the reluctance to take responsibility for processing claims to the insurance company illuminates the patient's feelings about the treatment, the therapist, or past significant relationships. If the issue of fee payment is clouded by complicated forms, bureaucratic procedures, or substantially delayed reimbursements, this aspect of treatment may not easily be understood in terms of communications by the patient. These issues are often clarified by having patients pay the therapist directly. Patients then can seek reimbursement from the insurance company themselves. Occasionally, however, patients are financially unable to manage this arrangement.

In addition to other carriers, NASW sponsors malpractice insurance coverage for clinical social workers. It is said that the following circumstances heighten the possibility of malpractice suits: lack of informed consent regarding treatment method, misusing the relationship to exploit the client, inappropriate treatment, faulty diagnosis, providing treatment without qualification, abandonment or premature termination of clients who still need service, and failure to warn others when the client has indicated intent to harm (Barker, 1987; Weill and Sanchez, 1983). Clinicians are increasingly facing ethical and legal liability dilemmas of premature termination brought about by treatment denials on the part of managed care.

Within these realities is the contractual arrangement between therapist and patient. The patient agrees to pay the practitioner for a service and the practitioner renders a service based on his or her clinical judgment and expertise. Thus, the primary differences between private practice and agency-based practice are the client's direct payment to the social worker and the social worker's ability to determine the conditions of work. This also means that the social worker has no one with whom to share responsibility. Missing is the comfort and support that one receives working with a team or being able to dash into the office of a supervisor or colleague, call on another worker with expertise in a particular area, or transfer or get direct and immediate help with a problem. Thus, the independent practitioner may spend more time pondering the client's problems away from the treatment situation than he or she might in an agency setting. This aspect of practice is a challenge. It sometimes indicates the need for a literature search and/or consultation. Issues of countertransference and transference may also emerge, providing another reason for private practice to be the bastion of the highly experienced and trained clinical social worker.

Referrals come primarily from other mental health professionals, former patients, and other professionals such as doctors, lawyers, and school counselors. Because of a long affiliation with the Reiss-Davis Child Study Center in Los Angeles, I have developed subspecialties of child and parent psychotherapy, couples therapy, and divorce work with children and parents. I have always maintained an avid interest in long-term therapy with individuals who would like to resolve conflicts and thereby have more contentment in their lives. Some of my clients/patients continue weekly therapy for three or four years. I screen out highly disturbed clients by referring them to a therapist who can provide hospitalization and medication. Cases referred to me are primarily young and middle-aged adults with problems including identity confusion, low self-esteem, anxiety, depression, relationship difficulties, and separation-individuation issues. Child referrals are usually presenting a variety of behavioral manifestations of anxiety and depression. According to Goldmeier, more than half of all patients seeking psychotherapy services are adults between the ages of 18 and 40. The three categories of mental disorder that are most prominent are anxiety disorders, adjustment disorders, and affective disorders (Goldmeier, 1986).

My office is located in a building with the offices of many other psychotherapists. Patients come to a comfortable waiting room and press a button that lights in my office to let me know they have arrived. With a number of comfortable chairs, I have several seating possibilities for individuals, couples, and families.

Client Description

The case I chose to present is a long-term treatment case that would not, most likely, have been authorized for long-term treatment under managed care. However, I believe that this client would not have been helped without an opportunity to have an extended therapeutic relationship that could shed light on her unconscious processes and give her a reparative emotional experience. She did not have insurance coverage, which freed us to develop a treatment contract without third-party intrusion. As she also had a limited income, we needed to arrive at a mutually acceptable fee, which meant a reduced fee.

At the time of referral, Nancy was a 31-year-old single woman who sought help for recurrent depression. One of many children in a rural family with a history of alcohol abuse and incest problems, Nancy felt isolated and unloved. Her mother was highly critical and her father favored her brothers. After an older sister left to marry, Nancy felt abandoned and alone. An early marriage to a self-centered and emotionally unavailable man was brief and unsatisfying. Recently, she had ended a relationship with a man who resembled her ex-husband.

A large, nice-looking woman, Nancy wept easily. She was intelligent, verbal, interesting, and had a warm sense of humor. When we began, Nancy was an assistant administrator in a small business and a postgraduate student. Depressed about her unsatisfactory relationships with men and a chronic weight problem, Nancy sometimes considered suicide. Having had previous psychotherapy experiences, Nancy was sophisticated about the role of unconscious processes in her difficulties.

Definition of the Client

In this situation, it was clear that the client was Nancy. Even if she had been married, had children, or had other significant biological or social relationships, Nancy's need to be viewed and valued as an individual would have indicated that she receive individual psychotherapy. Although the decision regarding definition of the client was clear, definition of the therapist was not. Patients assessed to be suicidal may be more appropriately treated by a psychiatrist who can medicate and hospitalize if necessary. After working together for several sessions, Nancy and I determined that she was not actively suicidal and that we could work well together.

Goals

Some initial goals were unarticulated at the beginning of treatment and were elaborated as work progressed. Nancy wanted to "feel better"" and we used the initial phases of treatment to identify and clarify the nature of her discomfort. Nancy recognized that feeling better was contingent upon gaining psychological insight and resolving conflicts especially regarding closeness and intimacy. She hoped that treatment would improve her self-esteem, allowing her to become involved in healthier relationships, and would reduce her depression and overeating. Each goal is observable or can be evaluated through self-report.

Contract

Our contract primarily involved the structure of treatment: session schedule, fee, insurance and billing arrangements, and cancellation policy (Rosen, Proctor, and Livne, 1985). Nancy did not have health insurance and had a limited income. Consequently, we negotiated a reduced fee that she believed she could manage and I found acceptable. Nancy was billed once a month. Agreement between patient and therapist about goals and methods unfolds as the therapist learns more about the patient. Areas for work are elaborated upon and reworked in the treatment process. Once treatment begins, patients frequently challenge the structure by not paying, canceling, requesting a change of time, or criticizing some aspect of the therapist's behavior. These may be manifestations of the patient's problems and can be used to help the patient to gain insight.

Use of Time and Meeting Place

At the beginning of treatment, Nancy and I agreed to meet weekly at a set time for a prescribed period. There was no discussion about the expected duration of treatment. It was clear that Nancy understood, perhaps as the result of a lengthy previous therapy experience, that treatment would take as long as she needed and that its duration would depend on her progress. We worked together for three years, always meeting in my office and assuming the same seats each week.

Treatment Modality

The primary treatment modality was psychoanalytic psychotherapy (Eagle, 1984; Strean, 1979). Psychoanalytic psychotherapy alleges that unless a person becomes aware of certain wishes, admonitions, and defenses, and recognizes that he or she is distorting the present and perceiving it as if it were part of his or her childhood, that person cannot be helped (Strean, 1979). Important in this modality are such concepts as the unconscious, resistance, defense mechanisms, and transference. Transferential reactions, for example, are unconscious attempts by the patient to recapitulate with the therapist types of interpersonal interaction similar to those he or she expressed with significant persons in the past. Transference suggests experiencing the therapist in terms of how one wishes the therapist to be and/or fears he or she might be (Strean, 1979). Here, a primary goal is insight about one's intrapsychic state and how situations affect one's responses.

Through exploration of Nancy's feelings, particularly those in the transference, we were able to relate many of her current difficulties to her early object relations. For example, during the first year of treatment, Nancy did not pay her bill for several months. In reality, she had a tight budget and had difficulty paying other bills as well; however, close scrutiny of her reactions to my inquiries about unpaid bills revealed underlying psychodynamics. Nancy resented my concern and interpreted it as distrust. After some exploration, it became evident that Nancy felt she had to pay me in order for me to care about her. By not paying, she was testing to see how long it would take for me to abandon her. As we gained more understanding about the meaning of the fee to Nancy, she managed payment more appropriately (Strean, 1979).

Stance of the Social Worker

My stance follows that of psychoanalytically oriented psychotherapy. It is primarily reactive and interpretive. I do not usually offer suggestions, but rather help the patient to explore the meanings and ramifications of his or her feelings, thoughts, and actions. Self-disclosure, advice-giving, and the use of outside resources or concrete services are not part of this stance.

Reassessment and Termination

Nancy recognized that her fears of rejection and criticism were feelings she frequently had as a child (Strean, 1979). She gained insight into her tendency to respond to earlier hurt and anger with depression and overeating. As her fears were understood, Nancy improved her ability to separate fantasy from reality. She developed a more realistic view of herself and was less fearful of intimacy. As her self-esteem improved, in an effort to be more attractive, she began to change her eating habits and lose weight. She experienced fewer and less intense depressions and had no serious periods of depression during her third year of therapy. At termination, Nancy was seriously involved in a gratifying relationship with an emotionally available, caring man.

Managed care would not have authorized this case for three years of open-ended psychoanalytic exploration. Case managers typically are mandated by their employers not to accept goals such as making the unconscious conscious or helping the patient achieve emotional growth, as these goals are not usually considered to be medically necessary. It appears that the cases that managed care will authorize for treatment are those with identifiable functioning and behavior impairments that can be addressed in brief, focused, and crisis intervention treatment models, as well as those treatable with medication. With the case summarized above, managed care might have authorized ten or twelve sessions of treatment and might have granted a brief extension or two. This certainly would have changed the nature of our work to that of a much more focused and problem-solving model. I believe that medication would have been recommended for treatment of her depression. The patient might have gained some minimum benefit from the treatment but much of the potential stability would have been left unachieved and, I believe, the patient would have continued to be at risk for suicide. Fortunately, this patient and therapist were able to arrive at a mutually agreeable reduced fee that removed them from the control of third-party payers and enabled the patient to have the time to reexperience her behavior patterns, to resolve underlying unconscious conflicts, and to learn new behaviors in the context of a safe, reliable, ongoing therapeutic relationship.

Practice in Context

Differentiating this kind of practice from others is the relative autonomy of the social worker to set the conditions of his or her own work. Unlike social workers in other contexts, in independent practice, barring the constraints of third-party insurers or managed care reviewers, one has the freedom and autonomy to select and screen cases and structure treatment as one wishes. Therapy decisions are guided by one's training and theoretical orientation and the particular needs of the individual case. Treatment is limited by the patient's ability to use this particular kind of therapy and to pay for services. Diminished organizational and policy constraints and the resultant heightened therapist-patient control of practice decisions is highly challenging and rewarding (Matorin et al., 1987).

BIBLIOGRAPHY

Alperin, R. M. (1994). Managed care versus psychoanalytic psychotherapy: Conflicting ideologies. *Clinical Social Work Journal, 22*(2), 137-148.

American Board of Examiners in Clinical Social Work (1995). *1995 Diplomate Directory.* Wilmington, DE: American Board of Examiners in Clinical Social Work.

American Psychiatric Association (1994). *Diagnostic and statistical manual for mental disorders,* DSM IV. Washington, DC: American Psychiatric Association.

Applebaum, P. S. (1993). Legal liability and managed care. *American Psychologist, 48*(3), 251-257.

Austad, C. S. and Berman, W. H. (Eds.). (1991). Psychotherapy in managed health care. Washington, DC: American Psychological Association.

Austad, C. S. and Hoyt, M. F. (1992). The managed care movement and the future of psychotherapy. *Psychotherapy, 29,* 109-118.

Barker, R. L. (1982). *The business of psychotherapy: Private practice administration for therapists, counselors, and social workers.* New York: Columbia University Press.

Barker, R. L. (1983). Supply-side economics in private psychotherapy practice: Some ominous and encouraging trends. *Psychotherapy in Private Practice, 1*(1), 71-81.

Barker, R. L. (1984). *Social work in private practice: Principles, issues, and dilemmas.* Silver Spring, MD: National Association of Social Workers.

Barker, R. L. (1987). Private and proprietary services. In A. Minahan (Ed.), *Encyclopedia of social work,* Eighteenth Edition. Silver Spring, MD: National Association of Social Workers, pp. 324-329.

Barker, R. L. (1992). *Social work in private practice.* Washington, DC: NASW Press.

Barker, R. L. (1995). Private practice. In Edwards, R. L. (Ed.) *Encyclopedia of social work,* Nineteenth Edition. Washington, DC: NASW Press, pp. 1905-1910.

Bernstein, B. E. (1981). Malpractice: Future shock of the 1980's. *Social Casework, 62,* 175-181.

Borenzweig, H. (1981). Agency vs. private practice: Similarities and differences. *Social Work, 26*(3), 239-244.

Brown, F. (1994). Resisting the pull of the health insurance tarbaby: An organizational model for surviving managed care. *Clinical Social Work Journal, 22*(1), 59-71.

Clifford, R., and Denkers, G. (1994). *A survey of psychologists' experiences with managed care.* CA: California Psychological Association, pp. 1-10.

Cutler, J. P. (1995). *Third-party reimbursement for clinical social work services.* Washington, DC: NASW Press.

DeAngelis, D. (1993). *State comparison of laws governing social work.* Washington, DC: NASW Press.

Dorwart, R. A. (1990). Managed mental health care: Myths and realities in the 1990s. *Hospital and Community Psychiatry, 41*, 1087-1091.

Eagle, M. N. (1984). *Recent developments in psychoanalysis: A critical evaluation.* New York: McGraw-Hill.

Esposito, G. (1995). *Managed care: (Still) arranging desk chairs on the Titanic (Special Report on Health Care).* Los Angeles, CA: California Society for Clinical Social Work.

Gibelman, M. and Schervish, D. (1993). *Who we are: The social work labor force as reflected in the NASW membership.* Washington, DC: NASW Press.

Goldman, C. (1995). Ninety percent rate managed care as negative. *California Society for Clinical Social Work: Clinical Update, 26*(3), 1-6.

Goldmeier, J. (1986). Private practice and the purchase of services: Who are the practitioners? *American Journal of Orthopsychiatry, 56*, 89-102.

Gothard, S. (1995). Legal issues: Confidentiality and privileged communication. In R. L. Edwards (Ed.), *Encyclopedia of social work*, Nineteenth Edition. Washington, DC: NASW Press, pp. 1579-1584.

Graham, S. (1992-1993). Managed care: The problem and solution. *The Psychotherapy Bulletin, 27*, 16-18.

Jackson, J. A. (1987). Clinical social work and peer review: A professional leap ahead. *Social Work, 32*(3), 213-220.

Johnson, D.A. and Huff, D. (1987). Licensing exams: How valid are they? *Social Work, 32*(2), 159-161.

Kelley, P. and Alexander, P. (1985). Part-time private practice: Practical and ethical considerations. *Social Work, 30*, 254-258.

Kelton-Locke, S. (1992). The ethical practitioner in the age of managed care. *The California Therapist*, 33-36.

Kurzman, P. A. (1995). Professional liability and malpractice. In R. L. Edwards (Ed.), *Encyclopedia of Social Work*, Nineteenth Edition. Washington, DC: NASW Press, pp. 1921-1927.

Land, H. (1987). The effects of licensure on student motivation and career choice. *Social Work, 32*(1), 75-77.

Lechnyr, R. (1984). Clinical social work psychotherapy and insurance coverage: Information on billing procedures. *Clinical Social Work Journal, 12*, 69-77.

Levin, A. M. (1984). *The private practice of psychotherapy.* NY: Free Press.

Matorin, S., Rosenberg, B., Levitt, M., and Rosenblum, S. (1987). Private practice in social work: Readiness and opportunity. *Social Casework, 68*(1), 31-37.

National Association of Social Workers. (1985). State comparisons of laws regulating social work. Silver Spring, MD: NASW Press.

Phillips, D. (1995). Professional standards and managed care. *N.F.S. Clinical Social Work: Progress Report, 13*(1).

Reamer, F. G. (1983). Ethical dilemmas in social work practice. *Social Work, 28*(1), 31-35.

Reamer, F. G. (1987). Ethics committees in social work. *Social Work, 32*(3) 188-192.

Reamer, F. G. (1994). *Social work malpractice and liability: Strategies for prevention.* New York: Columbia University Press.

Riemersma, M. and Leslie, R. (1992, November/December). Managed care in the 90s: A continuing education. *The California Therapist,* 9-15.

Rosen, A., Proctor, E. K., and Livne, S. (1985). Planning and direct practice. *Social Service Review, 59*(2), 166-177.

Scarf, M. (1996, June 16). Keeping secrets. *The New York Times Magazine,* 38-40.

Sharfstein, S.S., Maszynski, S., and Meyers, E. (1984). *Health insurance and psychiatric care: Update and appraisal.* Washington, DC: American Psychiatric Press.

Social workers vault into leading roles in psychotherapy. (1985, April 30). *The New York Times.*

Stern, S. (1993). Managed care, brief therapy and therapeutic integrity. *Psychotherapy, 30*(1), 162-175.

Strean, H. S. (1979). *Psychoanalytic theory and social work practice.* New York: The Free Press.

Tischler, G. L. (1990). Utilization management of mental health services by private third parties. *American Journal of Psychiatry, 147,* 967-973.

Wallace, M. E. (1982). Private practice: A nationwide study. *Social Work, 27,* 262-267.

Weil, M. and Sanchez, E. (1983). Impact of the Tarasoff decision on clinical social work practice. *Social Service Review, 57,* 112-124.

PART V:
CARE FOR THE FRAIL ELDERLY
AND HOSPICE CARE

Chapter 29

Hospital-Based Case Management for the Frail Elderly

Renee Weisman Michelsen
Toba Schwaber Kerson

CONTEXT

Description of the Setting

Morristown Memorial Hospital is a voluntary, nonprofit teaching hospital in Morristown, New Jersey. It consists of two divisions: a 558-bed acute care hospital and a 78-bed facility specializing in rehabilitation, subacute care, and short-term skilled nursing. The acute care facility serves as a level II trauma center and a medical/surgical regional referral center. Morristown Memorial Hospital is located in middle to upper-middle-class suburban Morris County; however, the patients served represent a variety of income levels.

The Elder Care Resource Center (the Center) is an independent department within the hospital; that is, it is not part of Social Work Services or Discharge Planning departments. The services provided span the senior population from the well and independent individual to the frail homebound senior. Services consist of (1) a senior membership program that provides wellness education, health screenings, and social events; (2) a hotline to provide information and referral for community members with concerns related to aging; (3) a corporate elder care resource and referral service for employees of member corporations; and (4) case management for the frail elderly. This article will focus on the case management service, defined here as assessment, care planning, service coordination, monitoring community services, and reassessment. The client may receive the service for as long as he or she requires it in order to remain in the community. The mission of the case management services is to improve access to community services for the frail elderly and their families through coordination of existing services via linkages with public and private agencies and informal service providers. Primary goals of the service are to identify service needs and gaps in the community and to work through coalition building to address these needs and develop new services. The overall goal is to promote community living and avoid premature or inappropriate admission to nursing homes.

Policy

The significant increase of Americans over age 65 and the development of health care policy are directly linked (Norris and Lampe, 1994). The 1990 U.S. census data reveal that nationwide, this segment of the population grew by 22 percent between 1980 and 1990 (Tudor and Carley, 1995). By the year 2000, it is estimated that those over 65 years of age will represent 13 percent of the nation's population (United States Public Health Service, 1992). The 1980 census recorded 51,900 residents of Morris County, New Jersey who were over 60 years of age, and the 1990 census recorded 63,000. This represents a 21.8 percent growth rate in the over-60 population. Elderly residents comprise 15 percent of the total county population. This demographic pattern results in greater demand for health care services and challenges the health care reimbursement system.

The policy issues affecting the Center and its clients have been closely linked with health care reimbursement since its inception. The Center was founded in 1984 during a time when the Medicare Prospective Payment System was changing the way that hospitals were reimbursed for the care of elderly patients. In 1984, the majority of states were phased into the federal DRG system. New Jersey, however, was one of the minority states that continued to operate under a model DRG waiver program that began in 1980. The DRG system mandated that hospitals be reimbursed based on the patient's diagnosis not the hospital's expenses. Historically, hospitals were reimbursed by Medicare and other insurers on a cost-plus basis. The DRG system challenged this method of payment and initiated a system in which the goal was to contain costs by reducing the patient's length of stay, thereby eliminating what was known as the "social admission." Social admissions consisted of those in which the patient was not acutely ill but was admitted to the hospital because other alternatives were unacceptable to the admitting physician. Such patients often lingered in the hospital at the expense of Medicare or another medical expense reimbursement system.

In the current health care arena, managed care contracts increasingly determine the levels of reimbursement that health care providers receive. The rising costs of health care, the growth in the elderly population, and the increasing utilization of hospital services by the elderly impose a heavy burden on the Medicare system. Managed Medicare is one current attempt to control these costs. Although the percentage of Americans in managed Medicare programs is only 2.4 million or 6.7 percent of the Medicare population (Findlay, 1995), the current trends in healthcare reform suggest that managed Medicare will continue to increase (Cafferky, 1995).

All of the incentives to reduce the length of stay in hospitals and avoid unnecessary admissions mean that frequently patients are more acutely ill when they are in the hospital and have greater needs when discharged (Simmons, 1994). Thus, community-based services that emphasize prevention and help to maintain the health and well-being of the frail population are increasingly important. In 1995, Medicare patients consumed 43 percent of acute care patient days at Morristown Memorial Hospital and 76 percent of days on the inpatient skilled nursing and rehabilitation units. Medicare patients represented 29.4 percent of total admissions. It is evident that the Medicare patients have longer lengths of stay than patients with other forms of insurance.

Morristown Memorial Hospital has provided community-based services for the frail elderly for more than a decade. The Elder Care Resource Center was founded in 1984, beginning with a grant from the Robert Wood Johnson Foundation. The purpose of the initial grant was to encourage hospitals to shift from their traditional acute care focus toward establishing a continuum of care that meets the chronic and long-term care needs of the elderly and that includes community-based services (Simmons, 1994). The Center has become a valuable resource to the hospital in the management of the chronically ill elderly patient partly because managed care systems emphasize community-based care. Hospitals are being challenged to become more involved in care beyond the walls of the institution.

The United States has not adopted a national long-term care policy. Long-term care refers to the combination of health and social services that are provided in a variety of institutional and noninstitutional settings, including the home, and are provided over an extended period of time to functionally impaired, chronically ill persons (Pollack, 1979). Medicare was designed to cover acute and not chronic custodial or long-term care. What long-term benefits and services exist vary from state to state and community to community.

Medicare HMOs do not address long-term care needs any more comprehensively than traditional Medicare, which provides indemnity, fee-for-service coverage, but these HMOs can be somewhat more flexible. Both reimburse for limited home care (nurse, home health aide, physical therapy, occupational therapy, speech therapy, dietitian, and social worker). Four conditions must be met to qualify for home care benefits under traditional Medicare: (1) the patient must need skilled nursing care or physical therapy, (2) the patient must be homebound, (3) a physician must order the service, and (4) the agency that provides the service must be a Medicare participating agency (Friedman, 1986). Under varying managed care plans, these conditions may be less firmly defined (Oliver, 1995), though payers recognize that home care is a less expensive alternative than inpatient care.

In many cases, neither the elderly nor their families understand traditional Medicare and HMO coverage regarding chronic illness. Many chronically ill people cannot perform the essential activities of daily living, such as bathing and dressing, but these functional difficulties do not qualify them for skilled nursing care because of the chronic nature of their problem. Medicare is designed to address acute illness and short-term rehabilitation. Home care agencies can only provide care for patients if their insurance or managed care plans approve the services or if the patient pays privately (Katz, 1983). Except for the rare patient who has purchased a private long-term care insurance policy, the client who needs financial assistance to pay for care will be at the mercy of a fragmented system of financially assisted services such as Medicaid, Medicaid waivers, state respite, and county programs.

Most of the clients of the Center are middle-income. These people do not meet the financial eligibility requirements of the Medicaid home care programs, yet many do not have the funds to pay for services over an extended period of time, as is often necessary with chronic illness. This group is in the precarious position of paying for long-term home care or institutional care until they impoverish themselves and must be supported by Medicaid for the first time in their lives. The frail elderly are being squeezed by a system in which acute inpatient days and public funding for community-based services are decreasing, and the private cost of in-home services is increasing. These circumstances challenge social work to reform policy as well as practice.

Technology

The elderly population in the United States is one of the largest consumers of health care services because more people are living longer with a variety of chronic illnesses. Forty percent of the elderly population suffer from some form of chronic illness, and this percentage increases with age. Although people are living longer, they often are faced with debilitation and dependency resulting from chronic disease.

Chronic illness often involves complicated "high tech" regimens and surgical and diagnostic procedures. These include nuclear medicine, dialysis and transplantation, joint replacements, bypass surgery, parenteral and enteral nutrition, chemotherapy, and respiratory therapy. Chronic illness can result in functional impairments in activities of daily living (ADLs) and instrumental activities of daily living (IADLs). ADLs include bathing, dressing, toileting and continence, transferring, eating, and walking. IADLs include shopping, meal preparation, housekeeping, laundry, medications, financial management, use of the telephone, and mobility outside the household. Technological advances in assistive devices such as bathroom equipment, incontinence products, stair gliders, ostomy products, and prostheses help the client cope with living with the disease.

The procedures, regimens and devices associated with chronic illness represent a level of technology unfamiliar to many clients and family members (Kerson and Kerson, 1985). Lechich (1984) points out that technology in home health care offers the client greater independence in the face of restrictive regimens, but each technology requires understanding to resolve the problems that the technology itself creates. Much case management intervention is focused on helping the client and family to cope with these aspects of life, as well as the fact that although the client undergoes many procedures and regimens, there is no cure for his or her ailment (Rothman, 1994).

Other aspects of technology that increase the efficiency of the Center and help the case manager, supervisor, and any covering workers include the use of a computerized database program to track clients and service utilization. These databases are useful for grant applications, creating reports requiring aggregate data on the clientele, and examining patterns of service utilization by diagnosis, age, and other client characteristics.

Organization

The Elder Care Resource Center is a hospital department composed of a director (MSW), a social worker (MSW), a case manager (BSW), a part-time secretary, and a variety of social work students. The composition of the staff and services provided have changed over time, reflecting the funding sources of the programs. Currently, the case management service is partially funded (60 percent) by a county grant. The remainder is funded by the hospital, contracts, and fee-for-service work done by the department staff.

Case management assumes responsibility for planning and oversight after the discharge planner has completed his or her work. The discharge planner, nurse, or physician identifies the frail patient who is likely to require multiple community services after discharge. Plans for services needed immediately after the patient leaves the hospital are made by the inpatient social worker who is increasingly challenged as many social work departments are recast and reduced in size. This, combined with the acuity level of the patients and the brevity of their stay, makes it harder for the inpatient worker to develop complex discharge plans. Collaborating with the inpatient social worker, the case manager ensures continuity of care by implementing the plan after the patient returns home and by monitoring progress.

Having a hospital-based case management program is beneficial to the organization in a variety of ways. A goal of case management is to reduce fragmentation. Case management helps to facilitate the discharge of elderly patients, which is critical in a managed care environment. When a case management client is readmitted, valuable data on prior functioning, service utilization, home environment, and emotional supports is readily available to facilitate discharge and provide appropriate patient care. Case management also relieves the patient of having to repeat information about him- or herself with each admission, provides necessary and plan information to the social worker, and prevents inappropriate readmissions through close monitoring of patient and situation.

In an effort to be valuable to all disciplines in the hospital system, referrals for case management can be made by acute care social workers, nurses, physicians, clergy, and other hospital staff. Family members, friends, and clients themselves can also request the service. Frail elderly individuals, not hospitalized but residing in Morris County, may also be referred for case management services. The grant received by the Center does not permit funds to be used to purchase home care services for clients. The goal is to coordinate and maximize existing resources, as well as to promote the development of new resources.

The Elder Care Resource Center is part of the community service delivery system. Over the last five years, a countywide case management system for the frail elderly has been established. The Center was the lead agency in developing the system along with the local area agency on aging (Tudor, 1995). The procedures, forms, and methods developed under the Robert Wood Johnson grant were the foundation for the present unique countywide New Jersey system.

PRACTICE DECISIONS

Description of the Client

Mrs. O'Malley is representative of an increasing population of elders over age 85 who reside alone and have minimal family support. According to 1990 census data, more than 1 million or 47.1 percent of persons over age 85 live alone (Burnette and Mui, 1994). Of the 63,000 people over age 50 in Morris County, 5 percent are women age 85 and over. Clients such as Mrs. O'Malley require long-term case management in order to be maintained in the community (Hammond, 1995).

Mrs. O'Malley, 85 years old and of Irish descent, was born in the United States. She has lived in a high-rise apartment in subsidized senior housing for 17 years. Her husband died 11 years ago, and she has lived alone since that time. She has no children and her only relative in the area is an elderly niece who has plans to move and is minimally involved. Mrs. O'Malley, as one of the building's first tenants, knows many people in her building and was previously socially active. In the last three years, as a result of many of her friends dying and her health declining, she has become more isolated (Kerson, 1989).

Mrs. O'Malley was referred to the Center by the social worker on the inpatient unit, who is responsible for discharge planning. She was admitted to the hospital with failure to thrive, congestive heart failure, and open leg ulcers due to edema. She also suffers from many chronic conditions such as diabetes, effects of polio, abdominal hernia, severe hearing loss, and arthritis. The client's physician was experiencing pressure to discharge her because her acute problem had been resolved. She spent three weeks in acute care and two weeks in subacute care, an unusually long length of stay, but the chronic nature of her disabilities made discharge complicated. She was weakened from her acute illness and prior to admission had been only marginally safe, with home-delivered meals and a home health aide four hours every day.

The referral to the Center for case management facilitated the patient's discharge. As Brody and Magel (1984) state, "Case management differs from discharge planning in that it assumes responsibility for mobilizing medical, social and health services to assure continuity of care as the patient returns to the community" (p. 677). The discharge planner confronted several obstacles to setting up the initial home care services. Agencies that had previously helped Mrs. O'Malley felt they could not serve her adequately because she had been a difficult client, other agencies felt the situation was too risky, and still others knew that she was hesitant to pay and did not have a guaranteed payer, such as a relative

(Rowland and Lyons, 1991). After great effort, the discharge planner was able to arrange the initial plan of services. The case manager visited the client in the hospital prior to discharge to introduce herself. The hospital staff was relieved and reassured by the fact that the Center would provide ongoing monitoring of this frail client.

Definition of the Client

The Center serves the frail elderly and their families. The criteria for eligibility for the case management service are that (1) the potential client must reside in our service area, (2) be 60 years of age or older, (3) and at risk of institutionalization. Often, the Center is contacted when the elderly person and/or his or her family is at the point of deciding if the person can remain at home alone, or if he or she should arrange for the client to go to a nursing home or move in with relatives. Such decisions are made even more complicated if the person has several chronic illnesses and disabilities as well as social and economic problems.

Goals, Objectives, and/or Outcome Measures

The client determines the development of case management goals and objectives. Mrs. O'Malley wanted to live independently and regain control over her environment. The goals of the case manager were to promote the client's independence and functional ability, prevent unnecessary readmission to the hospital and institutionalization, and, generally, to enhance the client's quality of life. Rashko (1985) cites these goals as fundamental components of case management with the frail elderly.

Many short-term objectives were identified during the course of intervention. In the beginning, a primary objective was to enable the client to accept help, especially from home health aides. In Morris County, there is not a distinction between homemaker and home health aide services. In the middle phase of work, a significant objective was to have the client become independent in personal care and in taking her medications. Now, objectives focus on helping the client to seek appropriate help prior to crisis and to maintain independence.

Use of Contract

Initially, establishing a contract with Mrs. O'Malley was difficult. When she went home from the hospital, being overwhelmed and frightened, she was anxious and suspicious of service providers. Although an initial relationship had been established between the client and the case manager, the client approached the alliance with hesitancy. After numerous episodes of the client "testing" the worker (for example not opening the door and being extremely uncooperative), Mrs. O'Malley began to realize the worker was going to be consistent, and a relationship evolved in which contracting was possible. Rashko (1985) discusses the need for case managers to be highly skilled in establishing positive relationships with the elderly to overcome initial resistance and fear. This relationship is the conduit for implementing a continuum of services. Mrs. O'Malley's situation verifies this concept.

The worker developed a care plan based on her assessment (see the section on treatment modalities for a detailed description of the assessment process). The client and worker established mutual goals, and the client initialed the care plan, which indicated that she was in agreement with the goals. To accomplish these mutual goals, verbal "subcontracts" were negotiated. The subcontracts were concrete in nature; for example, the case manager agreed to locate the home health aide and change the aide if the client wished, but the client had to inform the case manager of problems. Another subcontract involved transportation; the case manager helped the client arrange physician appointments and transportation, and the client had to be ready on time. This type of contracting gave the client structure, and helped her regain control over her environment.

Meeting Place

All sessions with Mrs. O'Malley were held in her apartment. This is necessary with most clients due to frailty and disability. Conducting sessions in the client's home has many advantages. The worker is able to fine-tune the service plan from observing the ways in which the client interacts and manages his or her environment. Environmental barriers may prevent the older person from functioning optimally in the home. In assessing an environment for an impaired elder, variables such as the ability to move safely around the home, get into and out of the bathtub, keep the house clean, prepare food, go up and down stairs, use the toilet, and operate needed appliances must be examined (Cannava, 1994). Relating to the client in his or her own environment is a luxury the hospital discharge planner does not have. In the home, the client feels more comfortable and much more in control (Rubinstein, Kilbride, and Nagy, 1992).

Use of Time

Initially, multiple home visits were made each week to assist the client through the crisis of returning home and accepting in-home services. A substantial amount of time was also spent with collateral contacts, such as home care providers, transportation services, physician, and housing manager, regarding the client. By the third month of contact, weekly visits were sufficient, although stressful events required additional interventions. In recent months, Mrs. O'Malley has required only monthly visits. The average length of time for each visit is one hour.

Primarily, progress is due to two factors: the client's improved health and the well-established relationship between the client and the worker. As Goldmeier (1985) describes, the work is " . . . time-limited in that it is focused on the problems of the moment and ongoing in terms of readiness to deal with the continuing problems of aging that do not end with one episode of case activity successful though it may be" (p. 323). The case manager became the client's anchor and the mortar that held the conglomeration of services together. In time, the client learned when to call the case manager, and the case manager became more familiar with the client's limitations and the specific areas in which she needed ongoing assistance.

Interventions

Case management is frequently used as an approach to caring for the multiple needs of the disabled (Rubin and Johnson, 1982), whether they are frail elders, the chronically mentally ill, or another population with multiple, ongoing needs. Exactly what comprises case management varies based on the needs of the population and the definition of the setting. Many agencies offer case management in that they coordinate the particular services they offer within their own setting. The Center's approach is a broader model of case management, which coordinates the formal services of multiple agencies as well as the informal services of family, friends, and volunteers.

Assessment

Case management involves assessment, care planning, arranging services, monitoring, and reassessment. On first visiting the client at home, the case manager assessed Mrs. O'Malley's biopsychosocial situation. The components of the comprehensive assessment are mental status testing, using the Short Portable Mental Status Questionnaire (SPMSQ) and the Geriatric Depression Scale (Gallo, Reichel, and Andersen, 1988); functional assessment (ADLs and IADLs); financial status and eligibility assessment for various entitlements; physical environment assessment; an analysis of social/support network; and a brief review of life history. Many workers, in an effort to assist the client efficiently and expeditiously, omit the review of the client's life history. It is through this reminiscence process that the case manager gets to know who the client was and gains insight into who the client is now. It is too easy to think of a client simply as a "fractured hip" or a "diabetic" and not see the total person in his or her situation (Beaver, 1991; Coleman, 1986; Kaminsky, 1984).

Mrs. O'Malley was much more alert and functional than she appeared to be in the hospital, as evidenced by her SPMSQ score of seven out of ten items correct (more than three errors indicate significant impairment). This screening tool is used because it is compact, easy to administer, and requires no special materials. It is a preliminary test, and if the client scores poorly, further cognitive testing is done, such as the Folstein Mini-Mental State Examination (Gallo, Reichel, and Andersen; 1988).

The client's ADLs are measured using the Katz Index of ADL (Katz et al., 1963). This screening tool helps to detect elders who are experiencing problems with the activities required for independence (Gallo, Reichel, and Andersen, 1988). Using the Katz Index, the case manager determines if the client is independent, needs assistance, or is dependent in the six essential ADLs (bathing, dressing, toileting, transferring, continence, and feeding). A similar scale is used to assess the client's level of independence in IADLs–shopping, meal preparation, housekeeping, medication, money management, use of the telephone, and mobility outside the home. Most often, a person's eligibility for assistance and severity of disability are described in terms of the number of his or her ADL and IADL limitations (Miller, 1995).

The analysis of Mrs. O'Malley's level of independence in ADLs and IADLs was critical in pinpointing the specific areas in which she was having problems and in targeting possible areas of intervention, such as obtaining a raised toilet seat or a large button phone (Fillit and Capello, 1994). Examination of the structural barriers to her receipt of care, such as not knowing how to access help, low income, and being unable to hear her doorbell, along with her beliefs about using help, were part of the initial assessment (Wallace, Campbell, and Lew-Ting, 1994). The initial assessment revealed that, with bathroom modifications, the client was independent in feeding, toileting, and transferring (that is, moving in and out of a bed or chair). She required assistance with dressing on occasion and was dependent in bathing. Her IADL abilities were much more severely impaired; she was dependent in shopping, meal preparation, housekeeping, financial management, and mobility outside the home, and she required some assistance in taking medications. With modified equipment, she was independent in using the telephone. The overall level of dependency in ADLs and IADLs, considering that Mrs. O'Malley had no nearby relatives or significant others assisting her, put her at a high risk for nursing home placement.

This level of dependency, especially not being able to cook her own meals, distressed Mrs. O'Malley considerably. She had been a private housekeeper and cook in her younger years, and she had enjoyed cooking for her husband and entertaining. She viewed food as an expression of herself and was saddened that her kitchen was no longer manageable. She was denied what had been a source of pleasure and identity (Modica, 1995). It was not her diseases that she identified as stresses, but her functional impairments resulting from the diseases, which resulted in reduced independence and social isolation (Backer, 1995).

Care Plan

The next phase of the process was care planning. The case manager worked with Mrs. O'Malley to develop a complex initial care plan involving formal and informal services to meet her diverse needs and that she would accept. The planning process emphasized the client's range of options and individual needs. As always, the care plan was a mutually agreed upon, written, concrete contract between the case manager and the client. After the care plan was negotiated, the case manager arranged services and provided ongoing monitoring via phone and visit contact with the client and phone contact with the service providers.

Many talents and skills are needed to put case management into action; it is not a simple mechanistic approach. An eclectic approach was taken with Mrs. O'Malley. She benefited greatly from behavioral techniques surrounding issues such as taking medication, meal preparation, and finances. Behavioral techniques helped her become incrementally more independent. Ongoing supportive counseling was needed to help Mrs. O'Malley work through her losses and regain control of her environment. When Mrs. O'Malley would begin to feel a loss of control over her environment, she would begin to show signs of depression, consistent with the Geriatric Depression Inventory (Gallo, Reichel, and Andersen, 1988). Many psychosocial factors contributed to Mrs. O'Malley's despair, including social isolation, chronic illness with functional impairment, and low-income status. This is consistent with the findings of Burnette and Mui (1994), who state that a sense of control in life was the most significant predictor of the client's depression.

Mrs. O'Malley also suffered from intermittent anxiety related to her situation. It was usually expressed in the form of increased calls to the case manager, during which the client would have a perceived increase in her hearing deficit and would moan and not be able to say why she had called. Often, the reassurance of the social connection to the case manager was enough to alleviate the anxiety. Burnette and Mui (1994) found that elders residing alone were more likely to experience symptoms of both depression and anxiety. The case manager was skilled in identifying and intervening with both depression and anxiety.

Reminiscence Therapy

Reminiscence therapy (Parker; 1995; Wallace, Campbell and Lew-Ting, 1992) helped Mrs. O'Malley adapt and alleviated situational depression. She seemed to be more satisfied as her self-concept strengthened and cognitive functioning improved. Reminiscence therapy also helped the case manager and client join in the therapeutic relationship. Such work can help in many ways, including coping; increasing relational intimacy; reducing interpersonal uncertainty; developing or reestablishing friendships; and more globally, exploring one's identity (Parker, 1995). Mrs. O'Malley had wonderful personal stories to tell, which fascinated the worker. The client developed a psychohistorical perspective integrating the past, present, and future (Kishton, 1994).

This reflective process provided important information on the client's past coping strengths and life experiences that had contributed to her personality, as well as her reaction to her current life situation. The worker was able to engage the client and help her deal with "unfinished business" using this technique. Having someone to listen to her stories made Mrs. O'Malley feel her life had been valuable and she had someone to whom she could pass along her wisdom.

Reminiscence therapy also added a dimension of trust to the relationship (Erikson, Erikson, and Kivnick, 1986). As Mrs. O'Malley's trust grew, she began to reveal more of herself in the relationship, and the case manager was able to switch from a problem-focused orientation to a "strengths perspective" (Perkins and Tice, 1995). The strengths of the client were employed to help her become more of a full partner in her care. The client's self-direction and determination to remain at home guided all of the interventions. Making her own personal choices about her daily life demonstrated her personal freedom, although it often angered service providers who felt that she needed to always have something with which she disagreed. The small-scale decision making was integral to the retention of her autonomy (Rubinstein, Kilbride, and Nagy, 1992).

Stance of the Social Worker

The case of Mrs. O'Malley is typical in that the worker assumes three roles: coordinator, advocate, and counselor. The roles are not mutually exclusive and the worker often finds herself performing them at the same time. In this case, balancing the three roles was often challenging.

The service coordinator role requires one to take a very active stance. The worker is responsible for setting up and maintaining all of the needed services. When Mrs. O'Malley experienced problems such as the home health aide being late, the home-delivered meals not arriving, or the walker needing to be replaced, the case manager investigated the circumstances and was responsible for resolving the problems.

In the role of coordinator, the case manager found that she needed to provide support for the cadre of aides serving the client. Frequent mediation sessions between the aide and the client were needed. Mrs. O'Malley would frequently complain that the aide did not do enough and the aide felt the client was too demanding.

The role of advocate is intertwined with that of coordinator, and is also one in which the worker needs to be direct. The case manager constantly argued for particular services in particular amounts at specific times. Often, there are many people competing for the same service, and it is up to the worker to present the client's care convincingly. Mrs. O'Malley also needed an advocate to speak to her physician regarding physical therapy, simplifying her medication regime, and other aspects of her care. The partnership between the primary care physician and the social worker are crucial (Dorfman et al., 1995).

In the role of counselor, the stance varied from directive behavioral therapy to therapeutic listening. Time and patience were essential to making counseling effective. At different points and in different roles, the case manager took a variety of stances ranging from very active to contemplative. The roles of coordinator and advocate require political savvy; the case manager is continually balancing her relationships with the client and the service providers, keeping together the client's vital support system.

Concrete Services

Services such as home health aide, visiting nurse, home-delivered meals, senior transportation, and chore service have made it possible for Mrs. O'Malley to remain in her apartment. An ". . . important aspect of the home for frail elders is the basic ability to command a territory" (Rubinstein, Kilbride, and Nagy, 1992, p. 82). The privacy of her home and the memories were very important to Mrs. O'Malley. During home visits, she would show the case manager different items of sentimental value or discuss how the table they were sitting at once was the center of special meals and parties. Her home helped preserve her identity (Rubinstein, Kilbride, and Nagy, 1992). "In-home and community based services enable the senior to age in place in familiar surroundings with optimal independence and dignity" (New Jersey Association of Area Agencies on Aging, 1995, p. 6).

Visiting Nurse and Home-Health Aide

Through contracting, the case manager and client agreed on the aide's schedule, which would be reviewed every other week. Over time, the client's service utilization patterns varied. When Mrs. O'Malley was discharged from the hospital, Medicare provided a visiting nurse and a home health aide for two weeks. The nurse monitored the client's physical status and instructed her on the new array of medications. Because Mrs. O'Malley qualified for this skilled level of care she was also entitled to a home health aide for two hours, three times a week. The client needed four hours daily of the aide service and paid privately for the additional hours.

After service under Medicare terminated, Mrs. O'Malley continued to need a home health aide to assist her with bathing, dressing, shopping, housekeeping, and meal preparation. It was difficult to persuade the client to pay for these services because she feared spending all her money. The relationship between the aide and the client became very important to the client. It was often her primary source of socialization and helped her readjust to being at home.

As Mrs. O'Malley's condition improved, the case manager decreased the frequency of her home health aide service. She continued to require chore services, transportation, and home-delivered meals. The Center provided a dedicated volunteer to assist her with tasks such as shopping and with companionship.

Reassessment

Reassessment is continual. A formal written reassessment reviewing functional ability, mental status, and utilization of services is conducted every six months and results in a renegotiated care plan. At the time of the six month reassessment, Mrs. O'Malley was eating, walking outside with a cane, bathing herself, and socializing more as her health improved. She scored 100 percent correct on the SPMSQ. Her neighbors and friends were no longer overwhelmed by her needs and spent more time with her.

The one-year reassessment verified ongoing progress. Mrs. O'Malley had become independent in taking her medication. She no longer needed a home health aide. Mrs. O'Malley was able to venture out to visit a friend in the neighboring building. She showed the ability to sustain the gains she had made over time. Mrs. O'Malley used more services to meet her IADL needs than ADLs (Mui and Burnette, 1994). Although she needed assistance with both ADLs and IADLs, as her situation stabilized, the need for ADL care diminished while IADL remained consistent as a function of not having a relative or spouse on whom to rely.

At the two-year marker, Mrs. O'Malley is reading the newspaper daily to keep up with current events. She requires less help with financial management. At times, she does her grocery shopping and goes to doctors' appointments by utilizing senior transportation. She has made significant progress and continues to demonstrate that returning to her apartment was the correct decision.

The collaborative efforts of the case manager and the client, the review and maximization of the client's strengths, and the worker serving as an advocate were the factors that contributed to the improvement in the client's quality of life. "The practitioner's knowledge of client strengths becomes invaluable in helping to construct the possibility of change, transformation, and hope" (Perkins and Tice, 1995, p. 87).

Transfer or Termination

Termination occurs when the client reaches the goal of functional independence. At this point, the client is able to sustain herself utilizing formal and informal networks without ongoing assistance. Termination also occurs if the client is placed in a nursing home or other facility. Mrs. O'Malley continues to require active assistance and support and therefore remains an open case.

Case Conclusion

Mrs. O'Malley is a success. The primary goal of restoring independent living through improving functional ability was achieved. Mrs. O'Malley's strong will to remain in the community motivated her to join in a partnership with the case manager. The client responded positively to the variety of approaches the worker implemented. The case manager helped her establish an environment that she could master, which in turn helped her to deal effectively with her feelings about aging and illness. Mrs. O'Malley's resilience, the case manager's efforts, as well as the formal and informal supports came together to make a fragile situation work.

Differential Discussion

Mrs. O'Malley needed an intense form of case management. Without the case management service, the conclusion to the case is likely to have been quite different. Mrs. O'Malley might have been placed in a nursing home. She also might have had numerous emergency room visits and potential inappropriate admissions to the hospital. The relationship with the case manager proved to be the conduit to the client's acceptance of help. In conjunction with professional training and experience, the case manager was courteous, compassionate, and innovative.

This is a classic case of an elderly person whose family is unable to provide day-to-day assistance. If the client had a primary caregiver, the social worker's approach would have varied. It has been the Center's experience that with ongoing support and guidance the caregiver can assume many of the tasks the social worker took on in the case of Mrs. O'Malley. In cases where there is a primary caregiver, case management service tends to be of a shorter duration. As the American population continues to age, society will be increasingly challenged to provide care. Although an array of public services turn caregiving into waged work (Leira, 1994), the majority of caregiving is provided by families and informal sources (Miller, 1995; Cohen and Eisdorfer, 1993).

The community in which the client lives shaped the outcome of the case. Morros County is a service-rich community, and Mrs. O'Malley's ability to pay for home care facilitated receipt of the service. Other help, such as chore service for which she waited a considerable period of time, also proved invaluable. The case manager can only manage the services that exist in the community and continually advocates for those in short supply.

Throughout the case, the flexibility the Center allotted the worker allowed her to be creative and perform many untraditional tasks. It has often been said around the office that case management is doing what no one else does. Case management cannot be accomplished in the confines of the weekly 50-minute hour.

Practice in Context

Over a decade ago, the Center adopted the mission of promoting a countywide case management system without the funds to purchase services for clients. Many community agencies were skeptical about the value of such a program. There were turf battles on many fronts. The inpatient social workers felt an encroachment on their territory, and the community agencies felt the hospital was trying to take over. The Center overcame these obstacles and accomplished its mission by becoming a resource to the key actors: clients, families, service providers, and the hospital. The Center added a dimension that had not previously existed and that facilitated continuity of care. It is now one of the lead agencies in the countywide case management system.

Currently, the Center operates within a grant that mandates that case management be done in the manner described throughout the chapter. The service is valuable to the hospital in accordance with managed care and the focus on shorter lengths of stay, prevention, and the need for a continuum of care to avoid inappropriate admissions.

Future funding will play a major role in defining the service and the number of clients served. County grants are directly affected by federal allocations of the Older Americans Act, which is frequently challenged. The hospital's mission and managed Medicare will also influence the Center's future. The Center helps the hospital achieve its goal of partnering with the community to improve overall health status. Care provided outside the walls of the institution will be increased, strengthening ties to the community, including seniors (Lumsdon, 1993). The hospital will continue to face increased competition, shorter lengths of stay, and an increase in patient acuity. As long as the Center is compatible with the political and reimbursement climate and remains a resource to the institution, the support for its services is likely to continue.

In some form or another, case management services will continue to be an essential component of the long-term care system, especially as the elderly population increases. This opens up a vast arena of opportunity for the profession of social work. The skills of psychosocial assessment, counseling, and community organization, combined with an unmatched ability to understand and negotiate the service delivery system, are unique. Historically, social workers have downplayed the concrete service element of practice, but it is this expertise that makes social workers unquestionably valued in the long-term care system. Social workers also have an opportunity to impact on the development of national health care and long-term care policies.

Hospital-based case management programs linking acute and non-acute care are likely to become more prolific. In 1984, Brody and Magel wrote, ". . . development and utilization of a short-term/long-term care system is more than a marketing idea, it is a strategy for hospital survival" (p. 678). In 1995, this is an even more poignant statement. A flexible case management program that provides the care coordination needed for older people with chronic health problems and that ensures continuity and appropriate provision of resources along the continuum of care will remain invaluable. "Social work leadership in the design and delivery of health care coordinated services is crucial to the future role of social work in health care" (Simmons, 1994).

REFERENCES

Backer, J. (1995). Perceived stressors of financially secure, community residing older women. *Geriatric Nursing, 16*, 155-159.

Beaver, M. L. (1991). Life review/reminiscent therapy. In P. K. H. Kim (Ed.), *Serving the elderly: Skills for practice*. New York: Aldine de Gruyter, pp. 67-88.

Brody, S. J. and Magel, J. S. (1984). DRG: The second revolution in health care for the elderly. *Journal of the American Geriatrics Society, 32*, 676-679.

Burnette, D. and Mui, A. C. (1994). Determinants of self-reported depressive symptoms by frail elderly persons living alone. *Journal of Gerontological Social Work, 22*, 3-18.

Cafferky, M. E. (1995). *Managed care and you: The consumer guide to managing your health*. New York: McGraw-Hill, Inc.

Cannava, E. (1994). "Gerodesign": Safe and comfortable living spaces for older adults. *Geriatrics, 49*, 45-49.

Cohen, D. and Eisdorfer, C. (1993). *Caring for your aging parents*. New York: G. P. Putnam and Sons.

Coleman, P. G. (1986). *Aging and reminiscence processes: Social and clinical implications*. New York: John Wiley & Sons.

Dorfman, R. A., Lubben, J. E., Mayer-Oakes, A., Atchison, K., Schweitzer, S. O., De Jong, F. J., and Matthias, R. E. (1995). Screening for depression among a well elderly population. *Social Work, 40*, 295-303.

Erickson, E. H., Erikson, J. M., and Kivnick, H. Q. (1986). *Vital involvement in old age*. New York: W. W. Norton.

Fillit, H. and Capello, C. (1994). Making geriatric assessment an asset to your primary care practice. *Geriatrics, 49*, 27-31.

Findlay, S. (1995). California: Edgy at the cutting edge. *Business and Health, 13*, 36-44.

Friedman, J. (1986). *Home Health Care*. New York: W. W. Norton.

Gallo, J. J., Reichel, W., and Andersen, B. (1988). *Handbook of Geriatric Assessment*. Rockville, MD: Aspen Publishers.

Goldmeier, J. (1985). Helping the elderly in times of stress. *Social Casework, 66*, 323-332.

Hammond, J. M. (1995). Multiple jeopardy or multiple resources? The intersection of age, race, living arrangements, and educational level and the health of older women. *Journal of Women and Aging, 7*(3), 5-24.

Kaminsky, M. (Ed.). (1984). *The uses of reminiscence: New ways of working with older adults*. Binghamton, NY: The Haworth Press, Inc.

Katz, S. (1983). Assessing self maintenance: ADLs. *American Geriatrics Society, 31*, 721-727.

Katz, S., Ford, A. B., Moskowitz, R. W., Jackson, B. A., and Jaffee, M. W. (1963). Studies of illness in the aged: The index of ADL. *Journal of the American Medical Association, 185*, 914-919.

Kerson, T. S. (1989). Women and aging: A clinical social work perspective. In J. D. Garner and S. O. Mercer (Eds.), *Women as they age: Challenge, opportunity and triumph*. Binghamton, NY: The Haworth Press, Inc, pp. 123-147.

Kerson, T. S. and Kerson, L. A. (1985). *Understanding chronic illness*. New York: The Free Press.

Kishton, J. M. (1994). Contemporary Eriksonian theory: A psychobiographical illustration. *Gerontology and Geriatrics Education, 14*, 81-91.

Lechich, A. (1984). High technology and home health care (Proceedings for 1983 The Pride Institute Conference). *Pride Institute Journal, 3*, 6-7.

Leira, A. (1994). Concepts of caring: Loving, thinking, and doing. *Social Service Review, 68*, 185-201.

Lumsdon, K. (1993). Patience and partnership. *Hospitals and Health Networks, December 20*, 26-28.

Miller, M. S. (1995). *Health care choices for today's consumer*. Washington, DC: Living Planet Press.

Modica, P. E. (1995). A simple glass of water is not simple for everyone–from a student's perspective. *Journal of Nutrition for the Elderly, 14*, 85-87.

Mui, A. C. and Burnette, J. D. (1994). A comparative profile of frail elderly persons living alone and those who live with others. *Journal of Gerontological Social Work, 21*, 5-26.

New Jersey Association of Area Agencies on Aging. (1995). Defining the vision for long term care in New Jersey. Unpublished conference report, New Jersey Association of Area Agencies on Aging. New Jersey Department of Labor, New Jersey Data Center (1991), 1990 Census of Population and Labor, Summary Tape File 1.

Norris, T. and Lampe, D. (1994). Healthy communities, healthy people. *National Civic Review, Summer-Fall*, 4-9.

Oliver, S. (1995, January 16). "All this for nothing?" *Forbes*, 56-57.

Parker, R. G. (1995). Reminiscence: A continuity theory framework. *The Gerontologist, 35*, 515-525.

Perkins, K. and Tice, C. (1995). A strengths perspective in practice: Older people and mental health challenges. *Journal of Gerontological Social Work, 23*, 83-97.

Pollack, W. (1979). *Expanding health benefits for the elderly, Volume I*. Washington, DC: The Urban Institute.

Raiff, N. R. and Shore, B. K. (1993). *Advanced case management: New strategies for the nineties*. Newbury Park, CA: Sage.

Rashko, R. (1985). Systems integration at the program level: Aging and mental health. *The Gerontologist, 25*, 460-463.

Rothman, J. (1994). *Practice with highly vulnerable clients: Case Management and community based service*. Englewood Cliffs, NJ: Prentice-Hall.

Rowland, D. and Lyons, B. (Eds.). (1991). *Financing home care: Improving protection for disabled elderly people.* Baltimore, MD: Johns Hopkins University Press.

Rubin, A. and Johnson, P. J. (1982). Practitioner orientation towards the chronically disabled: Prospects of policy implementation. *Administration in Mental Health, 10*(1), 3-12.

Rubinstein, R. L., Kilbride, J. C., and Nagy, S. (1992). *Elders living alone: Frailty and the perception of choice.* New York: Aldine de Gruyter.

Simmons, J. (1994). Community based care: The new health social work paradigm. *Social Work in Health Care, 20*, 35-46.

Tudor, R. K., and Carley, S. S. (1995). Time to choose. *Journal of Health Care Marketing, 15*, 48-53.

U.S. Bureau of the Census. (1990). America in transition: An aging society. *Current Population Reports*, Series P-23, 128. Washington, DC: U.S. Government Printing Office.

U.S. Public Health Service (1992). *Healthy People 2000* (Publication No. PHS 91-50212). Washington, DC: U.S. Government Printing Office.

Wallace, S. P., Campbell, K., and Lew-Ting, C. (1994). Structural barriers to the use of formal in-home services by elderly Latinos. *Journal of Gerontology: Social Sciences, 49*, S253-S263.

Chapter 30

Home Care

Nancy V. Lotz

CONTEXT

Description of the Setting

The Visiting Nurse Association of Greater Philadelphia (VNA) is a voluntary, nonprofit, Medicare-certified home health organization which provides multidisciplinary and specialty health services, including skilled nursing (which provides geriatric, pediatric, home infusion, psychiatric, AIDS and wound care), as well as maternal/child health, home hospice, and cardiopulmonary, oncology, diabetic, and asthma care. In addition, the VNA provides speech, physical and occupational therapies, medical social work, and home heath aide services, and can arrange for home medical equipment and supplies to its patients. Home health services are available 24 hours a day, seven days a week. The VNA serves 1,800 patients each month in four counties. Headquarters are in Philadelphia, the location of 90 percent of the VNA's patients; branch offices for field staff are located in the outlying counties. The VNA has approximately 550 full-time, part-time, and contract employees, of whom 200 are nurses.

The mission of the VNA is to provide comprehensive health care and related health programs and services of the highest quality to persons in their place of residence; to provide these services to all people, regardless of their ability to pay, in so far as it is financially feasible, while generating the resources to accomplish this; and to take a leadership role in support of public and professional education, research, and advocacy for home care. The primary health problems seen are cardiovascular disease, cancer, diabetes, fractures, and strokes. While the VNA has a large maternal/child health program, the majority of patients are at least 65 years old and female, with many being 75 to 84 years old. Forty-five percent of the patients are white, 45 percent are African American, and 10 percent are Hispanic and Asian, with the latter population growing rapidly.

Policy

In 1965, the Social Security Amendment, Title 18 (Medicare) allowed federal reimbursement of health care and social services. The Consolidated Omnibus Budget Reconciliation Act of 1981 (COBRA) allowed proprietary agencies to apply for Medicare certification in home health (Smith, 1987). The number of home health agencies in the Delaware Valley exploded, and competition for patients became a survival issue (Benjamin, 1986). The Tax Equity and Fiscal Responsibility Act of 1982 (TEFRA) changed the basis for reimbursement to hospitals. Before, it was the cost to the hospital of providing daily care for the patient. Now, it is the diagnostic category of the patient. The resultant system, the Medicare Prospective Payment System, established a patient classification system of 468 diagnosis-related groups (DRGs), which determine the amount that Medicare will reimburse the hospital for care of a patient (Livengood, Smith, and Hallstead, 1983; social security administration, 1983). Consequently, hospitalizations are shorter with patients being discharged in a more debilitated state (Feller, 1986).

Initially, home health referrals increased as a result of TEFRA and the DRGs, but as the census of hospitals began to decline, so did the number of referrals for home health (Lerman, 1987a, 1987b; Ingoldsby et al., 1994). Thus, competition for referrals was further escalated. Concerned about their own survival, hospitals began to diversify services and to form networks or joint ventures with other health organizations including home health organizations (Kuntz, 1983). Today, free-standing home health organizations such as the VNA are trying to increase referrals by appealing directly to the patient through community outreach programs.

The VNA bases its work on a medical model, and services are provided only by orders of a physician, which are certified every 60 days. Most referrals are made by area hospitals, other health organizations such as HMOs, the VNA's community outreach program, and physicians. Private individuals and community organizations can also initiate contact, but medical orders are required before services are rendered. Health insurance information is obtained as part of intake. All cases are initially assessed by a visiting nurse who decides if the patient will be admitted for service, and the nurse verifies the patient's health insurance. With the growing number of Medicare HMO subscribers, field staff are reminded to inquire every month about any insurance changes because each insurance contract, whether it be traditional Medicare or another form of insurance, dictates the amount of service a patient may receive. Medicare regulations specify conditions of eligibility as well as types of services. To receive services, a person must be homebound, in need of skilled, intermittent care, and not receiving such care from another health care organization.

According to Medicare regulations, nursing, physical therapy, and speech therapy are primary services, while social work, occupational therapy, and home health aide service are secondary. Social work referrals are made at intake or by field staff, especially nurses, after the case is opened. Social workers provide consultation to staff and direct service to patients and families (Hoffman, 1983; Dobrof, 1984; Williams, 1995). The code of federal regulations governing Medicare defines the employment qualifications for the Medical Social Worker in Home Health Care Section 405.1202 and Conditions of Participation for Social Service Section 405.1226 (Federal Health Insurance, 1987; Home Health Social Work Standards ..., 1987). Medicare's criteria for social workers in home health care are a master's of Social Work degree from an accredited institution and at least one year of experience in a health care setting (Jacobs and Lurie, 1984). The documentation of social work services must also comply with Medicare regulations in order for reimbursement to be approved (Holloway, 1984).

Reimbursement is made only for the period during which a primary service is involved, with the exception of occupational therapy, which may continue independently once all primary services end. Interdisciplinary coordination is essential in order to ensure that social work and home health aide services comply with this regulation. Other funding sources such as HMOs require prior authorization for any service being provided. All care decisions are made by the HMO care manager, who is the gatekeeper of funds and services. In each of these situations, if there is no authorization, no payment is made, and the VNA must absorb the cost.

In the late 1980s, the Health Care Financing Administration allowed Medicare HMOs in another effort to control costs while maintaining high quality care (Health Care Financing Administration, 1989a, b, c; 1990). In these instances, HMOs contract with Medicare to provide the full range of Medicare-covered services for a fixed monthly fee. The HMOs offer all Medicare services except hospice care, which is a separate Medicare benefit, and may additionally offer preventive services, vision and dental care, and prescription drug coverage. Using aggressive marketing campaigns, HMOs are rapidly enrolling new members. Traditionally, HMOs have provided care to healthy people focusing on preventive care. Treating the people who are chronically ill is very different and costly.

If a VNA patient is a member of an HMO, a VNA intake nurse acts as a mediator between field staff and the HMO care manager who authorizes frequency, number of home visits, and length of service. VNA staff can advocate for additional visits, but the HMO has the final say. The VNA's experience is that managed care plans drastically limit the number of visits by all disciplines to its subscribers. HMOs also reimburse for services at a much lower rate than it costs to provide these services; thus, fees must be subsidized through the VNA's Indigent Fund. Every dollar used to offset fees that are below the cost of the service means one less dollar for a truly indigent person.

Medicaid and many private insurances do not reimburse for social work services at all. With federal and state governments trying to control health care costs, there is little chance that coverage for social work will increase. Limited insurance coverage creates a dilemma for staff. Often, the only available options are extensive telephone contact or transfer of cases to long-term care management agencies or other health providers.

In 1985, the Health Care Financing Administration (which under the Department of Health and Human Services is responsible for Medicare, federal participation in Medicaid, and other health programs) created a uniform system for physicians' orders and a prodigious amount of paperwork. It introduced several new comprehensive forms for physicians' orders and treatment plans for Medicare patients, which must be completed by all disciplines after the initial visit, signed by the physician within 30 days, updated by staff, and recertified through new forms prior to the 60-day validity limit.

Criteria for Denial of Service

An elaborate system through intermediary insurance companies, which pays claims under contract to the federal government, monitors these forms and uses them to deny payment for services. A medical denial means that the service provided did not meet Medicare's requirement for skilled nursing services; a technical denial means that the physician did not sign the form, the form was completed incorrectly, or the patient was not homebound. Payment for part or all of the service period may be denied. Documentation recorded and processed in a timely manner is crucial to the total operations of the VNA. While Medicare Home Care is not a large percentage of health care dollars, Medicare Home Care expenditures are growing at an average annual rate of 25 percent. Knowing that changes are inevitable, the VNA is trying to position itself to remain proactive, viable, and competitive in the marketplace by developing critical pathways for specific diseases, exploring alternative models to maximize interdisciplinary coordination and planning, and other ways to maximize effectiveness and efficiency (Benjamin, 1986).

Reimbursement Changes May Support Social Work

Changes in reimbursement may have a positive outcome for social work. Current reimbursement is based on the number of visits made by the social worker. The VNA's productivity standard for a full-time, salaried social worker is three and one-third visits per day. Currently the only way to reduce cost per visit is to increase staff's productivity standard. Social work visits differ from all other disciplines in that much of the work is done pre- and post-visit. The social worker spends much time on the telephone, working with relatives or informal supports, contacting and networking with community agencies and other health providers, coordinating and facilitating community referrals, completing applications, and advocating for patients' rights and needs. Social workers also provide education and information to patients, families, and the team, and counsel patients about their disease. If reimbursement were a lump-sum payment or a flat payment for social work services, regardless of patients' needs, social workers would have the flexibility to determine the most efficient and economic way to provide social services. The number of home visits might decline, but the number of patients served would increase.

Technology

Technology has enabled the VNA of Greater Philadelphia to expand its services medically and professionally. The population of the United States is aging and people are living longer with chronic ailments. Hospital stays are shorter and patients are discharged to home "sicker and quicker" (United States House, Select Committee on Aging, 1985, 1986a, 1986b, 1987). While the number of patients being served by the VNA has increased, the services per patient have become more comprehensive. Providing 500,000 visits this year, the VNA is the largest "hospital without walls" in the region. An example of VNA expansion is the creation of the Infusion Program, which takes a nontraditional approach by structuring its multidisciplinary care process around a community health generalist nurse specializing in home infusion therapies. This approach, unique to home infusion programs, allows for unfragmented care that promotes a level of patient assessment and care provision unparalleled today. In certain situations, the visiting nurse meets the patient in the hospital to begin teaching infusion methods prior to discharge.

Living at home with advanced chronic illness or trauma convalescence often requires devices that reduce architectural or physical barriers. Patients' mobility and physical condition can be improved with equipment such as hospital beds, wheelchairs, walkers, commodes, raised toilet and bath tub seats, grab bars, stair lifts, ramps; assistive devices such as braces, long-handled tongs and sponges, button hookers and large print telephone dials or telephones with speed dialing; removal of architectural barriers such as throw rugs and some doors; and help with activities of daily living (Kerson and Kerson, 1985). Today with the introduction of new, lighter materials that are prefabricated and pliable, orthotics are readily available to disabled persons. These new splints and braces can prevent deformities or promote function. Some equipment is covered for payment by insurance plans, and when coverage is not available, families pay suppliers. When patients cannot afford equipment, referrals are made to social workers who then explore community resources to find alternative funding or negotiate financing. In some cases, patient do without needed equipment.

Providing service in the home calls for creativity and collaboration (Sitt, 1985; Weinstein, 1984; Zimner, Groth-Junker, and McCusker, 1985). Rehabilitation staff can often increase a person's functional ability and independence using everyday household items, such as an old handbag filled with canned goods used as a weight for exercises to strengthen arms and legs; physical therapists teach patient how to use a TENS (transcutaneous electrical nerve stimulation) to reduce pain without drugs or penetration of the body; nutritional supplements can often be made with low-cost ingredients when expensive prepackaged supplements are unaffordable; and nurses employ a variety of teaching techniques that address the patients physical or mental impairments. Technology has also improved internal operations at the VNA, as computers allow interagency communication to verify insurance coverage. All bills are now electronically transmitted. A voice-messaging system has been installed and personal beepers have improved access to field staff. Documentation is still done manually, but the VNA is currently exploring software that begins to address the clinical reporting needs of the staff.

Organization

Founded in 1886 as the Visiting Nurse Society of Philadelphia by Helen Furness Jenks, the VNA has a long and rich history. The VNA is governed by a board of trustees comprised of governmental, community, medical, and business representatives. Policy promulgation and performance monitoring are the primary responsibilities of the board. The VNA has a parent corporation, Philadelphia Home Care, and two affiliates: Home Care Specialists, which offers private pay nursing, homemakers, and companions; and the Hospice of the VNA, which is a Medicare-certified home health hospice program. The president/CEO and his executive staff implement the policies. Information is transmitted to staff by voice mail, a bimonthly newsletter, memos, team meetings, and general staff meetings. Expanding the VNA's network of services has enhanced patient care and provided the organization greater flexibility (Gilbride, 1983).

A part of the VNA for 20 years, social work has become an integral and respected member of the health care team (Berger and Anderson, 1984; Berger, 1988). Comprised of a director, who reports to the executive vice president/chief operating officer and 11 licensed social workers and who chairs the VNA's Ethics Committee, the department has doubled in size in the last year in response to the volume of referrals. Each social worker is assigned to a nursing team covering a specific geographic area. The goal of social work services in home health care is to improve or maintain the social, emotional, functional, and physical health status of the patient, as well as to enhance the coping skills of the family or their caregiver system (Banchard, Gill, and Williams, 1991; Pinkston and Linsk, 1984; Getzel, 1983). Services are available to all patients of the VNA with social or emotional problems that adversely affect their medical condition, treatment, or rate of recovery. The VNA has always taken pride in offering care to the indigent and others without health insurance. To maintain this mission, the VNA created the Indigent Care Program, which in 1995 raised more than $1,200,000. When social work service is deemed necessary and insurance does not cover the service, the director of social work can authorize visits to be covered by the Indigent Care Fund.

Attached to every social work referral is a face sheet that lists logistical, medical, and billing information. Upon receipt, the social worker contacts the referring nurse or therapist to notify him or her of social work involvement and may request additional pertinent information to prepare for the initial visit. Then the social worker schedules a home visit for psychosocial assessment and establishes goals and a treatment plan (Kirschner and Rosengarten, 1982). Social workers also orient new staff, provide in-service education, and serve on administrative committees.

DECISIONS ABOUT PRACTICE

Description of the Client

Miss Nettie Davis, age 92, is an African-American woman who never married and lives with her cats in an inner-city neighborhood. Her mind is sharp, but her body is weak and frail. She is strong-willed, distrustful of others, fiercely independent, but mellowing with age. Her primary diagnoses are spinal stenosis, degenerative joint disease, ambulation dysfunction, and hypertension. In June, Miss Davis fell in her kitchen and was found by her neighbor, after being on the floor for several hours. Emergency medical transport transported her to the closest hospital, and she was admitted. A CT scan proved negative for pathology and an X ray ruled out fractures, but her right side was bruised and she complained of pain. After a brief hospitalization, she was discharged to her home with a referral to the VNA for skilled nursing, home health aide support, and physical therapy evaluation (Gamer, 1984; Haug, 1985).

A social work referral was made after the nurse's initial assessment, and a verbal order was obtained. The referral reported the following: the patient lived alone with no visible support system except a neighbor; the nurse questioned the patient's safety and ability to manage; the patient potentially needed short- and long-term care planning; and the patient was hard of hearing, letting the telephone ring a long time. A visit was scheduled for the next afternoon.

Miss Davis' home is a small, two-story rowhouse. She resides on the first floor because she cannot climb stairs. A hospital bed and commode now sit in her dining room. She uses a cane to ambulate, but was discharged from the hospital with a walker to maximize her safety. Most of her friends and family have died. Her primary supports are her neighbor, Mrs. Johnson, who has a key to the house, stops in daily, and feeds her cats; a good friend, Mr. Gotham, who assists with bill paying, shopping, and running errands; and her married nephew who lives in New York City and visits infrequently. When he visits, he and his wife assume full caregiving responsibility. Miss Davis has declined her nephew's offer to move in with him. Frozen meals are delivered weekly through a local church, but she doesn't know who arranged the meals or how to contact the church. As Miss Davis grew stronger and was able to ambulate more freely with her walker, she resumed some activities of daily living. Mr. Gotham accompanied her to her doctor's appointment using paratransit for transportation. Miss Davis hand delivered medical forms to her doctor, and the social worker submitted these medical forms to the County Office on Aging (COA), requesting long-term homemaker services.

About six weeks later, Miss Davis fell again and was admitted to the hospital. Both the social worker and nurse contacted the hospital's social work department to notify them of Miss Davis' living situation and to refer her for discharge planning. Unfortunately, she was sent home without a discharge plan. Her neighbor, Mrs. Johnson, called the VNA to request that services be resumed. Miss Davis' physician was contacted, and he ordered home health services, including social work. The second fall affected Miss Davis physically and mentally. She appeared more frail, and her confidence was shaken. She now acknowledged that she needed daily care, and home health aide service twice a day was requested for two weeks. General caregiving fell to Mrs. Johnson who was reluctant to assume that level of responsibility, and Mrs. Johnson suggested that Miss Davis consider nursing home placement. Miss Davis' nephew was contacted and a family conference was conducted at Miss Davis' bedside to identify her care options. Personal assets determine a person's care options, so Miss Davis had to disclose her financial situation. Time was a concern because decisions and arrangements had to be made, the VNA would eventually be terminating service, and it would be months before long-term homemaker services, provided by COA, would be available. This demand for financial disclosure was the final assault on Miss Davis' fierce independence.

Definition of the Client and Goals

As defined by Medicare regulations, the patient is the client in all cases. Often, the social worker meets with the caregiver or people in the client's informal support system, so the client relationship is expanded to include them. Initially, Miss Davis was the focus, but when she required more assistance in order to maintain whatever independence her physical condition allowed, I turned to her nephew to assist with decision making and care arrangements. The social worker assesses the patient's needs, and together the social worker and patient establish a treatment plan that includes the goals of their work together. This process can be an ongoing one depending upon the patient's rate of recovery or adjustment to their illness. Treatment plans are written for a 60-day period and signed by the patient's physician. Goals are set and shared by each discipline.

Initially, Miss Davis' goal was to resume her former level of functioning. I coordinated appropriate community referrals that would allow her to be safe and maximally independent. Since she needed a new form of transportation to reach her doctor's office, I coordinated Miss Davis' enrollment with a paratransit service. I also counseled her on the benefits of renting and installing an emergency medical response system in her home, but she declined the suggestion, saying it was too expensive and she would rely on her neighbor's checking on her each day. A problem developed with her home-delivered meals, and I spent much time investigating which community agency provided these meals. Once this was accomplished, I then tried to rectify the delivery problem. On occasion, I picked up the meals and brought them to her. Meal preparation was an activity Miss Davis could no longer manage, and having prepared food was essential. From the onset, I recognized that Miss Davis would need ongoing homemaker services a few times a week. I coordinated the referral to COA. When problems continued with the delivery of her frozen meals, I referred her for hot, daily, home-delivered meals provided by the COA. Frail and infirm after her second fall, Miss Davis required a more intensive level of in-home services, and I requested an augmented treatment plan at the COA. My overall goal was the establishment of a workable care plan (Austin and Siedl, 1981).

Contract and Meeting Place

The contract was established when I met Miss Davis and she gave me permission to act on her behalf. It provided a framework for the client/social worker relationship and was altered as Miss Davis' home care needs changed. The VNA is a home-visiting agency; therefore, all contacts except discharge planning meetings, interdisciplinary team meetings, and professional conferences occur in the patient's home. Unless it has been prearranged to meet in a particular room, the meeting place is usually determined by the patient's location when the social worker arrives. When Miss Davis felt strong enough she would be out of bed sitting at her kitchen table; as she became more frail and confined to her hospital bed, our meetings were held in the dining room, which was near her bedroom.

Use of Time

Medicare regulations and VNA policy specify conditions of participation for the professional medical social worker. Patient contact is to be made within 48 hours of referral, and a home visit is to be made within five working days. The length and frequency of visits is set by the social worker and varies on a case-by-case basis. The duration of service is set by the nurse or therapist. Cases remain open only while skilled interventions are provided. Time spent with the patient is only part of the social worker's intervention. Telephone contacts, correspondence, and case reporting before and after the home visits are time-consuming. There is a direct correlation between time spent in pre- and post-activities and case complication. Initially, most visit time was spent gathering information with the patient and counseling her about community resources, and then making appropriate referrals. Later, when Miss Davis needed alternative care planning, a great deal of time was spent on the telephone mobilizing her support system and convincing her nephew to take a more active role with his aunt's care planning. Time was also spent sharing information and strategizing with Miss Davis' nurse and physical therapist.

Interventions and Stance of the Social Worker

Social work intervention follows a brief, crisis-oriented treatment model and requires knowledge of family systems theory. A social worker in home health must also possess strong relationship and direct practice skills. Specific modes of intervention, for Miss Davis and all other social work clients, include an amalgam of education, counseling, short-term therapy, advocacy, coordination of services, and referrals for concrete services, all related to the client's identified medical condition. Although physically compromised, Miss Davis was alert, oriented, and capable of making appropriate decisions for herself. A calendar on her kitchen wall identified our visit pattern, and the VNA's telephone number was on her refrigerator and taped to her bedside table. She was vague about her finances, saying a friend paid her bills, and she was not interested in purchasing additional in-home services. Other interventions have been previously discussed. My original stance was related to my initial goals: to complete a psychosocial assessment and win Miss Davis' trust. My stance changed as Miss Davis' physical condition deteriorated. At times, I was a supportive listener, an active participant in clarifying care options and pursuing community services, and a strong advocate.

Use of Outside Resources

Home health care social workers are community resource specialists. Knowledge of programs' eligibility criteria and application procedures is vital to our work. Providing information and coordinating referrals in a timely manner is essential because social work's service periods are short and usually crisis related. Frequently, patients have physical or mental impairments that require the social worker to manage the entire application process through the linkage and advocacy stage. When patients and families can share responsibility, follow-up is transferred to them. The most common types of community resource requests are long-term home health aide/homemaker services, nursing home placements or respite care, transportation to doctor's appointments, securing entitlements, adult day care programs, help with pharmaceutical and medical supplies, affordable and accessible housing, nutritional programs, especially home-delivered meals, home repair programs, and legal services. There are significant gaps in programs for the population under 60 years of age. For people over 60 years of age, the COA offers a broad spectrum of services, but access and availability of services is hindered by an overburdened centralized intake unit and long waiting lists. With Miss Davis, much of my time was spent gathering information, completing forms, and making and tracking referrals. Follow-up with these resources was crucial. Only Miss Davis' nephew would take on additional responsibility; her neighbor and good friend could do no more. Living alone with declining health meant Miss Davis would soon rely on outside resources to provide a safe and adequate level of care. The ecomap for Miss Davis outlines her network of resources (Figure 30.1).

Reassessment and Termination

Examples of reassessment occurred in three instances: (1) when problems with Miss Davis' home-delivered meals continued and she needed a referral to a different agency; (2) after she fell a second time and her informal supports could not assume more caregiving responsibility; and (3) when, as the nurse approached discharge, Miss Davis trusted me enough to share financial information with me so that I could show her that she could afford to buy in-home services or pay for nursing home placement (Liu, Manton, and Liu, 1985). Except when there is a sudden change in the patient's health status and discharge is immediate, VNA patient discharge is planned by all involved disciplines. At the time of discharge from the agency, Miss Davis was still at home finalizing plans with her nephew. I did discuss care options, their costs, and where to obtain services with Miss Davis and her nephew and felt confident that they would move ahead together to formulate the best plan for Miss Davis.

A NOTE ABOUT THE PROFESSION IN CONTEXT

Social work in home health care has come a long way since the Medicare program was enacted in 1965. As the role of social work in home health care has developed, so have its professional affiliations. In 1979, a local home health social worker's group formed to provide in-service education, peer support, supervision, and advocacy. In the mid 1980s, the National Association of Social Workers (NASW) established a home health care group (NASW makes point . . . , 1987; National Association of Social Workers, 1987). In 1986, the Social Workers in Home Health Care

FIGURE 30.1. Ecomap for Nettie Davis

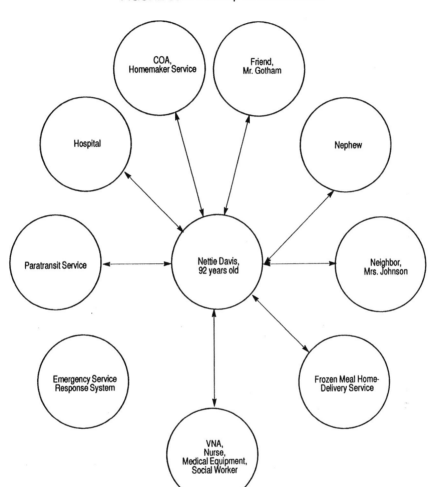

Coalition was created to interpret and influence new regulations. In January 1995, the American Network of Home Health Care Social Workers was founded, and its first national conference was held in 1996. Today business is booming and while many health care settings are experiencing a downsizing or restructuring, home health social work is growing (National Association of Social Workers, 1991; NASW Clinical Indicators . . . , 1995). The challenge for social workers is to assert a strong social work identity within the home health care organization and in the larger health care reform movement.

REFERENCES

Austin, C. D. and Seidl, F. W. (1981). Validation of professional judgment in a home care agency. *Health and Social Work, 6*(1), 50-56.

Benjamin, A. E. (1986). Trends and issues in the provision of home health care: Local governments in a competitive environment. *Journal of Public Health Policy, 7*(4), 480-494.

Berger, R. M. (1988). Making home health social work more effective. *Home Health Care Service Quarterly, 9*(1), 4-8.

Berger, R. M. and Anderson, S. (1984). The in-home worker: Serving the frail elderly. *Social Work, 29*(5), 456-461.

Blanchard, L., Gill, G., and Williams, E. (1995). *Guidelines and documentation requirements for social workers in home health care.* Home Health Line, March 27, 1995.

Dobrof, R. (Ed.). (1984). *Gerontological social work in home health care.* Binghamton, NY: The Haworth Press.

Eaton, B. J. (1984). Hospital improves service through diversification. *Home Health Journal, 5*(3), 9-10.

Everstine, D. S. and Everstine, L. (1983). *People in crisis: Strategic therapeutic interventions.* New York: Brunner/Mazel.

Federal Health Insurance for the Aged and Disabled: Conditions of Participation, Home Health Agencies, 42 C.F.R. 405.1202 and 405.1226 (1987).

Feller, B. A. (1986). *Americans needing home care.* U.S. National Center for Health Statistics, Program Division of Health Statistics. Pub. No. PHS 86-1581.

Gamer, J. D. (1984). From hospital to home care: Who goes there? A descriptive study of elderly users of home health care services post hospitalization. *Journal of Gerontological Social Work, 7*(4) 75-85.

Getzel, G. S. (1983). Social work with family caregivers to the aged. *Social Casework, 4*(9), 201-209.

Gilbride, N. (1983). Philadelphia home health expanding market boom. *Home Health Journal, 4*(9), 6, 15.

Haug, M. R. (1985). Home care for the ill elderly: Who benefits? (Editorial). *American Journal of Public Health, 75*(2), 127-128.

Health Care Financing Administration (1989a, April). *Medicare Home Health Agency Manual,* Publication No. 11, 206.3. Washington, DC: U.S. Government Printing Office.

Health Care Financing Administration (1989b, October). *Medicare Home Health Agency Manual,* Publication No. 11, 234.7. Washington, DC: U.S. Government Printing Office.

Health Care Financing Administration (1989c, October). *Medicare Home Health Agency Manual,* Publication No. 11, 234.8. Washington, DC: U.S. Government Printing Office.

Health Care Financing Administration (1990, June). *Medicare Home Health Agency Manual,* Publication No 11, 234.9. Washington, DC: U.S. Government Printing Office.

Hoffman, J. (1983). Medical social services offer agencies a greater flexibility in the provision of in-home services. *Home Health Journal, 4*(2), 13.

Holloway, V.M. (1984). Documentation: One of the ultimate challenges in home health care. *Home Healthcare Nurse, 2*(1), 19, 22.

Home health social work standards get NASW nod. (1987, July). *NASW News, 32,* 7, 10.

Ingoldsby A., Kuman N., Cohen M. A., Wallack, C. (1994). Medicare home health care: The struggle for definition. *Journal of Long-term Home Health Care, 13*(3), 6-13.

Jacobs, P. E. and Lurie, A. (1984). A new look at home care and hospital social worker. *Journal of Gerontological Social Work, 7*(4), 87-99.

Kaye, L. W. (1985). Home care for the aged: A fragile partnership. *Social Work, 30*(7), 312-317.

Kerson, T. and Kerson, L. (1985). *Understanding chronic illness.* New York: The Free Press.

Kirschner, C. and Rosengarten, L. (1982). The skilled social work role in home care. *Social Work, 27*(6), 527-530.

Kuntz, E. F. (1983). Alternative services: Hospitals move into home care by striking partnership deals. *Modern Health Care, 13*(12), 116-118.

Lerman, D. (1987a). Home care payer mix: Referrals need expansion. *Hospitals, 61*(2), 98.

Lerman, D. (1987b). Room to expand home care business in 1987. *Hospitals, 61,* (1), 51.

Liu, K., Manton, K. G., and Liu, B. M. (1985). Home care expenses for the disabled elderly. *Health Care Financing Review, 7*(2), 51-58.

Livengood, W. S., Smith, C., and Hallstead, S. (1983). The impact of DRGs on home health care. *Home Healthcare Nurse, 1*(1), 29-34.

National Association of Social Workers (1987). NASW standards for social work in health care settings. Silver Spring, MD: NASW Press.

National Association of Social Workers. (1991). *Social work speaks,* Second Edition. Silver Spring, MD: NASW Press.

NASW clinical indicators for social work and psychosocial services in home health care. (1995, June). NASW Task Force on Home Health Care. Washington, DC: NASW Press.

NASW makes point on nursing home, home health bills. (1987, July). *NASW News, 32*(7), 11.

Pinkston, E. M. and Linsk, N. L. (1984). *Care of the elderly: A family approach.* New York: Pergamon Press.

Silverstone, B. and Burack-Weiss, A. (1982). The social worker function in nursing homes and home care. *Journal of Gerontological Social Work, 5*(1/2), 7-33.

Sitt, G. (1985). Home health care innovations in health care delivery. *Hawaii Medical Journal, 44*(5), 168-169.

Smith, J. B. (1987). Home care is more than Medicare regulations. *American Journal of Nursing, 3*, 304-306.

Social Security Administration. (1983). *Medicare: Health insurance for the aged: Length of stay by diagnosis.* Washington, DC: U. S. Government Printing Office.

United States House, Select Committee on Aging. (1985, September 30). Home health care: Present and future options. Hearing, 99th Congress, 1st Session, Pub. No. 99-539.

United States House, Select Committee on Aging. (1986a, April 10). Out "sooner and sicker": Myth or Medicare crisis? Hearing, 99th Congress, 2nd Session, Pub. No. 99-591.

United States House, Select Committee on Aging. (1986b, August). The "black box" of home care quality: A report. 99th Congress, 2nd Session, Pub. No. 99-573.

United States House, Select Committee on Aging, Subcommittee on Human Services. (1987, January). Exploring the myths: Caregiving in America: A study. 100th Congress, 2nd Session, Pub. No. 99-611.

Weinstein, S. M. (1984). Specialty teams in home care. *American Journal of Nursing, 84*(3), 342-345.

Williams, E. (1995). Understanding social work in the home health care setting. *Home Health Care Practice, 7*(2), 12-20.

Zimner, J. G., Groth-Juncker, A. and McCusker, J. (1985). A randomized controlled study of a home health care team. *American Journal of Public Health, 75*(2), 135-141.

Chapter 31

A Support Group in a Home for the Elderly

Phyllis Braudy Harris

CONTEXT

Group work with residents in long-term care facilities is now recognized as viable and often a treatment of choice for many frail elderly. According to the geriatric social work literature over the past 15 years, the amount of reported social group work services with this population of elderly has increased dramatically. There seem to be two major reasons for this. First, the number of elderly in the population is growing rapidly. In 1975, the over-65 segment of the population comprised 23 million people (11 percent of the United States population), with the oldest segment of this group, the 85-and-over cohort, numbering 2 million, or .8 percent of the population. By the year 2050, there will be 67 million people (22 percent of the population) over 65, and the 85-and-over cohort will number 16 million (24 percent of the total elderly population in the United States. The "Greying of America" is upon us, with the oldest old (those 85 and older) increasing in the greatest proportions (U.S. Bureau of the Census, 1989; U.S. House Select Committee on Aging, 1987). The oldest old make up the majority of the nursing home population.

The second reason for this increase in social group work services with the elderly, especially in long-term care facilities, is the unique contribution of social group work. The central tenet of social group work is the concept of the group as a mutual aid system in which new behaviors, roles, and relationships can be explored in an accepting environment (Schulman, 1985). The opportunity this type of experience affords the elderly in long-term care facilities is extremely important, since as a function of reaching an advanced age with chronic health problems, many elderly have experienced a series of losses such as roles, home, health, friends, family, and finances (Horner, 1982; Wetzel, 1980). Participation in a social group work experience affords these elderly the possibility of redeveloping a new peer social support network. As Abels and Abels (1980) have stressed, the major focus of social group work should be the strengthening and development of social networks.

Group work has the advantage over other therapeutic interventions in that it can facilitate for the members an emotional closeness, encourage meaningful self-disclosure, and promote identification with the struggles of other people in similar situations (Corey and Corey, 1992). This treatment modality can give the elderly a chance to develop or relearn social interaction skills, to make new contacts, and to develop mutual aid peer support systems. It also offers the elderly a chance for therapeutic ventilation, for personal growth and development, and the opportunity to evaluate their own life situation in terms of comparable others (Lowy, 1982).

Groups with institutionalized elderly can be of different types. Burnside and Schmidt (1994) list some examples, such as (1) educational, (2) reality oriented, (3) remotivational, (4) support and self-help, (5) reminiscence, (6) psychotherapy, and (7) activity and social groups. Group work can also be a combination of different types, as will be illustrated by the case presented here, the "Being Old" group. This was a combination educational, support and self-help, social, and psychotherapeutic group. It gave cognitively alert elderly nursing home residents, with adequate social interaction skills, the opportunity to openly and honestly confront the problems they were having with aging. The group also provided these elderly residents with an opportunity to develop new peer social support networks. The name "Being Old" was given to the group in its first session by a participant who suggested we call the group what it really was: "We're old so the group should be called the 'Being Old' group."

Description of the Setting

The "Being Old" Group was held at the Jewish Home for the Aged, a 310-bed nursing home serving elderly Jewish residents in a midwestern state. The Jewish Home is a nonprofit organization that began in 1907 as a charitable burial society and evolved into a home for aged. It is an Orthodox institution that adheres to traditional Jewish laws and rituals while delivering state-of-the-art nursing care. It provides medical, educational, social, psychological, nutritional, recreational, religious, and cultural services for its residents and day-program participants, over 50 percent of whom are Medicaid recipients. The Jewish Home operates on a social, rather than a medical model, because it is a permanent residence for chronically ill elderly, not an acute care hospital. The social work department has always played an important role in the home.

Residents' ages range from 66 to 100, with 85 being the average age. The average length of stay is four and one-half years. Most of the population was born in Eastern Europe, coming to the United States in the pre- and post-World War I immigration waves. Though Yiddish is the native tongue, most of the residents speak English fluently. Not well-educated themselves, they see education as a very important family value, and most of their children are well-educated professional or businesspeople.

Policy

The Jewish Home receives federal funding through Title 18 (Medicare) and Title 19 (Medicaid). The home follows the regulations stipulated by these acts for skilled nursing facilities. One regulation that promotes social work practice in the home is the stipulation that social work services must be made available to nursing home residents. The medically related social needs of the residents are to be identified during admission, and services to meet these needs are to be provided during the resident's stay in the facility and in the planning of his or her discharge. This gives the social work department the legal mandate to provide services within the home, but it is up to the social workers to creatively and effectively use this sanction. The Medicaid and Medicare acts also put constraints upon the social worker in terms of the type of services and medical equipment they will fund (U.S. Department of Health and Human Services, 1981; Kaufman, 1980).

Licensed by the state, the Jewish Home for Aged also follows the laws and policies for the State Department of Public Health. These affect every area of the home's operation, from administration to the scheduling of machinery maintenance. The other state agency that influences the relationship of social worker and client is the state department of human services, which implements the reimbursement of federal and state monies and regularly monitors the type and quality of care each resident receives. It also evaluates whether the elderly patient could manage in a non-nursing home setting.

Technology

The technology of geriatric medicine and chronic illness also affects the relationship between social worker and client. Quite different from the acute care hospital setting in which the focus of medical care is on curing the patient, in the nursing home the goal is toward rehabilitation and maintaining the highest possible level of functioning. Therefore, a different approach is needed with geriatric patients. Geriatric medicine in the United States is still an unpopular specialty in hospitals and medical schools. Even with the recent emergence of geriatric assessment units in medical centers (47 percent of the 114 units in medical centers began during or after 1983), only 50 percent of the physicians primarily servicing these units are trained in geriatric medicine (Barry, 1994; Epstein et al., 1987). The limited interest and concern on the part of the medical community places a serious constraint and burden upon the geriatric social worker (Aging in the Eighties, 1986).

It is important for physician and social worker to allow extra time in work with geriatric patients. Patiently listening to complaints, aches, and pains allows the provider to understand the patient's needs. Especially important to consider when communicating with the elderly is their high incidence of impaired vision and hearing, which hampers their communication skills. Also, better patient education is needed in order for the elderly resident to have a clearer understanding of his or her chronic illness.

Organization

The Jewish Home's policies are determined by a board of directors that is comprised of 42 lay members of the Jewish community. The policies reflect the charter of the facility, which charges the directors to establish, provide, and maintain a Jewish Home in the state for the aged and chronically ill. An acceptable applicant must be Jewish, a resident of the state, and at least 65 years old. The person must be in need of 24-hour supervision and have a physician's statement that he or she is in need of closely supervised medical care. The applicant must not evidence signs of moderate or severe cognitive impairment at the time of admission and must be cognizant of the fact that he or she is moving into a home for the aged on a permanent basis. The admission policy limits access to those who are able to some extent to avail themselves of the social, recreational, educational, and religious services that the home provides.

One effect of this admission policy is to promote the use of social work services. The social worker meets the elderly resident and his or her family at a time when the resident is able to communicate to the social worker his or her needs and concerns and can begin to establish a relationship with the social worker. As the resident becomes more impaired and needs more supportive services, established relationships can promote a better understanding of the situation and more effective service delivery (Getzel and Mellor, 1982).

Factors within the organizational structure can also act as constraints or supports on social work practice, depending upon the social worker's approach (Peterson, 1986; Green and Monohan, 1982). Strong formal and informal structures within the Jewish Home for Aged affected the "Being Old" Group. Even though the nursing home is small in comparison to a hospital setting, the informal networks are important and require that the social worker understand them in order to be an effective mediator and advocate (Wells and Singer, 1985). Thus, it is essential for the social worker to establish a good rapport with the various department heads, charge nurses, and nurse's aides. More often than not, problems can be solved more quickly and effectively by using the informal networks than by going through bureaucratic channels. Mastery of these informal channels was quite useful in avoiding the scheduling of the "Being Old" Group members for activities such as baths, physical therapy, and beauty shop appointments at times when group meetings were held.

The formal organizational structure of the home supported the formation of the group. The executive director had a social work orientation and gave the social work department freedom and latitude in performing and implementing innovative therapeutic programs (Boissenau and Kirschner, 1983). This orientation was reinforced by the director of the Social Work Department, who also had considerable group work experience. Thus, this official philosophy of the nursing home created a positive environment that lent itself to the formation of a "Being Old" group. Thus, the home itself, as well as the state and federal governments, all create constraints and supports for the social worker and her relationship with the client. The social worker must learn to recognize and identify these constraints and supports, and to take a creative approach toward working within them.

PRACTICE DECISIONS

Definition of the Client

Only a small amount of group work that deals specifically with problems of aging has been done in most nursing homes. In this home, there were groups relating to orientation, diabetes, reality orientation, and a resident council, but nothing that specifically gave the elderly nursing home residents the opportunity to openly discuss and confront the problems they were having with being old (Boling, 1987; Scharlack, 1985). After talking with different residents, I decided such a group was needed.

The residents who could best participate in and benefit from this type of confrontation group were those who were most alert and who had adequate social interaction skills and limited sensory impairment. Since a great many sensory deficits in group members will greatly affect the expectations and goals of the group, I kept this in mind as I chose group members (Ebersole, 1976).

I invited the registered occupational therapist to assist in leading the group, because some of the discussions would concern physical health issues in which the therapist had expertise. Together, the occupational therapist and I decided on the group's composition. Thirty-five prospective group participants were selected, and these people were approached by one of the group leaders, interviewed, and invited to join the group. Only a small group of participants was expected because this type of group would not appeal to all the invited residents, and many programs and activities occurred at the nursing home at any given time. We also decided that the group sessions would be announced over the public address system and that anyone else who wanted to attend would be welcome, because only the most motivated and interested residents would be likely to respond to such an announcement. A total of 28 people came to the group, but the usual attendance was 9 to 12 people, consisting mostly of a constant core of the same 9 persons. Attendance was completely voluntary, and approximately one-third of the people who attended at least one session continued to come regularly. The age range of the participants was 69 to 91. That the majority of participants were women was reflective of the higher percentage of women in the home's total population.

In terms of composition, groups ideally require homogeneity (stability) and heterogeneity (diversity) (Gitterman, 1982). Homogeneity refers to common background: age, sex, ethnic and religious backgrounds, comparable life experiences, and also common personality capacities and capabilities. These commonalities tend to stabilize a group and help in the quick development of group identity and cohesiveness. Too much homogeneity can also be a problem reflected in the lack of diversity and vitality in the group. Gitterman states that groups that are overly homogeneous do not create the necessary tension for change to take place or provide the necessary models for alternate attitudes and behaviors.

Goals

The goals of the group were briefly explained to each resident in the individual interview sessions. They were explained in detail at the first session and reiterated again during that session and later ones. As Toseland (1990) advises, the group leader needs to state clearly the purpose and the function of the group. The goals of the group were the following: (1) to encourage verbalization of fears, feelings, and problems of old age; (2) to encourage group members to share feelings and experiences; (3) to develop the beginnings of a peer support system; (4) to encourage self-help among the participants; (5) to provide educational information that would clear up misinformation and misunderstandings about physical and mental health problems of old age; and (6) to help the members as a group and as individuals come to some self-realization and acceptance of the aging process. These goals were reassessed at various times by the leaders in their post-group evaluation meetings and with the participants themselves. This helped the residents see that progress was being made within the group.

Contract, Meeting Place, and Time Period

The group contracted in the first session to meet for a short period every week for 20 weeks. The leaders felt that this would be sufficient to discuss the issues they and the residents might wish to cover. Each session lasted 45 minutes to an hour. The meeting place chosen by the leaders was the board room of the home. This was an area of the building to which the residents do not usually have access, and the leaders felt that meeting there would lend the group prestige and status. The room contained a substantial conference table and chairs; it was quite businesslike and relayed the message to the group participants that serious work was going to take place here. The room was also directly across the hallway from the executive director's office, so its location reflected his support of these sessions.

Interventions and Stance of the Social Worker

Aging is a very broad topic to discuss, so the leaders chose as general topics for discussion the five main problem areas for the elderly as outlined in the Older Americans Resources and Service (OARS) Program's Multidimensional Functional Assessment Questionnaire (Pfeiffer, 1975). The areas are physical health, emotional health, social resources, financial resources, and independence versus dependence. Each topic could have been discussed for months, but the leaders chose the problems that the nursing home residents most commonly experienced in each area. The occupational therapist led the discussions in the area of physical health, which covered, among other topics, cardiovascular disease, arthritis, diabetes, and sensory loss. The book *Aging and Mental Health* (Butler, Lewis, and Sunderland, 1991) was used as a reference for the discussion on emotional health, which dealt with the attitude of giving up, loneliness and losses, ageism, mental impairment, death and dying, and coping mechanisms. The discussion of social resources included such topics as sexuality, loss of friends, family, status, and prestige in the community. Financial resources included the topics of retirement and lack of financial reserves. The last problem area discussed was independence versus dependence. This dealt with the elderly persons' increased dependencies on their adult children and the institution.

The stance the leaders decided to take with the group greatly influenced the progress of the group itself. From the beginning, the tone of the group was one of warmth and acceptance. This helped the residents feel more comfortable in expressing their thoughts and feelings. The leaders also stated in the first session that they would be active members and give the group a great deal of support and direction, but it was expected that as the group evolved and coalesced, group members would become increasingly active. It was hoped that the residents' conversations would become more directed toward one another and that perhaps they would eventually initiate topics for discussion and lead the group through them (Weiner, 1986; Yalom, 1985).

At times, the leaders felt it would be appropriate and help stimulate discussion if they expressed their own feelings about aging and related life experiences. Corey and Corey's modeling technique was quite beneficial in moving the group along when members were stuck or exhibited a great deal of resistance (Corey and Corey, 1992). A great many of the Rogerian person-centered therapeutic procedures of positive, supportive, empathic listening were also used, although at times the leaders became more directive than traditional Rogerian models would advocate in order to stimulate discussion. The technique of confronting certain feelings was also used at certain times in the group sessions, though it needed to be done with the elderly in a gentle, accepting manner. Appropriate reminiscing was also an important technique used throughout the session.

William Schwartz suggests that the best way to understand the movement of a group is to examine the group process by dividing it into four separate phases (Schwartz and Zalba, 1971): the first phase is a preparatory phase that the worker carries out in organizing the group; during the second phase, the worker helps the group to begin; the third phase is the work phase, containing the essential happenings of the group; and the final phase tends toward separation and termination. The "Being Old" Group followed these phases in its evolution.

The first, or preparatory, phase was described above. The second phase was embodied in the first three meetings of the "Being Old" Group.

These initial meetings were the most difficult sessions for the leaders to control for a number of reasons. First, the participants, though familiar with each other's faces since they resided together, were for all practical purposes strangers to each other. Second, they felt uncomfortable sharing feelings and ideas with strangers. Third, many of members had never participated in a group such as this before and were unclear about what to expect. Fourth, there is a social taboo among the elderly about talking openly about such subjects as death, dementia, and sexuality. Also, there is such a negative stereotype about old age that it also presented an area of social taboo not easily discussed. Finally, there was a fear that if they did open up and discuss such topics, they would meet rejection and ridicule. As Lawrence Schulman (1979) discusses, each group member brings to the group the norms of behavior and taboos that exist in his culture. One of the tasks of the group leader is to help members develop new norms and feel free to challenge some taboos so that the group can become more effective. The leaders used this technique, and from this beginning came important statements that laid the foundations for the later stages. One woman named the group, saying, "Let's say it as it is. We are old. People talk but never listen to each other; here we should be willing to listen to each other." Another woman confided, "I was a very independent person once; I never understood how many problems old people had until I became old." Group participants displayed their various coping mechanisms, but no one denied that they had problems with growing old.

By the fourth session, the group had moved into the third stage of the process, the work phase. Group cohesion had begun to develop, and members were ready to open up and discuss their feelings more freely. They were willing to share feelings and take risks, as was demonstrated by one woman expressing her feelings on the topic of sexuality:

> Is there anything wrong with having a certain person of the opposite sex that you enjoy just talking with, just sitting together and conversing with? Is there anything wrong with it? I have done nothing I would be ashamed of, but as I sit in the lobby or walk through the halls, people talk about me as if I have done a terrible thing, and it hurts me.

Other participants reacted to this woman's statement, some supportive of her and others not (Walz and Blum, 1987). There was definite movement toward conversation with each other and away from directing the conversation toward the group leaders. In later sessions dealing with ageism and society's attitude toward old people, the members shared their feelings and were quite supportive of each other. One participant vented angry feelings:

> I never felt old and I don't feel old now at 87 years old. Yes, I feel weak, unsure of my footing, but I don't feel old and I don't like being stereotyped. I'm younger than a lot of young people. You see a lot of young people who are old, absolutely old, because their minds are asleep.

During this stage, members emerged as group leaders and took responsibility for running some of the sessions and bringing topics to the group for discussion. One member asked, "What as residents can we do to help people who have given up?" The underlying feeling of the group was, "Yes, I am my brother's keeper." As another member stated, "It is the responsibility of everyone living here at the home to help each other. It makes a difference when we old people try to help each other in any way and as much as we are capable of."

The termination phase, according to Schwartz, deals with the member's development of self-realization and acceptance of aging, with its fears and joys (Simons and West, 1984-1985). In relation to the topic of mental impairment–the most difficult for the elderly group members to discuss–one participant stated, "I can't go visit the people on the third floor (the section of the building where the most mentally impaired residents reside) because it upsets me too much. I go up there and get sick of it, and I must come down."

Another member stated, "What is most frightening is that this may happen to any of us. A close friend of mine became senile." Unlike earlier sessions, most of the group members were willing to admit their fears of this aspect of aging and be supportive of each other. The final session dealt with acceptance of the aging process and with positive aspects of it. The member who emerged as the group leader remarked that at age 87, there were less societal expectations placed upon her and she felt a new degree of personal freedom and expression.

Outcomes and Case Conclusion

A number of significant outcomes resulted from the "Being Old" Group. One was the establishment of a camaraderie and closeness among its members that carried beyond the group sessions. A new peer social support network was established. This is a definite accomplishment in a nursing home setting where the atmosphere generally promotes self-preoccupation and an unhealthy competition for attention.

Another significant outcome was the "Positive Aspects of Being Old" bulletin board. The member who developed into the group leader came to the author with the suggestion of placing a bulletin board in the lobby of the home, where all the residents, staff, and visitors could see it. She was specifically aiming it toward the resident population, which she labeled as having given up. This was a board that she, a resident, would take the responsibility of maintaining. She would find articles about the positive aspects of being old, put them on the bulletin board, and write captions underneath them, changing them regularly. She wanted to reach and educate as many people as possible. She asked the author to help her arrange for the bulletin board and get administrative support for it. She stated she did not want the effect of the "Being Old" Group just to fade away after the group ended.

The most important outcome, though, was that through the group work process, elderly people who at first showed great resistance to sharing their feelings and talking about being old progressed to the point of sharing feelings, supporting each other, and accepting responsibility for themselves and others. The participants had to examine, share, work through, and come to terms with their feelings about being old. The leaders felt the goals of the group were reached and that the "Being Old" Group was a successful experience for the elderly nursing home residents. Other nursing home residents have asked the leaders to run another "Being Old" Group at a different time so they, too, can have the opportunity of this experience.

Differential Discussion

The "Being Old" Group was a positive social work group experience for these institutionalized elderly. In rethinking possible explanations for this group's success, a number of reasons emerge. Also, some problems in the running of the group must be examined.

A number of decisions made by the group's leaders contributed to its success. First of all, the group's goals were relevant for its members and met their needs, aspirations, and capabilities. As Louis Lowy (1982) discusses, there are differential needs within the life span of an older person that social group work can address. Included in these needs are coping needs, which come into play as the older person adapts to changes in him- or herself and the social environment; expressive needs, which are those strivings associated with fulfilling oneself by participating in activities for one's own sake; contributory needs, that is, wanting to give to others; and the need to exert some degree of influence over conditions in one's environment. The "Being Old" Group addressed these needs and gave members a better understanding of the problems associated with aging, as well as a chance to express their fears and realities.

A second reason for the group's success was its ability to discuss significant topics that are considered taboo for the elderly, such as sexuality and dementia, in an accepting, nonthreatening atmosphere. An unstated norm of behavior existed in the nursing home, mirroring the society at large, which prohibited an open and honest discussion of these topics (MacLean and Bonar, 1983). The mutual expressing and sharing of feelings about such topics allows group members to be in touch with their feelings and to confront them, which is necessary for continued growth and development (Shulman, 1985).

Third, group composition positively affected the nature of the group's development. The "Being Old" Group, with its constant core of nine people, was able to fulfill both the heterogeneous and homogeneous needs for group composition, which aided the group in meeting its goals. Another structural aspect from which the group benefitted was the decision by the leaders to have a time-limited group formed for a specific purpose with the time length specified in advance to the members (Alissi and Casper, 1985). This type of group structure fostered a sense of urgency and immediacy within the group, which helped give it an impetus and pushed it forward.

The decision to have two leaders from complementary professional disciplines also aided the process. Since the size of the group was not predetermined and the leaders wanted members to have the opportunity for maximum participation, it was decided two leaders would be necessary. A given rule of thumb in group work is not to have more than seven members for one group leader. This decision worked for this group because the few times one of the leaders was absent, the group did not run as smoothly. Having an occupational therapist and a social worker lead the group led to a more thorough and accurate discussion of the various topics, since the leaders were experts in different areas.

Perhaps the final reason for the group's success was its group work approach. This focused on group process and stages of group development. Issues and problems were handled by discussion and confrontation, rather than by structured tasks involving role-play and learning techniques. The techniques of reflection, clarification, reminiscence, and support were used. It was an effective method for helping the institutionalized elderly to develop mutual support and manage some of their concerns and fears. This approach appears to be a very effective way of treating the cognitively alert elderly (Toseland, 1990).

Two major limitations must be addressed. First, this type of discussion confrontation group was directed toward the highest functioning residents in the home. Thus, the leaders were directing their group membership toward a very select group of clients, whose capacity and capability to benefit from a social group work experience were enormous. Whether this type of group experience would be effective with less capable institutionalized elderly needs to be further explored. The second limitation was the high dropout rate. Only one-third of the people who attended the sessions remained as active group members. People dropped out for such reasons as ill health, prior commitments because of scheduling in the nursing home, and the inability to face the subjects being discussed. The leaders talked individually with the elderly residents who dropped out and extended an open invitation for them to come back. However, there was not a concerted effort by those who left to rejoin the group. Perhaps if there had been, more people would have benefited from the group experience (Carlton, 1986).

PRACTICE IN CONTEXT

Any social work practice is affected by the environment in which it practices. In terms of the "Being Old" Group, the group was strongly influenced by the agency's policies, organizational structure and philosophy, and geriatric technology. The Jewish Home for Aged was established as a nonprofit nursing home to provide a full spectrum of sociomedical care to the elderly and chronically ill, which has been this facility's building block. Within this framework, all aspects of the home are guided by state and federal legislation, which places both inhibiting and promoting factors on social work practice.

The "Being Old" Group did have the agency's administrative support to establish this type of social group work for the residents, an important impetus for group progress. This sanction was reflected by the use of the home's board room for the group sessions. Thus, the formal organizational structure did have a crucial positive impact upon this group. In addition, by using the informal organizational network, the leaders were able to obtain support for the group on all organizational levels and assure that group members would be available at the time of the group meetings. Thus, a clear working knowledge of the organization's formal and informal structures was imperative in order to be effective in the role of resident advocate, therapist, and mediator.

The area of technology most influencing resident care is the specialty of geriatric medicine. In addition to the specialized knowledge needed about certain medical procedures with the elderly patient and the different effects of certain drugs, a whole different doctor-patient manner and approach is needed in dealing with the geriatric patient. This understanding has to be incorporated into the nursing home's total resident care plan. Geriatric medicine is lagging behind other specialties in its knowledge base and in the number of physicians specializing in this area. This affects the geriatric social worker's role with the client (Solde and Manton, 1985; Green and Monahan, 1981).

Thus, three major contextual factors hindered or supported the "Being Old" Group. It is within this context that the social group work experience took place. It was a successful group work experience for the nine regularly attending members. Group goals were met, and a peer social support network was established among the members. The "Being Old" Group clearly demonstrates that given the opportunity, cognitively alert elderly in long-term care facilities have the ability for continued learning, individual growth and development, the capacity to confront their fears constructively and to adjust to new life situations, and lastly the ability to give and care about others.

REFERENCES

Abels, S. and Abels, P. (1980). Social group work's contextual purposes. *Social Work with Groups, 3*(3), 25-37.

Aging in the eighties. (1986). Advanced data from vital health statistics. Hyattsville, MD: National Center for Health Statistics.

Alissi, A. S. and Casper, M. (1985). Time as a factor in group work. *Social Work with Groups, 8*(2), 3-16.

Barry, P. P. (1994). Geriatric clinical training in medical schools. *American Journal of Medicine, 97*(4a), 8-9.

Boissoneau, R. and Kirshner, A. N. (1983). The behaviorally-oriented long-term care administrator. *Journal of Long-Term Care Administration, 11*(1), 15-20.

Boling, T. E. (1987). Growing old: Adjustments to change. *Nursing Homes, 36*(2), 20-23.

Burnside, I. and Schmidt, M. G., (Eds.). (1994). *Working with older adults: Group process and techniques.* Boston: Jones and Bartlett Publishers.

Butler, R., Lewis, M., and Sunderland, T. (1991). *Aging and mental health.* New York: Macmillan Publishing Company.

Carlton, T. O. (1986). Group process and group work in health social work practice. *Social Work with Groups, 9*(2), 5-20.

Corey, G. and Corey, M. S. (1992). *Groups: Process and Practice*, Fourth Edition. Pacific Grove, CA: Brooks/Cole.

Ebersole, P. (1976). Group work with the aged: A survey of literature. In I. M. Burnside (Ed.), *Nursing and the aged.* New York: McGraw-Hill.

Epstein, A.M., Hall, J. A., Besdine, R., Cumella, E., Feldstein, M., McNeil, B. J., and Rowe, J. W. (1982). The emergence of geriatric assessment units. *Annals of Internal Medicine, 106*, 299-303.

Getzel, G. S. and Mellor, M. J. (1982). Gerontological social work practice in long-term care. *Journal of Gerontological Social Work, 5*(1/2), 1-4.

Gitterman, A. (1982). The use of groups in health settings. In A. Lurie, G. Rosenberg, and S. Pinsky (Eds.). *Social work with groups in health settings*. New York: Watson Academic Publications, Inc.

Greene, V. L. and Monahan, D. J. (1981). Structural and operational factors affecting quality of patient care in nursing homes. *Public Policy, 29*(4), 399-415.

Horner, J. (1982). *That time of year: A chronicle of life in a nursing home.* Amherst, MA: University of Massachusetts Press.

Huttman, E. D. (1985). *Social services for the elderly*. New York: The Free Press.

Kaufman, A. (1980). Social policy and long-term care of the aged. *Social Work, 25*(2), 133-137.

Lowy, L. (1982). Social group work with vulnerable older persons: A theoretical perspective. *Social Work with Groups, 5*(2), 21-32.

MacLean, M.J. and Bonar, R. (1983). The normalization principle and the institutionalized elderly. *Canada's Mental Health, 31*(2), 16-18.

Peterson, K. J. (1986). Changing needs of patients and families in long-term care facilities: Implications for social work practice. *Social Work in Health Care, 12*(2), 37-49.

Pfeiffer, E. (1975). *OARS multidimensional functional assessment questionnaire.* Durham, NC: Duke University Center for the Study of Aging and Human Development, Older Americans Resources and Services Program.

Scharlach, A. E. (1985). Social group work with institutionalized elders: A task-centered approach. *Social Work with Groups, 8*(3), 33-47.

Schulman, L. (1979). *The skills of helping: Individuals and groups.* Itasca, IL: F.E. Peacock Publishers.

Schulman, L. (1985). The dynamics of mutual aid. *Social Work with Groups, 8*(4), 51-59.

Schwartz, W. and Zalba, S. R. (Eds.). (1971). *The practice of group work.* New York: Columbia University Press.

Simons, R. L. and West, G. E. (1984-1985). Life changes, coping resources, and health among the elderly. *International Journal of Aging and Human Development, 20*(3), 173-189.

Toseland, R. (1990). *Group work with the older adults.* New York: New York University Press.

U.S. Bureau of the Census. (1989). Projections of the population of the United States by age, sex, and race: 1988-2080. *Current Population Reports*, Series, P.25, No. 1018. Washington, DC: U.S. Government Printing Office.

U.S. Department of Health and Human Services, Health Care Financing Administration, (1981). *Long-term care: Background and future directions.* Washington, DC: U.S. Government Printing Office.

U.S. House Select Committee on Aging. (1987). *Exploding the myths: Caregiving in America.* (CP No. 99-611). Washington, DC: U.S. Government Printing Office.

Walz, T. and Blum, N. (1987). *Sexual health in later life.* Lexington, MA: Lexington Books.

Weiner, M. (1986). Group treatment with the aged. *Journal of Jewish Communal Service, 62*(4), 307-317.

Wells, L. M. and Singer, C. A. (1985). A model for linking networks in social work practice with the institutionalized elderly. *Social Work, 30*(4), 318-322.

Wetzel, J. W. (1980). Interventions with the depressed elderly in institutions. *Social Casework, 61*(4), 234-239.

Yalom, I. D. (1985). *The theory and practice of group psychotherapy,* Third Edition. New York: Basic Books.

Chapter 32

Alzheimer's Disease: Intervention in a Nursing Home Environment

Susan O. Mercer
Betsy Robinson
Toba Schwaber Kerson

CONTEXT

Alzheimer's disease (AD) is a progressive, relentless dementia characterized by cognitive impairment, disorientation, personality changes, and ultimately death (Sandson, Sperling, and Price, 1995; Terry, Katzman, and Bick, 1995; Update on Alzheimer's Disease, Parts 1 and 2, 1995; Zandi, 1994). It is rapidly becoming one of the nation's most heart-rending and expensive diseases. It affects an estimated 2,500,000 Americans, causes 150,000 deaths annually, is the fourth leading cause of death, and usually strikes persons over age 65. The prevalence of the disease at age 65 is 10.3 percent; over age 80, the prevalence rises to 47 percent (Corrada, Brookmeyer, and Karnas, 1995). Annually, 2.6 percent of those over 65 develop the disease (Rowland, 1995). As the proportion of older Americans rises, the absolute number of people with Alzheimer's disease will increase. The annual U.S. bill for the disease is estimated to be greater than $20 billion.

There are only hypotheses as to the cause, including the possibility of a genetic factor, and there are no known cures. Ante-mortem diagnosis is an exclusionary process (Corey-Bloom et al., 1995; Forstl and Hertschel, 1995; Klatka et al., 1996; Sandson, Sperling, and Price, 1995). That is, a complete neurological, physical, and psychiatric evaluation should rule out other conditions associated with dementia. A detailed social and medical history will help reveal whether there has been an insidious onset and gradual progression of symptoms that suggest AD.

There are stages and phases of Alzheimer's disease (Gruetzner, 1992; Volicer and Hurley, 1995). The disease typically begins with memory loss, mistakes in judgment, and affect changes (Mega et al., 1996). The person may lose car keys, leave the stove on, or generally appear absent-minded. As the dementia progresses, all the senses are affected. If the person lives long enough, complete disorientation will occur, in addition to night restlessness, increased aphasia, failure to recognize family, general loss of socially acceptable behaviors, and perseveration. Eventually, the symptoms progress to a point where the person is bedridden, incontinent, unresponsive, and mute (Van-Ort and Phillips, 1992). The disease may progress from 2 to 14 years or more. Eventually, the person requires total nursing care (Allen, 1992; Kerson, 1985).

Description of the Setting

The case intervention occurred with a resident placed at Riley's Oak Hill Manor South in Little Rock, Arkansas. Riley's, Inc., the parent corporation, also owns a nursing home in North Little Rock, which participates in third-party payment and has a retirement center adjacent to Riley's South Nursing home. Retirement center residents are provided short-term care at the nursing home as needed. Riley's South is a 224-bed, private-pay, for-profit, modern, skilled-care nursing home that primarily serves the elderly residents of the state. Riley's can accommodate the ambulatory resident who needs regular medication and minimal supervision as well as the resident requiring intensive care. The one-level facility is 17 years old, 63,000 square feet in area, and purpose-built. In the minimum care wing, residents require little supervision, may bring their own furniture, and may come and go as they please. The intermediate and skilled care wings provide a more structured environment (Hampel and Hastings, 1993; Savishinsky, 1992; Stahlman, 1992). There are four intensive care beds for residents who must be monitored 24 hours a day or who require intravenous feeding; five furnished patios for visiting and outside activities; and three large day rooms for activities, meals, and socialization. A large central dining room serves cafeteria-style meals and is also used for activities. There is a large, well-equipped physical therapy room, as well as an arts and crafts center where residents can pursue ceramics, painting, and woodworking. One section of the yard is fenced to provide a safe "wandering" space for residents. The facility is centrally and conveniently located in the state and community. It is within five minutes of the four major hospitals and medical centers, and yet it is at the end of a private cul-de-sac, surrounded by piney woods. The average age of the resident population is 80, with the ages ranging from 28 to

100. Eighty-three percent are women. About 40 percent of the residents experience dementia and confusion with a variety of diagnoses and etiologies. The average length of stay is one year, which is considerably lower than the national average. Approximately 62 percent of the discharged residents return to alternate care settings, such as their family's homes with health aide assistance. Many residents and families take advantage of the respite care and short-stay options.

Policy

The home is regulated and licensed as a skilled care facility by the Arkansas Office on Long-Term Care. Since it is private pay, there are no federal or state monies involved. The home's policies are established by the governing board, the president of the corporation, the director of operations, and the administrator. The social work profession has always played an important role in the policies and practices of the home. The standards of excellence go well beyond federal and state requirements. Since its inception, the facility has had a full-time master's-level social worker as well as a consultant with a doctor of social work degree. The MSW was recently promoted to the administrator's position and a new MSW was hired. The home has also routinely provided field placement and supervision opportunities for two first-year MSW students. Riley's is unique in the state for the quality and quantity of professional social workers. We are not too humble to tout the "social work power," and believe the social work presence has made a positive difference in the level of care and quality of life for the residents, families, and staff.

The admissions policy does not discriminate on the basis of sex, race, religion, or ethnic background. The home may refuse admission to persons who are currently abusing alcohol or drugs, anyone under age 18, persons who are actively psychotic, have a known communicable disease, require a respirator, or require a liquid narcotic administered through an IV. The administrator and social worker reserve the right to evaluate each applicant on an individual basis. The resident's rights are strictly adhered to, and the resident and family are provided a copy of the bill of rights upon admission. Staff are trained and involved in the implementation of the policies and procedures. Living wills are available for the resident to discuss and complete with her family and physician (Volicer and Hurley, 1995). Upon request from the resident, the facility will maintain a confidential file for this advance directive (Soskis and Kerson, 1992). The admissions packet is detailed and outlines all the services and conditions of the facility. The home provides medical nursing, pharmacy, nutritional/dietary, housekeeping/laundry, beauty shop, recreational/activity, religious, and social work services. Dental, occupational therapy, speech pathology, and physical therapy services are available on a contract basis.

Technology

Technology can be addressed in a variety of ways. There is technology related to mechanical, structural, and architectural advances. The facility is responsive to whatever the physician requests in terms of special devices or beds. For example, there are clinatron beds that aid in recovery from decubitus. As well, for stroke patients who no longer have "internal thermometers" operating, there is a machine that monitors internal body temperature and adjusts a cooling pad accordingly. A computer at the facility is linked to the computers in the corporate office, and stores a variety of medical records, such as medications, physicians' orders, admission and discharge documentation, care plans, and social histories.

The home is receptive to advances in the ways to best manage residents with Alzheimer's disease. This includes indoor and outside free "wandering" space, the need for increased exercise, and minimal physical restraints. The facility is exploring the feasibility of developing a specialized Alzheimer's wing. The activity director has special expertise in working with the visually impaired, and these skills are particularly utilized during resident orientation. The staff have regular in-service training sessions, which are led by full-time supervisory staff, as well as by consultants.

Technology can also be measured by the facility's responsiveness to knowledge advances in geriatrics and gerontology. Riley's merits a high rating here also. The home is affiliated with the Graduate School of Social Work at the University of Arkansas at Little Rock; the Geriatrics Department and the School of Nursing at the University of Arkansas Medical Sciences Campus; and the geriatrics unit of the Veterans' Administration Medical Center. The pharmacology consultant specializes in geriatrics and is affiliated with the Department of Pharmacy at the University Medical Center. Nursing students from the various university programs also rotate through the facility for training. The facility has permitted carefully monitored research projects to be completed. For example, the senior author obtained an Arkansas Endowment for the Humanities grant to fund a 12-month poetry writing project. A recent interdisciplinary study (by the senior author and nurse colleagues) examined the results of a cognitive skills remediation training program on Alzheimer's disease residents (Heacock et al., 1991). The residents and staff benefit from such projects through exposure to technical expertise, model interventions, and community visibility. Riley's philosophy is "resident-first care," and administration places resources and actions behind the slogan.

Organization

The administrator, an LCSW, has the overall responsibility for the operations of the home. The social worker, director of nursing, medical records supervisor, and dietary manager all report directly to her. The assistant administrator reports directly to the administrator and has housekeeping/laundry and the maintenance supervisor under her direction. There are 4 RNs, 16 LPNs, and 48 nurse's aides under the supervision of the center's nursing director. The administrative and supervisory staff have been stable, experiencing little turnover since the home's inception. This continuity contributes to an informal aspect of organization, which makes for comfortable and trusting relationships, minimal bureaucracy, and easy, frequently quick, decision making.

The master's-level social worker manages all admissions and coordinates room assignments, internal reassignments or reclassification of levels of resident care, and payment rates. She completes all social histories on residents, is responsible for planning social work intervention with residents and families, coordinates the interdisciplinary care plan committee, is responsible for keeping the policy and admission manual updated, and coordinates the work of the activity director and her assistant (both are full-time positions). The activity personnel plan and supervise daily activities such as exercise classes, cultural events, shopping activities, arts and crafts, book rentals, and special events/parties. Also, the activity director coordinates the resident council and the monthly publication of resident events and news.

DECISIONS ABOUT PRACTICE

Client Description

Emma Brown is a well-dressed, white female who looks younger than her 80 years. She is generally alert, but frequently confused. She sometimes exhibits agitation and suspiciousness, but is generally pleasant and cooperative (Bahro, Silber, and Sunderland, 1995; Deutsch and Rovner, 1991). Immediate family live nearby and include her sister, Mary Jones, and her niece (Mary's daughter Sarah) (Kuhn, 1990; Monaha, 1995; Wright et al., 1995). A stepdaughter and two stepsons, who live 90 miles away, write, and send gifts, but do not visit.

Mrs. Brown was admitted to Riley's in the spring, following hospitalization for a broken clavicle, which she suffered in a motor vehicle accident. She was en route to visit her sister who was in the hospital following a stroke. Details of the accident are sketchy. She was driving alone, apparently became confused and lost, and was in a "trance-like daze" when her car struck another vehicle (Bloedow and Adler, 1992; Rees, Bayer, and Phillips, 1995). Following extensive testing, she was diagnosed with Alzheimer's disease. Her history reflects that she had an active, healthy life. Surgeries included a hysterectomy and, most recently, cataract removal. She smoked for 15 years, but stopped smoking many years ago. Her alcohol intake was minimal. She was treated for anemia and resulting peptic disease four years ago. There is no evidence of hypertension or cardiovascular or central nervous system impairment. A detailed social history revealed that memory loss predated the car accident. In the fall before her admission to Riley's, she relocated to an apartment complex for the elderly because of forgetfulness and mild confusion (Binetti et al., 1996). She felt the move would help her cope and provide additional security (Cotrell and Lein, 1992-1993). However, she soon became unable to find her sister's home or other familiar places. Instead of helping, the move seemed to exacerbate her memory impairment.

Mrs. Brown was discharged from the hospital at the same time that her sister Mary was released for post-stroke recuperation. They were placed together at Riley's in the minimal care unit. Her sister recovered well and was discharged in two months. Emma, on the other hand, remained confused and began to wander, particularly at night (Williams and Trubatch, 1993). She spoke frequently of having to go home, and her wandering seemed to focus around this theme. During her night wandering, Emma supposedly began to fall. The staff would find her sitting on the floor unable to tell them what had happened. Her sister and niece felt Emma's problems were a result of the difficulty of being alone in the nursing home. In November, Emma was relocated to her sister's home. Unfortunately, this change did not alter the wandering or the forgetfulness. Emma's behavior became quite disruptive and unmanageable for her sister. She rummaged through drawers and closets, searching for mysterious, lost items. Her sister's frustration was heightened when she began to hoard and scatter clothes as well (Monaha, 1995). Following a brief hospitalization for a severe rash, Emma was readmitted to Riley's nursing home in December for long-term, intermediate-level nursing care.

Emma Brown was the youngest of two daughters. After graduation from high school, she went to work as a bank clerk. In her mid-twenties she married and moved to California with her husband, a vaudeville performer. They divorced after a stormy three years. She returned to Arkansas to live with her parents and work as a secretary in a public school. Soon after her parents' deaths, she married a widower who had three children. They had a satisfactory marriage prior to his death ten years later. She returned to work until her retirement at age 65. Church work, family, and friends remained important to her.

The initial evaluation upon readmission to Riley's revealed symptoms consistent with the early stages of Alzheimer's disease (Brechling and Schneider, 1993). Although the family had been given the diagnosis, little information had been provided and few attempts had been made to discuss with them her poor prognosis and the inevitable progressive decline (Duncan and Morgan, 1994; DuMars and DuMars, 1994; Walker et al., 1994). Emma was alert and ambulatory, with some insight intact, and was able to hide her cognitive impairments through a social facade. In fact, she experienced marked confusion, time and spatial disorientation, frequent periods of anxiety and agitation, and occasional paranoia regarding the staff.

Activity staff reported inconsistent participation levels, largely due to her inability to remember when and where activities took place. She exhibited increased wandering and agitation at night, a condition commonly referred to as sundowning (Exum et al., 1993; Little et al., 1995). She suffered occasional nighttime incontinence. Her affect appeared sad and hinted of her continual frustration of feeling lost and needing to "go home." She rummaged through her closet and drawers as well as those of her roommate, was completely unable to find her way to her room or other relevant locations in the facility, was often found sitting and blankly staring into space, and would inappropriately respond to staff initiatives.

Emma's family visited weekly. Their primary concerns centered on her reports of items being stolen and other tales she would recount about strange people, peculiar activities, and unusual demands placed on her. They said that their visits with Emma were not satisfactory, and they seemed unsure and uncomfortable in relating to her and her changing mental status.

Three assessment scales were administered (Kane and Kane, 1988). The Mini-Mental State (MMS) revealed a score of 20 out of a possible 30 (Folstein, Folstein, and McHugh, 1975; Agostinelli et al., 1994). She scored lowest in the areas of orientation and recall, and scored average in registration, attention, and calculation. She did well on questions dealing with language. The Beck Depression Inventory revealed only mild depression with a score of 10 (Beck and Beamesderfer, 1974). The areas of concern noted were feelings of disappointment, punishment, self-blame, level of irritation, decision making, appearance, and interest in sex. An evaluation of her performance on activities of daily living (ADL) revealed independence in all but bathing, dressing, and continence. Difficulty in these areas stemmed from the need for assistance in focusing her activities, making decisions, remembering instructions, and other relevant facts surrounding the activity (Corcoran and Gitlin, 1992).

Because of Emma's verbal accessibility and her reasonably high MMS, she was assessed as a good candidate for social work interventions. Generally, these were designed to alleviate the behavioral problems associated with the early stages of Alzheimer's disease, and the specific problems noted in ADL activities (Clark, 1995; Lund et al., 1995; Orange et al., 1995; Teri et al., 1992).

Goals and Interventions

The treatment approach was eclectic. It included strategies from crisis intervention (with family and staff), basic problem solving, and behavioral techniques such as modeling and the principle of successive approximation or reinforcing successive steps to the final desired behavior (Gugel, 1994; Lord and Garner, 1993; McGrowder and Bhatt, 1988; Teri et al., 1992; Wells and Singer, 1988).

A primary goal for Emma was reducing her anxiety and the resulting wandering, rummaging, and suspiciousness. Frequent, routine contacts with the social worker were established during the day. Sessions were kept brief and focused, with little decision making required of her. Reassurance of continued care and praise for her intact, positive attributes were a major theme in all contacts. A daily log was maintained to systematically observe and record the timing and events surrounding her anxiety. Definite patterns were observed. For example, she had increased confusion and agitation following time spent trying to converse with more severely confused and disoriented residents (Mor et al., 1995). Her wandering behavior increased when she had to urinate, and she had heightened confusion and fear following an episode of nighttime incontinence. Her fear increased when more than one staff member approached her at once, and her confusion increased during periods of high noise levels (Taft et al., 1993).

Staff were instructed regarding the effects of the situations described above and were oriented in specific ways they could work to prevent such accidents. (Bonder, Miller, and Linsk, 1991; Brannon, Streit, and Smyer, 1992; Kruzich, 1995; Pietrukowicz and Johnson, 1991; Pray, 1993). When such episodes occurred, Emma was taken out of the area and her attention was diverted in various ways. Once she attended a music concert in the activity area. Snack breaks and escorted walks outside were also helpful. The social worker used reality orientation and reminiscence techniques to lessen her agitation and stimulate cognitive functioning. Care was taken to listen closely to the content of her conversation and make verbal connections with her whenever possible.

The second major goal was increasing her ability to perform selected activities of daily living, including dressing herself and being able to find her room. Signs were made noting where to find particular pieces of clothing. The steps necessary to appropriate dressing were outlined on a poster along with corresponding pictures. Care was taken to use language and incorporate preferences familiar to her. Clothes were inventoried and placed in groups. This was redone as Emma's rummaging necessitated. The social worker was present each morning as Emma dressed, in order to note problems, progress, and provide continued reassurance. Her progress was rewarded with verbal reinforcement, snacks, and afternoon walks. It became evident that part of Emma's difficulty in dressing was due to the type and amount of clothing she had. Her niece assisted by removing duplicate items and clothing that was too difficult to fasten. All remaining outfits were clustered so that choosing one hanger would eliminate further decision making.

To enable Emma to find her room, a technique called backward chaining was used (Harrell et al., 1980). Emma's family made a wreath for her room door that included blue ribbons, her favorite color. Emma and the social worker spent two days talking about and admiring the wreath to establish that it would serve the purpose of distinguishing her room for her. Following this, she was worked backward from her room to other major areas in the building. As Emma was able to consistently find her room from one location, the same process was attempted from further away. Repeated focus was placed on landmarks along the route in order to help her encode and recall. The landmarks were chosen according to her particular memory capabilities; colors and objects were easier to retain and locate than numbers or letters. In one instance, a landmark was created by placing a blue arrow on one wall to indicate the direction she should take.

The third and final major goal regarded Emma's family; specifically, increasing their knowledge and awareness of Alzheimer's disease, suggesting ways to make their visits more rewarding, and dealing with their feelings about the diagnosis (Bonder, Miller, and Linsk, 1991; Duncan and Morgan, 1994; Kerson, 1985; Walker et al., 1994; Zarit, Orr, and Zarit, 1985). They were asked to come to the facility on specific days each week, and to permit the social worker to be with them during their visit with Emma. In addition, the niece, Sarah, was counseled individually by the social worker. She was given materials to read and discuss. She and her mother were made aware of specific ways in which their behaviors might exacerbate Emma's anxiety. Through modeling and counseling, they were taught to defuse Emma's agitation over "tales" by responding to her feelings and the parts of her conversation that were reality-based. It was important that they respond to her but not become frustrated themselves and compound the problem by asking for details of stories and events that were largely unreal and delusions. Since they were involved in some of the interventions, they felt a part of the process. One of the most difficult tasks for the family was to lower their expectations of Emma and to allow her to be "different" than they had known her (Wuest, Ericson, and Stern, 1994). They had to let the old Emma go in order to make contact with the new Emma. In particular, they had to accept that she could no longer handle dressing in the more sophisticated style of clothing she had previously worn. They had to modify their image of her to accommodate her needs and abilities. This meant modifying the places they took her on outings from the nursing home.

Use of Contract and Time

The interventions took place over an eight-week period. Because of the nature of the facility and the particular case goals, sessions took place where and when they were deemed appropriate. Contacts were made in Emma's room, the day area, the social worker's office, or other sites, depending on the purpose of the encounter. Emma was seen at regular times throughout each day to establish a predictable routine. The intervention goals were explained to her and accepted. Emma's family, particularly her niece, was asked to commit to regular sessions during this time to facilitate goal achievement. The primary care-providing staff were consulted at weekly intervals to record observances, note progress and problems, and recruit their assistance in meeting goals (Henderson, 1994).

Stance of the Social Worker

Emma and her family were open to interventions. The frustration level of each individual was high, and they were motivated to participate in anything that might prove helpful. Strategies were planned from broad to specific. Initially, their level of frustration dictated my stance in this case. I began by presenting myself as a primary means of support, and it was necessary to come back to this supportive role frequently. Because of Emma's confusion and cognitive impairment, I was firm and direct in guiding her, careful to be specific, simple, and concrete in my requests, and always positive and complimentary. Her niece's and sister's lack of knowledge regarding Alzheimer's disease required direct and straightforward education (Kuhn, 1990). As their reluctance to allow her a different image became apparent, I had to become increasingly firm and, at times, gently confrontative in sessions with them.

Lowering the family's anxiety while giving them more information and support was chosen as a goal because of its importance in decreasing Emma's anxiety and providing her with positive, life-enhancing supports. Furthermore, a knowledgeable and supported family had fewer negative interactions with staff over misunderstood and unexpected events (Duncan and Morgan, 1994). Likewise, I worked to decrease Emma's anxiety so that she would more readily accept and succeed at other goals. It was important to use Emma's strengths to the best advantage. Since her language and appearance were reasonably intact, these became central components to the overall intervention. It was important to remain flexible. A sense of humor also helped sustain us through some of the more painful moments.

Case Conclusion and Reassessment

It was no surprise to observe Emma becoming dependent on the support and attentions of the social worker. Each morning she would wait anxiously for my arrival to her room for our lessons, as she referred to them. Initially, our morning meetings seemed to generate a fear in Emma of failure or of appearing crazy. The consistency and trust established within the relationship, as well as her own satisfaction at the increasing number of successful attempts at dressing herself with the resulting positive rewards, served to allay these fears. Though Emma is still not totally independent in dressing, she does average three days a week in which she is able to manage her own dressing unassisted. Staff is conscientious in complimenting her on her actions. Her frustration about inability to do things is no longer a daily occurrence; she now refers to having some problems from time to time. Overall, she has expressed pleasure and enjoyment at the strategies.

Recently, Emma's roommate began to chatter incoherently during the session. Emma turned to her and remarked, "Please be quiet, we are working on my lessons and they are important." On another occasion, Emma's sister and niece were present in the room as the groupings of clothes on a hanger were explained. The sister was confused about the activity. After her sister asked the same question for the third time, Emma remarked, "If you can't understand any better than that, maybe you should get lessons, too."

Sarah, who was the primary caregiver to her mother in addition to looking after Emma's needs, responded well also. She not only gained much in the way of information and support, but was able to learn more effective ways of interacting with her aunt. As a result, she did not become overly concerned with Emma's confused stories and was able to defuse potentially cata-strophic situations. This made her visits with Emma more enjoyable and she no longer confronted the staff about allegedly stolen items. She has also gained skills to help her with her mother who exhibits periods of marked confusion. The efficacy of the interventions is most clearly seen in her relaxed demeanor; her verbal expressions of satisfaction with Emma, herself, and the facility; and in the fact that the weekly number of visits to Emma have doubled.

Emma is now able to find her room successfully from the hallway in all but a few instances. She still has difficulty on occasion finding the correct hallway and frequently becomes lost when venturing past the day area of her wing. She has been able to retain the knowledge that the various landmarks we have chosen along the way will help her, but is unable at times to find them.

Emma still wanders at night, but does so less often. She continues to be anxious at times, but is easily diverted to more pleasant encounters. The social worker and staff continue to sort out the reality-based pieces of her conversation, and this technique appears to lessen her anxiety and confu-sion. It was evident that careful attention to her loose verbal associations or seemingly nonsensical words would often point to an opportunity to connect to her intact parts. For example, "a crispy piece" was her way of asking for a Nestlé Crunch Bar. Reminiscence about her gardening efforts led her to a discussion of "erps." Through imagination, effort, and pic-tures it was eventually determined that she was referring to Burpee's seedless cucumbers.

Emma is not "cured," but the goals that were specific to her capabili-ties and needs were achieved. Unfortunately in Alzheimer's disease, pro-gressive deterioration is inevitable. The social worker's support and efforts will continue and even increase as the disease inexorably prog-resses. New goals and strategies will be developed, and it is possible that future interventions will include group contact for socialization and addi-tional reality orientation. As Emma's dementia advances, her family will need even greater support and assistance.

Differential Discussion

Despite the poor prognosis associated with Alzheimer's disease, many interventions can make life more bearable for the person with the disease and her family. As with the case described, basic education and support, along with careful attention and mapping of the resident's behavior and needs, produce almost immediate benefits to all involved. Too many times we seem reluctant to discuss the particulars of Alzheimer's disease and its devastating diagnosis. That reluctance extends to physicians as well. The devastation of the disease can be offset for residents and families by active intervention to prolong and celebrate the intact functioning in addition to creating concrete strategies to reach new levels—in other words, to be the eternal optimist.

Consistency is important in any intervention. To accomplish this, cooperation among the entire staff, including all shifts, is necessary. Although efforts to consult, educate, and support staff were helpful in reaching the goals, there was still evidence of inconsistencies between different staff members and different shifts. For example, the grouping of clothing needed consistent follow-through from staff in nursing, housekeeping, and laundry. This was difficult to achieve and required considerable time. In retrospect, a more thorough way to ensure this consistency would have been to schedule facility-wide inservice training to explain, model, and support the strategies.

Staff approaches were sometimes counter to the interventions. On several occasions, wandering behavior was handled as a crisis in which all available staff rushed to stop and lead her back to safety. It is clear that a standardized policy regarding wandering and catastrophic reactions needs to be in place. All residents and staff would benefit from such a policy protocol, which would be reinforced through frequent training sessions.

Although the design of the nursing home follows the current architectural model for long-term care facilities, the wings made Emma's attempts to find her room more difficult. There are two clusters of symmetrical wings at either end of the building. Once the correct wing is located, four identical hallways extend from the nursing station like spokes on a wheel. The halls are labeled with a letter on one wall, but it can only be seen from one angle. Like Emma, many residents have lost the capacity to read or interpret the letter. The physical environment plays an important part in assisting with resident orientation. In any facility, the environment should be examined closely as to whether it supports or hinders the programs. The use of wall color or colored lines on the floor, for example, would be helpful in delineating the wings and halls.

A deliberate effort was made to include the family in goal setting and intervention strategies. This was important for their well-being as well as for the achievement of the goals. As is often the case, Emma's family felt guilty about placing her in the facility. Some of their initial efforts to be helpful and show concern only served to complicate Emma's life and behavior. I used their feelings and energy and focused them in ways that would be more beneficial. In retrospect, I could have involved them further. For example, they could have done any necessary regrouping of clothing. Even though they did sit in on many of the reminiscence sessions, more would have been helpful. The opportunities for modeling would have thereby increased. Participation in a family group and the statewide Alzheimer's organization could have added to their support, understanding, and involvement (Wasow, 1986).

Inadvertently, the interventions to help Emma dress independently probably caused some additional stress. For example, in spite of her desire to please, she let it be known that the first printed signs were too complicated because they still required too many decisions. The independent dressing strategy had to be modified twice to accommodate her abilities. In order to prevent unnecessary pressure, more time should have been spent exploring what her ability level was prior to any intervention.

Emma's dementia has already had a profound effect on her and her family. Assuming she lives long enough, she will reach the unresponsive, mute stage of Alzheimer's disease. Despite the poor prognosis, some well-considered interventions targeting specific behaviors and concerns can ease the burden and improve the quality of life. Such interventions must be based on a thorough assessment of the problem, its context, and identifiable patterns. Emma was assisted in maintaining some of the intact dimensions of her personality and relationship abilities. She has an advocate, a listener, someone to remain in dialogue with her, and she is not alone in her confusion and anxiety.

PRACTICE IN CONTEXT

Nursing homes are a diverse grouping of institutions that are designed and licensed to care for frail, older people. Some like Riley's are excellent, others are adequate, and some are quite inadequate. They basically operate on a medical model, and this model defines much of the care priorities and practice. Although few professional social workers would deny the importance, relevance, or need for social work in nursing homes, few are drawn to work in this area. All institutions are governed by policies, organizational structure, technology, and philosophy of care. Riley's South is no exception; yet it is a first-class operation, far from the typical nursing home. The large number of residents presents a different practice constraint on the social worker. While its private, for-profit status affords many additional resources, it sometimes limits practice because the institution exists because it generates income. While admission of those who can pay is paramount, the facility's willingness to employ a full-time professional social worker to direct admissions and manage casework, an administrator who is also an MSW, and a social work consultant are all indications of its commitment to the psychosocial needs of the residents and families. In fact, this commitment assures a more smoothly run nursing home in which the psychosocial needs of patients, families, and staff are taken into consideration (Heiselman and Noelker, 1991). Policy affects practice, but the inverse is also true. The analysis of the case described herein is leading to two changes within the facility: a standardized policy regarding dealing with wandering and catastrophic reactions, and a change in identification of the wings and hallways to better accommodate the confused residents. Thus, a practice intervention has led to a policy change. The process is circular, dynamic, as it should be.

REFERENCES

Agostinelli, B., Demers, K., Garrigan, D., and Waszynski, C. (1994). Targeted interventions: Use of the mini-mental state exam. *Journal of Gerontological Nursing, 20*, 15-23.

Allen, J. E. (1992). *When memory fails: Helping the Alzheimer and dementia patient.* New York: John Wiley & Sons.

Bahro, M., Silber, E., and Sunderland, T. (1995). How do patients with Alzheimer's disease cope with their illness? A clinical experience report. *Journal of the American Geriatric Society, 43*(1), 41-46.

Beck, A. T. and Beamesderfer, A., (1974). Assessment of depression: The depression inventory. In P. Pichot (Ed.), *Psychological measurement in psychopharmacology.* Switzerland: Karger.

Binetti, G., Magni, E., Padovani, A., Cappa, S. F., Bianchetti, A., and Trabucchi, M. (1996). Executive dysfunction in early Alzheimer's disease. *Journal of Neurology, Neurosurgery and Psychiatry, 60*(1), 91-93.

Bloedow, R. A. and Adler, G. (1992). Driving and dementia: Perspectives from an outpatient clinic. *Social Work in Health Care, 17*(3), 31-43.

Bonder, B. R., Miller, B., and Linsk, N. (1991). Who should do what? Staff and family responsibilities for persons with Alzheimer's disease in nursing homes. *Clinical Gerontologist, 10*(4), 80-84.

Brannon, D., Streit, A., and Smyer, M. (1992). The psychosocial quality of nursing home work. *Journal of Aging and Health, 4*(3), 369-389.

Brechling, B. G. and Schneider, C. A. (1993). Preserving autonomy in early stage dementia. *Journal of Gerontological Social Work, 20*, 17-33.

Clark, L. W. (1995). Interventions for persons with Alzheimer's disease: Strategies for maintaining and enhancing communicative success. *Topics in Language Disorders, 15*(2), 47-65.

Corcoran, M. A. and Gitlin, L. N. (1992). Dementia management: An occupational therapy home-based intervention for caregivers. *American Journal of Occupational Therapy, 46*(9), 801-808.

Corey-Bloom, J., Thal, L. J., Galasko, D., and Folstein, C. (1995). Diagnosis and evaluation of dementia. *Neurology, 45*(2), 211-218.

Corrada, M., Brookmeyer, R., and Karnas, C. (1995). Sources of variability in prevalence rates of Alzheimer's disease. *International Journal of Epidemiology, 24*(5), 1000-1005.

Cotrell, V. and Lein, L. (1992-1993). Awareness and denial in the Alzheimer's disease victim. *Journal of Gerontological Social Work, 19*, 115-129.

Deutsch, L. H. and Rovner, B. W. (1991). Agitation and other noncognitive abnormalities in Alzheimer's disease. *Psychiatric Clinics of North America, 14*(2), 341-351.

DuMars, R. C. and DuMars, H. B. (1994). Counseling and guidance approaches with the family of the client with Alzheimer's disease. *Journal of Rehabilitation Counseling, 25*(4), 36-39.

Duncan, M. T. and Morgan, D. L. (1994). Sharing the caring: Family caregivers' views of their relationships with nursing home staff. *Gerontologist, 34*(2), 235-244.

Exum, M. E., Phelps, B. J., Nabers, K. E., and Osborne, J. G. (1993). Sundown syndrome: Is it reflected in the use of PRN medications for nursing home residents? *The Gerontologist, 33*(6), 756-761.

Folstein, M. F., Folstein, S. E., and McHugh, P. R., (1975). Mini-mental state: A practical method for grading the cognitive state of patients for the clinician. *Journal of Psychiatric Research, 12*, 189-198.

Forstl, H. and Hertschel, F. (1995). Contribution to the differential diagnosis of dementias II: Neuroimaging. *Reviews in Clinical Gerontology, 4*(4), 317-341.

Gruetzner, H. (1992). *Alzheimer's: A caregiver's guide and sourcebook.* New York: John Wiley & Sons.

Gugel, R. N. (1994). Behavioral approaches for managing patients with Alzheimer's disease and related disorders. *Medical Clinics of North America, 78*(4), 861-867.

Hampel, M. J. and Hastings, M. M. (1993). Assessing quality in nursing home dementia special care units: A pilot test of the joint commission protocol. Special Section: Aging and mental health services. *Journal of Mental Health Administration, 20*(3), 236-246.

Harrell, T., Smith, C., Piroch, H., and Goldstein, R., (1980). ADL: Level II. Department of Aging and Mental Health, Florida Mental Health Institute, University of South Florida.

Heacock, P., Walton, C., Beck, C., and Mercer, S. (1991). Caring for the cognitively impaired: Reconceptualizing disability and rehabilitation. *Journal of Gerontological Nursing, 17*(3), 22-26.

Heiselman, T. and Noelker, L. S. (1991). Enhancing mutual respect among nursing assistants, residents, and residents' families. *The Gerontologist, 31*(4), 552-555.

Henderson, J. N. (1994). The culture of special care units: An anthropological perspective on ethnographic research in nursing home settings. *Alzheimer's Disease and Associated Disorders, 8*(Suppl. 1), S410-6. Tampa, FL: Department of Community and Family Health, Suncoast Gerontology Center.

Kane, R. and Kane, R. (1988). *Assessing the elderly: A practical guide to measurement.* Lexington, MA: The Rand Corporation.

Kerson, T. S. (1985). *Understanding Chronic Illness.* New York: The Free Press.

Klatka, L. A., Schiffer, R. B., Powers, J. M., and Kazee, C. (1996). Incorrect diagnosis of Alzheimer's disease: A clinicopathologic study. *Archives of Neurology, 53*(1), 35-42.

Kruzich, J. M. (1995). Empowering organizational contexts: Patterns and predictors of perceived decision-making influence among staff in nursing homes. *The Gerontologist, 35*(2), 207-216.

Kuhn, D. R. (1990). The normative crises of families confronting dementia. *Families in Society, 71*(8), 451-460.

Little, J. T., Satlin, A., Sunderland, T., and Volicer, L. (1995). Sundown syndrome in severely demented patients with probable Alzheimer's disease. *Journal of Rehabilitation Counseling, 25*(4), 36-39.

Lord, T. R. and Garner, J. E. (1993). Effects of music on Alzheimer patients. *Perceptual and Motor Skills, 76*(2), 451-455.

Lund, D. A., Hill, R. D., Caserta, M. S., and Wright, S. D., (1995). Video respite-super (TM): An innovative resource for family, professional caregivers and persons with dementia. *The Gerontologist, 35*(5), 683-687.

McGrowder, L. R. and Bhatt, A. (1988). A wanderer's lounge program for nursing home residents with Alzheimer's disease. *The Gerontologist, 28*(5), 607-609.

Mega, M. S., Cummings, J. L., Fiorello, T., and Gombein, J. (1996). The spectrum of behavioral changes in Alzheimer's disease. *Neurology, 46*(1), 130-135.

Monaha, D. J. (1995). Informal caregivers of institutionalized dementia residents: Predictors of burden. *Journal of Gerontological Social Work, 23*(3-4), 65-82.

Mor, V., Branco, K., Fleishman, J., Hawes, C., Phillips, C., Morris, J., and Fries, B. (1995). The structure of social engagement among nursing home residents. *Journal of Gerontology, 50*(B), P1-8.

Orange, J. B., Ryna, E. B., Merideth, S. D., and MacLean, M. J. (1995). Application of the communication enhancement model for long-term care residents with Alzheimer's disease. *Topics in Language Disorders, 15*(2), 20-35.

Pietrukowicz, M. E. and Johnson, M. M. (1991). Using life histories to individualize nursing home staff attitudes toward residents. *The Gerontologist, 31*(1), 102-106.

Pray, J. E. (1993). Fostering effective interaction between nursing home staff and residents experiencing Alzheimer's related dementia. Dissertation.

Rees, J., Bayer, A., and Phillips, G. (1995). Assessment and management of the dementing driver. *Journal of Mental Health, 4*(2), 165-175.

Rowland, L. P. (Ed). (1995). *Merritt's textbook of neurology.* Baltimore, MD: Williams and Wilkins.

Sandson, T. A., Sperling, R. A., and Price, B. H. (1995). Alzheimer's disease: An update. *Comprehensive Therapeutics, 21*(9), 480-485.

Savishinsky, J. (1992). *The ends of time: Life and work in a nursing home.* Westport, CT: Gergin and Garvey of Greenwood Publishing Group.

Soskis, C. and Kerson, T. S. (1992). The Patient Self-Determination Act: Opportunity knocks again. *Social Work in Health Care, 16*(4), 1-18.

Stahlman, S. D. (1992). Nursing homes. In R. L. Schneider and N. P. Kropf (Eds.), *Gerontological social work: Knowledge, service settings and special populations* (pp. 237-273). Chicago: Nelson-Hall Publishers.

Taft, L. B., Delaney, K., Seman, D., and Stansell, J. (1993). Dementia care: Creating a therapeutic milieu. *Journal of Gerontological Nursing, 19*(10), 30-39.

Teri, L., Rabins, P., Whitehorse, P., Berg, L., Reisberg, B., Sunderland, T., Eichelman, B., and Phelps, C. (1992). Management of behavior disturbance in Alzheimer's disease: Current knowledge and future directions. *Alzheimer's Disease and Associated Diseases, 6*(2), 77-88.

Terry, R. D., Katzman, R., and Bick, K. L. (Eds.). (1995). *Alzheimer disease.* New York: Raven Press.

Update on Alzheimer's Disease. (1995). Part 1. *Harvard Medical Letter, 11*(3), 1-5.

Update on Alzheimer's Disease. (1995). Part 2. *Harvard Medical Letter, 11*(9), 1-5.

Van-Ort, S. and Phillips, L. (1992). Feeding nursing home residents with Alzheimer's disease. *Geriatric Nursing, 13*(5), 249-253.

Volicer, L. and Hurley, A. (1995). Protecting self-determination of dementia patients. *Journal of the American Geriatric Society, 43*(8), 938.

Walker, R. J., Pomeroy, E. C., McNeil, J. S., and Franklin, C. (1994). A psychoeducational model for caregivers of patients with Alzheimer's disease. *Journal of Gerontological Social Work, 22*(1-2), 75-91.

Wasow, M. (1986). Support groups for family caregivers of patients with Alzheimer's disease. *Social Work, 31*(2), 93-97.

Wells, L. M. and Singer, C. (1988). Quality of life in institutions for the elderly: Maximizing well-being. *The Gerontologist, 28*(2), 266-269.

Williams, J. K. and Trubatch, A. D. (1993). Nursing home care for the patient with Alzheimer's disease: An overview. *Neurology, 43*(8, Suppl.4), S20-S24.

Wright, L. K., Hickey, J. W., Buckwalter, K. C., and Clipp, E. C. (1995). Human development in the context of aging and chronic illness. *International Journal of Aging and Human Development, 41*(2), 133-150.

Wuest, J., Ericson, P. K., and Stern, P. N. (1994). Becoming strangers: The changing family caregiving relationship in Alzheimer's disease. *Journal of Advanced Nursing, 20*(3), 437-443.

Zandi, T. (1994). Understanding difficult behaviors of nursing home residents: A prerequisite for sensitive clinical assessment and care. *Alzheimer Disease and Associated Disorders. 8* (Supplement 1), S345-354.

Zarit, S. H., Orr, N. K., and Zarit, J. M. (1985). *The hidden victims of Alzheimer's disease: Families under stress.* New York: New York University Press.

Chapter 33

Hospice Care for a Widowed Mother of Six Children

Sylvia Ziserman
Martin B. Millison
Bonnie Carolan-McNulty

CONTEXT

In the mid 1960s, ideas about how the terminally ill should be cared for were being challenged in the United States and Great Britain. Out of this controversy, the hospice movement was born. This movement, which was once an "alternative institution," has now become part of the mainstream in health care (Gummer, 1988). The term "hospice" relates back to medieval times, when hospices were way stations for travelers on their journeys through life. Liegner (1975) describes hospices as places that teach a new attitude toward death and dying, with the conscious acceptance of death as a part of birth and the struggle of life. Hospice care is a philosophy and a system of care for the terminally ill patient that accepts death in an affirmative way (Plumb and Ogle, 1992).

Hospice philosophy combines medical knowledge, reverence for life, and efficient management with the emphasis on patient goal achievement (McDonnell, 1986). Since hospice is basically a system of care, its practical application can be carried out in a variety of settings. In 1967, St. Christopher's Hospice in England became the first freestanding hospice program. By the early 1970s, the hospice concept moved across the Atlantic to Canada, where it was established as a part of a hospital structure. In 1974, the New Haven Hospice opened. It varied from its predecessors in that the care was provided in patients' homes. Since that beginning in New Haven, hospice in the United States has grown from a grass roots movement supported by volunteer staff and charity-based budgets to an established part of the health care delivery system. Through the efforts of the National Hospice Organization and the results of three major studies (Buckingham and Leiper, 1982; Greer and Mor, 1981; Wilson and English, 1980), Congress expanded Medicare coverage to include hospice in 1983. The number of Medicare-certified hospices grew from 31 in 1984 to 1,459 in 1994. Medicare hospice regulations are standard throughout the nation (Tierney and Wilson, 1993).

Description of the Setting

The Palliative Care Service of the Fox Chase Cancer Center was started in 1982 as a small program of a hospital-based cancer center. Over the years, the program worked with local community visiting nurses agencies until Fox Chase established its own home care program. In 1989, the Palliative Care Center was certified as a hospice program by Medicare and the Pennsylvania Medical Assistance Program. It is an established resource for many other insurance programs as well. The mission of the hospice is consistent with the cancer center in that the entire patient population all suffers from cancer-related illnesses. Referrals come from the Fox Chase system and the community. The hospice will serve anyone from the state of Pennsylvania living within a one-hour drive from its office.

The average daily census is 20 active patients and approximately 150 families in bereavement. Because of the research emphasis at Fox Chase, the average length of stay per patient is 40 days, lower than the national average of 65 days. The typical patient is over 60 years old and Caucasian. Ninety-eight per cent of patient deaths occur at home.

Policy

Federal acceptance of hospice laid the groundwork for state legislatures to address hospice licensure and reimbursement (Joint Commission on Accreditation of Hospitals, 1986). States have varied in their response, though strong recognition of the importance of hospice exists in almost every state. Still, in this era of cost containment, hospice is vulnerable to the cutback initiatives of the current Congress. In the private sector, hospice has also received wide acceptance. With the current focus on health care reform, less hospitalization, and less duplication of services, hospice serves as a model because of its goal-directed and cost-efficient nature.

Hospice is an excellent example of managed care. In fact, in many ways hospice care was a forerunner of managed care in that its programs are given a specified reimbursement per patient, and the hospice determines how to spend the money for patient care. This avoids duplication of services and expensive procedures. Still, cost-effective management remains a challenge (Baker, 1992).

Hospice care is provided in a variety of settings. Under the Tax Equity and Fiscal Responsibility Act (TEFRA) of 1982, hospice was defined as a comprehensive home care program (McDonnell, 1986). This point is emphasized by the requirement that home care days be 80 percent of the services provided by hospice (Department of Health and Human Services, 1984). As society changed and the availability of at-home caretakers decreased, "home" has been redefined to include the nursing home as one's primary residence. Therefore, terminal patients who live in a private home or in a nursing home may receive hospice services under Medicare. Another uncommon, but often needed hospice setting, is the inpatient hospice facility, where care is provided under the hospice model. An inpatient hospice may be free standing, or may be part of a nursing home or hospital.

The Medicare hospice benefits are designed to incorporate the needs of the patient and family at different levels. The most commonly used level is routine care, in which care is provided by the hospice team at the patient's place of residence. The continuous care level provides increased nursing care on an hourly basis to address an acute medical crisis in the home. The general inpatient care level provides similar care but in an inpatient setting. Both of these levels are very short-term and medically oriented in their provision of care. The last of the four levels primarily offer relief for the caregiver by providing respite care for the patient in a facility other than the home.

The hospice is expected to assume responsibility for the care of the terminally ill person until his or her death. Each insurance provider varies in coverage of hospice benefits. In most cases, including Ann's, the insurer permits the hospice to extend its services beyond the expected six-month prognosis.

Technology

Medical advances have lengthened the time between the diagnosis of a terminal illness and the actual death. As a result, the patient has more time to develop pain, fear, unwanted dependency, and feelings of dehumanization (Blues and Zerwekh, 1984). At a time when other health care services decide that they have no treatment left to offer, hospice becomes the treatment of choice. At a time when the patient is experiencing a sense of loss in the physical, social, psychological, and spiritual aspects of life, hospice can help that person gain and maintain some control over the life that remains (Kemp, 1994).

Cancer is the disease most identified with hospice, because of the ability to predict the length of illness. "Terminal" has been defined as having a prognosis of six months or less to live before death. As our medical technology has become more sophisticated, a growing number of cardiac, respiratory, and neuromuscular diseases that reach the terminal stages are appearing as part of the hospice population. The largest new population in hospice today are those patients with an end-stage AIDS diagnosis. These patients present special challenges to hospice, complicated by multiple psychosocial and practical needs in addition to the traditional symptom management and terminal care issues. The National Hospice Organization has recently published medical guidelines to help physicians determine the appropriateness of noncancer diseases for admission to hospice (National Hospice Organization, 1995).

The primary goals of hospice are to (1) control pain and manage symptoms while enabling the patient to remain alert to his or her environment and (2) provide support to patients and family, thereby enhancing the quality of remaining life. Technology is concerned with patient and family comfort. Pain can be managed by a variety of medications that differ in strength, depending upon individual need. After the appropriate medication is determined, a schedule of administration is planned and implemented with dosage adjusted as needed. Radiation and chemotherapy are sometimes used, but primarily for palliative reasons.

In recent years, the technology of symptom management has advanced. Hospice professionals use this and other medical developments to help families and other caregivers perform tasks necessary for patient care. For the social worker, it means helping the family to deal with their feelings in a constructive manner, find concrete resources, and facilitate communication between family members (Levitt, 1986). Families can learn to perform highly technical tasks when provided with proper training, reinforcement, and support (Buckingham, 1983).

Organization

Hospice care is provided by an interdisciplinary team because the needs of the dying patient and his or her family are multifaceted (Kilburn, 1988). The four core team professionals are a physician, registered nurse, social worker, and a pastor or other counselor. All four core service providers are employees of the hospice, while other required services such as home health aides, therapists, and homemakers may be provided under contract. The hospice program is directed by a master's-level, hospice-certified registered nurse. The staff consists of three registered nurses and one master's-level social worker (McDonald, 1991). The medical director is an oncologist who also serves as director of home care and the pain management center at Fox Chase Cancer Center. The volunteer director and chaplain hold hospital-wide positions as well.

Referrals are made by physicians, other health care workers, or the family themselves. The multifaceted process of dying must be addressed by a team working together. The terminally ill patient helps to define the role of the team and its members. The medical director determines each patient's appropriateness for hospice. Each situation is evaluated by a registered nurse, who visits the home and explains the program and available services. Patients are seen on an average of twice a week by the nurse who becomes the care manager. Addressing the physical process of dying is mainly the responsibility of the physician and the nurse. Home health aides are assigned as needed, averaging two to five visits per week. They may visit up to seven days a week if the situation warrants it. The social worker visits within the first two weeks of service. Regular visits are scheduled based upon priority of need. The chaplain contacts families within the first three weeks of service. Volunteers are available as soon as service begins and continue based on the patient's needs and desire for such contact. Volunteers are unpaid, nonprofessionals who have completed a training course directed by the Fox Chase Cancer Center. The team meets weekly to discuss each patient and update the care plan.

The assurance of adequate pain control, bowel function, respiratory relief, and disease-specific symptoms, cannot be accomplished when the patient/family is overwhelmed by financial concerns, past losses, or failed relationships. The social worker's intervention through supportive counseling, advocacy, and grief work is essential to overall hospice care (Worden, 1991; Kulys and Davis, 1986; Simos, 1979). The social work assessment is an integral part of the care plan. Guidelines for social work intervention in hospice has been recently published by the National Hospice Organization (1994).

Since the unit of care is the patient and family, the resolution of shared concerns is the key to achieving a sense of peace at the time of death. The role of the chaplain or pastoral counselor is to assess spiritual needs and to be available to assist with resolution of past issues and future fears. There are often spiritual issues that other members of the hospice team feel either inadequate or reluctant to address. Also, the hospice volunteer provides companionship and practical support, and eases the burden on families and caregivers by providing respite for the family and assistance in running errands. Medicare mandates that at least 5 percent of the patient care budget be allocated for volunteer activity.

Finally, hospice offers bereavement services for which the social worker is often the key staff member. The family's work of grieving begins when the patient is still alive, and hospice offers bereavement services addressing such issues as loss and separation, loneliness, and resolution for one year after the death. Bereavement services include exploring the survivor's ability to cope, assessing risk factors, and making appropriate referrals. Bereavement support is provided through support groups, memorial services, individual visits, mailings, and referral to other agencies.

Overall, the personal and professional composition of the team is the true measure of the success of any hospice program. Effective teams comprise dedicated professionals who share an awareness of their own values and beliefs toward death and demonstrate an expertise in the care of the dying (Todek and Jacobs, 1983). They also share a basic philosophy and modes for working together to achieve the stated goals. Being an employee of the hospice program helps to affirm investment and interest. Ongoing group development nurtures accountability to one another and the program.

DECISIONS ABOUT PRACTICE

Client Description

The client, Ann, was a recently widowed 55-year-old mother of six, with children ranging in age from 15 to 35 years. Her husband had died nine months earlier, two months after she was diagnosed with colorectal cancer. At the time of diagnosis, the cancer had metastasized to Ann's liver. She rejected the treatment option of a liver resection, choosing to receive chemotherapy. After six months of chemotherapy, Ann's condition deteriorated. She refused second-line chemotherapy as well as experimental protocols. Hospice care was offered and accepted, and the family became the client. Ann's family was Italian Catholic, deeply rooted in their ethnic heritage and strongly connected to their church. All of her children and grandchildren either attended or graduated from parochial school. The family's close-knit relationship was demonstrated by frequent visits to Ann's home by her 6 children and 14 grandchildren. Her only surviving sibling was also involved in her care.

The patient and her family were quite open in discussing her diagnosis and prognosis. Her children were very supportive and involved in her disease progression and in the decision-making process. As the family began to explore Ann's future needs and discuss who would be available to help, many ongoing problems became known to the hospice social worker. The second-oldest daughter had a drug problem, two failed marriages, and had lost custody of her children; the teenage daughter had been hospitalized for a suicide attempt, but was not currently in treatment; and the oldest son, who was looked upon to "keep the family together," was having severe financial and legal problems. Once these problems were disclosed, the hospice team could better understand and respond to some of the anger that emerged when care issues and finances were explored. Luckily, one daughter, Lisa, was available to Ann, from early morning after her children went to school until the evening. Lisa would paint the kitchen, shop for groceries, clean the house, and manage many other tasks. Since Lisa lived within a block of Ann, she became the primary caregiver. Other children were available to help, but it was Lisa who assumed the major responsibility. Mother and daughter had a long-term symbiotic relationship. Ann's intention was to have Lisa inherit the house upon her death.

Ann's eldest son, Joe, had been expected to carry much of the financial burden of care, but his own problems made that impossible. This became a family crisis until other children offered to assist with household expenses. As her disease progressed, Ann experienced greater pain. Ann was placed on long-acting morphine medication with the availability of a short-term breakthrough medication as needed for pain. When the pain increased, medications were adjusted accordingly. Through adjustments in her medication and increased socialization with her assigned volunteer, Ann's quality of life improved and she was able to resume her role in the family (Davis, Eshelman, and McKay, 1989).

The social worker met with the family as a whole on several occasions to (1) explore their awareness of Ann's disease progression and needs at each stage, (2) explore available family supports, (3) educate them about and refer them to resources, and (4) help them to accept Ann's imminent death and cope with the loss. The meetings occurred through Ann's death and into the bereavement period. As Ann's disease progressed, her family continued to deny the gravity of the situation and needed considerable support to be able to cope with their impending loss.

Definition of the Client

The unit of care in hospice is comprised of the patient and the family. Families often rally around the dying patient in times of crisis (Rosen, 1990). The term "family" is used here to denote the key persons who provide support or care to the terminal patient. As previously stated, the client in this case consisted of Ann, her children, sister, and to some extent her grandchildren. Although the family unit was considered the client, psychosocial interventions were carried out primarily with the patient, two of her daughters, and her eldest son.

Goals, Objectives, and/or Outcome Measures

Social work goals were to (1) allow Ann to remain at home, (2) facilitate grief work related to the death of Ann's husband, (3) assist Ann and the family in understanding the physical and emotional changes she was experiencing, (4) assist Lisa and other family members in caring for Ann, (5) help the family cope with Ann's increased dependency needs and her impending death, (6) to assist the family with anticipatory grief work, and (7) help the family with issues of grief, loss, and separation after the death.

Use of Contract

At the initial assessment, the patient and family consented to the full range of hospice care, which includes social work services, by signing a formal consent agreement. Although no written contract existed between social worker and client, the social worker committed herself to regular visits in the client's home, and the client agreed to be involved with the social worker for concrete needs and emotional support. In addition, a number of family meetings were held in which available family members participated.

Meeting Place

Traditionally, hospice care in America is home-based, unlike the institution-based model of Europe (Hayslip and Leon, 1992). The Fox Chase Hospice Program is an in-home-based service as opposed to a freestanding hospice or a hospice program that utilizes a certain number of beds in a hospital. The in-home hospice allows the patient the enjoyment and comfort of familiar surroundings. All meetings with Ann and her family were held at home. By visiting Ann at home, the social worker had the opportunity to observe her interacting with those who were important to her. Also, the home setting was more conducive to open communication than would be the case at a hospital or inpatient setting.

Use of Time

Time is a very important dimension in hospice care. Often the patient is not referred to hospice until he or she is actively dying. Sometimes the social worker sees the patient only once or twice before the patient dies. Since a referral to hospice means that the individual has six months or less to live, the family or the physician is often reluctant to refer to hospice. When they do refer, the patient often has an even shorter life expectancy. Ann was a hospice patient well beyond six months. This gave the social worker ample time to intervene knowledgeably. Initially, the social worker visited Ann every two weeks, but as her conditioned worsened, meetings were held weekly. The initial social work intervention focused on the completion of a psychosocial assessment. The needs of the unit of care, which in hospice is the patient and the family/caregivers, are paramount. Families find themselves in a state of disequilibrium when one of them is dying (Rosen, 1990). The system is dealing with issues of loss, separation, and grief. This particular family had additional concerns as they had only recently faced the unexpected loss of Ann's spouse. It can be assumed that they had not sufficiently grieved his death before being confronted with Ann's impending death. Both deaths occurred within one year. Kastenbaum (1978) refers to this condition as bereavement overload, that is, the inability or lack of opportunity to work through feelings of pain and sorrow at the loss of one close relationship because of the death of another close relationship. This plight often occurs with the elderly who experience multiple losses in a short period of time.

Interventions

While the social worker worked actively in this case, much of the intervention occurred between the family, the patient, and members of the hospice team of physician, nurse, social worker, representative of the clergy or counselor, and volunteer. What follows is a brief description of interventions by the social worker, volunteer, and chaplain. The interventions demonstrate ways in which the hospice team works together with patient and family to help the final days be less painful, less stressful, and less dehumanizing.

Social Work

Social work intervention in this case focused on anticipatory grief work for Ann and her family. The family needed to explore and resolve feelings related to Ann's terminal prognosis and plan for her care and eventual death. Additionally, because of the recent death of the patient's spouse, bereavement issues had to be addressed. One form of social work intervention was the family meeting. During meetings, some of the issues discussed were (1) Ann's need for constant companionship; (2) finding activities that would give her pleasure in her remaining days; (3) financial and insurance concerns; (4) age-appropriate interventions for Ann's grandchildren, related to grief, bereavement, and the funeral; and (5) improved family relationships. An example of one tangible result of the family meetings was the agreement to inform the youngest daughter's school about her mother's terminal illness as a way of helping them to better understand her behavior.

Another major intervention was to help patient and family accept the reality of the situation. A great deal of denial occurred as the patient lived beyond the medical expectations. Initially, the family engaged in grief work, but as Ann's condition stabilized, family members began to deny that their mother was going to die. At this juncture, the social worker met with family members individually and in a group to help them to see that remission was not the same as cure. This was beneficial to family members, because when Ann's condition worsened, they were better able to cope with the idea that death was near.

Another critical intervention occurred when Ann's health deteriorated and she contemplated suicide. During in-depth discussions, the social worker helped the client sort out her fears. Ann drew upon her faith as she grappled with the decision that suicide was not the answer for her. The guilt that she would bear in relation to God and to her children would not allow her to take that step. As a result of the discussions regarding suicide, her children committed themselves to making sure that Ann was not left alone. The older grandchildren were included in the scheduling.

As death became more imminent, the family, with the help of the social worker, was able to discuss Ann's will, funeral arrangements, living arrangements for the teenage daughter, and age-appropriate interventions with the grandchildren. Life review was an important intervention for the entire family (Pickrel, 1978). As her illness progressed, Ann was encouraged to think of a way to initiate closure with her family and friends. She chose to have a family gathering and invited extended family and a few close friends. The gathering included much picture-taking and videotaping. The event gave her many hours of pleasure, and she spoke of that day for weeks after the party and viewed the videotape with anyone who would watch. The party occupied her thoughts and helped her think about things other than illness. It also helped Ann's extended family share some special time with her. The memory of the party and the videotape ultimately were gifts to the family. The social worker also encouraged Ann to make a videotape for the family that would help the younger children know her better and provide all the family with a lasting memory. The taping was an opportunity for Ann to leave a special message. This was her last gift to the family. Each child was given a copy of the tape. All reported that although the tape was painful to view, they were thankful for this gift.

Grief work with the grandchildren became a part of family work. The children accepted the social worker's presence. Together, the social worker and the children engaged in age-appropriate conversation, play, writing, and drawing. These interventions facilitated closure and prepared the grandchildren for Ann's death. As a result of the interaction, the children were able to attend the viewing and the funeral without fear.

Volunteer

A hospice volunteer was assigned to Ann. Sally, the volunteer, visited Ann weekly and became well integrated into the patient's extended family system. She also had regular telephone contact with Ann during the week. As time progressed, the telephone calls became longer and dealt with issues and concerns of the patient. Often family members were home when Sally visited, while at other times Ann and Sally were alone. Sometimes, Sally and Ann took care of Lisa's children, while Lisa shopped or went to a PTA meeting. Often volunteer and patient would play cards or talk about issues of the day. Ann did a lot of life review, talking about her husband, his death, and their relationship. In Sally, Ann gained a new friend, someone who had the time and the interest in being with her.

Chaplain

Spirituality plays an important part in the care of the terminally ill (Bollwinkel, 1994; Millison and Dudley, 1992). Thus, the hospice chaplain is an important member of the hospice team. After Ann became too ill to attend church, the hospice chaplain paid a visit to her. Noticing her strong faith and her belief in Catholicism, the chaplain notified her church of her desire to speak to a priest. A priest visited monthly administering the sacraments and helping her deal with spiritual issues concerning her death and her husband's.

Stance of the Social Worker

In hospice work, the stance of the social worker often depends on the time available to the client, the desire of the client to engage with the social worker, and the support of the caregiver/family. In this particular case, the elements were all there for social work involvement directly and indirectly. Most hospice patients do not live very long, and many are too ill to engage in a relationship with a social worker. Because of the long period of time Ann spent as a hospice patient, extensive counseling was possible for patient and family. There was ample time to engage Ann and to deal with issues such as loss, finances, grief, suicide, and funeral arrangements. Also, because a large, close-knit family was present, family sessions were held throughout hospice service. Also, the social worker was able to assist Ann in planning a deeply meaningful activity. In addition to direct service work, the social worker helped Ann obtain important concrete services, intervened on her behalf with other hospice team members, and even encouraged the family to advocate on behalf of Ann's teenage daughter with her school.

Use of Outside Resources

Most of the concrete services relate directly to necessary equipment for care at home. Hospital beds, wheelchairs, bedside commodes, walkers, and dressings are frequently needed. It is also important to review insurance to determine benefits. All of this became a part of the work with Ann.

Reassessment

Reassessment is part of hospice care; daily assessments are made between social worker and physician, nurse, clergy, volunteer, and others who may be involved. Cases are also reviewed in weekly team meetings. Changes in physical condition dictate modifications in the approach. Ann lived as a hospice patient for 13 months—seven months beyond the medical guidelines for hospice eligibility. Reassessment had to be undertaken to assess her continued eligibility for hospice. As changes occur in the patient and the hospice, the participants join together to bring about a satisfactory fit between the person needing the care and the environment. By anticipating the needs of the terminally ill person, the social worker assists in "orchestrating proactive interventions" throughout the continuum of hospice care (Rusnak, Schaefer, and Moxley, 1990).

Transfer and Termination

In hospice cases there are two termination occasions. The first occurs around the death of the client and the second occurs when the survivors no longer receive bereavement services. Transfer is rare because almost every hospice client dies while actively receiving service. Bereavement services end either when the survivors are ready or at one year after the death. Thirteen months after being admitted to hospice, Ann died at home with her sister and her children by her side. In the latter stages of her illness, she declined rapidly. She accepted a hospital bed and a commode in her home. Her home was her "turf," where she lived and where she died. She spent her last year surrounded by family.

For surviving family members, bereavement is an integral aspect of hospice. Bereavement addresses such issues as loss and separation, and feelings of loneliness and isolation (Mors and Masterson-Allen, 1987). A bereavement assessment evaluates risk factors as well as survivors' ability to cope and makes appropriate referrals. The hospice team follows the family for twelve months after the death of the loved one. During that time period, bereavement support can be provided through support groups, memorial services, individual visits, mailings, and, when necessary, referral to other services. Bereavement work was done with two of Ann's daughters and some of the grandchildren. The social worker attended both the funeral and the viewing. Most family members attended the memorial service held one month after Ann's death. Two of Ann's daughters attended a ten-week support group led by the social worker, and daughter Lisa met with the social worker several times for individual counseling. The final formal contact was a memorial service one year after Ann's death.

Case Conclusion

Ann and her family were accepting of all hospice supports and services. Her extended life gave the social worker the opportunity to engage in anticipatory grief work with patient and family. The patient had ample time to discuss and to plan her final days, as well as her funeral. The family was attentive and supportive to the patient. All of the family, including the grandchildren, attended the viewing and the funeral.

This case was selected because it demonstrates what hospice can offer when there is time, an accepting patient, and an involved family (Goddard, 1993). The patient's extended life allowed the social worker to observe and understand family dynamics. As the work with Ann and the family progressed, it became obvious that this outwardly loving family had deep emotional problems. They had resisted dealing with their problems in the past, and continued to do so as Ann was dying. The hospice social worker, therefore, became the appropriate professional to assist the family with their problems, including their issues of loss and grief. The patient's physical and emotional needs were met, and she was able to spend her last year of life in her home, surrounded by her family. She had the opportunity to come to closure in many aspects of her life. Ann died with dignity and in control of her life until the end. The hospice team helped Ann and her family to achieve their goals and Ann to achieve "a good death."

Differential Discussion

In reviewing the work with Ann and her family, we are grateful for the extended time with the patient and her family. It enabled effective relationships to be built not only with Ann and her primary caregiving daughter but with her other children and grandchildren as well. Counseling in a time-limited situation often constrains the depth of the work with a multi-problem family.

Hospice care allows the social worker the freedom to assist the family to cope and deal with anticipatory grief and closure issues. Had Ann died within the anticipated time, the social worker may not have been able to complete the bereavement work related to her husband's death or the anticipatory grief work with her children and grandchildren. A shorter time period would not have allowed time for bereavement work. This would have made the bereavement process more difficult for the family, particularly because of the earlier death of Ann's husband. The family was well-invested in caring for the patient, compliant with the care plan, and accepting of all facets of Hospice Services. They used social work services appropriately and encouraged intervention with the grandchildren. Social work with this family was intense, difficult, sad, frustrating and very gratifying. The family coped adequately during Ann's terminal period despite their problems. Family members who accepted support throughout the bereavement process worked through their grief and came to appropriate resolution within time.

REFERENCES

Baker, M. (1992). Cost-effective management of the hospital-based hospice program, *Journal of Nursing Administration, 22*(1), 40-45.

Blues, A. and Zerwekh, J. (1984). *Hospice and palliative care nursing.* Orlando, FL: Green and Stratton.

Bollwinkel, E. (1994). Role of spirituality in hospice care. *Annals of the Academy of Medicine, 25*(2), 261-263.

Buckingham, R. (1983). *The complete hospice guide.* New York: Harper & Row.

Buckingham, R. and Leiper D. (1982). A comparative study of hospice services in the United States. *American Journal of Public Health, 72*(5), 455-463.

Davis, M., Eshelman, E. R., and McKay, M. (1989) *The relaxation and stress reduction workbook*, Third Edition. Oakland, CA: New Harbinger Publications.

Department of Health and Human Services, Health Care Financing Administration (1984). Conditions for hospice benefit under Medicare. *Federal Register*, publication no.: Health Care Financing Administration 02154.

Goddard, M. (1993). The importance of assessing the effectiveness of care. *Journal of Social Policy, 22*(1), 1-17.

Greer, D. and Mor, V. (1981). *Evaluating the impact of hospice care: The national hospice study design.* Paper presented at the Annual Meeting of the American Public Health Association, Los Angeles, California.

Gummer, B. (1988). The hospice in transition: Organizational and administrative perspectives. *Administration in Social Work, 12*(2), 31-43.

Hayslip, B. and Leon, J. (1992). *Hospice care*. Newbury Park, CA: Sage Publications.

Joint Commission on Accreditation of Hospitals (1986). *Hospice standards manual.* Chicago, IL: Joint Commission on Accreditation of Hospitals, 6-7.

Kastenbaum, R. (1978). Death, dying, and bereavement in old age: New developments and their positive implications for psychosocial care. *Aged Care and Service Review, 1,* 1-10.

Kemp, C. (1994). Spiritual care in terminal illness. *The Journal of Hospice and Palliative Care*, March/April, 31-36.

Kilburn, L. (1988). *Hospice operations: A comprehensive guide to organization development, management, care planning, regulatory compliance, and financial services.* Arlington, VA: National Hospice Organization.

Kulys, R. and Davis, M. (1986). An analysis of social services in hospice. *Social Work, 31*(6), 448-458.

Levitt, J. (1986). The conceptualization and assessment of family dynamics in terminal care. *The Hospice Journal, 2*(4), 1-19.

Liegner, L. (1975). Care of the dying patient. *Journal of the American Medical Association, 234*, 1047-1048.

McDonnell, A. (1986). *Quality hospice care*. Owings Mills, MD: Rynd Communications.

Millison, M. and Dudley, J. (1992). Providing spiritual support: A job for all hospice professionals. *The Hospice Journal, 8*(4), 49-66.

Mors, V. and Masterson-Allen, S. (1987). *Hospice care systems: Structure, process, cost and outcomes.* New York: Springer.

National Hospice Organization. (1993). *Standards of a hospice program of care.* Arlington, VA: National Hospice Organization.

National Hospice Organization (1994). *Guidelines for social work in hospice.* Arlington, VA: National Hospice Organization.

National Hospice Organization. (1995). *Medical guidelines for determining programs in selected non-cancer diseases.* Arlington, VA: National Hospice Organization.

Pickrel, J. (1978). Tell me your story: Using life review in counseling the terminally ill. *Death Studies, 13*(3), 127-135.

Plumb, J. and Ogle, K. (1992). Hospice care. *Primary Care: Clinics in Office Practice, 19*(4), 807-820.

Rosen, E. (1990). *Families facing death: Family dynamics of terminal illness.* Lexington, MA: Lexington Books.

Rusnack, B., Schaefer, S. M., and Moxley, D. (1990). Hospice: Social worker's response to a new form of social caring. *Social Work in Health Care, 15*(2), 95-119.

Simos, B. (1979). *A time to grieve: Loss as a universal human experience.* New York: Family Service Association of America.

Tierney, J. and Wilson, D. (1993). The effect of Medicare regulations on hospice practice: Enhancing staff performance. *American Journal of Hospice and Palliative Care, 10*(2), 26-31.

Todeck, C. and Jacobs, S. (1983). Perspectives on hospice. *Cancer Nursing, 6*(3), 183-187.

Wilson, D. C. and English, D. J. (1980). An assessment of the existing staffing patterns and personnel required in a hospice to deliver interdisciplinary patient care and the problems related to delivering humanistic care to hospice patients. Hyattsville, MD: Human Resources Administration.

Worden, W. (1991). *Tasks of grief: Grief counseling and grief therapy.* New York: Springer.

Index

Page numbers followed by the letter "f" indicate figures.

Order Your Own Copy of
This Important Book for Your Personal Library!

SOCIAL WORK IN HEALTH SETTINGS
Practice in Context, Second Edition

_____ in hardbound at $59.95 (ISBN: 0-7890-6018-3)

_____ in softbound at $29.95 (ISBN: 0-7890-6019-1)

COST OF BOOKS_____

OUTSIDE USA/CANADA/
MEXICO: ADD 20%_____

POSTAGE & HANDLING_____
*(US: $3.00 for first book & $1.25
for each additional book)
Outside US: $4.75 for first book
& $1.75 for each additional book)*

SUBTOTAL_____

IN CANADA: ADD 7% GST_____

STATE TAX_____
*(NY, OH & MN residents, please
add appropriate local sales tax)*

FINAL TOTAL_____
*(If paying in Canadian funds,
convert using the current
exchange rate. UNESCO
coupons welcome.)*

☐ **BILL ME LATER:** ($5 service charge will be added)
(Bill-me option is good on US/Canada/Mexico orders only;
not good to jobbers, wholesalers, or subscription agencies.)

☐ Check here if billing address is different from
shipping address and attach purchase order and
billing address information.

Signature_____

☐ **PAYMENT ENCLOSED: $**_____

☐ **PLEASE CHARGE TO MY CREDIT CARD.**

☐ Visa ☐ MasterCard ☐ AmEx ☐ Discover
☐ Diner's Club

Account #_____

Exp. Date_____

Signature_____

Prices in US dollars and subject to change without notice.

NAME_____

INSTITUTION_____

ADDRESS_____

CITY_____

STATE/ZIP_____

COUNTRY_____ COUNTY (NY residents only)_____

TEL_____ FAX_____

E-MAIL_____
May we use your e-mail address for confirmations and other types of information? ☐ Yes ☐ No

Order From Your Local Bookstore or Directly From
The Haworth Press, Inc.
10 Alice Street, Binghamton, New York 13904-1580 • USA
TELEPHONE: 1-800-HAWORTH (1-800-429-6784) / Outside US/Canada: (607) 722-5857
FAX: 1-800-895-0582 / Outside US/Canada: (607) 772-6362
E-mail: getinfo@haworth.com
PLEASE PHOTOCOPY THIS FORM FOR YOUR PERSONAL USE.

BOF96